ORAL PATHOLOGY
for the
DENTAL HYGIENIST

With General Pathology Introductions

ORAL PATHOLOGY
for the
DENTAL HYGIENIST

SEVENTH
EDITION

With General Pathology Introductions

Olga A.C. Ibsen, RDH, MS

Adjunct Professor
Department of Oral and Maxillofacial Pathology, Radiology and Medicine
New York University
College of Dentistry
New York, New York;
Adjunct Professor
University of Bridgeport
Bridgeport, Connecticut

Joan Andersen Phelan, MS, DDS

Professor and Chair
Department of Oral and Maxillofacial Pathology, Radiology and Medicine
New York University
College of Dentistry
New York, New York;
Diplomate, American Board of Oral and Maxillofacial Pathology

ELSEVIER

ELSEVIER

3251 Riverport Lane
St. Louis, Missouri 63043

ORAL PATHOLOGY FOR THE DENTIAL HYGIENIST:
WITH GENERAL PATHOLOGY INTRODUCTIONS,
SEVENTH EDITION

ISBN: 978-0-323-40062-6

Notices

Knowledge and best practice in this field are constantly changing. As new research and experience broaden our understanding, changes in research methods, professional practices, or medical treatment may become necessary.

Practitioners and researchers must always rely on their own experience and knowledge in evaluating and using any information, methods, compounds, or experiments described herein. In using such information or methods they should be mindful of their own safety and the safety of others, including parties for whom they have a professional responsibility.

With respect to any drug or pharmaceutical products identified, readers are advised to check the most current information provided (i) on procedures featured or (ii) by the manufacturer of each product to be administered, to verify the recommended dose or formula, the method and duration of administration, and contraindications. It is the responsibility of practitioners, relying on their own experience and knowledge of their patients, to make diagnoses, to determine dosages and the best treatment for each individual patient, and to take all appropriate safety precautions.

To the fullest extent of the law, neither the Publisher nor the authors, contributors, or editors, assume any liability for any injury and/or damage to persons or property as a matter of products liability, negligence or otherwise, or from any use or operation of any methods, products, instructions, or ideas contained in the material herein.

Previous editions copyrighted 2014, 2009, 2004, 2000, 1996, 1992

International Standard Book Number: 978-0-323-40062-6

Senior Content Strategist: Kristin Wilhelm
Content Development Manager: Ellen Wurm-Cutter
Senior Content Development Specialist: Rebecca Leenhouts
Publishing Services Manager: Jeff Patterson
Senior Project Manager: Jodi M. Willard
Design Direction: Bridget Hoette

Printed in China

Last digit is the print number: 9 8 7 6 5 4 3 2 1

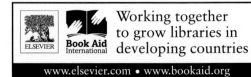

Personal Dedication

To
Our husbands
Lawrence *and* **Jerry**

For their years of support and encouragement of all our professional endeavors, especially each and every edition of Oral Pathology for the Dental Hygienist: With General Pathology Introductions. *They have assisted us in innumerable ways, and we are most grateful to them. We appreciate their dedication to us and, ultimately, to the profession.*

With our love,
Olga *and* **Joan**

Professional Dedication

We dedicate this edition of Oral Pathology for the Dental Hygienist: With General Pathology Introductions *to the faculty who have chosen this text over the past 25 years and to past, present, and future students who have used or will use this text. Our goal in developing this text has been to enhance patient care by providing dental hygienists with a comprehensive knowledge of oral pathology. We encourage you to join us in using this knowledge to provide optimal care to the patients we serve.*

Olga A.C. Ibsen, RDH, MS
Joan Andersen Phelan, MS, DDS

Contributors

Olga A.C. Ibsen, RDH, MS
Adjunct Professor
Department of Oral and Maxillofacial Pathology, Radiology and
  Medicine
New York University
College of Dentistry
New York, New York;
Adjunct Professor
University of Bridgeport
Bridgeport, Connecticut

Joan Andersen Phelan, MS, DDS
Professor and Chair
Department of Oral and Maxillofacial Pathology, Radiology and
  Medicine
New York University
College of Dentistry
New York, New York;
Diplomate, American Board of Oral and Maxillofacial
  Pathology

Margaret J. Fehrenbach, RDH, MS
Dental Hygiene Educational Consultant
Dental Science Technical Writer
Seattle, Washington

Kenneth E. Fleisher, DDS
Clinical Associate Professor
Oral and Maxillofacial Surgery
New York University
College of Dentistry
New York, New York;
Diplomate, American Board of Oral and Maxillofacial Surgery

Anne Cale Jones, DDS
Distinguished Teaching Professor
Department of Pathology
School of Medicine
The University of Texas Health Science Center at San Antonio
San Antonio, Texas;
Diplomate, American Board of Oral and Maxillofacial
  Pathology

John E. Kacher, DDS
JKJ Pathology
The Woodlands, Texas;
Diplomate, American Board of Oral and Maxillofacial
  Pathology

Heddie O. Sedano, DDS, Dr Odont
Professor Emeritus
University of Minnesota School of Dentistry
Minneapolis, Minnesota;
Lecturer, Section of Pediatric Dentistry
School of Dentistry and Craniofacial Clinic
Department of Pediatrics, School of Medicine
University of California, Los Angeles
Los Angeles, California;
Diplomate, American Board of Oral and Maxillofacial
  Pathology

Anthony T. Vernillo, DDS, PhD, MBE
Professor
Oral and Maxillofacial Pathology, Radiology and Medicine
New York University
College of Dentistry
New York, New York

Preface

Welcome to the seventh edition of *Oral Pathology for the Dental Hygienist: With General Pathology Introductions!*

Knowledge of oral pathology is an essential component of dental hygiene practice. The seventh edition of *Oral Pathology for the Dental Hygienist: With General Pathology Introductions* is an optimal resource for achieving success in applying this knowledge to patient care. Our objectives have always been to facilitate both the teaching and learning of oral pathology. It is our goal that the dental hygiene student will learn to recognize lesions and conditions, describe them using professional terminology and, through data collection, assist in the preliminary diagnosis of the lesion/condition identified. The text is supported by full-color illustrations.

Although the intended audience is the dental hygiene student, this text is also an excellent reference for dental students and practicing dental hygiene professionals. It covers the pathologic conditions likely to be encountered in private practice and integrative health care settings. Furthermore, it can provide an introduction to oral disease for other health professionals, such as nurses, physician assistants, and medical technologists.

Importance to the Profession

Oral pathology is one of the most significant subjects in the dental hygiene curriculum. One person dies every hour of every day from oral cancer; this statistic has not changed in over 40 years. Clinicians need to understand oral pathology to provide thorough extraoral and intraoral examinations that will ensure identification of abnormal conditions as early as possible.

The student's ability to recognize the slightest deviation from normal is the first step in the evaluation process. The diagnostic principles described in this text should be applied to every lesion or condition identified. The application of these principles should begin at the student's very first clinical experience. As clinical experience increases, the student will become more proficient in the data collection process. In addition to recognizing abnormal findings while doing a clinical examination, students must develop the skills necessary to obtain more information from the patient. This is an important component of the diagnostic process. Besides providing a resource to identify abnormalities clinically, the information in this text will enhance the student's ability to ask appropriate questions.

Clinical faculty will also find this text helpful when describing the clinical characteristics of oral lesions and conditions encountered in the clinic. It is a very helpful resource, and the earlier students become familiar with the content, the more proficient they will become when describing a lesion using professional terminology.

About This Edition

The text is divided into 10 chapters. Chapter 10 has been revised and expanded to include additional conditions. Several chapters begin with a general pathology introduction that will assist the student in understanding the pathologic processes discussed within the chapter. The seventh edition includes a variety of **learning features** to help students achieve the best possible outcomes in both the classroom and clinical setting.

- Each chapter begins with a **list of objectives** that provides an overview of the topics covered in the chapter. These objectives clearly define what the student is expected to learn and guide the faculty in test question preparation.
- A **detailed vocabulary list** with definitions and pronunciations is presented at the beginning of each chapter. This list helps students learn essential new dental terminology so they can more effectively describe lesions and conditions in the classroom and in the clinical setting.
- Useful **synopsis tables** provide the student with a quick overview of lesions, conditions, and diseases covered in the chapter. They summarize in outline format the main features of each chapter and include the diagnostic processes used to make the final diagnosis of the lesion. They are also very handy and quick reference guides for the clinical practitioner.
- **New emphasis on Differential Diagnoses.** For most but not all lesions/conditions in the synopsis tables, two or three conditions that could be considered in the differential diagnosis of the lesion are listed.
- **Review questions** at the end of each chapter help students test their knowledge of the chapter material and serve as excellent practice for taking the National Board Dental Hygiene Exam (NBDHE). Several additional questions have been added to each chapter— for a total of 500—and the answers are included in the text.
- A **list of references** appears at the end of each chapter. This provides the student with additional study resources. The references have been updated in each chapter. Some classic references remain. New research is also reflected in the references.
- A **comprehensive glossary** at the end of the text provides easy access to the definitions of all the bolded words in the text.

New to This Edition

Although for this edition we have added the subtitle "With General Pathology Introductions," this topic, in most chapters, has been a part of the text since the first edition. General pathology introductions have helped the student comprehend the pathologic process of oral lesions and conditions. We have never included systems pathology because those conditions are covered in other courses.

Chapter 10, now entitled "Orofacial Pain and Temporomandibular Disorders," has been completely revised. At the request of faculty and clinicians, this chapter now includes Burning Mouth Disorder, Trigeminal Neuralgia, Bell's Palsy, and Temporomandibular Disorders.

In this edition, you will find additional vocabulary words and several new illustrations. Each chapter has been thoroughly reviewed and updated. The glossary has been expanded to include all of the bolded terminology within the chapters, making it an even more valuable reference.

All of the chapter review questions offer four answer selections, which clearly reflect the design and format of most NBDHE questions. This format change will assist faculty in preparing students for the NBDHE, course reviews, and curriculum examinations.

About Evolve

An Evolve website offers a variety of additional learning tools and greatly enhances the text for both students and instructors.

For the Student

Evolve Student Resources offer the following:

- **Case Studies.** More than 50 case studies with questions, answers, and rationales, which are set up in the format of the NBDHE. These provide a case-based format that will assist the student with the critical thinking skills necessary for national board examinations as well as for clinical practice.
- **Practice Exam.** A 200-question practice exam is designed to help students prepare for the NBDHE as well as for course exams.
- **Printable Versions of the Synopsis Tables.** The printable versions allow students to print out these helpful tables for inclusion with notes and make it easy to transport them from class to class.

For the Instructor

Evolve Instructor Resources offer the following:

- **Test Bank in ExamView.** A test bank containing more than 750 questions divided by chapter is included along with rationales for all answer choices. The questions can be sorted by chapter or randomly, making the creation of quizzes and exams much easier for the instructor.
- **Image Collection.** This image collection includes every illustration from the book, making it easy for the instructor to incorporate a photo or drawing into a lecture or quiz.
- **TEACH Instructor's Resource** with the following assets:
  - **TEACH Lesson Plans** organize chapter content into 50-minute class times and map it to CODA educational standards and to chapter learning objectives.
  - **TEACH PowerPoints** provide lecture presentations with talking points for discussion, all mapped to chapter learning objectives.
  - **TEACH Student Handouts** are PDFs of the lecture presentations for easy posting and sharing with students.

From the Authors

Oral Pathology for the Dental Hygienist: With General Pathology Introductions has been written specifically for dental hygiene students and dental hygiene practitioners. Our goal for this new edition has been to continue to provide the highest standard oral pathology textbook. We strongly encourage instructors to continue to use the text in other courses, such as radiology, oral histology, and clinical courses. Dental hygienists have earned a reputation for excellence in identifying abnormal oral findings. The integration of oral pathology throughout the dental hygiene curriculum ensures more comprehensive patient care by the student and the dental hygiene practitioner.

Olga A.C. Ibsen, RDH, MS
Joan Andersen Phelan, MS, DDS

Acknowledgments

Through the years, many individuals have contributed to the success of *Oral Pathology for the Dental Hygienist: With General Pathology Introductions*.

Our former editors at Elsevier have included Shirley Kuhn, who was with us through the first four editions; Content Strategy Director Penny Rudolph, who also guided us through the fourth edition; John Dolan, who directed us through the fifth edition; and Kristin Wilhelm, Senior Content Strategist, who assisted us with the sixth edition. We sincerely appreciated their encouragement, support, and direction.

This seventh edition was directed and supported by Kristin Wilhelm, Senior Content Strategist; Becky Leenhouts, Senior Content Development Specialist; and Jodi Willard, Senior Project Manager. They guided us through all the stages of production, and we thank them for their encouragement and attention to this outstanding text, especially their insight into the needs of the Evolve site.

We also appreciate all of the contributions from Dr. Joan M. Iannucci at Ohio State University. Dr. Iannucci contributed to the first five editions of this text.

We will always be grateful to our oral pathology teachers: Drs. Melvin Blake, Ernest Baden, Leon Eisenbud, Paul Freedman, Stanley Kerpel, Harry Lumerman, Michael Marder, James Sciubba, Philip Silverstein, Marshal Solomon, David Zegarelli, and Edward V. Zegarelli. Olga A.C. Ibsen is especially grateful to two individuals who influenced her personal and professional life: her dad, the late Dr. Joseph A. Cuttita, and her godfather, the late Dr. Edward V. Zegarelli. All of these individuals strongly influenced our passion for pathology!

Gloria Turner of the Diagnostic Pathology Laboratory at NYU College of Dentistry prepared most of the slides used for the color photomicrographs that have enhanced each edition of *Oral Pathology for the Dental Hygienist: With General Pathology Introductions*. We extend our sincere appreciation for her outstanding work. Additional color photomicrographs were provided by Oral Pathology Laboratory, Inc., Flushing, New York.

We are proud to present the seventh edition of *Oral Pathology for the Dental Hygienist: With General Pathology Introductions*.

Olga A.C. Ibsen, RDH, MS
Joan Andersen Phelan, MS, DDS

In Memoriam

It is with sadness that we report the death of Dr. Heddie Sedano in October 2016. He was an oral pathologist with a special interest and knowledge in oral and maxillofacial genetics. Dr. Sedano was the author of the Genetics chapter in all seven editions of *Oral Pathology for the Dental Hygienist: With General Pathology Introductions*. He generously provided his expertise to faculty and students who used this text and who learned from his unique knowledge. We sincerely appreciate his contributions to the profession. We extend condolences to his family and other colleagues in the profession.

Contents

ORAL PATHOLOGY
for the
DENTAL HYGIENIST

With General Pathology Introductions

1

Introduction to Preliminary Diagnosis of Oral Lesions

OLGA A.C. IBSEN

OBJECTIVES

After studying this chapter, the student will be able to:

1. Define each of the words in the vocabulary list for this chapter.
2. Do the following related to the diagnostic process:
   - List and discuss the eight diagnostic categories that contribute to the diagnostic process.
   - Name a diagnostic category and give an example of a lesion, anomaly, or condition for which this category greatly contributes to the diagnosis.
   - Describe the radiographic appearance and historical data (including the age, sex, and race of the patient) that are relevant to periapical cemento-osseous dysplasia (cementoma).
   - Define leukoplakia and erythroplakia.
   - For the following lesions, state all of the diagnostic categories that can contribute to the diagnosis: tori, squamous cell carcinoma, linea alba, erythema migrans, leukoplakia, nutritional deficiencies, angular cheilitis, and necrotizing ulcerative gingivitis (NUG).

3. Do the following related to variants of normal:
   - Define "variant of normal" and give three examples of these lesions involving the tongue.
   - Describe the clinical appearance of Fordyce granules (spots), torus palatinus, mandibular tori, melanin pigmentation, retrocuspid papilla, lingual varicosities, linea alba, and leukoedema and identify them in the clinical setting or on a clinical illustration.
   - Describe the clinical and histologic differences between leukoedema and linea alba.
4. Do the following related to other benign conditions with unique clinical features.
   - Define lingual thyroid and list three symptoms associated with it.
   - List and describe the clinical characteristics and identify a clinical picture of median rhomboid glossitis (central papillary atrophy), erythema migrans (geographic tongue), fissured tongue, and hairy tongue.

❖ Vocabulary

Clinical Appearance of Soft Tissue Lesions

Bulla (adjective, bullous; plural, bullae) A circumscribed, elevated lesion that is more than 5 mm in diameter, usually contains serous fluid, and looks like a blister.

Lobule (adjective, lobulated) A segment or lobe that is a part of the whole; these lobes sometimes appear fused together (Fig. 1.1).

Macule An area that is usually distinguished by a color different from that of the surrounding tissue; it is flat and does not protrude above the surface of the normal tissue. A freckle is an example of a macule.

Papule A small, circumscribed lesion usually less than 1 cm in diameter that is elevated or protrudes above the surface of normal surrounding tissue.

Pedunculated Attached by a stemlike or stalklike base similar to that of a mushroom (Fig. 1.2).

Pustules Variously sized circumscribed elevations containing pus.

Sessile Describing the base of a lesion that is flat or broad instead of stemlike (Fig. 1.3).

Vesicle A small, elevated lesion less than 1 cm in diameter that contains serous fluid.

Soft Tissue Consistency

Nodule A palpable solid lesion up to 1 cm in diameter found in soft tissue; it can occur above, level with, or beneath the skin surface.

Palpation The evaluation of a lesion by feeling it with the fingers to determine the texture of the area; the descriptive terms for palpation are soft, firm, semifirm, and fluid filled; these terms also describe the consistency of a lesion.

Color of Lesion

Colors Red, pink, salmon, white, blue-black, gray, brown, and black are the words used most frequently to describe the colors of oral lesions; they can be used to identify specific lesions and may also be incorporated into general descriptions.

Erythema An abnormal redness of the mucosa or gingiva.

Erythroplakia A clinical term used to describe an oral mucosal lesion that appears as a smooth red patch or granular red and velvety patch.

Leukoplakia A clinical term for a white plaquelike lesion on the oral mucosa that cannot be rubbed off or diagnosed as a specific disease.

Pallor Paleness of the skin or mucosal tissues.

Size of Lesion

Centimeter (cm) One-hundredth of a meter; equivalent to a little less than one-half inch (0.393 inch) (Fig. 1.4). If a lesion is described as being 3 cm in size, it is really about one and one-half inches.

Millimeter (mm) One-thousandth of a meter (a meter is equivalent to 39.3 inches); the periodontal probe is of great assistance in documenting the size or diameter of a lesion that can be measured in millimeters (general terms such as small, medium, or large are sometimes used, but these terms are not as specific) (Fig. 1.5).

Surface Texture

Corrugated Wrinkled.

Fissure A cleft or groove, normal or otherwise, showing prominent depth.

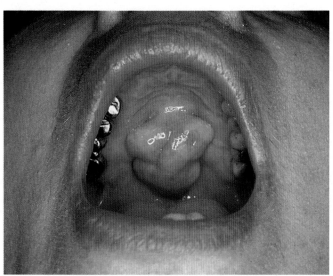

• **Figure 1.1** Lobulated torus palatinus.

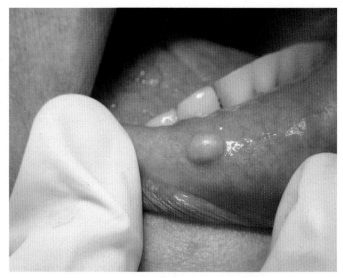

• **Figure 1.3** Fibroma with a sessile base.

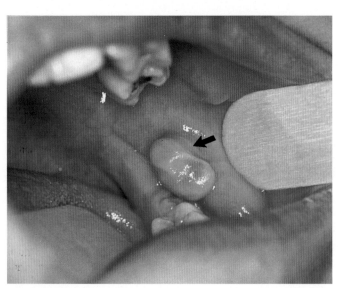

• **Figure 1.2** Fibroma with a pedunculated base. Arrow points to the stemlike base.

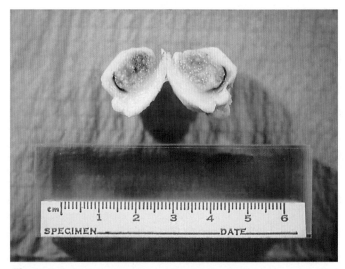

• **Figure 1.4** A ruler measuring centimeters is used to measure all specimens submitted for microscopic examination.

Papillary Resembling small, nipple-shaped projections or elevations found in clusters.

Smooth, rough, folded Terms used to describe the surface texture of a lesion.

Radiographic Terms Used to Describe Lesions in Bone

Coalescence The process by which parts of a whole join together, or fuse, to make one.

Diffuse Describes a lesion with borders that are not well defined, making it impossible to detect the exact parameters of the lesion; this may make treatment more difficult and, depending on the biopsy results, more radical (Fig. 1.6).

Multilocular Describes a lesion that extends beyond the confines of one distinct area and is defined as many lobes or parts that are somewhat fused together, making up the entire lesion; a multilocular radiolucency is sometimes described as resembling soap bubbles; an odontogenic keratocyst often presents as a multilocular, radiolucent lesion (Fig. 1.7).

Radiolucent Describes the black or dark areas on a radiograph; radiant energy can pass through these structures; less dense tissue such as the pulp is seen as a radiolucent structure (Fig. 1.8).

Radiolucent and radiopaque Terms used to describe a mixture of light and dark areas within a lesion, usually denoting a stage in the development of the lesion; for example, in a stage I periapical cemento-osseous dysplasia (cementoma) (Fig. 1.9A), the lesion is radiolucent; in stage II it is radiolucent and radiopaque (Fig. 1.9B).

Radiopaque Describes the light or white area on a radiograph that results from the inability of radiant energy to pass through the structure; the denser the structure, the lighter or whiter it appears on the radiograph; this is illustrated in Fig. 1.10.

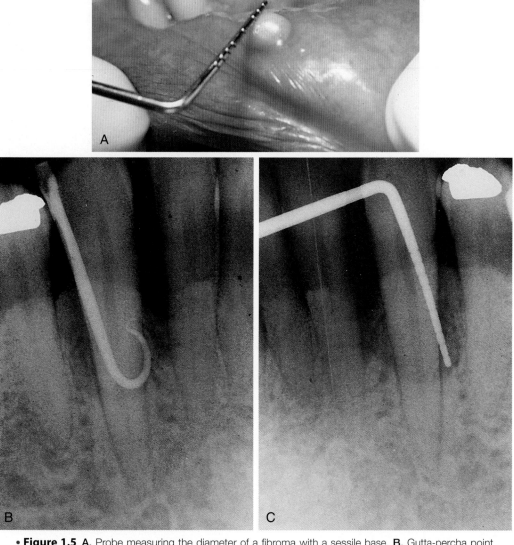

• **Figure 1.5 A,** Probe measuring the diameter of a fibroma with a sessile base. **B,** Gutta-percha point used to explore a radiographic defect. **C,** Periodontal probe placed before a radiograph.

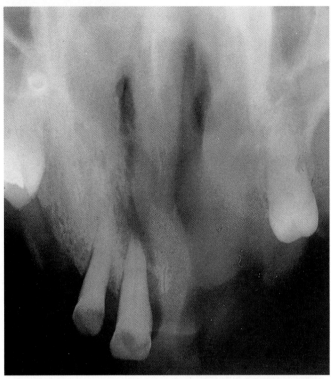

• **Figure 1.6** Squamous cell carcinoma involving the alveolar bone and hard palate showing diffuse borders. (Courtesy Drs. Paul Freedman and Stanley Kerpel.)

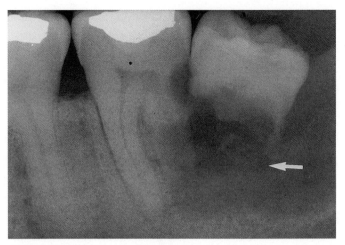

• **Figure 1.7** Odontogenic keratocyst (*arrow*), illustrating a multilocular lesion. (Courtesy Dr. Victor M. Sternberg.)

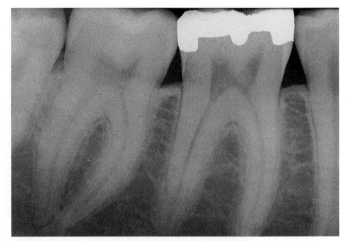

• **Figure 1.8** Prominent pulp chambers, horns, and canals in mandibular molars.

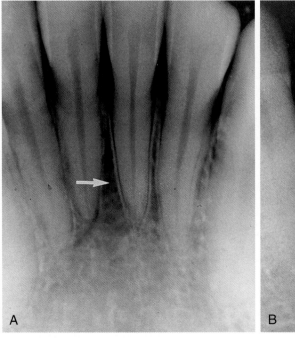
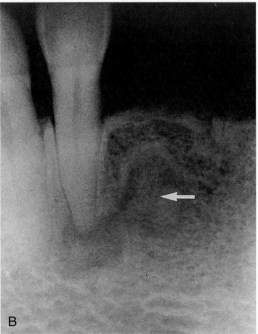

A   B

• **Figure 1.9** A, Stage I periapical cemento-osseous dysplasia (cementoma). B, Stage II periapical cemento-osseous dysplasia (cementoma).

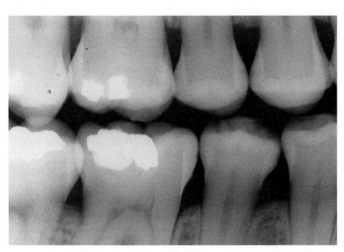

• **Figure 1.10** Amalgam restorations on the occlusal surfaces of the maxillary and mandibular molars.

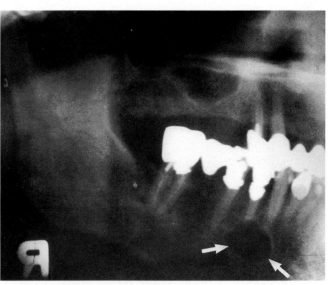

• **Figure 1.12** Traumatic bone cyst (*arrows*) around the roots. (Courtesy Drs. Paul Freedman and Stanley Kerpel.)

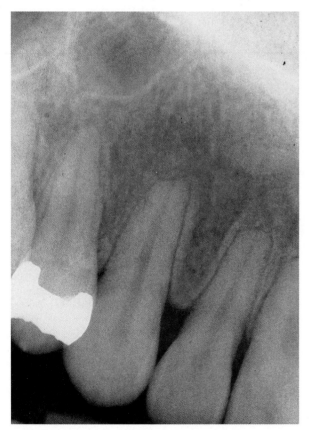

• **Figure 1.11** Resorption of the roots on maxillary anteriors as a result of rapid orthodontic movement.

Root resorption Observed radiographically when the apex of the tooth appears shortened or blunted and irregularly shaped; occurs as a response to stimuli, which can include a cyst, tumor, or trauma; Fig. 1.11 illustrates resorption of the roots as a result of a rapid orthodontic procedure (see Fig. 1.26); external resorption arises from tissues outside the tooth such as the periodontal ligament, whereas internal resorption is triggered by pulpal tissue reaction from within the tooth; in the latter the pulpal area can be seen as a diffuse radiolucency beyond the confines of the normal pulp area.

Scalloping around the root A radiolucent lesion that extends between the roots, as seen in a traumatic bone cyst; this lesion appears to extend up the periodontal ligament (Fig. 1.12).

Unilocular Having one compartment or unit that is well defined or outlined, as in a simple radicular cyst (Fig. 1.13).

Well circumscribed Term used to describe a lesion with borders that are specifically defined and in which one can clearly see the exact margins and extent (Fig. 1.14).

Additional Vocabulary Words

Anomaly Something that deviates from what is standard or normal.

Dysphagia Difficulty swallowing.

Dysphonia Difficulty speaking.

Dyspnea Difficulty breathing.

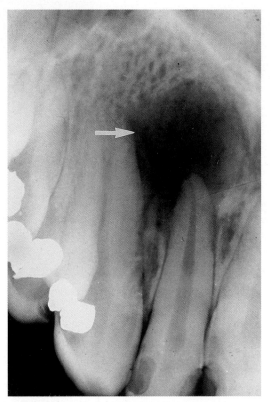

• **Figure 1.13** Radicular cyst (*arrow*) at the apex of the maxillary lateral incisor, illustrating a unilocular lesion.

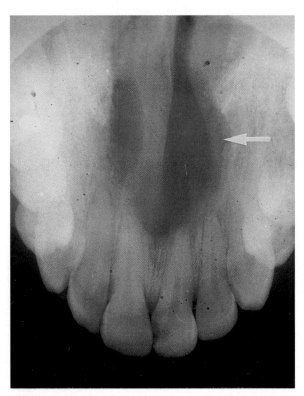

• **Figure 1.14** Well-circumscribed median palatal cyst (*arrow*).

To understand the material in this text, it is imperative that the reader approach it in a systematic manner. Significant time is spent in the dental hygiene curriculum identifying and describing normal structures. Before one can identify the abnormal condition, it is necessary to have a solid understanding of the basic and dental sciences such as human anatomy and physiology, histology, and dental anatomy. Once one has a solid understanding of normal structures and those that are variants of normal, findings that deviate from normal and pathologic conditions are recognized more easily. The preliminary evaluation and description of these lesions are within the scope of dental hygiene practice and are truly among the most challenging experiences in clinical practice.

In the first part of this chapter the definitions of commonly used terms that describe the clinical and radiographic features of a lesion, including terms used for normal, variants of normal, and pathologic conditions discussed throughout this text, are presented. The reader is encouraged to use these terms in the clinical setting so that they become part of an everyday professional vocabulary, thereby facilitating communication between the hygienist and other dental practitioners in the clinical setting.

The second part of this chapter focuses on the eight diagnostic categories that provide a systematic approach to the preliminary evaluation of oral lesions. These diagnostic categories are used in the synopsis tables for every lesion or condition covered in the text. Each area is described, and the strength of that area in the diagnostic process is illustrated using specific examples of lesions.

The final part of the chapter includes conditions that are considered variants of normal and those that are benign conditions of unknown cause. Most are diagnosed from their distinct clinical appearance and history.

The Diagnostic Process

Making a Diagnosis

How is a diagnosis made? What are the essential components? The answers to these questions begin with data collection. The process of diagnosis requires gathering information that is relevant to the patient and the lesion being evaluated; this information comes from various sources.

Certain distinct diagnostic categories should be thought of as pieces in a puzzle, with each piece playing a significant role in the final diagnosis. The eight categories that contribute segments of information leading to the definitive or final diagnosis are (1) clinical, (2) radiographic, (3) historical, (4) laboratory, (5) microscopic, (6) surgical, (7) therapeutic, and (8) differential findings. It is important to note that usually one area alone does not provide sufficient information to make a diagnosis; the strength of the diagnosis is often derived from one, two, or even three areas. As the dental hygienist becomes more aware of the diseases and conditions discussed in this text, it will be most helpful to use the diagnostic categories as a guide to evaluating lesions.

Clinical Diagnosis

Clinical diagnosis suggests that the strength of the diagnosis comes from the clinical appearance of the lesion. By observing the area in a well-illuminated clinical setting and palpating it if necessary, the clinician can establish a diagnosis for some lesions on the basis of color, shape, location, and history of the lesion. When a diagnosis can be made on the basis of these unique clinical features, biopsy or surgical intervention is not necessary. Examples

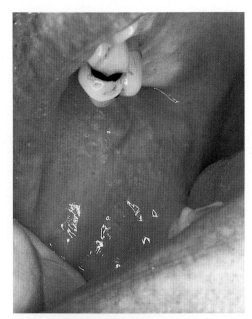

• **Figure 1.15** Fordyce granules.

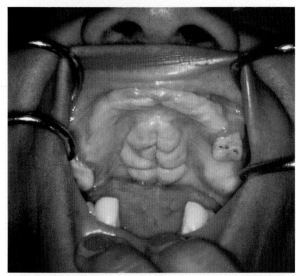

• **Figure 1.16** Lobulated torus palatinus. (Courtesy Dr. Edward V. Zegarelli.)

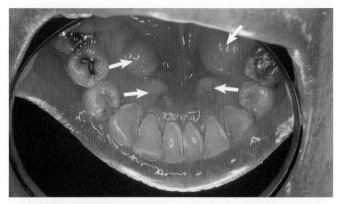

• **Figure 1.17** Arrows point to lobulated mandibular tori.

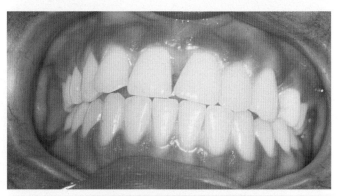

• **Figure 1.18** Melanin pigmentation.

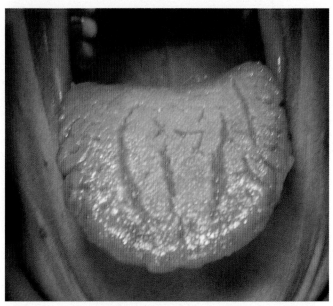

• **Figure 1.19** Fissured tongue.

of lesions that can be clinically diagnosed are Fordyce granules (Fig. 1.15), torus palatinus (Fig. 1.16), mandibular tori (Fig. 1.17), melanin pigmentation (Fig. 1.18), retrocuspid papillae (see Fig. 1.51), and lingual varicosities (see Fig. 1.52). These lesions are described later in this chapter.

Other benign conditions of unknown cause that are recognized by their distinct clinical appearance include fissured tongue (Fig. 1.19), median rhomboid glossitis (central papillary atrophy) (Fig. 1.20), erythema migrans (Fig. 1.21), and hairy tongue (Fig. 1.22). These conditions are also discussed later in this chapter.

Sometimes the diagnostic process requires historical information in addition to the clinical findings. For example, an amalgam tattoo (focal argyrosis) can be observed as a blue-to-gray patch on the gingiva or mucosa where an amalgam restoration is or has been located (Fig. 1.23A). Although this condition is usually easily observed and a clinical diagnosis made, any history involving the area can still be very helpful in confirming the clinical impression. The patient in Fig. 1.23A had root canal therapy

and a retrograde amalgam on a deciduous tooth. The amalgam tattoo is observed in the apical area of the permanent central incisor; no evidence of an amalgam restoration exists in the entire anterior area. The history helped confirm the clinical diagnosis. The diagnosis of herpes zoster (shingles) caused by varicella zoster virus is also made from the clinical and historical features. A prodromal period of pain is followed by the eruption of vesicles with a unilateral distribution along a sensory nerve (Fig. 1.23B) (see Chapter 4).

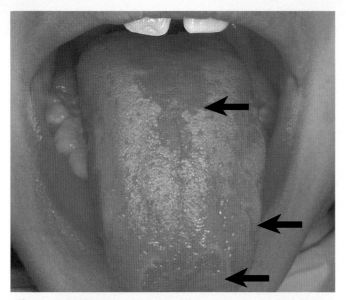 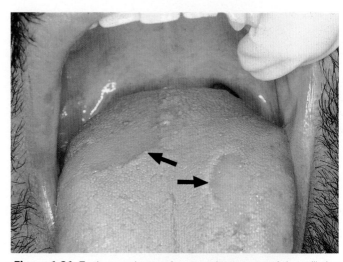

• **Figure 1.20** Median rhomboid glossitis (*top arrow*) and erythema migrans (*bottom arrows*).

• **Figure 1.21** Erythema migrans. Arrows point to areas of depapillation.

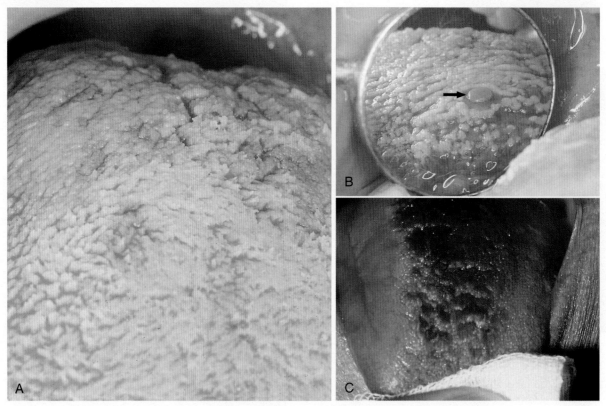

• **Figure 1.22** **A,** White hairy tongue. **B,** White hairy tongue showing a circumvallate papilla (*arrow*). **C,** Black hairy tongue.

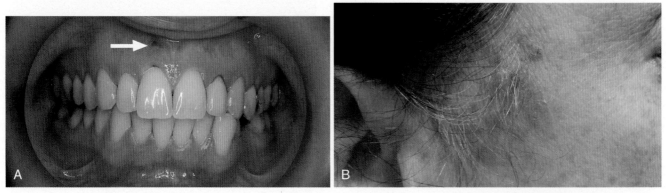

• **Figure 1.23** **A,** Arrow points to an amalgam tattoo at the apical area of the patient's maxillary right central incisor. This patient had a root canal procedure on a deciduous tooth. No other amalgam restoration is in the area; thereforev it was helpful to know the patient's past dental history to confirm this diagnosis. **B,** Patient with herpes zoster (shingles) involving the ophthalmic branch of the trigeminal nerve.

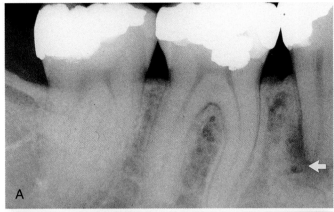

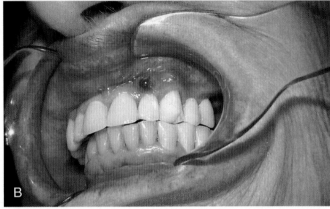

• **Figure 1.24 A,** Periapical pathosis (PAP); a radiolucency is seen at the apex of the mandibular second premolar (*arrow*). **B,** In another patient a fistula is seen on the maxillary lateral incisor. A fistula is usually an indication of PAP. When a fistula is observed clinically, a radiograph is necessary for diagnostic and treatment purposes.

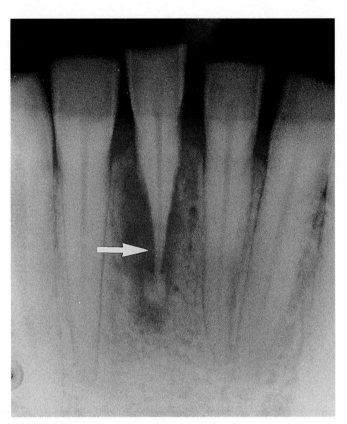

• **Figure 1.26** Arrow points to external resorption on a mandibular central incisor. (Courtesy Dr. Gerald P. Curatola.)

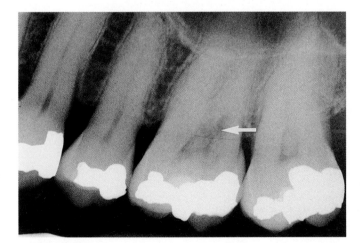

• **Figure 1.25** Arrow points to the area of internal resorption on the maxillary first molar.

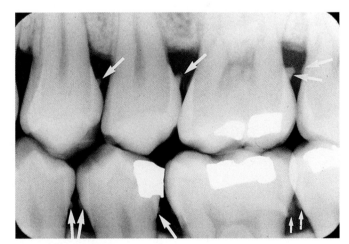

• **Figure 1.27** Arrows point to heavy interproximal calculus.

Radiographic Diagnosis

In a radiographic diagnosis the radiograph provides sufficient information to establish the diagnosis. Although additional clinical and historical information may contribute, the diagnosis is obtained from the radiograph. Conditions for which the radiograph provides the most significant information include periapical pathosis (Fig. 1.24), internal resorption (Fig. 1.25), external resorption (Fig. 1.26), heavy interproximal calculus (Fig. 1.27), dental caries (Fig. 1.28), compound odontoma (Figs. 1.29 and 1-30A), complex odontoma (Fig. 1.30B), supernumerary teeth (Fig. 1.31), impacted or unerupted teeth (Fig. 1.32), and calcified pulp (Fig. 1.33). Normal anatomic landmarks are also easily observed radiographically. In some cases the radiographic image may show very distinct and well-defined structures such as the

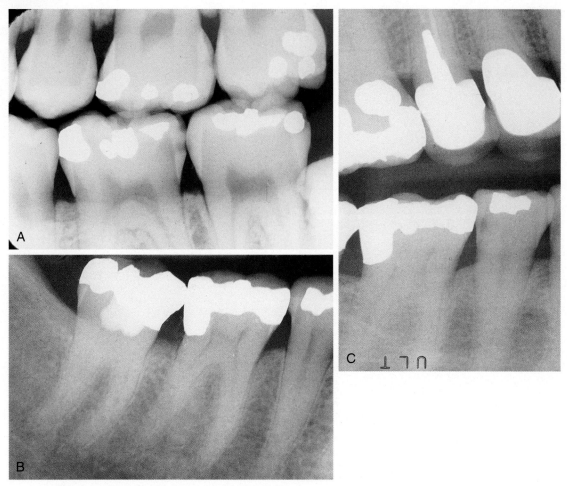

• **Figure 1.28** **A,** Dental caries. The reader should observe the interproximal radiolucencies. Clinical examination is necessary to confirm the involvement of some of the areas. **B,** Periapical radiograph showing a subtle carious area on the distal aspect of the mandibular second premolar. **C,** The patient in (B) was seen a year later. During the scaling procedure a defect on the distal aspect of the mandibular second premolar was detected. This vertical bitewing radiograph was taken. The reader should note the definite radiolucent, carious area on the distal aspect of the mandibular second premolar. This example emphasizes the need for careful clinical and radiographic evaluation. (**B** and **C** courtesy Dr. Victor M. Sternberg.)

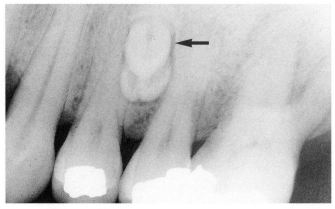

• **Figure 1.29** Arrow points to compound odontoma.

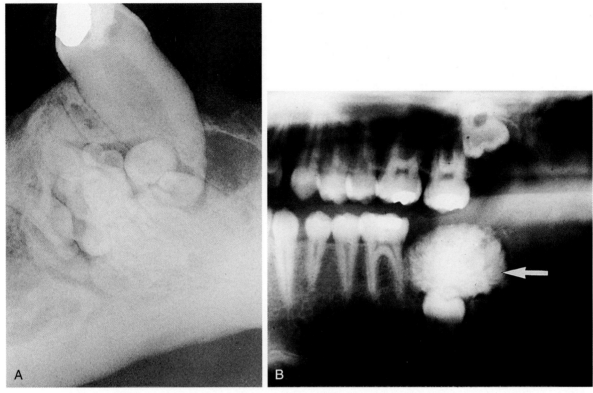

• **Figure 1.30 A,** Compound odontoma rather easily diagnosed from the radiograph alone. **B,** Complex odontoma (*arrow*) confirmed by histopathologic examination. (**B** courtesy Drs. Paul Freedman and Stanley Kerpel.)

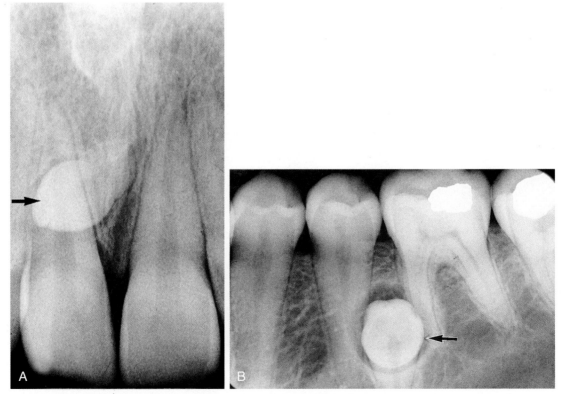

• **Figure 1.31 A,** Mesiodens (*arrow*). A supernumerary tooth is located between the maxillary central incisors. **B,** A radiograph showing a supernumerary mandibular premolar (*arrow*) surrounded by a radiolucent area diagnosed as a dentigerous cyst. Clinically this area was thought to be a mandibular torus until the radiograph was taken.

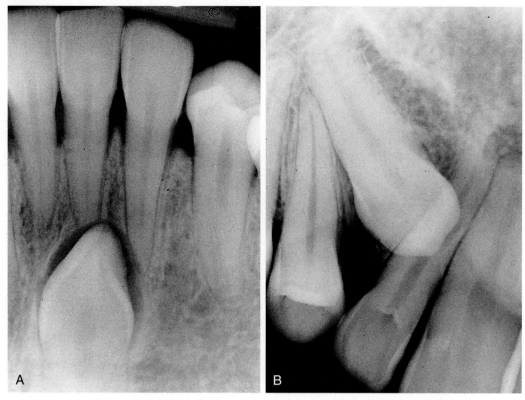

• **Figure 1.32 A,** Impacted mandibular cuspid. **B,** Impacted maxillary cuspid.

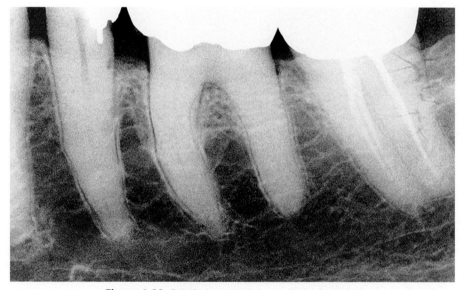

• **Figure 1.33** Calcified pulp in the mandibular first molar.

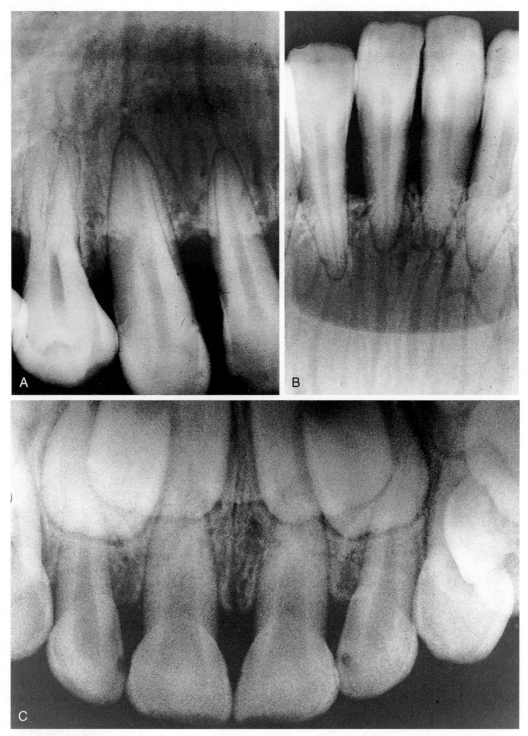

• **Figure 1.34** **A,** Nutrient canals in the anterior maxillary arch. **B,** Nutrient canals in the mandibular anterior area. **C,** The mixed dentition of a 5-year-old child is observed in this radiograph.

nutrient canals seen in Fig. 1.34A-B and the mixed dentition seen in Fig. 1.34C. Unusual radiographic findings are illustrated in Fig. 1.35 A-K.

Historical Diagnosis

Historical data constitute an important component in every diagnosis; occasionally when historical data are combined with observation of the clinical appearance of the lesion, the historical information constitutes the most important contribution to the diagnostic process. Personal history, family history, past and present medical and dental histories, history of drug ingestion, and history of the presenting disease or lesion can provide information necessary for the final diagnosis. Thorough medical and dental histories must be a part of every patient's permanent record.

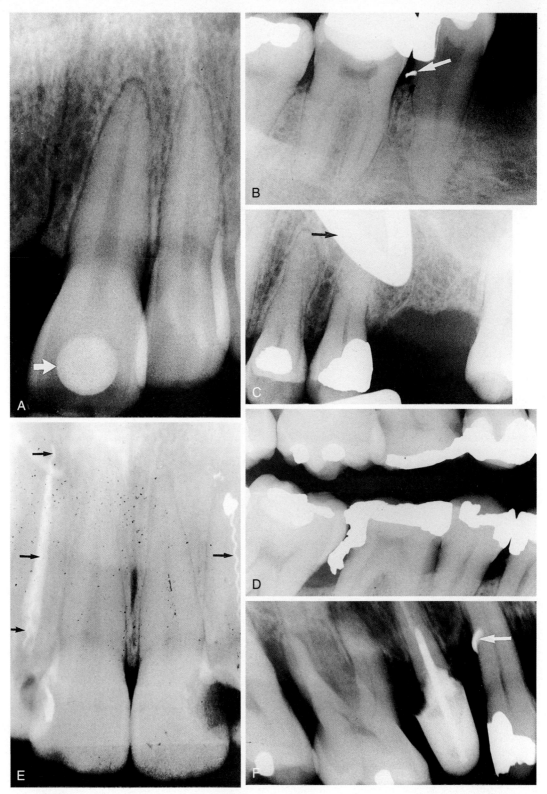

• **Figure 1.35** **A,** Arrow points to a 7-carat cubic zirconia (a round stone) that was glued to this patient's maxillary left central incisor. **B,** The radiopaque area on the distal aspect of the mandibular second premolar (*arrow*) is an amalgam fragment. There was a subtle clinical amalgam tattoo in the interproximal papilla that was not detected or charted on initial examination, which included a full-mouth series of radiographs and incomplete scaling. When the radiographs were viewed after the patient was dismissed, the radiopaque area was thought to be the tip of a broken instrument. Further evaluation of the instruments used at that appointment ruled out the possibility of a broken instrument. When the patient returned for an additional appointment 2 weeks later, another radiograph, using the same long cone and precision Rinn instruments, was taken of the area. The radiopaque fragment remained in the exact same place. Clinically, a very close look at the interproximal papilla in the area then revealed a subtle bluish-black area. The dentist surgically slit the papilla on the buccal aspect and revealed the amalgam particle. **C,** This patient wore wide-framed eyeglasses during the radiographic procedure. The arrow points to a U-shaped radiopacity from the eyeglass frame. **D,** This radiograph reveals an obvious radiopaque overhang from the amalgam restoration on the distal aspect of the mandibular first molar. **E,** Instruments from a root canal procedure were broken in these two maxillary lateral incisors (*arrows*). **F,** The broken tip of a curette (*arrow*) is observed as a radiopaque area on the distal aspect of the maxillary first premolar.

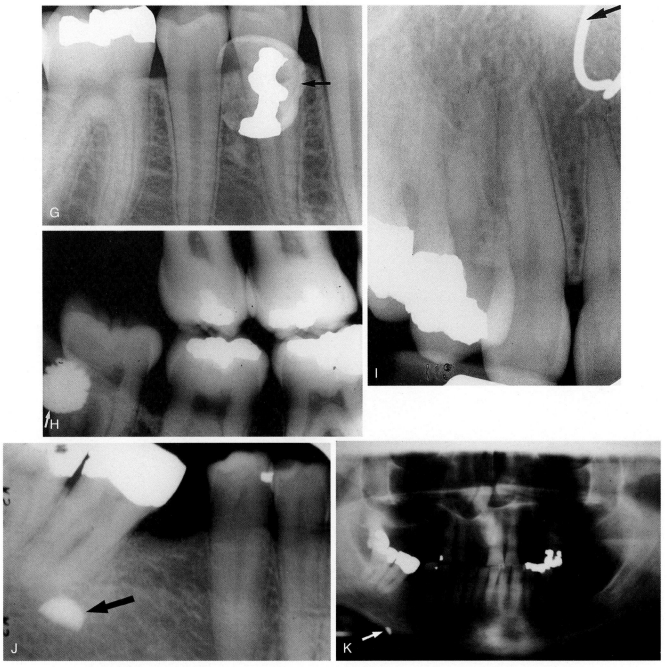

• **Figure 1.35, cont'd** **G,** Arrow points to a retained deciduous tooth with an amalgam restoration. **H,** Arrow points to a radiopaque area that identifies a retained shotgun pellet on the distal aspect of the mandibular third molar. **I,** Arrow points to a radiopaque circular area that is a nose ring. **J,** Periapical radiograph showing a radiopaque area at the apex of the mesial root of the mandibular second molar. This object was a retained piece of shrapnel. **K,** Panoramic radiograph of the same patient showing the same object (*arrow*). This radiograph gives a more accurate view of the location of the object. It was found to be in the soft tissue in the area and not within bone.

The clinician should review these documents carefully and update them with the patient at each visit.

Pathologic conditions in which the family history contributes a significant role in the diagnosis include amelogenesis imperfecta (Fig. 1.36), dentinogenesis imperfecta (Fig. 1.37), and many other genetic disorders. In addition, clinical findings and radiographs provide significant assistance to the diagnostic process of these conditions.

A patient's medical or dental status, including drug history, can also contribute significant information to a diagnosis. For example, a history of Crohn disease or ulcerative colitis may contribute to the diagnosis of oral ulcers (Fig. 1.38A), which

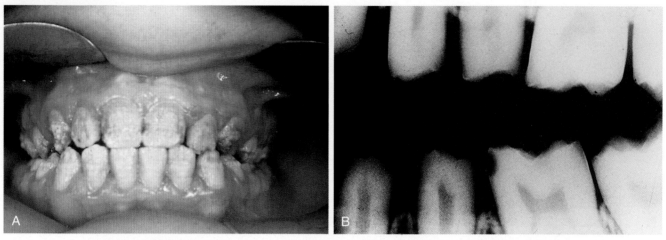

• **Figure 1.36 A,** One of the clinical appearances of amelogenesis imperfecta. **B,** The radiographic aspect of amelogenesis imperfecta. (Courtesy Dr. Edward V. Zegarelli.)

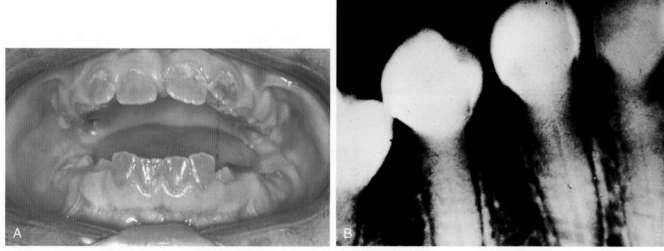

• **Figure 1.37 A,** Clinical appearance of dentinogenesis imperfecta. **B,** Radiographic appearance of dentinogenesis imperfecta. (Courtesy Dr. Edward V. Zegarelli.)

could be related to these medical conditions. Another example of the value of this type of information is the patient in Fig. 1.38B, who experienced gingival enlargement; drug history revealed that the patient was taking a calcium channel blocker. Allergic reactions may also be a part of the patient's medical history. Urticaria (hives) (see Chapter 3) is an immediate response to an allergen. Ingested allergens are often the cause of urticaria, but other causes include insect venom, drugs, topical agents, or systemic disease. Although the cause cannot always be identified, urticaria appears as well-demarcated areas of swelling on the skin, often erythematous (Fig. 1.38C-D). Sometimes hypersensitivity reactions may be delayed. However, in any case, each time the patient comes in contact with the allergen, the reaction may be more severe.

A history of a skin graft from the hip to the ridge and mucobuccal fold area in the anterior mandible in a patient can provide significant information relevant to the diagnosis of a white- or brown-pigmented area on the mandibular anterior ridge and vestibule (Fig. 1.39).

Periapical cemento-osseous dysplasia (cementoma) is another lesion in which the patient's personal history contributes significantly. It is found most frequently in black women in the third decade of life. Other characteristics of the lesion reveal that it is asymptomatic and that the teeth involved are vital (see Fig. 1.9). No treatment is necessary.

Laboratory Diagnosis

Clinical laboratory tests, including blood chemistries and urinalysis, can provide information that contributes to a diagnosis. An elevated serum alkaline phosphatase level is significant in the diagnosis of Paget disease of bone. This feature, in addition to a distinctive radiographic appearance that includes a "cotton-wool

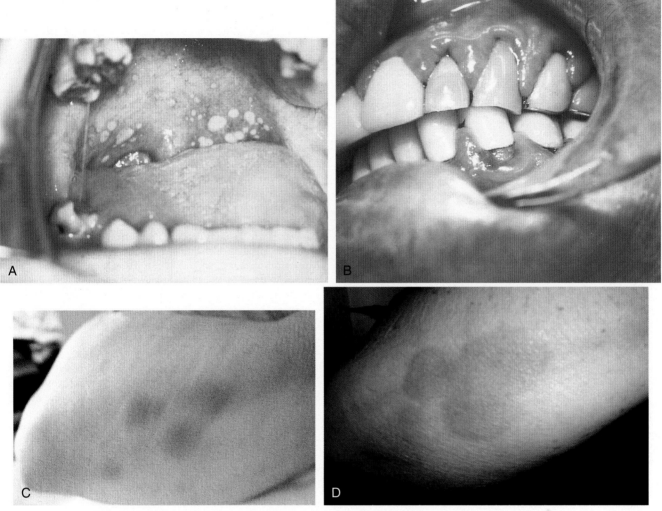

• **Figure 1.38 A,** Oral ulcers on the soft palate associated with ulcerative colitis. **B,** Gingival enlargement seen in a patient taking nifedipine, a calcium channel blocker. **C** and **D,** Urticaria. **D,** Same patient as in (C) 8 hours later. (**A** courtesy Dr. Edward V. Zegarelli.)

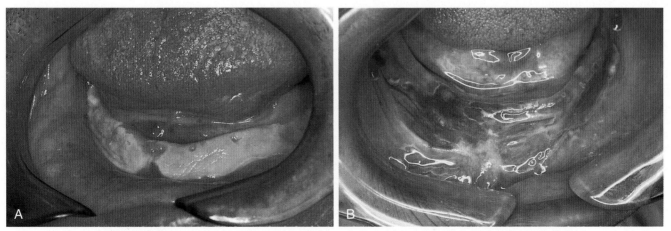

• **Figure 1.39** Skin grafts performed to enhance the mandibular ridge in **(A)** a white patient and **(B)** a black patient. Without the patients' past medical and dental histories, it would be difficult to diagnose this anomaly.

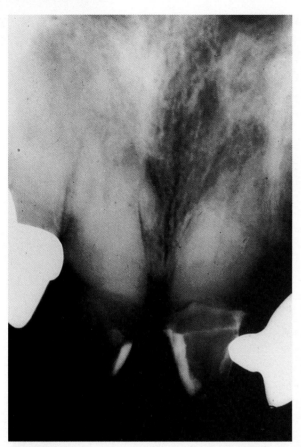

• **Figure 1.40** Radiographic appearance of Paget disease of bone, showing the traditional irregular radiopacities ("cotton-wool effect") in bone and hypercementosis of roots characteristic of this disease.

effect" (Fig. 1.40) and hypercementosis, provides conclusive information for a definitive diagnosis (see Chapter 8). Laboratory cultures are also helpful in determining the diagnosis of oral infections.

Microscopic Diagnosis

Microscopic examination is of particular importance in the diagnostic process and therefore, although it is a form of laboratory diagnosis, it is discussed separately from laboratory diagnosis. The microscopic examination of the biopsy specimen (via scalpel biopsy) taken from the lesion in question contributes significant information. This procedure is often the main component of the definitive diagnosis. However, the skill of the practitioner performing the biopsy is of equal importance. It is most important that an adequate tissue sample be removed for microscopic evaluation. If other diagnostic information such as clinical features or history of the lesion indicates the strong possibility of malignancy and the biopsy report does not concur, a second biopsy should be performed.

Additional screening technologies can also be used to detect changes in tissues. Some include brush testing and light-based systems that can contribute to the diagnosis. However, scalpel biopsy is considered the "gold standard" procedure used to provide the microscopic analysis that will establish the definitive diagnosis of a lesion.

A white lesion (**leukoplakia**) (Fig. 1.41A) cannot be diagnosed on the basis of its clinical appearance alone. *Leukoplakia* is a clinical term for a white lesion that cannot be rubbed off and cannot be diagnosed through clinical characteristics alone. The microscopic appearance of this type of white lesion can vary from a thickening of the epithelium or surface keratin layer to all levels of epithelial dysplasia, which can be premalignant. Fig. 1.41B illustrates hyperkeratosis and mild epithelial dysplasia. In addition, squamous cell carcinoma can be the diagnosis.

Erythroplakia is a clinical term for a red lesion that cannot be diagnosed on the basis of clinical features alone (Fig. 1.41C). Most erythroplakias (90%) are microscopically diagnosed as severe epithelial dysplasia (premalignant) or squamous cell carcinoma (see Chapter 7).

There are more than 130 types of the human papillomavirus (HPV). Some are very low risk, and others are high risk. Those associated with squamous cell carcinoma are high-risk types (HPV types 16 and 18). Others, such as those causing verruca vulgaris (the common wart), are low-risk types. Examples of low-risk types are HPV types 2, 6, 11, 27, and 57. Verruca vulgaris exhibits microscopic features that are characteristic of HPV infection (see Chapter 4). The squamous papilloma (see Chapter 7) has also been associated with low-risk types of HPV.

Surgical Diagnosis

The strength of a surgical diagnosis comes from surgical intervention. For example, diagnosis is made using the information gained during the surgical procedure for the traumatic bone cyst shown in Fig. 1.42. A traumatic or simple bone cyst will appear as a radiolucency that scallops around the roots. Surgical intervention provides conclusive evidence when the lesion is opened and an empty void within the bone is found. The void usually fills with bone and heals after the surgical procedure. Lingual mandibular bone concavity, also referred to as a *static bone cyst* or *Stafne bone cyst* (Fig. 1.43), is a developmental anomaly that is often bilateral. The radiolucent area is oval or elliptical in shape and is found anterior to the angle of the ramus and inferior to the mandibular canal. A computed tomography scan would further confirm the diagnosis, showing the invagination of the lingual aspect of the mandible. However, if the radiolucency is not in the classic location, surgical examination and biopsy would be necessary to confirm the diagnosis. There is no treatment necessary for lingual mandibular bone concavity.

Therapeutic Diagnosis

Nutritional deficiencies are common conditions to be diagnosed by therapeutic means. Although angular cheilitis (Fig. 1.44) may be associated with a deficiency of the B-complex vitamins, it is most commonly a fungal condition and responds to topical application of an antifungal cream or ointment such as nystatin. A thorough patient history should be obtained to rule out a contributory nutritional deficiency.

Necrotizing ulcerative gingivitis (NUG) has distinct clinical features (Fig. 1.45) and constitutional signs. It responds to hydrogen peroxide rinses because the anaerobic bacteria that cause NUG cannot survive in an oxygenated environment. Prescribing hydrogen peroxide rinses and observing the results without culturing the bacteria applies the principle of therapeutic diagnosis because it is based solely on clinical and historical information with confirmation by the response of the condition to therapy. Antibiotic therapy can also be used in the treatment of NUG.

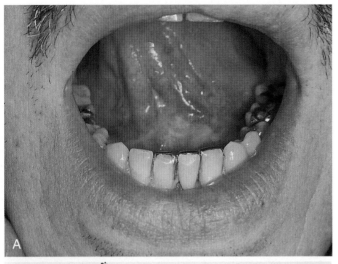

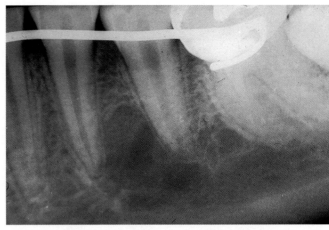

• **Figure 1.42** Traumatic bone cyst. (Courtesy Dr. Edward V. Zegarelli.)

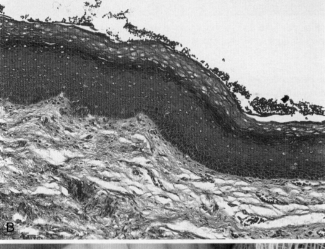

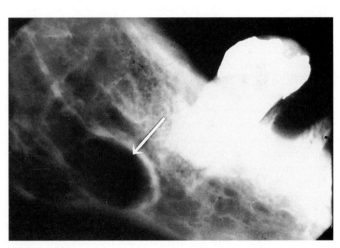

• **Figure 1.43** Arrow points to a static (Stafne) bone cyst. (Courtesy Dr. Edward V. Zegarelli.)

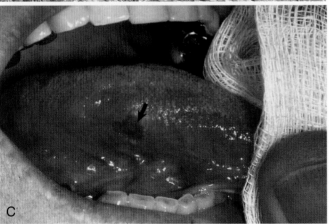

• **Figure 1.41** **A,** A white lesion is seen on the anterior floor and ventral surface of the tongue. **B,** Microscopic examination of the white lesion showed a thickened keratin layer, called *hyperkeratosis,* and some atypical changes in the basal layer of the epithelium (mild epithelial dysplasia). **C,** Erythroplakia (*arrow*) in this case diagnosed microscopically as squamous cell carcinoma. (C, Reprinted with permission from Savvy Success, Flanders, NJ.)

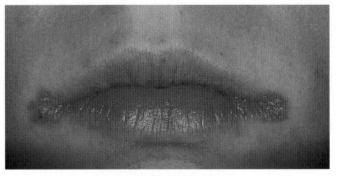

• **Figure 1.44** Angular cheilitis.

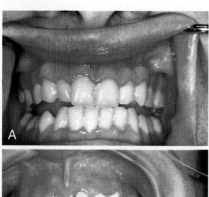
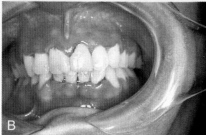

• **Figure 1.45 A,** Necrotizing ulcerative gingivitis (NUG). **B,** Another example of NUG. The clinician should note the gingival contours and punched-out, blunted papillae.

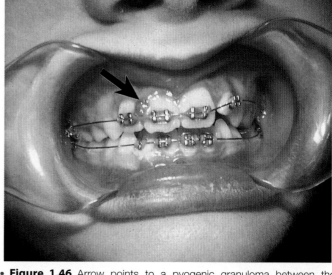

• **Figure 1.46** Arrow points to a pyogenic granuloma between the patient's right maxillary central and lateral incisors. (Courtesy Dr. Victor M. Sternberg.)

Differential Diagnosis

The differential diagnosis is that point in the diagnostic process when the practitioner decides which test or procedure is required to rule out the conditions originally suspected and to establish the definitive or final diagnosis. All previously discussed components are applied to the differential diagnosis. The final diagnosis emerges from a thorough evaluation of the suspected lesions (Box 1.1; Fig. 1.46).

To arrive at a diagnosis, data collection included the patient's medical and dental health histories, the history of the lesion in question, a clinical description and evaluation, and biopsy and microscopy reports. Box 1.1 illustrates the fact that arriving at a diagnosis involves a process. As stated previously, the diagnostic process can be thought of as a puzzle because the information from each diagnostic category becomes part of it. In Box 1.1 the microscopic examination contributed most significantly to the definitive or final diagnosis. The differential diagnosis included three possible diagnoses; the biopsy and microscopic examinations provided conclusive information in the diagnostic process.

The hygienist can be effective in the preliminary evaluation of the lesion by calling it to the attention of the dentist and then gathering and preparing all the data for the clinician who will perform the biopsy. In addition, it is both challenging and stimulating to discuss diagnostic impressions with other professionals on the basis of the data available before biopsy.

Variants of Normal

Fordyce Granules

Clusters of ectopic sebaceous glands are called **Fordyce granules.** They are most commonly observed on the lips and buccal mucosa. Clinically they appear as tiny yellow papules in clusters and are usually distributed over the buccal mucosa or vermilion border of the involved lips. The surrounding tissue is normal. Because more than 80% of adults over 20 years of age have Fordyce granules, they are considered developmental and a variant of

---

BOX 1.1

Case Study

The following case study illustrates how the diagnostic processes work together and how the differential diagnosis is used.

An 11-year-old white girl came to the dental office with her mother. The mother was concerned about the interdental papilla on the child's labial aspect between the maxillary right central and lateral incisors (Fig. 1.46). Nothing in the medical history explained the condition; the child had been wearing orthodontic appliances for about 1 year.

Clinically, the interdental papilla was enlarged and had a papillary surface that bled easily when probed. The sessile lesion measured 5 mm cervicoincisally by 3 mm mesiodistally. No pain was felt in the area. Information pertinent to the history of the lesion was secured from the mother. The lesion had been there for about 1 year and was first noticed around the time the child began wearing braces. At times tags of the lesion or pieces of it "fell off" during brushing. The orthodontist "pulled most of it off" at one point, but it was never surgically removed or submitted for microscopic examination and seemed to grow back. Additional questioning revealed that the child had a wart on her foot within the last year. A biopsy was performed, and the tissue sample was placed in formalin and sent to an oral pathology laboratory with the following differential diagnoses:

1. **Pyogenic granuloma:** The spongy inflammatory tissue was possibly caused by mechanical irritation from the orthodontic bands, thereby causing pyogenic granuloma.
2. **Papilloma:** On the basis of the papillary surface texture of the lesion, it was thought it could be a papilloma.
3. **Verruca vulgaris:** Because the child had a wart on her foot and could have spread the virus by self-innoculation, verruca vulgaris was suggested. In addition, histologically a wart has lateral lipping, and it was thought that this could explain why pieces of the lesion fell off periodically during brushing. However, the surface of a verruca vulgaris is usually keratinized and therefore whiter than the lesion illustrated in Fig. 1.46 (see Chapters 4 and 7).

The microscopic examination revealed stratified squamous epithelium covering a core of loose and edematous fibrous connective tissue. The stroma contained numerous endothelium-lined, blood-filled capillaries and a dense infiltrate of lymphocytes, plasma cells, and neutrophils.

The definitive or final diagnosis was pyogenic granuloma.

normal. Microscopically, Fordyce granules appear as normal sebaceous glands. They are asymptomatic and require no treatment (Fig. 1.47).

Torus Palatinus

Torus palatinus or palatal torus, an example of exostosis, is an exophytic growth of normal compact bone. It is benign. Palatal tori occur more frequently in women (2:1). They are more common in Asians, Native Americans, and the Inuit. Current research reports include both genetic and environmental influences in the pathogenesis. They are asymptomatic, develop gradually, and are observed clinically in the midline of the hard palate. Palatal tori may take on various shapes and sizes, may be lobulated, and are covered by normal soft tissue. It is not unusual for the palatal torus to be traumatized, which can cause discomfort and possible ulceration on the surface of the torus. The diagnosis of torus palatinus is made on clinical examination. When the torus is large, it may be seen as a radiopaque mass on a radiograph. No treatment is indicated unless the torus interferes with speech, swallowing, or a prosthetic appliance (Fig. 1.48).

Mandibular Tori

Outgrowths of normal dense bone found on the lingual aspect of the mandible in the area of the premolars above the mylohyoid ridge are **mandibular tori.** They are bilateral in more than 90% of cases, often lobulated, can appear fused together, and have a slight predilection for males. As with palatal tori, they are more common in Asians, Native Americans, and the Inuit. Diagnosis of mandibular tori is made on clinical examination. Mandibular tori usually do not require treatment unless the patient needs a

prosthodontic appliance (denture) and the tori interfere with proper fabrication and placement (Fig. 1.49).

Melanin Pigmentation

Melanin is the pigment that gives color to the skin, eyes, hair, mucosa, and gingiva. **Melanin pigmentation** of the oral mucosa

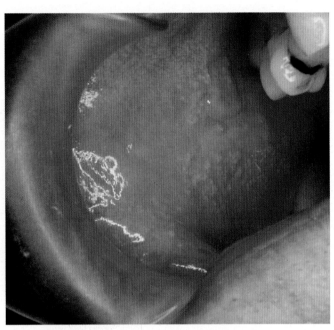

• **Figure 1.47** Fordyce granules on the buccal mucosa.

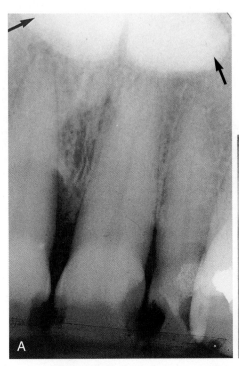

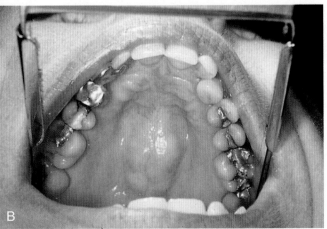

• **Figure 1.48 A,** Radiopaque appearance of torus palatinus (*arrows*). **B,** Clinical appearance of torus palatinus.

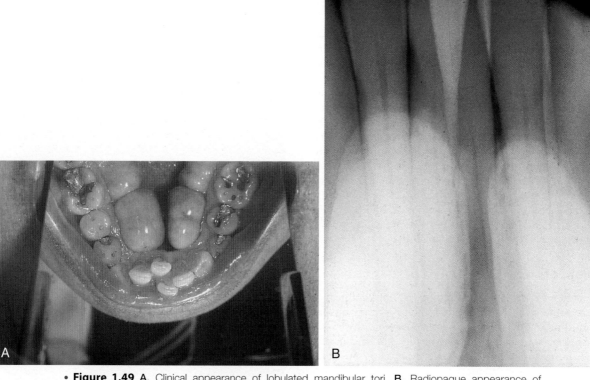

• **Figure 1.49 A,** Clinical appearance of lobulated mandibular tori. **B,** Radiopaque appearance of mandibular tori in same patient. (Courtesy Dr. Edward V. Zegarelli.)

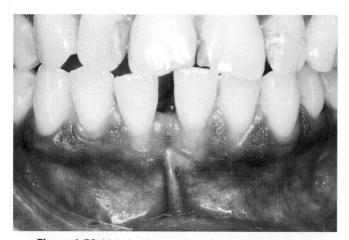

• **Figure 1.50** Melanin pigmentation of the mandibular gingiva.

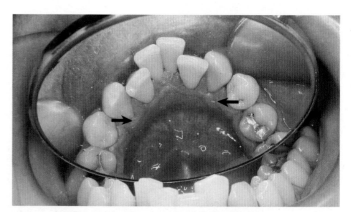

• **Figure 1.51** Arrows point to the retrocuspid papillae on the gingival margin of the lingual aspect of the mandibular cuspids.

or gingiva is most commonly observed in dark-skinned individuals (Fig. 1.50; and see Fig. 1.18).

Retrocuspid Papilla

A **retrocuspid papilla** is a sessile papule found on the gingival margin of the lingual aspect of the mandibular cuspids (Fig. 1.51). It is only a few millimeters in size. It is observed more often in the young and resolves with age.

Lingual Varicosities

Prominent lingual veins, called **lingual varicosities,** are usually observed on the ventral and lateral surfaces of the tongue. Clinically, red-to-purple enlarged vessels or clusters are seen. A relationship between varicosities in the legs and prominent lingual veins has been reported. A recent study suggested that they may be associated with a history of smoking or cardiovascular disease. Lingual varices are most commonly observed in individuals older

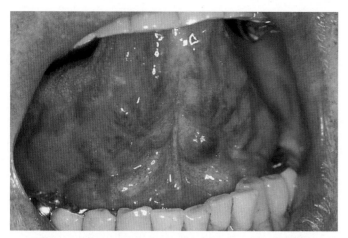

• **Figure 1.52** Lingual varices. (Courtesy Dr. David Zegarelli.)

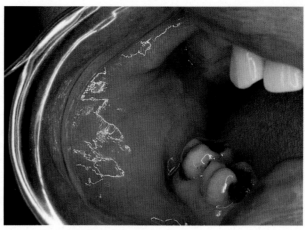

• **Figure 1.54** Leukoedema of the buccal mucosa, showing an opalescent, velvety texture.

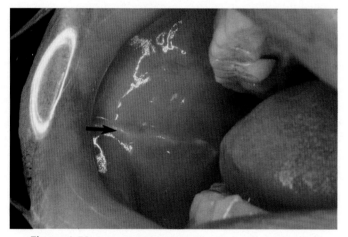

• **Figure 1.53** Arrow points to linea alba on the buccal mucosa.

than 60 years of age and therefore are thought to be related to the aging process (Fig. 1.52).

Linea Alba

Linea alba is a "white line" that extends anteroposteriorly on the buccal mucosa along the occlusal plane. It may be bilateral and can be more prominent in patients who have a clenching or bruxing habit (Fig. 1.53).

Leukoedema

A generalized opalescence is imparted to the buccal mucosa by **leukoedema.** It is most commonly observed in black adults (up to 90%), suggesting an ethnic predisposition. Leukoedema can also be seen in white and Hispanic individuals. Clinically, a gray-white opalescent appearance is diffused throughout the buccal mucosa, giving the mucosa an opaque quality. If the mucosa is stretched, the opalescence becomes less prominent. The condition becomes more pronounced in smokers and less obvious when the patient stops smoking. The opalescence is an integral part of the buccal tissue and cannot be removed. Histologically significant intracellular edema in the spinous cells and acanthosis of the epithelium are seen. It is a benign condition that is a variant of normal and requires no treatment (Fig. 1.54).

Other Benign Conditions With Unique Clinical Features

Lingual Thyroid

The thyroid gland begins to develop during the first month of fetal life and is located initially in the area of the foramen cecum on the posterior tongue. In normal development the thyroid gland descends to its normal location in the neck. When thyroid tissue either does not descend or remnants become entrapped in the tissue that makes up the tongue, a developmental anomaly called a **lingual thyroid** results. Research has indicated a high predilection in females, and studies have linked the emergence of a lingual thyroid with hormonal changes because it appears to be associated with puberty, pregnancy, and menopause. Clinically, lingual thyroid is observed as a mass in the midline of the dorsal surface of the tongue posterior to the circumvallate papillae between the foramen cecum and the epiglottis The lesion usually has a sessile base and is 2 to 3 cm in width. Clinical symptoms can include **dysphasia**, **dysphonia**, and **dyspnea**. The lingual thyroid is composed of normal thyroid tissue and may be the patient's functioning thyroid. A thyroid scan should be performed to determine the diagnosis. No treatment is required if lingual thyroid is the patient's only functioning thyroid.

Median Rhomboid Glossitis (Central Papillary Atrophy)

The cause of **median rhomboid glossitis** (central papillary atrophy) is not clear. It was at one time thought to be developmental. Research has suggested that it may be associated with a chronic fungal infection by *Candida albicans*. Some authors refer to it as a form of erythematous candidiasis. Clinically, median rhomboid glossitis appears as a flat or slightly raised oval or rectangular erythematous area in the midline of the dorsal surface of the tongue, beginning at the junction of the anterior and middle thirds and extending posterior to the circumvallate papillae. It is devoid of filiform papillae; therefore its texture is smooth. If the remaining surface of the tongue is coated, the area appears more prominent. No specific treatment exists; however, the lesion may resolve with topical antifungal treatment, confirming a therapeutic diagnosis of candidiasis. On occasion the condition spontaneously resolves (Fig. 1.55).

Erythema Migrans (Geographic Tongue)

The cause of **erythema migrans**, or **geographic tongue** (erythema areata migrans, benign migratory glossitis), is not clear. The familial occurrence of erythema migrans suggests that genetic factors play a role. Some investigators suggest that it is exacerbated by stress, and studies exist that associate the histologic findings with those found in psoriasis. The characteristic clinical appearance involves the anterior two-thirds of the dorsal and lateral borders of the tongue. Diffuse areas devoid of filiform papillae can be observed. These areas appear as erythematous patches that are surrounded by a white or yellow perimeter. The fungiform papillae appear distinct within the erythematous patch. The condition does not remain static; remission and changes in the depapillated areas may occur every few days. Erythema migrans is usually asymptomatic

and discovered by the dental hygienist or dentist on a routine oral mucosal examination. Usually no treatment is indicated. The diagnosis is a clinical one based on its appearance. On occasion a patient complains of a burning discomfort or sensitivity to spicy foods. If the burning discomfort becomes severe, topical corticosteroid treatment may be helpful (Fig. 1.56A).

Ectopic geographic tongue is the term used to describe erythema migrans when it is found on mucosal surfaces other than the tongue. In Fig. 1.56B it is seen in the mandibular anterior mucobuccal fold.

Fissured Tongue

The cause of **fissured tongue** is unknown. It is seen in about 5% of the population. Familial patterns of occurrence suggest that genetic factors are probably involved. There is a slight predilection in males. Clinically, the dorsal surface of the tongue appears to have deep fissures or grooves from 2 to 6 mm that may become irritated if food debris collects in them. The diagnosis of fissured tongue is a clinical one based on the appearance. About one third of patients with fissured tongue have erythema migrans as well. It is asymptomatic, and no treatment is indicated for the condition. However, a patient with a fissured tongue may be advised to brush the tongue gently with a soft toothbrush to keep the fissures clean of debris and irritants (Fig. 1.57; and see Fig. 1.19). Tongue scraping may remove surface debris, but does not reach the depth of the deep grooves and fissures present in fissured tongue.

Hairy Tongue

Hairy tongue is a condition in which the patient has an increased accumulation of keratin on the filiform papillae that results in a white, "hairy" appearance. This may be the result of either an increase in keratin production or a decrease in normal desquamation. Unless otherwise pigmented, the elongated filiform papillae are white (Fig. 1.58). In the condition known as black hairy tongue, the papillae are a brown-to-black color because of chromogenic bacteria (Fig. 1.59). Tobacco and certain foods may also

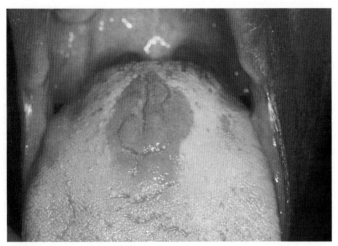

• **Figure 1.55** Median rhomboid glossitis (central papillary atrophy). (Courtesy Dr. Edward V. Zegarelli.)

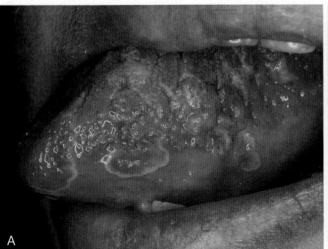

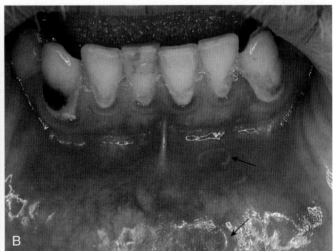

• **Figure 1.56** **A,** Erythema migrans (geographic tongue). **B,** Erythema migrans observed in the mandibular anterior mucosa.

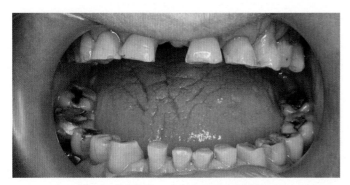

• **Figure 1.57** Fissured tongue and attrition.

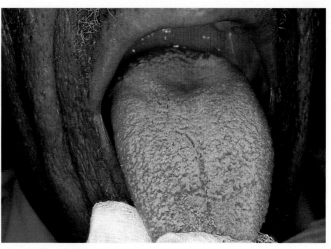

• **Figure 1.58** White hairy tongue.

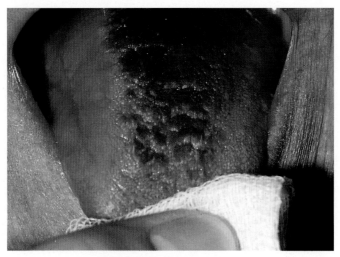

• **Figure 1.59** Black hairy tongue.

discolor the papillae. Although the cause is unknown, hydrogen peroxide, bismuth subsalicylates for upset stomach, alcohol, or chemical rinses have been suggested to stimulate the elongation of the filiform papillae that results in the appearance of hairy tongue.

Treatment involves directing the patient to brush the tongue gently with a soft toothbrush (wet with water only) to remove debris. If the causative agent is identified, the patient should be advised to discontinue its use. The condition usually clears completely but may recur.

Selected References

Books

Darby ML: *Darby's comprehensive review of dental hygiene*, ed 8, St. Louis, 2016, Elsevier. Inc.

Langlais RP, Miller CS, Gehrig JS: *Color atlas of common oral diseases*, ed 5, Philadelphia, 2017, Wolters Kluwer.

Neville BW, Damm DD, Allen CM, et al: *Oral and maxillofacial pathology*, ed 4, St Louis, 2016, Elsevier.

Regezi JA, Sciubba JJ, Jordan RCK: *Oral pathology: clinical pathologic correlations*, ed 7, St Louis, 2017, Elsevier.

Stedman's Medical Dictionary for the Dental Professions, ed 2, Philadelphia, 2011, Lippincott Williams & Wilkins.

Journal Articles

Bouquot JE, Gundlach KKH: Odd tongues: the prevalence of common tongue lesions in 23,616 white Americans over 35 years of age, *Quintessence Int* 17:719, 1986.

Brannon RB, Pousson RR: The retrocuspid papillae: a clinical evaluation of 51 cases, *J Dent Hyg* 77:180, 2003.

Chapnick L: External root resorption: an experimental radiographic evaluation, *Oral Surg Oral Med Oral Pathol* 67:578, 1989.

Comfort M, Wu PC: The reliability of personal and family medical histories in the identification of hepatitis B carriers, *Oral Surg Oral Med Oral Pathol* 67:531, 1989.

Daley TD: Pathology of intraoral sebaceous glands, *J Oral Pathol Med* 22:241, 1993.

Ibsen OAC: Diagnosing smoking-related lesions, *Dimens Dent Hyg* 2:32–35, 2004.

Ibsen OAC: Putting the pieces together, *Dimens Dent Hyg* 2:3–10, 2004.

Ibsen OAC: Oral cancer: incidence, the diagnostic process, and screening techniques, *Dimens Dent Hyg* 4:4, 2006.

Ibsen OAC: The missing link, *Dimens Dent Hyg* 6:28–31, 2008.

Kalan A, Tarig M: Lingual thyroid gland: clinical evaluation and comprehensive management, *Ear Nose Throat J* 78:340, 1999.

Kaugars GE, Miller ME, Abbey LM: Odontomas, *Oral Surg Oral Med Oral Pathol* 67:2172, 1989.

Lydiatt DD, Hollins RR, Peterson GP: Multiple idiopathic root resorption: diagnostic considerations, *Oral Surg Oral Med Oral Pathol* 67:208, 1989.

McCann AL, Wesley RK: A method for describing soft tissue lesions of the oral cavity, *J Dent Hyg* 60:304, 1986.

Neupert EA, Wright JM: Regional odontodysplasia presenting as a soft tissue swelling, *Oral Surg Oral Med Oral Pathol* 67:193, 1989.

Pogrel MA, Cram D: Intraoral findings in patients with psoriasis with a special reference to ectopic geographic tongue (erythema circinata), *Oral Surg Oral Med Oral Pathol* 66:184, 1988.

Rosen DJ, Ardekian L, Machtei EE, et al: Traumatic bone cyst resembling apical periodontitis, *J Periodontol* 68:1019, 1997.

Suzuki M, Sakae T: A familial study of torus palatinus and torus mandibularis, *Am J Phys Anthropol* 18:263, 1960.

Review Questions

1. After arriving at a differential diagnosis, information from which one of the following categories will best establish a final or definitive diagnosis?
   a. Clinical
   b. Historical
   c. Microscopic
   d. Radiographic

2. The descriptive term that would best be used for a freckle is a:
   a. Bulla
   b. Vesicle
   c. Lobule
   d. Macule

3. Which one of the following terms describes the base of a lesion that is stalklike?
   a. Sessile
   b. Lobule
   c. Pedunculated
   d. Macule

4. Clinical diagnosis can be used to determine the final or definitive diagnosis of all of the following *except:*
   a. Fordyce granules
   b. Unerupted supernumerary teeth
   c. Mandibular tori
   d. Erythema migrans

5. Radiographic diagnosis would contribute to the definitive diagnosis of all of the following *except:*
   a. Internal resorption
   b. Periapical cemento-osseous dysplasia
   c. Odontomas
   d. A retained deciduous tooth

6. To determine the presence of blood dyscrasias, which one of the following would provide the most definitive information?
   a. Laboratory blood tests
   b. Bleeding during probing
   c. Pallor of the gingiva and mucosa
   d. Patient complaint of weakness

7. When an antifungal ointment or cream is used to treat angular cheilitis, which one of the following diagnostic categories is being used?
   a. Clinical
   b. Therapeutic
   c. Laboratory
   d. Differential

8. Yellow clusters of ectopic sebaceous glands commonly observed on the buccal mucosa and evaluated through clinical diagnosis are most likely:
   a. Lipomas
   b. Fibromas
   c. Fordyce granules
   d. Linea alba

9. A slow-growing, bony, hard, exophytic growth on the midline of the hard palate is developmental and hereditary in origin. The diagnosis is determined through clinical evaluation. You suspect:
   a. Torus palatinus
   b. Mixed tumor
   c. Palatal cyst
   d. Nasopalatine cyst

10. The "white line" observed clinically on the buccal mucosa that extends from anterior to posterior along the occlusal plane is:
    a. Leukoedema
    b. Leukoplakia
    c. Linea alba
    d. Lichen planus

11. Which one of the following occurs as an erythematous area, is devoid of filiform papillae, is oval to rectangular in shape, does not change its characteristics, and is located on the midline of the dorsal surface of the tongue?
    a. Median rhomboid glossitis
    b. Erythema migrans
    c. Fissured tongue
    d. Lingual thyroid

12. Which one of the following diagnostic categories would the dental hygienist most easily apply to the preliminary evaluation of oral lesions?
    a. Microscopic
    b. Clinical
    c. Therapeutic
    d. Differential

13. These examples of exostoses are found on the lingual aspect of the mandible in the area of the premolars. They are benign, bony, hard, and require no treatment. Radiographically they appear as radiopaque areas and are often bilateral. You suspect:
    a. Retrocuspid papilla
    b. Lingual mandibular bone concavity
    c. Genial tubercles
    d. Mandibular tori

14. Which one of the following terms is most often used when describing mandibular tori?
    a. Bullous
    b. Lobulated
    c. Sessile
    d. Pedunculated

15. Which of the following conditions is a benign anomaly, has a diffuse gray-to-white opaque appearance on the buccal mucosa, and is most commonly seen in adult black individuals?
    a. Leukoedema
    b. Linea alba
    c. Erythema migrans
    d. Leukoplakia

16. A patient has the clinical signs of necrotizing ulcerative gingivitis. The hygienist has the patient begin hydrogen peroxide rinses without culturing the bacterial flora. This action applies to which one of the following diagnostic categories?
    a. Therapeutic
    b. Microscopic
    c. Clinical
    d. Final or definitive

17. A small circumscribed lesion usually less than 1 cm in diameter that is elevated and protrudes above the surface of normal surrounding tissue is called a:
    a. Bulla
    b. Macule
    c. Vesicle
    d. Papule

18. The base of a sessile lesion is:
    a. Broad and flat
    b. Stemlike
    c. Corrugated
    d. Lobulated

19. The identification of which one of the following is *not* determined by clinical diagnosis?
    a. Fordyce granules
    b. Tori
    c. Compound odontoma
    d. Retrocuspid papilla

20. Another term for erythema migrans is:
    a. Allergic tongue
    b. Median rhomboid glossitis
    c. Geographic tongue
    d. White hairy tongue

21. The cause of supernumerary teeth is most likely:
    a. Genetic
    b. Traumatic
    c. Cystic
    d. Systemic

22. Historical diagnosis can include the patient's:
    a. Age and sex
    b. Family history
    c. Medical history
    d. All of the above

23. Which condition is most often seen on the buccal mucosa?
    a. Melanin pigmentation
    b. Fordyce granules
    c. Nicotine stomatitis
    d. Angular cheilitis

24. Which one of the following is *not* considered a variant of normal?
    a. Migratory glossitis
    b. White hairy tongue
    c. Fissured tongue
    d. Hairy leukoplakia

25. Which cyst is often described as a radiolucency that scallops around the roots of the teeth involved?
    a. Stafne bone
    b. Traumatic bone
    c. Radicular
    d. Residual

26. What percentage of erythroplakias is diagnosed as severe epithelial dysplasia or squamous cell carcinoma?
    a. 10%
    b. 25%
    c. 60%
    d. 90%

27. Which of the following best describes the number of types of HPV? More than:
    a. 35
    b. 75
    c. 100
    d. 130

28. Which one of the following terms best defines leukoplakia?
    a. Clinical
    b. Histologic
    c. Historical
    d. Microscopic

29. Gingival enlargement is caused by which of the following groups of drugs?
    a. Antiviral
    b. Calcium channel blockers
    c. Antibiotics
    d. Hypersensitivity medications

30. Because it is associated with candidiasis, an antifungal medication is used sometimes to help in the diagnosis or treatment of:
    a. Lingual thyroid
    b. Erythema migrans
    c. Central papillary atrophy
    d. Black hairy tongue

31. The best way to determine whether lingual thyroid contains the patient's functioning thyroid tissue is:
    a. Thyroid scan
    b. Blood test
    c. Biopsy
    d. Medication

32. Retrocuspid papillae are found on the:
    a. Lingual gingiva between maxillary centrals
    b. Buccal mucosa
    c. Lingual aspects of mandibular canines
    d. Lateral border of the posterior tongue

Chapter 1 Synopsis

Condition/Disease	Cause	Age/Race/Sex	Location
Fordyce granules	Variant of normal	Adults	Most common on the buccal mucosa and lips
Torus palatinus *Pleomorphic adenoma*	Genetic	More common in females Develops after age 13 yr Increased prevalence in Native Americans	Midline of palate
Mandibular tori	Genetic	Develops after age 13 yr	Lingual mandibular premolar area
Melanin pigmentation	Variant of normal	Increased prevalence with increased skin pigmentation	Gingiva and oral mucosa Most prominent in dark-skinned individuals
Retrocuspid papillae *Fistula*	Developmental	N/A	Lingual gingival margin of the mandibular cuspids
Lingual varicosities	Aging process	Older adults	Most common on ventral and lateral surfaces of the tongue
Linea alba *Lichen planus*	Clenching/bruxing habit	N/A	Buccal mucosa at occlusal plane

NOTE: Items listed in *italics* under a specific condition/disease should be considered in a differential diagnosis.
N/A, Not applicable.

33. The benign stratified squamous cell papilloma is considered low risk and is associated with which types of HPV?
    a. 16 and 18
    b. 2 and 3
    c. 6 and 11
    d. 1 and 9

34. The most common location for lingual thyroid is:
    a. Ventral tongue
    b. Dorsal of anterior third of tongue
    c. In the neck
    d. Between the foramen cecum and epiglottis

35. Which of the following is characterized by symptoms including dysphagia, dysphonia, and dyspnea?
    a. Median rhomboid glossitis
    b. Erythema migrans
    c. Lingual thyroid
    d. Fissured tongue

36. All of the following are characteristics of periapical cemento-osseous dysplasia except one. Which one is the exception?
    a. Black women
    b. Vital teeth
    c. Mid thirties
    d. Elevated serum alkaline phosphatase

37. All of the following are diagnosed without biopsy except one. Which one is the exception?
    a. Fissured tongue
    b. Erythroplakia
    c. Central papillary atrophy
    d. Erythema migrans

38. A lesion is measured at 6 cm. What is the approximate size of the lesion?
    a. 6 inches
    b. 3 inches
    c. 100 mm
    d. 10 mm

Clinical Features	Radiographic Features	Microscopic Features	Treatment	Diagnostic Process
Tiny, yellow lobules in clusters	N/A	Normal sebaceous gland lobules	None	Clinical
Bony hard exophytic structure	Radiopaque	Compact bone	None	Clinical
Bony hard exophytic structures	Radiopaque	Compact bone	None	Clinical
Most prominent in dark-skinned individuals Brown to gray-black pigmented mucosa	N/A	Melanin pigment in the basal cell layer of the epithelium and subjacent connective tissue	None	Clinical
Red, sessile nodule	N/A	Fibrous connective tissue with large stellate-shaped cells	None	Clinical
Red-to-purple enlarged blood vessels	N/A	Thick-walled blood vessels	None	Clinical
Anterior-posterior white line	N/A	Epithelial hyperplasia and hyperkeratosis	None	Clinical

Continued

Chapter 1 Synopsis—cont'd

Condition/Disease	Cause	Age/Race/Sex	Location
Leukoedema	Unknown	Black	Buccal mucosa
Lingual thyroid	Developmental thyroid tissue entrapped in posterior dorsal tongue	Affects women more than men	Between foramen caecum and epiglottis
Median rhomboid glossitis	Unknown, associated with *Candida*	Rare in children Adults	Midline of dorsal tongue
Erythema migrans	Genetic Associated with stress Some cases associated with psoriasis		Dorsal and lateral borders of tongue
Fissured tongue	Unknown; genetic factors associated	N/A	Dorsal tongue
Hairy tongue	Unknown Associated with smoking, peroxide rinses, alcohol		Dorsal midposterior tongue

NOTE: Items listed in *italics* under a specific condition/disease should be considered in a differential diagnosis.
N/A, Not applicable.

Clinical Features	Radiographic Features	Microscopic Features	Treatment	Diagnostic Process
Gray-white film that gives the mucosa an opalescent quality	N/A	Intracellular edema and acanthosis of the epithelium	None	Clinical
Exophytic mass Symptoms: dysphagia, dysphonia, and dyspnea	N/A	Normal thyroid tissue	None	Clinical (Thyroid scan may be necessary)
Flat or slightly raised erythematous, rectangular area anterior to the circumvallate papillae	N/A	Epithelial hyperplasia	None	Clinical
Erythematous, depapillated areas with white borders Occasional complaint of burning discomfort	N/A	Epithelial hyperplasia with tiny collections of neutrophils near the surface	None Avoid spicy foods	Clinical
Deep fissures or grooves	N/A		Gently brush tongue without toothpaste	Clinical
Elongated filiform papillae (e.g., black, white, yellow)	N/A	N/A	Gently brush tongue without toothpaste	Clinical

2

Inflammation and Repair

MARGARET J. FEHRENBACH, JOAN ANDERSEN PHELAN, AND OLGA A.C. IBSEN

OBJECTIVES

After studying this chapter, the student will be able to:

1. Define each of the words in the vocabulary list for this chapter.
2. Do the following related to inflammation:
   - Describe the differences between acute and chronic inflammation.
   - List and describe the major local and systemic clinical signs of inflammation.
   - Describe how the microscopic events are associated with each of the major clinical signs of inflammation.
3. List the white blood cells that are involved in the inflammatory response and describe how each is involved.
4. List and describe the biochemical mediators involved in inflammation.
5. List and describe the four major systemic clinical signs of inflammation.
6. Discuss chronic inflammation, as well as antiinflammatory therapy.
7. Define and contrast hyperplasia, hypertrophy, and atrophy.
8. Do the following related to regeneration, repair, and microscopic events during repair:
   - Compare and contrast the concepts of regeneration and repair.
   - Describe the microscopic events that occur during repair in the oral cavity.
   - Describe the microscopic events that occur during healing in bone.

- Describe and contrast healing by differing intentions.
- List local and systemic factors that can impair healing.
9. Do the following related to traumatic injuries to teeth:
   - Describe and contrast attrition, abrasion, and erosion.
   - Describe the relationship between bruxism, abrasion, and abfraction.
   - Describe the pattern of erosion seen in bulimia.
10. Describe the cause, clinical features, and treatment of each of the following: oral mucosal burns, aspirin burns, phenol and other chemical burns, electric burns, thermal burns, lesions from cocaine use and self-induced injuries, hematomas, traumatic ulcers, frictional keratosis, linea alba, and nicotine stomatitis.
11. Describe the clinical features, cause (when known), treatment, and microscopic appearance of each of the following: traumatic neuroma, amalgam tattoo, melanosis, oral and labial melanotic macule, solar cheilitis, mucocele, ranula, sialolith, necrotizing sialometaplasia, sialadenitis, pyogenic granuloma, peripheral giant cell granuloma, chronic hyperplasic pulpitis, irritation fibroma, denture-induced fibrous hyperplasia, gingival enlargement, and chronic hyperplastic pulpitis.
12. Describe and differentiate among a periapical abscess, a periapical granuloma, and a radicular cyst.
13. Discuss tooth resorption, both external and internal.
14. Discuss the causes and diagnosis of focal sclerosing osteomyelitis and alveolar osteitis.

❖ Vocabulary

Abscess (ab′ses) A collection of purulent exudate that has accumulated in a contained space formed by the surrounding tissue.

Actinic (ak-tin′ic) Relating to or exhibiting chemical changes produced by radiant energy, especially the visible and ultraviolet parts of the spectrum; relating to exposure to the ultraviolet rays of sunlight.

Acute (ah-kūt′) An injury or course of inflammation that is of short duration.

Angiogenesis (an″je-o-jen′ə-sis) The formation and differentiation of blood vessels.

Atrophy (at′rə-fe) The decrease in size and function of a cell, tissue, organ, or whole body.

Biochemical mediators (bi″o-kem′-əkəl me′de-a′tors) Chemicals in the body that activate responses.

Central (sen′trəl) In the context of oral lesions, *central* indicates that the lesion is within bone.

Chemotaxis (ke″mo-tak′sis) The movement of white blood cells, as directed by biochemical mediators, to an area of injury.

Chronic (kron′ik) An injury or course of inflammation that is of long duration.

C-reactive protein (se-re-ak′tiv pro′ten) A nonspecific protein, produced in the liver, that becomes elevated during episodes of acute inflammation or infection.

Cyst (sist) An abnormal sac or cavity lined by epithelium and surrounded by fibrous connective tissue.

Cytolysis (si-tol′ə-sis) The dissolution or destruction of a cell.

Demastication (de″ mas tĭ-ka′shun) When tooth wear is increased by chewing an abrasive substance.

Edema (ə-de′mə) An excess level of plasma or exudate in the interstitial space that results in tissue swelling.

Emigration (em″i-gra′shən) The passage of white blood cells through the walls of small blood vessels and into injured tissue.

Epithelialization (ep″i-the″le-əl-ĭ-za′shən) The process of renewal of a new surface layer of epithelium.

Erythema (er″ə-the′mə) The redness of the skin or mucosa.

Exudate (eks′u-dāt) A body fluid with a high protein content that leaves the microcirculation during an inflammatory response that consists of serum that contains white blood cells, fibrin, and other protein molecules.

Fever (fe′vər) An elevation of body temperature to greater than the usual level of 37° C (98.6° F).

Fibroblasts (fi′bro-blasts) The cells that form fibers as well as intercellular substance.

Fibroplasia (fi″bro-pla′shə) The formation of fibrous tissue as usually occurs in healing.

Fistula (fis′tu-lə) An abnormal passage that leads from an abscess to the body surface.

Granulation tissue (gran″u-la′shən) The initial connective tissue formed in healing.

Granuloma (gran″u-lo′mə) A lesion composed of a collection of macrophages usually surrounded by a rim of lymphocytes that is a form of chronic inflammation.

Hyperemia (hi″pər-e′me-ə) An excess of blood within blood vessels in a part of the body.

Hyperplasia (hi″pər-pla′zhə) An enlargement of a tissue or organ resulting from an increase in the number of cells; the result of increased cell division.

Hypertrophy (hi″pər′tro-fe) An enlargement of a tissue or organ resulting from an increase in the size of its individual cells, but not in the number of cells.

Inflammation (in″flə-ma′shən) A nonspecific response to injury that involves the microcirculation and its blood cells.

Injury An alteration in the environment that causes tissue damage.

Keloid (kē′-lŏid) The excessive scarring that mainly occurs in skin in some cases with healing.

Leukocytosis (loo″ko-si-to′sis) An increase in the number of white blood cells circulating in blood.

Leukopenia (lü-kə-′pē-nē-ə) A decrease in the number of white blood cells circulating in blood.

Local (lo′kəl) A disease process that is confined to a limited location in the body that is not general or systemic.

Lymphadenopathy (lim-fad″ĕ-no-p′ə-the) The abnormal enlargement of a lymph node or nodes.

Macrophage (mak′ro-fāj) The second type of white blood cell to arrive at a site of injury that was originally a monocyte; it participates in phagocytosis during inflammation and continues to be active in the immune response.

Margination (mahr″jĭ-na′shən) A process during inflammation in which white blood cells tend to move to the periphery of the blood vessel at the site of injury.

Microcirculation (mi″kro-sur″ku-la′shən) The small blood vessels, including arterioles, capillaries, and venules of the vascular system.

Myofibroblasts (mi″o-fi′bro-blasts) Fibroblasts that have some of the characteristics of smooth muscle cells, such as the ability to contract.

Necrosis (nə-kro′sis) The pathologic death of one or more cells, or a part of tissue, or an organ that results from irreversible damage to cells.

Neutrophil (noo′tro-fil) The first white blood cell to arrive at a site of injury; the primary cell involved in acute inflammation; also called a *polymorphonuclear leukocyte.*

Opacification (o-pas″ĭ-fĭ-ka′shən) The process of becoming opaque.

Opsonization (op″sə-nĭ-za′shən) The enhancement of phagocytosis by a process in which a pathogen is marked, with opsonins, for destruction by phagocytes.

Osteoblast (os-te-o′-blast) The cell that forms bone.

Pavementing (pāv″mənt-ing) The adherence of white blood cells to blood vessel walls during inflammation.

Peripheral (pə-rif′ər-əl) In the context of oral lesions, peripheral indicates that the lesion is within the gingival tissue or alveolar mucosa.

Phagocytosis (fag″o-si-to′sis) The ingestion and digestion of particulate material by cells.

Purulent exudate (pu′roo-lənt eks′u-dāt) An exudate containing or forming pus.

Pyrogens (pi′ro-jen) The fever-inducing substances produced from either white blood cells or pathogenic microorganisms.

Radicular (rə-dik′u-lər) Pertaining to the root of a tooth.

Regeneration (re-jən″ər-a′shən) The process by which injured tissue is replaced with tissue identical to that present before the injury.

Repair (rə′per) The restoration of damaged or diseased tissue by cellular change and growth.

Serous exudate (sēr′əs eks′u-dāt) An exudate that has a watery consistency. The consistence resembles that of serum.

Systemic (sis-tem′ik) Pertaining to or affecting the body as a whole, as well as a disease process pertaining to or affecting the body as a whole.

Transudate (trans′u-dāt) The extravascular fluid component of blood that passes through the endothelial cell walls of the microcirculation.

White blood cells The cells within the blood and surrounding tissue, also called *leukocytes,* that are involved in the inflammatory and immune responses.

Traumatic injury (trə-mat′ik) A disease process that results from injury that causes tissue damage.

Waldeyer's ring (wal·dey·er′s ring) The ring of lymphatic tissue formed by the two palatine tonsils, the pharyngeal tonsil, the lingual tonsil, and intervening lymphoid tissue.

Inflammation, immunity, and repair are the body's responses to injury. Inflammation allows the body to eliminate injurious agents and injured tissue, to contain or control injuries, and to begin the process of healing. This chapter begins with a description of injury, the inflammatory response, and tissue regeneration and continues with a description of oral lesions that occur in response to injury. Many of these lesions caused by injury are quite common and are likely to be encountered when the dental hygienist examines the hard and soft tissues of the oral cavity and the skin of the face. Immune responses and oral lesions that occur as a result of destruction through activity of immune responses are described in Chapter 3. Orofacial lesions that occur as a result of infection are included in Chapter 4.

Injury

Injury is the result of an alteration in the environment that causes tissue damage. Severe injury may result in **necrosis,** the pathologic death of one or more cells or a part of tissue or an organ that results from irreversible damage to cells. Less severe injury may result in reversible cellular responses such as hyperplasia, hypertrophy, and atrophy, which are described later in this chapter.

Injury to orofacial tissue may have different causes such as physical injury, chemical injury, infection, nutritional deficiencies, and toxicities. Physical injury can affect teeth, soft tissue, and bone. Chemical injury can occur from the application of caustic substances. Microorganisms can cause injury by invading orofacial tissue and causing infections. Nutritional deficiencies can render orofacial tissue more susceptible to injury from other sources, and toxic overdoses of some nutrients can also cause tissue damage.

Innate Defenses

The body has a number of innate or natural defenses to protect against injury. These inborn defenses are present from birth and include intact skin or mucosa that acts as a physical barrier to injury, cilia and mucus in the respiratory system that serve as a mechanical defense system, and stomach acid that kills most of the microorganisms that are taken into the body through the mouth. The flushing action of tears, saliva, urine, and diarrhea removes foreign substances. Components of saliva and tears have antimicrobial activity, and the resident microbiota on the skin and mucosal tissue prevents colonization by pathogens. The process of inflammation and its white blood cells that are brought to the area of injury are innate responses to injury.

Inflammation

Inflammation is a nonspecific response to injury and occurs in the same manner, regardless of the nature of the injury. The extent and duration of the injury determine the extent and duration of the inflammatory response. The inflammatory response may be **local** and limited to the area of injury, or it may become **systemic,** involving the whole body, if the injury is extensive. Inflammation of a specific tissue is denoted by the suffix *-itis* combined with the name of the tissue, such as in *tonsillitis, pulpitis,* and *gingivitis.*

The inflammatory response may be acute or chronic. If the injury is minimal and brief and its source is removed from the tissue, it is considered **acute.** The duration of the acute inflammatory response is short, lasting only a few days. The tissue may return to its original state, or repair of the tissue may begin immediately.

If injury to the tissue continues and the inflammatory response is longer lasting, it is referred to as **chronic;** the duration of chronic inflammation may last weeks, months, or even indefinitely. Because of its prolonged duration, chronic inflammation produces more extensive tissue destruction, heals less readily, and is associated with more serious functional deficiencies than an acute inflammation.

The inflammatory response is a dynamic process, continually changing in response to injury and repair. Transitional stages exist during which the response is changing from one type of inflammation to the next and from an innate inflammatory response to an immune response (see Chapter 3). An acute inflammatory response may be superimposed over a chronic inflammatory response. Inflammation may mask the correct diagnosis upon biopsy of a lesion.

On occasion, an overwhelming inflammatory response may lead to further injury. Repair of the tissue occurs only if the persistent source of injury is removed. Studies now show the importance of the inflammatory process because without inflammation, infection and wounds would not heal, the tissue would become more and more damaged, and the body, or any organism, would eventually undergo destruction. Health professionals traditionally try to control inflammation to encourage healing. However, the stringent level of this control may be changing to allow some amount of inflammation in order to promote healing.

Current research is also demonstrating that chronic inflammation is a major component of the pathogenesis of common disorders such as atherosclerosis, insulin resistance, and Alzheimer disease, as well as cancer; inflammation could be a common link in the pathogenesis of these diseases, because these degenerative disorders often exhibit high levels of proinflammatory markers in their blood, such as C-reactive protein (CRP), as discussed later.

Microscopic Events of Inflammation and Clinical Signs

Microscopic events occur within the injured tissue during both acute and chronic inflammation. These events cause changes that can be observed clinically. The local clinical changes at the site of injury are considered the major (or cardinal) clinical signs of inflammation and include redness, heat, swelling, pain, and loss of the usual level of tissue function (Table 2.1). In addition, systemic clinical signs of inflammation may be present when the response is more extensive; these major systemic clinical signs are discussed later in this chapter.

The microscopic events of inflammation involve the small blood vessels, or **microcirculation.** These include arterioles, capillaries, and venules in the area of injury, as well as red blood cells, white blood cells, and chemicals produced in the body called **biochemical mediators** (Fig. 2.1).

Normally, blood, and the cells it contains, flows easily through the microcirculation. Exchange of oxygen and nutrients needed for the health of the surrounding tissue occurs as plasma fluid passes between the endothelium lining the vessel walls of the arterioles and capillaries. Plasma is the fluid component of blood in which the blood cells are suspended; it is composed mainly of water and proteins. Most of the plasma that leaves the microcirculation reenters the circulation through the venules. The lymphatic vessels carry away any excess plasma that does not reenter the blood vessels.

During inflammation, the status quo of the body undergoes a change, with underlying microscopic events proceeding faster than the visible clinical changes. The sequence of events is shown in Box 2.1.

The first microscopic event of the inflammatory response is a brief, immediate reflex constriction of the microcirculation in the area of the injury. This is followed, within seconds, by a dilation of the same small blood vessels. This dilation leads to an increase in the diameter of the blood vessels and is caused by biochemical mediators that are released at the time of the injury. Dilation of

TABLE 2.1 Major Local and Systemic Clinical Signs of Inflammation and Associated Microscopic Events

Clinical Feature	Associated Microscopic Events
Major Localized Clinical Signs of Inflammation	
Redness or erythema and heat	Hyperemia resulting from dilation of the microcirculation
Swelling	Permeability of the microcirculation leads to exudate formation in the tissue
Pain	Pressure on nerves by exudate formation and release of biochemical mediators
Loss of the usual level of tissue function	Events associated with swelling and pain
Major Systemic Clinical Signs of Inflammation	
Fever	Production of pyrogens affects the hypothalamus, which increases body temperature
Leukocytosis	An increase in the number of white blood cells circulating in the blood
Lymphadenopathy	Hyperplasia and hypertrophy of lymphocytes
Elevated C-reactive protein	A nonspecific protein produced in the liver and elevated in the circulating blood when inflammation is present in the body

• BOX 2.1 Inflammatory Response: Sequence of Events

1. Constriction of the small blood vessels of the microcirculation occurs.
2. Dilation of the same small blood vessels of the microcirculation occurs.
3. Vessels of the microcirculation increase in permeability.
4. Plasma with low protein content leaves the microcirculation as a transudate.
5. Blood in the microcirculation increases in viscosity.
6. Blood flow through the microcirculation slows down.
7. White blood cells marginate and pavement along the vessel walls.
8. White blood cells emigrate from the microcirculation, disrupting the basement membrane surrounding endothelial cells and increasing vascular permeability.
9. Plasma with high protein content leaves the microcirculation as an exudate.
10. White blood cells ingest foreign substances during phagocytosis.

the microcirculation results in increased blood flow through the blood vessels. The increased blood flow that fills the capillary beds in the injured tissue is called **hyperemia.** Hyperemia is responsible for two local clinical signs of inflammation: erythema and heat. **Erythema,** or redness, is easily visible in most inflamed orofacial tissue. However, local increased temperature changes may be more difficult to recognize.

While hyperemia is occurring, the permeability of the vessels of the microcirculation also increases and the blood vessels become "leaky." The endothelial cells contract, and spaces form between the cells. As a result the plasma fluid with a low protein content that contains no cells passes between the endothelial cells and

enters the tissue. This extravascular fluid is called a **transudate** and is the same type of fluid that usually moves from the microcirculation to the tissue as a result of imbalanced hydrostatic and osmotic pressures to supply oxygen and nutrients.

The loss of fluid within the microcirculation leads to increased blood viscosity. The blood becomes thicker and cannot flow as easily. This eventually results in decreased flow through the microcirculation. As the blood flow slows down, the red blood cells begin to pile up in the center of the blood vessels, and the white blood cells are displaced to the periphery of the blood vessels. This movement of the white blood cells to the periphery is called **margination.** The white blood cells are now in position to adhere themselves to the inner walls of the injured blood vessels, which have become "sticky" because of specific factors on the surfaces of the cells. This lining of the walls by white blood cells is called **pavementing** (Fig. 2.2).

After pavementing the vessel walls, the white blood cells begin to escape from the blood vessels through the walls, along with more fluid, and enter the injured tissue. This process by which the white blood cells escape from the blood vessels is called **emigration.** Emigration occurs as a result of opening of the cellular junctions of the endothelial cells lining the blood vessels; these cells contract in size in response to biochemical mediators.

As the white blood cells, primarily neutrophils, emigrate through the blood vessel walls and surrounding basement membrane, they further increase the permeability of the microcirculation and allow larger molecules and other cells to escape. The fluid that now flows into the injured tissue due to inflammation is called an **exudate.** This fluid contains cells and a higher concentration of protein molecules than in a transudate. The presence of transudate and exudate in the injured tissue helps to dilute injurious agents that may be present and carries injurious agents through the lymphatic vessels to the lymph nodes, where an immune response is stimulated (Chapter 3).

As transudate escapes into the tissue, excess fluid collects in the fibrous connective tissue at the site. This excess level of fluid in the interstitial space is called **edema** and results in localized enlargement or swelling of the tissue, another clinical sign of inflammation (Fig. 2.3). If the swollen tissue area is injured further, exudate may flow out of the tissue as either a thin clear fluid that is called a **serous exudate** or as a thick white-to-yellow pus, or *suppuration,* that contains tissue debris and many white blood cells that is called a **purulent exudate.** An **abscess** is a collection of purulent exudate that has accumulated in a contained space formed by the surrounding tissue.

The formation of exudate may be so excessive that it interferes with repair of the tissue. The injured tissue may allow the excess exudate to drain by formation of a drainage passage that bores through the tissue, allowing drainage to the outside. This channel through the tissue is called a **fistula** or fistulous tract; it is formed at the expense of healthy functioning tissue in the area that is lost as the tissue undergoes necrosis or cell death (Fig. 2.4). In some cases, excessive exudate in damaged tissue must be drained mechanically by making an incision in the surface of the swollen area and, often, by placing a drainage tube in the site of the incision (Fig. 2.5). This procedure of incision and drainage may be accompanied by the administration of medications to reduce inflammation and possibly an antibiotic, if there is evidence of infection.

As the exudate presses on sensory nerves in the area, exudate formation results in pain, another clinical sign of inflammation. Some biochemical mediators present in inflamed tissue can add

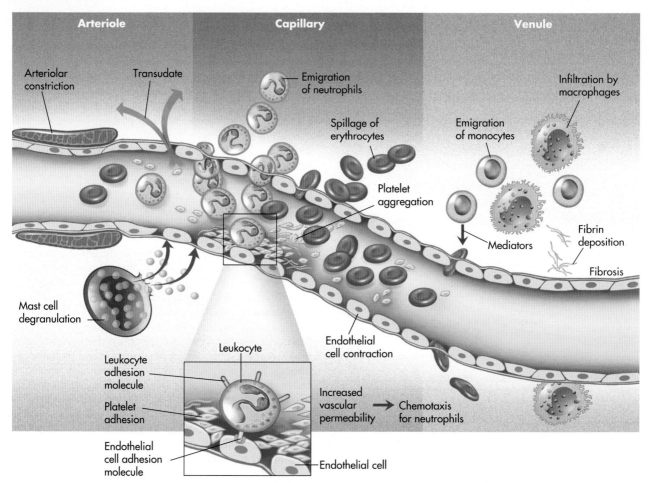

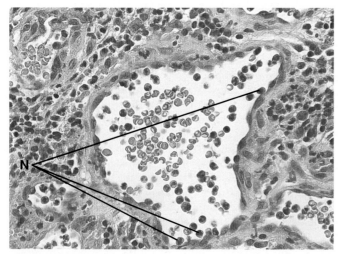

• **Figure 2.1** Microscopic events during inflammation. (From McCance K, Huether S: *Pathophysiology*, ed 7, St. Louis, Mosby, 2014.)

• **Figure 2.2** Microscopic view of a blood vessel showing margination and pavementing of neutrophils (*N*) at the periphery of a small blood vessel during inflammation.

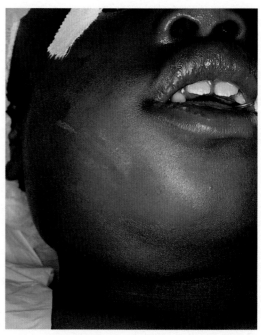

• **Figure 2.3** Swelling caused by increased local edema associated with a dental infection. The patient was hospitalized for treatment of the swelling. (Courtesy Dr. Sidney Eisig.)

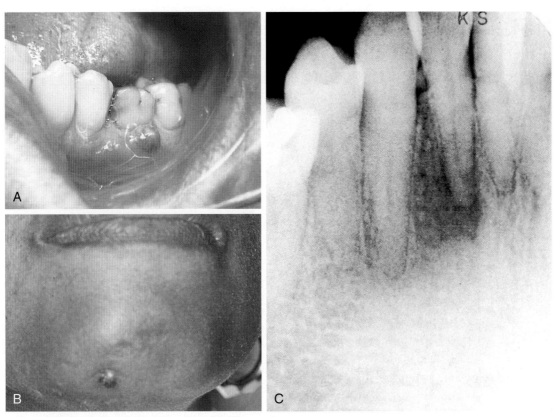

• **Figure 2.4** Fistulas formed from periapical abscesses. **A,** A fistula formed from an abscess associated with a mandibular first molar. **B,** The opening of a fistulous tract from a mandibular incisor is noted on the skin of the chin. **C,** A periapical radiolucency at the area of abscess causing the fistula to the skin in **B.**

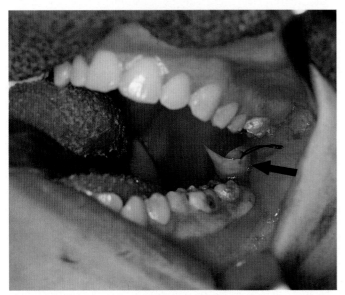

• **Figure 2.5** An intraoral abscess has been incised, and a drain (*arrow*) placed to allow the escape of purulent exudate from the tissue. (Courtesy Dr. Sidney Eisig.)

to the pain level. The swelling and pain in tissue resulting from the inflammatory process may then cause a loss of the usual level of tissue function, another clinical sign of inflammation.

This directed movement of white blood cells toward the site of the injury is called **chemotaxis;** biochemical mediators that enhance this directed movement are *chemotactic factors.* Emigration and chemotaxis of white blood cells to the area of injury allow these cells to be mobilized in the defense against the injury.

At first these cells try to wall off the site of the injury from the surrounding healthy tissue. Later, in the injured tissue, the white blood cells also try to remove foreign substances from the site by ingesting and then digesting them, thus undergoing **phagocytosis** (Fig. 2.6). The foreign substances may include pathogenic microorganisms or tissue debris. The presence of these substances may interfere with the repair process; in most cases, they must be removed for the inflammation to resolve and any necessary tissue repair to proceed. Recent studies show that the inflammatory process ends with the departure of macrophages through the lymphatics.

White Blood Cells in the Inflammatory Response

Emigration of **white blood cells,** or **leukocytes,** from the blood vessels into the site of injury and subsequent chemotaxis and phagocytosis are important components of the process of inflammation. As inflammation begins and continues over the 2 weeks after an injury, changes take place in the relative numbers of white blood cell populations present in the tissue (Fig. 2.7).

All white blood cells are derived from stem cells (Fig. 2.8). Hematopoietic stem cells (HSCs) are undifferentiated multipotent cells produced in the spongy tissue of the bone marrow found in the interior of certain long and flat bones, such as the bones of the pelvis and sternum.

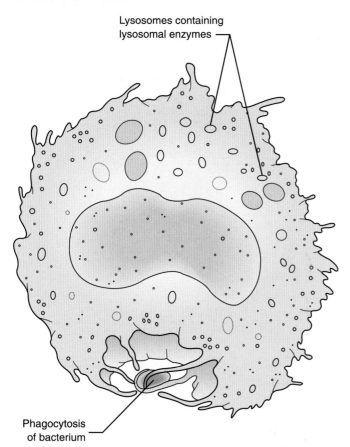

• **Figure 2.6** Phagocytosis of a foreign substance, a bacterium, by a white blood cell. The foreign substance will later be destroyed by digestion within the cell by lysosomal enzymes that are contained within lysosomes.

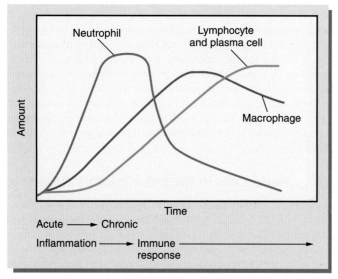

• **Figure 2.7** Changes in the white blood cell population of injured tissue over time, starting with acute inflammation, continuing to chronic inflammation, and extending to the beginning of the immune response.

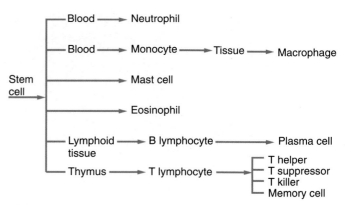

• **Figure 2.8** Derivation of white blood cells from a stem cell in the bone marrow.

The two types of white blood cells initially involved in the inflammatory response are the neutrophils and the monocytes (or macrophages in tissue). These two white blood cells are discussed in this chapter. Other cells within the blood and tissue, such as lymphocytes, plasma cells, eosinophils, and mast cells, participate in both inflammatory and immune responses. These cells are mainly involved in the immune response and are discussed in Chapter 3.

The neutrophil is the first type of white blood cell to arrive at the site of injury and is the most common inflammatory cell present during acute inflammation (Fig. 2.9). The second type of white blood cell to arrive at the site of injury is the monocyte, which becomes a macrophage as it enters the surrounding tissue. As inflammation continues, the number of neutrophils decreases. If the injury persists and chronic inflammation occurs, macrophages, lymphocytes, and plasma cells replace the neutrophils, with these additional cells becoming the most prevalent white blood cells present in the tissue (Fig. 2.10).

Neutrophils

The **neutrophil** is the first type of white blood cell recruited into the area of injury in response to chemotactic factors. Neutrophils constitute 60% to 70% of the entire white blood cell population. Neutrophils are produced throughout life and are mobile cells. The main function of the neutrophil is phagocytosis of substances such as pathogenic microorganisms and tissue debris. Microscopically, neutrophils possess a multilobed nucleus, which is why they are called *polymorphonuclear leukocytes,* and a granular cytoplasm that contains lysosomal enzymes (Fig. 2.11).

Lysosomal enzymes contained within vacuoles in the cell cytoplasm destroy substances after the cell has engulfed them. Removal of these substances from the site of injury is necessary to allow the process of repair. Neutrophils die shortly after phagocytosis. As a result, lysosomal enzymes and other damaging cellular substances that were meant only for intracellular destruction of foreign substances are released from the dying cells. This release can cause further tissue damage to the site when large numbers of neutrophils die.

Macrophages

The monocyte is the second type of white blood cell to emigrate from the blood vessels into the injured tissue, where it becomes a **macrophage**. As a macrophage, it responds to chemotactic factors, is capable of phagocytosis, is mobile, and has lysosomal enzymes

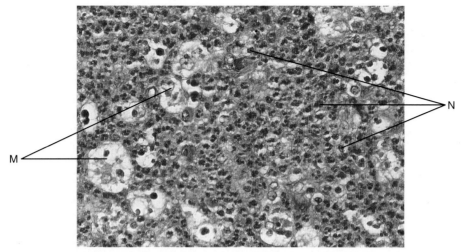

• **Figure 2.9** Microscopic view of acute inflammation, showing an increase in the number of neutrophils **(N)**. Macrophages **(M)** are also present (at medium magnification).

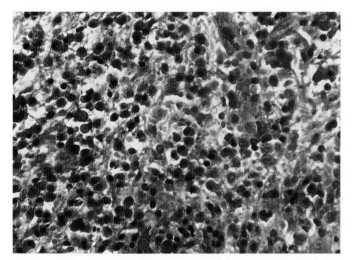

• **Figure 2.10** Microscopic view of chronic inflammation and the beginning of the immune response, mainly showing lymphocytes and plasma cells (at medium magnification).

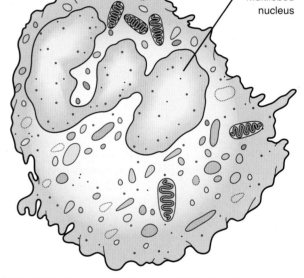

• **Figure 2.11** A neutrophil has a multilobed nucleus and granular cytoplasm.

in its cytoplasm that assist in the destruction of foreign substances within the cell.

The macrophage is larger than its monocytic precursor in the blood. The cell in all its forms constitutes 3% to 8% of the entire white blood cell population. Microscopically, it has a single round nucleus and does not have granular cytoplasm (Fig. 2.12). The macrophage has a somewhat longer life span than the neutrophil. In addition to its role in phagocytosis during inflammation, the macrophage is an important cell during the immune response (see Chapter 3).

Biochemical Mediators Involved in Inflammation

From the earlier discussion, it can be seen that chemical agents called *biochemical mediators* cause many of the events involved in the inflammatory response. Biochemical mediators are essential to the inflammatory response and can stimulate or amplify the response. During the response, basic mediators of inflammation can recruit other mediators and immune mechanisms, thus escalating the overall process. Some biochemical mediators are circulating in blood, some come from endothelial cells, some from white blood cells, and some from platelets; others are produced by certain pathogenic microorganisms as they injure the tissue.

The kinin system, the clotting mechanism, and the complement system are three systems of plasma proteins that are biochemical mediators of inflammation circulating in the blood. These may be activated during inflammation. The activation of each of these plasma protein systems involves a sequential cascade of events. These systems are interrelated; interaction among the systems takes place during their activation, among their products, and within their various actions.

Newer studies are also identifying other biochemicals that actively promote resolution and tissue repair without

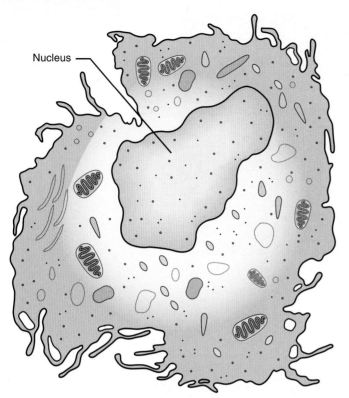

Nucleus

• **Figure 2.12** A macrophage. This cell was a monocyte when circulating in the blood.

compromising host defense. The resolution phase of inflammation is just as actively orchestrated and carefully choreographed as its induction. This includes specialized proresolving lipid mediators (SPMs) that are endogenous autacoids, biologic factors that are similar to hormones and serve to actively promote resolution of inflammation. In the future, drugs that induce resolution may be actively used during antiinflammatory therapy, including in periodontal disease.

Kinin System

The kinin system biochemically mediates inflammation by causing increased dilation and increased permeability of the blood vessels at the site of injury. This system is rapidly activated both by substances present in plasma and by those present in injured tissue. Its role is limited to the early phases of inflammation. Components of the kinin system also induce pain. The primary kinin is bradykinin. In order to limit the extent of inflammation, kinins are rapidly degraded by kininases, enzymes present in plasma and tissue.

Clotting Mechanism

The clotting mechanism functions primarily in the clotting of blood, which helps stop bleeding at the site of injury. The clotting mechanism forms a fibrinous meshwork at the site of injury that protects adjacent tissue and keeps foreign substances corralled at the site. It also biochemically mediates inflammation because certain of its products that are activated when tissue is injured cause local vascular dilation and permeability by also activating the kinin system. Later it will be shown that the clotting mechanism is also important in tissue repair, because it forms the future framework for the repair process.

Complement System

The complement system is composed of a series of plasma proteins that are activated in a cascading fashion, with one protein activating the next in the series. Various components of the complement system function during both the processes of inflammation and immunity. Complement components can cause mast cells to release granules from their cytoplasm that contain the biochemical mediator histamine and other mediators into the surrounding tissue. Mast cells are active during certain inflammatory reactions. They are usually located in large numbers in the loose connective tissue of the skin and mucosal tissue.

When histamine is released from mast cells, it causes an increase in vascular permeability and vasodilation (see Fig. 2.1). Other components of the complement system can cause cell death or necrosis by creating holes in the cell membrane called **cytolysis.** Complement proteins can also attach to the surface of bacteria, stimulating white blood cells to phagocytize them, a process called **opsonization.**

Other Biochemical Mediators of Inflammation

In addition to the biochemical mediators derived from circulating blood, other biochemical mediators can be involved during inflammation. These include prostaglandins, released white blood cell lysosomal enzymes and endotoxins, and lysosomal enzymes from pathogenic microorganisms. Prostaglandins are derived from cell membranes. They function by biochemically mediating the inflammatory response and causing increased vascular dilation and permeability, erythema, and pain, as well as changes in connective tissue. The lysosomal enzymes that are released from the granules within white blood cells act as chemotactic factors and can cause damage to connective tissue and to the clot that has formed at the site of injury.

Endotoxin and lysosomal enzymes released by pathogenic microorganisms may also serve as biochemical mediators. Endotoxin, produced from the cell walls of gram-negative bacteria, can serve as a chemotactic factor, activate complement, and function as an antigen and damage bone tissue. The lysosomal enzymes released from pathogenic microorganisms during infection are similar in chemical composition and action to those released by white blood cells.

Cell products from lymphocytes, such as cytokines, can also affect the inflammatory response. The cytokines are described in Chapter 3, because they participate in the immune response.

Systemic Clinical Signs of Inflammation

In addition to the major local clinical signs of inflammation, the four major systemic clinical signs that may occur are fever, an increase in the number of white blood cells or **leukocytosis,** enlargement of lymph nodes or **lymphadenopathy,** and elevated levels of C-reactive protein (CRP) (see Table 2.1).

Fever

Body temperature is controlled by a regulatory center in the brain, the hypothalamic thermoregulatory center. **Fever** is a body temperature higher than the usual level of 98.6° F (37°C) and is associated with a systemic inflammatory response. White blood cells and pathogenic microorganisms produce fever-inducing substances known as **pyrogens.** Pyrogens produce fever by increasing the synthesis and release of prostaglandins in the hypothalamus. Measuring body temperature with a thermometer is helpful in assessing whether a systemic inflammatory response is present.

The function of this increased body temperature by a fever is not clear. A moderately high fever may be helpful in combating some infections because increased temperature slows the growth of many pathogenic microorganisms. However, the body cannot tolerate an extremely high fever for very long, and such fever could prove fatal. Drugs can be given to reduce high fever by reducing systemic inflammation.

Leukocytosis

Leukocytosis is an increase in the number of white blood cells, or *leukocytes,* circulating in blood. The usual level is 4000 to 10,000/mm³. During a systemic inflammatory response, particularly a response to infection, leukocytosis occurs and the numbers increase to 10,000 to 30,000/mm³. This increase in white blood cells primarily involves neutrophils and occurs by increasing their formation and releasing immature forms from the bone marrow into the circulating blood. Leukocytosis occurs in response to biochemical mediators and is an attempt to provide more cells for phagocytosis. It occurs as a protective response to physiologic stressors, such as infection and pregnancy, but also with pathologic conditions, such as cancer and hematologic disorders.

In contrast, **leukopenia** is a decrease in the number of white blood cells circulating in blood. A white blood cell count of 4000 cells/mm³ or lower is considered a low white blood cell count. Leukopenia can be caused by radiation exposure, anaphylactic shock, autoimmune diseases, and immunodeficiency, as well as exposure to certain drugs or chemotherapeutic agents. As a result, there is a high risk for life-threatening infections.

A complete blood count (CBC) is a laboratory blood test that can be used to evaluate a patient for infection or a blood disorder. It can also include a "differential" white blood cell count, which measures the proportion of each white blood cell type. This can be useful in distinguishing a viral infection from a bacterial infection. In a viral infection there is characteristically an increase in lymphocytes, whereas in a bacterial infection there is an increase in neutrophils. In addition, in an allergic reaction there may be an increase in eosinophils. These results provide a useful tool for generally evaluating patients, but do not indicate the particular cause or site of inflammation within the body.

Lymphadenopathy

During the inflammatory process the lymph nodes enlarge. This enlargement of the lymph nodes is referred to as **lymphadenopathy** (Fig. 2.13). The enlarged lymph node, if located superficially, can be palpated as a pea- to grape-sized mass in the area of inflammation and possibly along the associated lymphatic drainage route, such as during a head and neck examination by a dental hygienist (Fig. 2.14). When palpated, the involved node feels not only firmer and larger than usual, but may also be tender. Deeper lymph nodes may also be enlarged, but these cannot be palpated during an examination.

Lymphadenopathy results from changes in the lymphocytes that reside in the lymph node. Lymphocytes are white blood cells that mature in lymphoid tissue and are the main white blood cells of the immune response. Lymphocytes travel from the lymph node to the tissue through the circulation where they are involved in the immune response. The role and maturation of lymphocytes is described in detail in Chapter 3.

The changes in the lymphocytes result in the change in size of the lymph nodes, causing them to enlarge during lymphade-

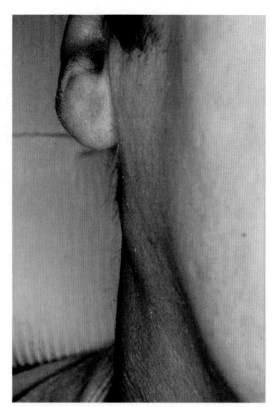

• **Figure 2.13** Enlarged cervical lymph node.

nopathy. These changes include an increase in the number of cells that is considered hyperplasia, resulting from increased cell division, and an enlargement of individual cells that is considered hypertrophy, resulting from cellular maturation. These changes in the lymphocyte population usually occur during chronic inflammation. The lymphoid tissue in **Waldeyer's ring** that includes the palatine, lingual, and pharyngeal tonsillar tissue may also undergo lymphoid hyperplasia and hypertrophy, which need to be monitored and possibly referred for medical consultation.

Elevated Levels of C-Reactive Protein

C-reactive protein (CRP) is a nonspecific protein produced in the liver; it plays an important role in interacting with the complement system, as well as in the clotting mechanism. Measurement of CRP is a diagnostic test associated with inflammation. For the most part, low levels of CRP circulate in the blood. Elevated levels of CRP are present during episodes of acute inflammation or infection and may continue at high levels with chronic inflammation. A concentration greater than 10 mg/L is usually considered a high level for CRP; most infections and episodes of inflammation result in levels of CRP at 100 mg/L. These higher levels of the protein then drop to the usual lower levels when inflammation subsides.

A high-sensitivity CRP (hs-CRP) assay is now available using a laser nephelometer (an instrument for measuring the size and concentration of particles suspended in a liquid or gas). The level of CRP can be used to help assess conditions such as rheumatoid arthritis and systemic lupus erythematosus and to determine whether a medication that has been taken is effective. It may be used to monitor tissue healing and as an early detection system for possible infections in patients who have had surgery, organ transplants, or severe burns. A chronically elevated level of CRP is associated with an increased risk for cardiovascular disease.

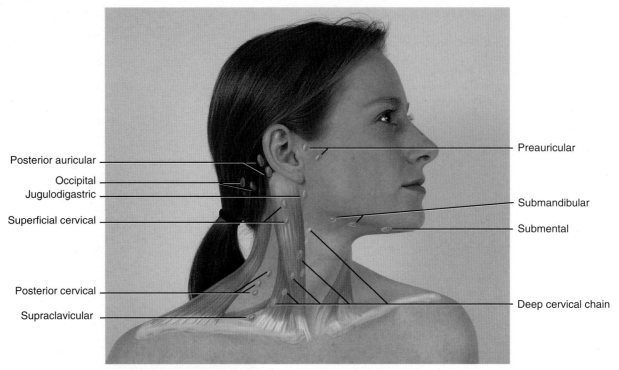

• **Figure 2.14** Location of lymph nodes in the head and neck that can be palpated after undergoing lymphadenopathy. (From Jarvis C: *Physical examination and health assessment,* ed 7, St. Louis, Saunders, 2015.)

Researchers are also exploring its role as a biochemical marker of periodontal disease activity. However, it is important to note that higher levels of CRP are still a nonspecific biochemical marker of inflammation levels for the entire body.

Chronic Inflammation

Chronic inflammation results from injuries that persist, often for weeks or months, even indefinitely. In addition to neutrophils and monocytes, other white blood cells are involved, as is the proliferation of fibroblasts. The cells involved in chronic inflammation include macrophages, lymphocytes, and plasma cells. Repair takes place at the same time that chronic inflammation proceeds, but it cannot be completed until the source of the injury is removed.

Granulomatous inflammation is a distinctive form of chronic inflammation. It is characterized by the formation of a **granuloma,** which contains microscopic groupings of macrophages usually surrounded by lymphocytes and occasional plasma cells. The macrophages within the granuloma become larger as they group together with their multiple nuclei and become multinucleated giant cells. Foreign substances in tissue and certain systemic infections such as tuberculosis tend to stimulate the formation of multiple granulomas. The body, which is unable to destroy the offending substances, tries to enclose them instead in these masses of inflammatory cells.

The formation of a granuloma is not preceded by an acute, neutrophil-mediated inflammation. Instead, it may be caused by antigens that evoke a cell-mediated hypersensitivity reaction or by antigens that persist at the site of inflammation. Granulomas destroy the surrounding tissue and tend to persist for a long time.

Antiinflammatory Therapy

Antiinflammatory drugs block or inhibit the inflammatory response during treatment, preventing or reducing the clinical signs of inflammation and adverse reactions to the injury. Diseases and conditions related to the inflammatory process such as asthma, arthritis, organ transplantation, and surgical trauma are treated with steroidal or nonsteroidal antiinflammatory agents. The steroidal antiinflammatory agents exert their analgesic effects by inhibiting the synthesis of prostaglandin, which if not inhibited could have served as a biochemical mediator of inflammation. Prednisone is an example of a steroidal antiinflammatory drug.

Nonsteroidal antiinflammatory agents also exert their analgesic effects by inhibiting the synthesis of prostaglandin. Examples of nonsteroidal antiinflammatory drugs (NSAIDs) include acetylsalicylic acid (aspirin) and ibuprofen. Another group of drugs, antihistamines, reduces the effects of the biochemical mediator histamine that is released in allergic responses.

Medications that are traditionally used to treat cancer such as methotrexate, sulfasalazine, leflunomide, cyclophosphamide, and mycophenolate are now being used to treat inflammatory diseases because they suppress the inflammatory response. The doses are significantly lower, and the risk of side effects tends to be considerably less than when prescribed in higher doses to treat cancer.

In some cases complete control of inflammation so that it is eliminated may not be the clinically effective therapy. Instead, patients may be closely monitored to allow the initial benefits of inflammation. These findings may in the future be applied to orofacial inflammation.

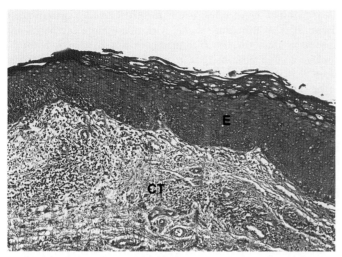

• **Figure 2.15** Microscopic appearance of epithelial hyperplasia (at low magnification). The epithelium (*E*) is thickened because of an increase in the number of cells in the spinous layer. CT, underlying connective tissue.

Reactive Tissue Responses to Injury

The cells in a tissue or organ may respond to injury by undergoing an adaptive response such as hyperplasia, hypertrophy, or atrophy. **Hyperplasia** is defined as an increase in the number of cells in a tissue or organ, with a consequent increase in size of the tissue or organ, in response to conditions that cause cellular stress. Pathologic hyperplasia frequently occurs in orofacial tissue. In the oral cavity an increase in the number of epithelial cells and an increased thickness of the epithelium commonly occur in response to chronic injury (Fig. 2.15). As surface epithelial cells are lost, division of deeper basal epithelial cells increases to replace the lost cells. With hyperplasia, the production of new cells exceeds the original number of cells lost; thus the epithelium becomes thickened, and the tissue appears paler or whiter.

When the injury subsides, the proliferation ceases. With time, the epithelium usually returns to its usual size, and the color of the tissue returns to its usual color. However, in some cases, the hyperplastic tissue persists even after the irritation is discontinued. Deeper hyperplasia of fibrous connective tissue may also occur in response to chronic injury and is commonly noted with lesions of the orofacial region. Orofacial lesions caused by epithelial and fibrous hyperplasia are described later in this chapter.

Hypertrophy is a response to cellular stress that is defined as an increase in the size of a tissue or organ because of an increase in the size of individual cells, not the number. For example, hypertrophy occurs in the smooth muscles of the uterus and the mammary glands in response to pregnancy, in cardiac muscle in response to long-standing high blood pressure, and in skeletal muscle in response to increased exercise. Hyperplasia and hypertrophy are often present together as a tissue or organ responds to the injury. Lymphadenopathy is an example in which both the size and number of cells increase.

In contrast to hyperplasia and hypertrophy, **atrophy** is the decrease in size and function of a cell, tissue, organ, or the whole body in response to certain conditions of cellular stress. Atrophied cells are capable of increasing to their usual size after the stress is removed. Atrophy can be present in the muscular wasting that occurs in some chronic diseases that do not allow mobility and function, as well as with overwhelming infections such as with the human immunodeficiency virus. It can also happen with changes in cellular growth, malnutrition, ischemia with its disruption of blood supply, or hormonal changes.

Tissue Repair

With resolution of the inflammatory response, the injured tissue undergoes repair as either regeneration or the formation of scar tissue. When tissue damage has been slight, the inflamed area may return completely to its usual structure and usual level of function. This is called **regeneration** and is the most favorable resolution of acute inflammation. Regeneration involves complete removal of all cells, by-products, and inflammatory exudate that entered the tissue during inflammation and return of the microcirculation to its preinflammatory state. In contrast, the process of scar formation takes place when complete return of the tissue to its usual structure and usual level of function is not possible because the damage has been too great. The damaged tissue is replaced by dense, fibrous connective tissue *(scar)*. Some tissue types such as epithelium, fibrous connective tissue, and bone have the ability to undergo repair. Other tissue types such as enamel do not.

Repair is the final defense mechanism of the body in its attempt to restore injured tissue to its original state. During the repair process cells and associated tissue that have undergone necrosis are replaced with live cells and new tissue components. However, the repair process cannot be completed until the source of injury is removed or the injurious agents are destroyed. Repair is not always a perfect process. Functioning cells and tissue components are often replaced by nonfunctioning scar tissue.

Research studies are currently investigating ways to enhance the repair process. Research on stem cells is at the core of a new field called *regenerative medicine.* Stem cells are characterized by their self-renewal properties and by their natural capacity to generate differentiated cell lineages. There is hope that stem cells might be harnessed and one day be used to repair damaged tissue, such as heart, brain, liver, skeletal muscle, and orofacial tissue structures.

Microscopic Events During Repair

After an injury occurs microscopic events occur in both the epithelium and connective tissue (Fig. 2.16). These events are different for each of these tissue types, but occur almost simultaneously and are dependent on each other for optimal healing. If the source of the injury is removed, the repair process for both types of tissue is usually completed within 2 weeks. The repair process is slightly different in the oral cavity than in skin because mucosal tissue is moist and a scab does not form. The three phases of the repair process that occur during these 2 weeks are inflammation, proliferation, and maturation.

Day of Injury

Immediately after the injury, a clot forms as blood flows into the injured tissue. The clot is produced in the area of injury as a result of activation of the clotting mechanism. The clot consists of a meshwork structure composed of locally produced fibrin, aggregated red blood cells, and platelets.

Along with the other contents of the clot, platelets are cellular fragments found in the blood and are extremely important in the formation of a clot. There are 250,000 to 400,000 platelets/mL^3 within the blood. The number of platelets is measured within the panel of the CBC. Hereditary factors, drugs, extensive injury, or

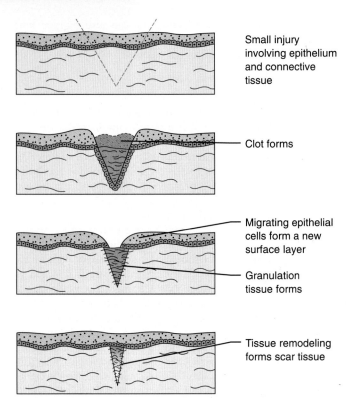

Small injury involving epithelium and connective tissue

Clot forms

Migrating epithelial cells form a new surface layer

Granulation tissue forms

Tissue remodeling forms scar tissue

• **Figure 2.16** Underlying microscopic events of the repair process from the day of injury to 2 weeks later.

certain diseases may affect red blood cells, platelets, and other factors involved in the formation of the clot and thus prevent or delay tissue repair.

Day After Injury

The day after the injury, acute inflammation is taking place in the area of future repair. Neutrophils emigrate from the microcirculation into the injured tissue, and phagocytosis of foreign substances and necrotic tissue with its dead cells occurs as part of the inflammatory response.

Two Days After Injury

Within 2 days of the injury, monocytes begin to emigrate from the microcirculation into the injured area as macrophages. Macrophages continue phagocytosis in a manner similar to that of the remaining neutrophils. However, neutrophils are reduced in number as the chronic inflammatory process proceeds. **Fibroblasts** proliferate within the injured connective tissue in response to biochemical mediators from macrophages. Fibroblasts become the most important cells during healing as they begin to produce and secrete new collagen fibers, using the fibrinous meshwork of the clot as a scaffold. This process is called **fibroplasia** and can occur within the process of healing and can also occur in abnormal levels as a result of injury. Examples of lesions illustrating abnormal healing are discussed later in this chapter.

Because an ample blood supply is necessary to sustain new tissue growth, the microcirculation begins to establish itself in the immature connective tissue or type 1 collagen. Macrophages, in addition to removing tissue debris by phagocytosis and promoting fibroblast levels, secrete growth factors to stimulate the growth of new blood vessels. This process is called **angiogenesis.**

The initial connective tissue formed is called **granulation tissue.** It is an immature tissue, with many more capillaries and fibroblasts than the usual connective tissue so that it clinically appears a vivid pink or red. It consists of immature type 1 collagen that is laid down in a haphazard disorganized fashion. In some cases, the growth of this tissue is excessive (or exuberant) and may interfere with the repair process until it is removed surgically.

If the surface epithelium has been destroyed by the injury, the epithelial cells create a new surface at the same time that granulation tissue forms in the injured connective tissue. The epithelial cells from the borders of the healing injured area lose their cellular junctions and become mobile. They then divide and migrate across the injured tissue, using the fibrinous meshwork of the clot as a guide to form a new surface layer. This process is called **epithelialization.**

In addition to serving as a guide for migrating epithelial cells and as a scaffold for forming connective tissue, the fibrinous meshwork of the clot serves to protect these two newly formed deeper tissue types from further injury. Thus it is important for the clot to remain in place during this healing time to allow optimal repair in the tissue. With some injuries, dressings placed over the clot may prove beneficial to the healing process (e.g., periodontal pack over a surgical site of the periodontium).

At the end of 2 days, lymphocytes and plasma cells begin to emigrate from the surrounding blood vessels into the injured area as chronic inflammation and an immune response begin. The macrophages already present in the area now assist the lymphocytes in the immune response occurring at the site of injury.

Seven Days After Injury

If the source of the injury has been completely removed, the inflammatory and immune responses in the tissue are completed 1 week after the injury. The fibrinous meshwork of the clot is digested by tissue enzymes and sloughs off, and the initial repair of the tissue is completed. Clinically the surface of the repaired injury remains redder than usual because of the thinness of the new surface epithelium and the increased vascularity of the new underlying connective tissue.

It is important to note that the immature type of collagen fibers found in granulation tissue is still present and remains fragile and at risk of reinjury. During this time fibroblasts differentiate into a subset of cells, the **myofibroblasts,** which are cells similar to smooth muscle cells, and the tissue in the site begins to contract. This contracting peaks 5 to 15 days after the injury and continues until the site is completely reepithelialized.

Two Weeks After Injury

Two weeks after the injury, the initial granulation tissue and its fibers have been remodeled, giving the tissue its full strength. This matured fibrous connective tissue is now called *scar tissue;* it clinically appears whiter or paler at the surface of the repaired injury because of the increased number of collagen fibers and decreased vascularity. A stronger type of collagen, type 3 collagen, now has replaced the immature type 1 collagen, and the collagen tissue overall becomes more organized.

Types of Repair

The amount of scar tissue remaining after an injury depends on many factors such as heredity, the strength and flexibility needed in the tissue, the tissue type involved, and the type of repair that

Sutured injury

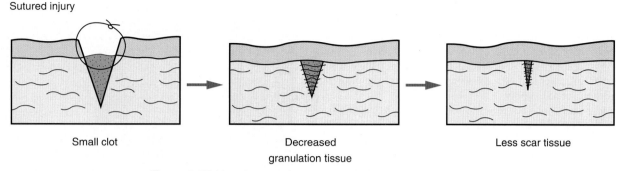

Small clot   Decreased   Less scar tissue
                granulation tissue

• **Figure 2.17** Use of sutures to encourage healing by primary intention.

Large injury

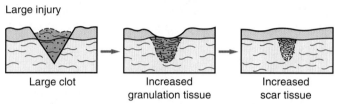

Large clot   Increased   Increased
                granulation tissue scar tissue

• **Figure 2.18** Healing by secondary intention without the use of sutures in a large injury.

has occurred. The oral mucosa is less prone to scar formation than skin. The three types of repair that can occur are healing by primary intention, healing by secondary intention, and healing by tertiary intention.

Healing by Primary Intention

Healing by primary intention refers to the healing of an injury in which little loss of tissue takes place, such as in a surgical incision. In this type of healing the clean edges of the incision are joined with sutures to form only a small clot, and very little granulation tissue forms (Fig. 2.17). Thus less scar tissue forms, and the uninjured tissue is retained. The use of sutures is an attempt to try to join the edges of the injury surgically so that healing by primary intention occurs and scarring is minimized.

Healing by Secondary Intention

Healing by secondary intention involves injury in which tissue is lost; thus the edges of the injury cannot be joined during healing. A large clot slowly forms, resulting in increased formation of granulation tissue (Fig. 2.18). Healing of a tooth extraction site is an example of healing by secondary intention. After healing, scar tissue increases, and the usual level of tissue function is greatly reduced.

However, this scar tissue formation can be so excessive that surgical correction is needed in some cases. A **keloid** is excessive scarring that mainly occurs in skin and appears raised and extends beyond its original boundaries. Individuals with pigmented skin are more likely to form a keloid, and a familial tendency to keloid formation has been reported (Fig. 2.19).

Healing by Tertiary Intention

If infection occurs at the site of a surgical incision that is healing by primary intention, healing by tertiary intention may result. This transformation occurs because of an enlargement of the injured area and an increase in the magnitude and duration of the inflammatory and immune responses triggered by the presence of pathogenic microorganisms. In some cases an infected injury is

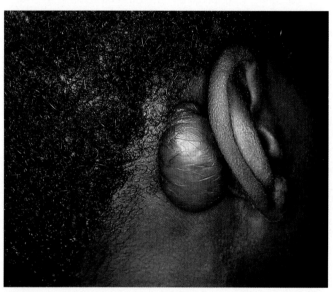

• **Figure 2.19** Example of keloid formation with excessive scar tissue formation after an injury. (Courtesy Dr. Harold Baurmash.)

left open, and the edges are not surgically joined until the infection is controlled.

Bone Tissue Repair

Repair of a bone injury is similar to the process that takes place in fibrous connective tissue except that it involves the creation of bone tissue. Tissue damage with bleeding leads to clot formation. Cellular proliferation occurs, converting the clot to granulation tissue. The granulation tissue forms a matrix on which bone-forming cell, called an **osteoblast**, lays down immature bone called *osteoid*. The osteoblasts are located on the viable bone at the periphery of the injury site. Over time, the immature bone becomes more calcified and the area of tissue damage is replaced by viable bone trabeculae. This process of bone tissue repair is the same process that occurs when an implant is placed and osseointegration takes place.

As with other tissues of the body, the factors of nutrition, age, and tobacco use can influence the repair process in bone. At the site of the injury blood supply and growth factors can further modulate the process. Removal of osteoblast-producing tissue and excessive movement of the bone can interrupt healing. Inadequate movement of bone during the healing process can also adversely affect repair. Injury, edema, or infection in the involved bone can delay repair.

Factors That Impair Healing

Certain local factors impair healing; these include bacterial infection, primarily by *Streptococcus* or *Staphylococcus* species; tissue destruction and **necrosis,** as discussed earlier; hemorrhage into the tissue, causing a hematoma; excessive movement of the injured tissue; and poor blood supply.

Systemic factors such as those resulting from malnutrition, especially when protein, zinc, calcium, and vitamin C are severely reduced in the diet, can also impair healing. The recent emergence of resistant strains of pathogenic microorganism is now more commonly preventing the resolution of the infectious process.

If the body is undergoing immunosuppression because of steroid use or chemotherapy, healing is also impaired. Certain genetic connective tissue disorders such as osteogenesis imperfecta (see Chapter 6) and metabolic disorders resulting from age, renal failure, and diabetes mellitus (see Chapter 9) can reduce the effectiveness of the natural healing mechanism. Tobacco use and recreational drug and alcohol abuse have also been shown to impair healing. Newer studies are looking at physical activity for promotion of healing and how obesity may prove to delay it.

Traumatic Injuries to Teeth

Traumatic injury to the teeth includes attrition, abrasion, abfraction, and erosion. Interactions between different types exist, and in many cases determining the primary cause is difficult. Identifying early signs of trauma to the teeth before any complications occur may prevent the need for advanced major rehabilitative treatment.

Attrition

Attrition is the wearing away of tooth structure during tooth-to-tooth contact or mastication. It involves the incisal, occlusal, and proximal surfaces of the teeth and is rarely seen on any other tooth surfaces unless teeth are abnormally placed in the arch (Fig. 2.20). Attrition occurs in both primary and permanent dentitions; it is usually a slow process that starts as soon as the teeth are in contact and continues over the lifetime of the dentition.

The first sign of attrition is the disappearance of the mamelons on the anterior teeth and the flattening of the occlusal cusps on molar teeth, causing wear facets (Fig. 2.21). The wear "matches" the opposing teeth. The rate of attrition is influenced by diet; a diet of more fibrous food causes greater attrition. Bruxism, the use of chewing tobacco with its abrasive sand content, and certain occupations and environments in which abrasive dust particles enter the mouth accelerate attrition. The term **demastication** may be used to describe this accelerated tooth loss because the patient may have both attrition and abrasion. Attrition also increases as patients grow older. The rate of attrition has been reported to be greater in men than in women.

Bruxism is the grinding of the teeth together for nonfunctional purposes. The signs and symptoms resulting from bruxism and their extent are related to the intensity of the grinding. These are varied and include wear facets visible on masticatory surfaces, an abnormal rate of attrition (Fig. 2.22), hypertrophy of masticatory muscles (especially the masseter muscle), increased muscle tone, muscle tenderness, muscle fatigue, cheek biting, pain in the temporomandibular joint area (see Chapter 10), tooth mobility, and pulpal sensitivity to cold.

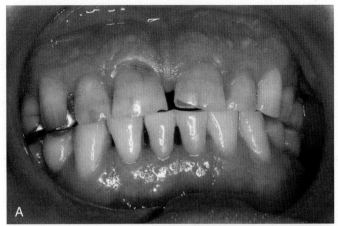

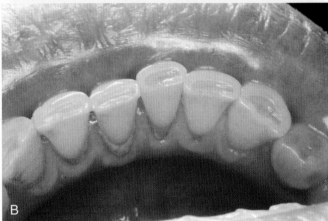

• **Figure 2.20** **A,** Attrition of adult dentition. **B,** Attrition of adult dentition (incisal view).

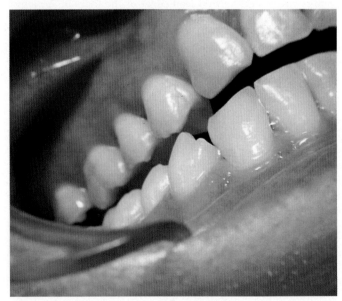

• **Figure 2.21** Attrition has caused the flattening of the cusps (wear facets) of both the maxillary and mandibular cuspid teeth.

The incidence of bruxism varies greatly according to the population studied. In studies of patients with periodontal disease, 60% to 90% of patients had evidence of bruxism. In children ages 2 to 5 years, the average prevalence reported was 20% to 30%, and the highest prevalence reported was 78%. Many children

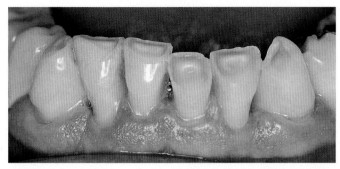

• **Figure 2.22** Attrition of the mandibular anterior teeth resulting from bruxism.

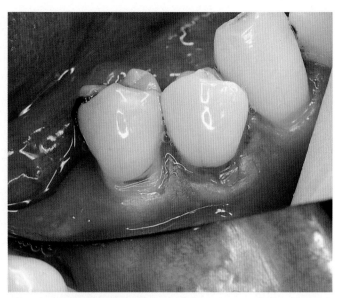

• **Figure 2.23** Abrasion at the cervical area of mandibular bicuspids caused by toothbrushing.

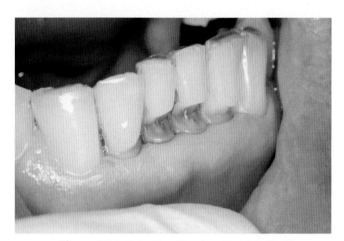

• **Figure 2.24** Abfraction. (Courtesy Dr. Mark Wolff.)

seem to outgrow these high levels of bruxism and resulting attrition seen in the primary dentition.

The cause of bruxism is unclear. Local factors such as occlusal interferences in combination with stress and tension are considered to be triggering factors. Certain conditions such as seizure disorders have been related to bruxism. The higher prevalence of bruxism reported in certain occupations is possibly related to the amount of stress associated with those occupations.

Management of the individual with bruxism includes eliminating the occlusal interferences through occlusal adjustments and protecting the teeth and periodontium from further destruction by fabricating an acrylic splint that can be worn as a protective device.

Abrasion

Abrasion is the pathologic wearing away of tooth structure or a restoration that results from a repetitive mechanical habit. It is most commonly seen on exposed root surfaces because the cementum and dentin are not as hard as enamel; however, abrasion also occurs on enamel surfaces. The process of abrasion is usually slow, and the dentin responds by laying down an inner protective layer of secondary dentin. Therefore pulpal exposure does not usually result.

Abrasion most frequently presents as horizontal wear on the cervical aspect of the root surface in areas of gingival recession and may occur from an improper toothbrushing technique, most commonly a back-and-forth scrubbing motion using excessive pressure. The use of an abrasive toothpaste or a hard toothbrush may accelerate abrasion (Fig. 2.23). However, most dentifrices manufactured in the United States have a very low abrasive index, and toothbrushes with soft bristles are now recommended. Other causes of abrasion include habits such as opening bobby pins with the teeth or holding needles or pins in the teeth. These practices result in a notching on the incisal edges of the maxillary incisors. Musicians who play wind instruments may also exhibit forms of abrasion of the teeth in the area of the mouth where the instrument is placed, and pipe smokers may show evidence of abrasion in the area of pipe placement. Abrasion may also result from porcelain crowns, bridges, or denture materials on surfaces of opposing teeth (unrestored, amalgam, resins, etc.), as well as the sand in smokeless tobacco. Abrasion may lead to exposed dentin resulting in hypersensitivity and an increased risk of caries.

The diagnosis of abrasion can often be made by correlating the clinical appearance of the lesions with information gained from questioning the patient about possible factors that may be causing

the lesions. The patient should be informed of the cause of the abrasion, and corrective measures should be taken to prevent further destruction of tooth structure. Restorative dental treatment to repair the defect may be appropriate.

Abfraction

Abfraction typically appears as a wedge-shaped defect at the cervical area of teeth, especially premolars (Fig. 2.24). These lesions occur in adults; the cause is related to microfracture of tooth structure in areas of concentration of stress. This may be related to fatigue, flexure, fracture, and deformation of tooth structure as the result of biomechanical forces on the teeth. The weakened tooth structure is more susceptible to abrasion, particularly toothbrush abrasion. Sometimes these lesions can be seen subgingivally in areas where abrasion and erosion do not occur. The lesions may be treated with composite or glass ionomer materials, but the forces on the teeth may result in dislodging of the restorations or cause additional damage to the abfracted area. Prevention may involve fabricating an acrylic splint.

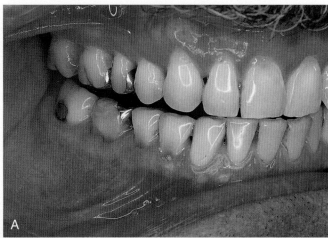

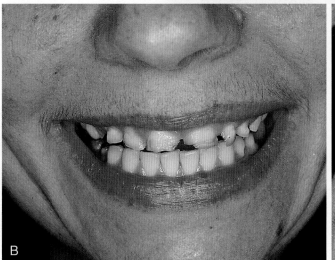

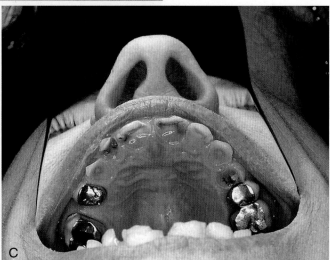

• **Figure 2.25** **A,** Erosion of buccal and labial surfaces of teeth that occurred as a result of accidental exposure to sulfuric acid. Erosion caused by bulimia: **B,** Decreased tooth size. **C,** Erosion of maxillary lingual surfaces.

Erosion

Erosion is the loss of tooth structure resulting from chemical action without bacterial involvement. The loss may occur on the smooth facial or lingual surfaces of the teeth and on the proximal and occlusal surfaces (Fig. 2.25A). The area of erosion appears smooth and polished and is usually extensive, involving several teeth. If erosion occurs in an area where restorations exist, the tooth structure is lost around the restoration, making the restoration appear raised from the surrounding demineralized tooth structure. This phenomenon is not seen in abrasion or attrition because in those cases the restoration is worn down along with the tooth surface.

Erosion may be seen in individuals who work in industries in which acid is used, such as battery manufacturing, plating companies, and soft-drink manufacturing, because the workers breathe the acid in the air. Erosion of teeth associated with intraorally applied cocaine hydrochloride drug abuse has been reported. Because of their low pH, overuse of soft drinks, especially diet formulations, is also strongly implicated in dental erosion and can be noted in some cases of early childhood caries when these drinks

are placed in the baby bottle. In addition, erosion of the facial surfaces of the teeth may occur as a result of frequent sucking on lemons. Erosion of the lingual surfaces of the teeth may occur as a result of chronic vomiting.

The location of erosion and abrasion cannot reliably identify the cause. The patient's history must be correlated with the location and cause.

Bulimia is an eating disorder characterized by food binges, usually of very high caloric intake, followed by self-induced vomiting. The frequent vomiting in an individual with bulimia results in generalized erosion of the lingual surfaces of teeth (Fig. 2.25B-C). The dental hygienist may be the first health care professional to identify a patient with bulimia and may assist in encouraging the patient to seek treatment. Bulimia differs from **anorexia nervosa,** another eating disorder, which is characterized by intense fear of gaining weight and self-imposed starvation. Vomiting after eating is a component of bulimia, but not of anorexia nervosa. The patient with bulimia maintains a normal body weight but is secretive about eating habits. Electrolyte imbalance and signs of malnutrition may be present. Irritation of the oral mucosa and lips may occur, and there may be traumatic

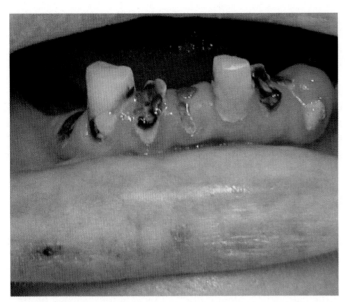

• **Figure 2.26** Extensive dental destruction related to methamphetamine abuse. (Courtesy Dr. Bobby Collins.)

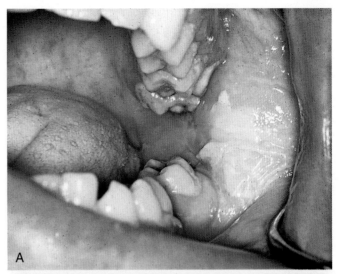

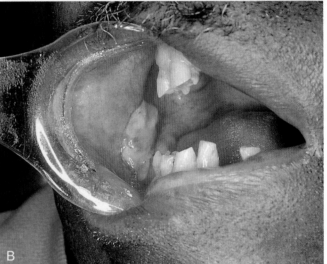

• **Figure 2.27 A** and **B,** Aspirin burns.

lesions on the backs of the fingers caused by their continual use to induce vomiting.

Dental management of patients who vomit frequently includes an effort to minimize the effects of acid on tooth enamel by encouraging the daily use of fluoride rinse, fluoride prescription pastes and gels and over-the-counter toothpaste containing fluoride. Rinsing the mouth with water after vomiting episodes also lessens the effects of acid. Brushing immediately after vomiting should be avoided, and patients with this disorder should be encouraged to use a toothbrush with very soft bristles: the mineralized tooth structure has been affected by acid, and the friction of brushing may increase the loss of tooth structure. Patients with severe bulimia-associated erosion may require full-coverage restorative dental treatment for esthetics and function.

Recently the oral manifestations of **methamphetamine** abuse have been described. The acid content of methamphetamine, decreased salivary flow, and craving for high sugar–containing beverages combined with lack of oral hygiene care result in the extensive and rapid destruction of teeth that is called "**meth mouth**" (Fig. 2.26).

Injuries to Oral Soft Tissue

Oral Mucosal Burns

Oral mucosal burns are common lesions. Some can be very serious because of the amount of tissue damage involved. Questioning the patient should reveal the cause of the lesion. Several different types of burns may involve the oral mucosa. These include aspirin burn, phenol and other chemical burns, electric burn, and thermal burn from hot foods. Mucosal burns can also be caused by hydrogen peroxide or tooth-whitening products. Additionally, endodontic materials such as formocresol or sodium hypochlorite can cause mucosal necrosis if they leak onto soft tissue. Use of a rubber dam can prevent these tissue injuries.

Aspirin Burn

An **aspirin burn** generally occurs when a patient with a toothache places an aspirin tablet directly on the painful tooth and adjacent mucosal tissue instead of swallowing it. Aspirin (acetylsalicylic acid) is an analgesic (pain reliever) and antiinflammatory agent that must be ingested to be effective. Topical application is a common misuse of aspirin. As a result of placing the aspirin on the mucosal tissue, the tissue becomes necrotic and appears white. The lesion is painful, and the necrotic tissue may separate from the underlying connective tissue and slough off, resulting in a large ulcer (Fig. 2.27). Questioning the patient should reveal the cause of the lesion, and the diagnosis is generally made without the need for biopsy and microscopic examination of the tissue. An aspirin burn is painful and heals slowly because of the extent of destruction. The ulcer usually heals spontaneously in 7 to 21 days. The patient requires appropriate treatment of the painful tooth and analgesic medication for symptomatic relief of pain until the ulcer heals.

Phenol and Other Chemical Burns

Phenol is used in dentistry as a cavity-sterilizing and cauterizing agent. When phenol comes into contact with the soft tissue, a whitening of the exposed area occurs as a result of tissue destruction. The surface tissue may slough off, exposing the underlying connective tissue (Fig. 2.28A). The resulting ulcer is painful, and the duration of healing depends on the extent of the destruction. The phenol should be removed immediately to minimize the destruction. If phenol is ingested, the patient should drink large amounts of water and be referred for medical evaluation. Several other chemicals used in dental treatment have been reported to cause necrosis when they come in contact with mucosal tissue. These include sodium hypochlorite, ferric sulfate, formocresol, and eugenol.

Phenol is also a component of some over-the-counter products that are advertised for relief of oral pain. Patients frequently misuse these preparations for oral ulcers, and the resulting destruction, in addition to being quite painful, may mask the clinical and microscopic diagnostic characteristics of the original ulcer. Over-the-counter products containing hydrogen peroxide or eugenol can also cause mucosal necrosis. Frequent use of hydrogen peroxide can delay healing.

Electric Burn

Electric burns in the oral area are usually seen in infants and young children who have bitten or chewed a live electric cord or have inserted something into an electric socket. The electric current can cause a great deal of destruction to oral tissue. Any tissue in the area may be damaged, including the permanent tooth buds. Permanent disfigurement and scarring may result from this type of injury. Treatment may require a multidisciplinary approach that includes plastic surgery, oral surgery, and orthodontic therapy.

Thermal Burns

Oral mucosal burns from hot food or liquid are common. They occur most often on the palate and tongue (Fig. 2.28B). Foods prepared in a microwave oven can cause thermal burns because the external food temperature may be cooler than the internal temperature.

Lesions Associated With Cocaine Use

Lesions located at the midline of the hard palate that vary from ulcers to keratotic lesions to exophytic reactive lesions have been reported to result from the smoking of crack cocaine (Fig. 2.28C). Palatal perforation has also been reported. When crack cocaine is smoked, the crack pipe directs extremely hot smoke to this part of the hard palate. Identification of these lesions is based on their location and the history of recent smoking of crack cocaine. Necrotic ulcers of the tongue and epiglottis related to smoking freebase cocaine have also been reported.

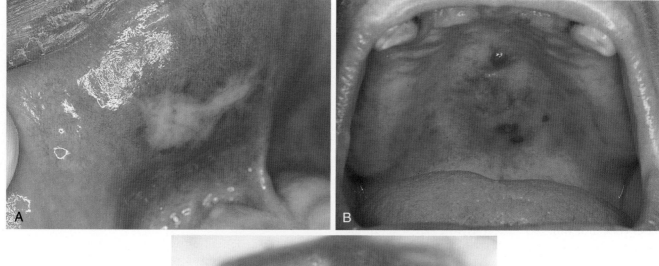

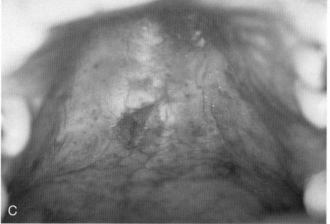

• **Figure 2.28** Mucosal burns. **A,** Chemical burn caused by contact with caustic material during endodontic treatment. **B,** Thermal burn of palate caused by contact with hot soup. **C,** Ulcer of midline of palate caused by heat generated during the use of crack cocaine. (Reprinted by permission of ADA Publishing Co., Inc. from Mitchell-Lewis DA, Phelan JA, Kelly RB, et al: Identifying oral lesions associated with crack-cocaine use, *J Am Dent Assoc* 125:1104, 1994. Copyright 1994, American Dental Association.)

Lesions From Self-Induced Injuries

Habits of which the patient may or may not be aware can cause injury. These lesions range from ulceration to epithelial hyperplasia and hyperkeratosis. Trauma to the gingiva by a fingernail or ulceration caused by a denture or chronic lip, cheek, or tongue biting (see Fig. 2.31) are examples of habits that may cause oral ulcers. Ulcers caused by continual self-induced injuries may be of long duration and require biopsy and microscopic examination to confirm the diagnosis and rule out neoplasia. See Fig. 2.31 for examples of epithelial hyperplasia and frictional keratosis from chronic trauma. Treatment of self-induced lesions depends on the amount and type of destruction and may involve psychotherapy.

Traumatic Ulcer

A **traumatic ulcer** occurs as a result of some form of trauma most commonly to the tongue, lips, or buccal mucosa (Fig. 2.29). Sources of trauma vary. Biting the cheek, lip, or tongue may result in a traumatic ulcer, as can irritation from a complete or partial denture or mucosal injury from sharp edges of food. The rapid removal of a dry cotton roll from the oral tissue after a dental procedure can cause a traumatic ulcer, and it is not uncommon to see a patient present for a dental hygiene appointment with a traumatic injury to the gingival tissue or vestibular mucosa that results from overzealous brushing before the appointment.

Traumatic ulcers are usually diagnosed on the basis of the relationship of the history to the lesion. Healing is usually uneventful and occurs in 7 to 14 days unless the trauma persists. If trauma persists, ulcers may last for weeks to months. The patient is monitored until healing is ensured. If an ulcer does not heal in 7 to 14 days, a biopsy and microscopic examination are usually indicated to rule out a more serious lesion such as neoplasia. Persistent trauma may result in a hard (indurated), raised lesion called a **traumatic granuloma** (see Fig. 2.29D). Clinically these lesions may resemble squamous cell carcinoma; therefore biopsy and microscopic examination of these ulcers is important. A traumatic ulcerative granuloma with stromal eosinophilia (TUGSE) is a type of traumatic ulceration with a unique microscopic appearance. This lesion appears microscopically as an ulcer with an underlying inflammatory infiltrate that contains numerous eosinophils. Persistent traumatic granulomas often heal rapidly after biopsy.

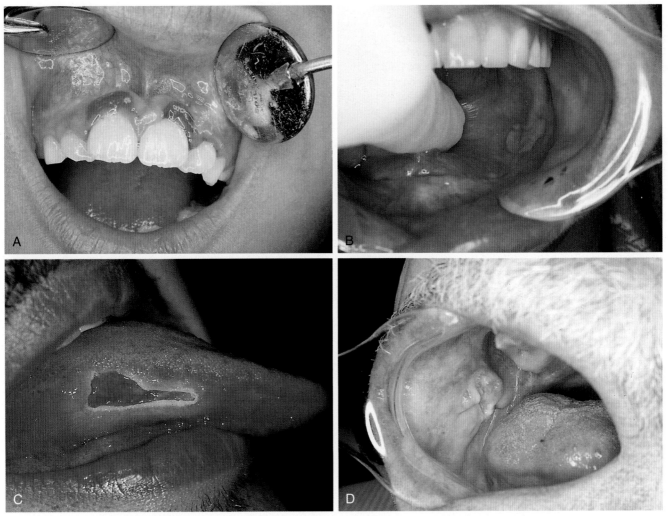

• **Figure 2.29 A,** Traumatic ulceration caused by irritation of gingiva by fingernails. **B,** Traumatic ulcer caused by denture. **C,** Traumatic ulcer on lateral tongue caused by chronic trauma to tongue by teeth. **D,** Traumatic ulcer (traumatic granuloma) of buccal mucosa.

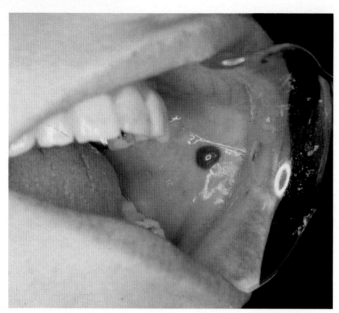

• **Figure 2.30** Hematoma on the buccal mucosa.

Hematoma

A **hematoma** is a lesion that results from the accumulation of blood within tissue as a result of trauma. In the oral cavity a hematoma appears as a red to purple to bluish-gray mass and is most frequently seen on the labial or buccal mucosa (Fig. 2.30). The size may vary from small to large, depending on the extent of the trauma. The trauma may be due to extensive biting or chewing of the oral tissue, from the administration of a local anesthetic, or surgical trauma. No treatment is required if the lesion is small because the lesion will spontaneously resolve; however, the patient should be advised of its presence. Larger lesions may require pressure on the site and the placement of ice on the site immediately after the trauma.

Frictional Keratosis

Chronic rubbing or friction against an oral mucosal surface may result in hyperkeratosis, a thickening of the keratin on the surface. This results in an opaque, white appearance of the tissue and represents a protective response, analogous to a callus on the skin. An example of frictional keratosis is an increase in surface keratin that results from chronic cheek and tongue chewing (Fig. 2.31) and chewing on edentulous alveolar ridges. There may be areas of ulceration or hematomas present. Frictional keratosis is not associated with malignancy.

The diagnosis of frictional keratosis is made by identification of the trauma causing the lesion, elimination of the cause, and observing resolution of the lesion. The keratosis may take a while to disappear on keratinized surfaces such as the hard palate and attached gingiva. Those on the buccal mucosa may resolve more rapidly.

Frictional keratosis must be distinguished from other white lesions. White lesions that are not caused by trauma and arise spontaneously are called **leukoplakia** or **idiopathic leukoplakia.** Leukoplakia may be a premalignant lesion (see Chapter 7). Scalpel biopsy and microscopic examination are necessary to establish the diagnosis of any white lesion for which a specific cause cannot be identified.

Linea Alba

Linea alba is a white raised line that forms most commonly on the buccal mucosa at the occlusal plane (Fig. 2.32). In some patients the line becomes prominent as a result of a teeth-clenching habit. The line follows the pattern of the adjacent teeth at the level of the occlusal plane. Although it is most commonly seen on the buccal mucosa, linea alba may form on the labial mucosa as well. Microscopically the white raised line is caused by epithelial hyperplasia and hyperkeratosis. No treatment is indicated. The prominence of linea alba may be helpful in evaluating the severity of a clenching habit.

Nicotine Stomatitis

Nicotine stomatitis is a benign lesion on the hard palate most typically associated with heavy, long-term pipe and cigar smoking, and is due to the effect of heat on the palatal mucosa; it may also be associated with cigarette smoking. Because of the decreased use of cigars and pipes, nicotine stomatitis is seen less frequently than previously. The initial response of the palatal mucosa to the heat from these substances is an erythematous appearance, with hyperkeratosis and **opacification** increasing over time. After the increase in keratinization, raised red dots are seen at the openings of the ducts of the minor salivary glands on the palatal surface (Fig. 2.33). The minor salivary glands become inflamed as a result of obstruction by keratin at the mucosal opening of the ducts. The palate may develop a very similar clinical appearance as a result of the chronic intake of very hot liquids. This condition is reversible if the irritant is removed.

Smokeless Tobacco Keratosis (Tobacco Pouch Keratosis, Spit Tobacco Keratosis)

Individuals who use smokeless tobacco in any of its many forms may develop a white lesion, **smokeless tobacco keratosis,** which is also called **tobacco pouch keratosis,** in the area where the tobacco is habitually placed. The mucobuccal fold is the most common location. The epithelium usually has a white, granular, or wrinkled appearance in early lesions. Long-standing lesions may be more opaquely white and have a corrugated surface (Fig. 2.34). Microscopically the epithelium may show changes that vary from hyperplasia and hyperkeratosis to atypical premalignant changes that are called **epithelial dysplasia** (see Chapter 7).

The lesion caused by smokeless tobacco often disappears when the tobacco is no longer placed in the area. Long-term exposure to smokeless tobacco has been associated with an increased risk of squamous cell carcinoma. Biopsy and microscopic examination of these lesions is indicated if the habit and lesion persist. In addition, the patient with this habit has an increased risk of caries, periodontal disease, attrition, and staining. Verrucous carcinoma has been associated with smokeless tobacco.

Traumatic Neuroma

A **traumatic neuroma** is a reactive lesion caused by injury to a peripheral nerve. It appears as a smooth nonulcerated nodule. Nerve tissue is encased in a sheath composed of Schwann cells and their fibers. When this sheath is disrupted, the nerve loses its framework. When a nerve and its sheath are damaged, the proximal end of the damaged nerve proliferates into a mass of nerve and Schwann cells mixed with dense fibrous scar tissue. In the

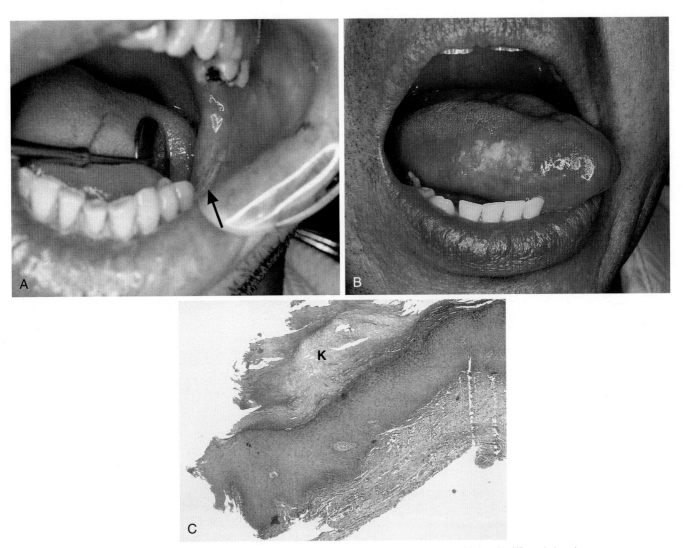

• **Figure 2.31** Frictional keratosis (indicated by *arrow*) caused by an opposing third molar **(A)**, and chronic tongue chewing **(B)**. **C,** Microscopic appearance of hyperkeratosis (low magnification) showing an increase in surface keratin (*K*).

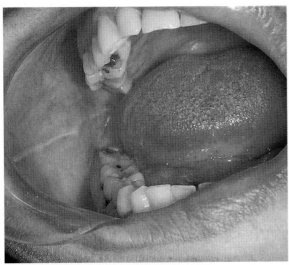

• **Figure 2.32** Linea alba.

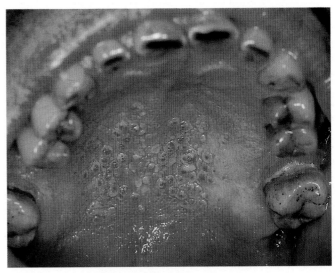

• **Figure 2.33** Nicotine stomatitis.

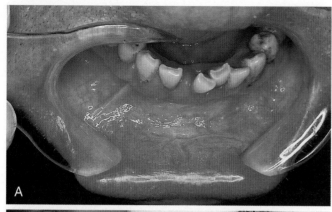

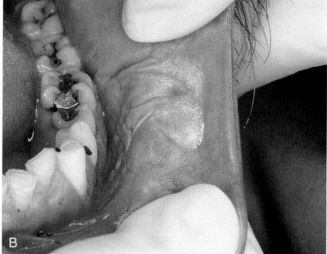

• **Figure 2.34** Smokeless tobacco–associated keratosis. Note the rough texture of the surface. **A,** Labial mucosa. **B,** Anterior buccal mucosa.

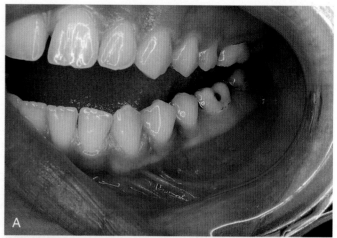

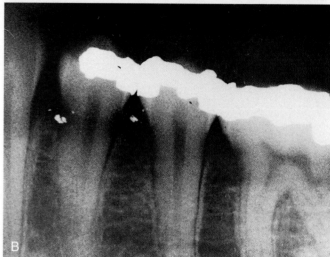

• **Figure 2.35 A,** This bluish-gray pigmentation of the gingiva is an amalgam tattoo. **B,** Periapical radiograph showing amalgam particles in the gingival tissue.

oral cavity injury to a nerve may occur from injection of local anesthesia, surgery, or other sources of trauma.

Traumatic neuromas are often painful. The pain may range from pain on palpation to severe and constant pain. Most traumatic neuromas occur in adults, and involvement of the mental nerve in the area of the mental foramen is the most common location. However, a traumatic neuroma may occur in other locations as well. Although the clinical features, particularly the pain that is characteristic, may suggest that a lesion is a traumatic neuroma, the diagnosis is made on the basis of a biopsy and microscopic examination. Traumatic neuromas are treated by surgical excision, and recurrence is rare.

The **palisaded encapsulated neuroma (PEN)**, also called a *solitary circumscribed neuroma,* is a benign lesion that has microscopic features similar to those of a traumatic neuroma. The PEN presents clinically as a painless mucosal nodule and has a distinct microscopic appearance. Unlike the traumatic neuroma, which exhibits a proliferation of small nerves, the PEN is a well-circumscribed lesion composed of nerve tissue partially surrounded by fibrous connective tissue. The nose and cheek are the most commonly reported sites on the skin of the face; intraorally, the most commonly reported sites are the palate, gingiva, and labial mucosa. Although the pathogenesis of the PEN is not clear, it has been considered a reactive and hyperplastic, rather than neoplastic, lesion. A history of trauma is usually not identified. However, these do not recur even if not completely removed.

Amalgam Tattoo

An **amalgam tattoo** is a flat, bluish-gray lesion of the oral mucosa that results from the introduction of amalgam into oral tissue (Fig. 2.35A). This may occur at the time of placement or removal of an amalgam restoration or at the time of tooth extraction if fragments of amalgam fracture off a restoration and remain in the tissue. The metallic particles disperse in the connective tissue and result in a permanent area of pigmentation. Over time the mercury-silver-tin amalgam changes, and it is mainly silver that remains in the tissue.

Amalgam tattoos may be seen in any location in the oral cavity, but are most commonly found on the gingiva or edentulous alveolar ridge. The posterior region of the mandible is the most common location.

An amalgam tattoo is usually diagnosed on the basis of clinical appearance of the pigmented area. If the amalgam fragments are large enough, they may be seen as radiopacities on a periapical or panoramic radiograph (Fig. 2.35B). As amalgam particles diffuse in the tissue over time, the size of the amalgam tattoo may increase. Biopsy and microscopic examination may be necessary to distinguish an amalgam tattoo from a melanocytic lesion, particularly if it is located in an area other than the gingiva or

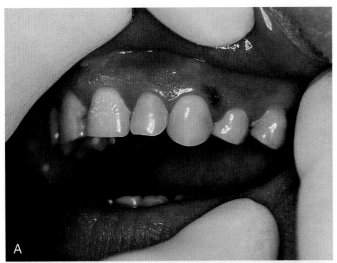

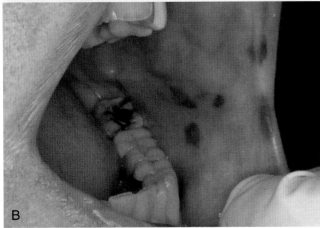

• **Figure 2.36** **A,** Posttraumatic melanin pigmentation: area of melanin pigmentation on the gingiva after healing of a traumatic injury. **B,** Oral melanotic macules on the buccal mucosa. (**B** courtesy Dr. A. Ross Kerr.)

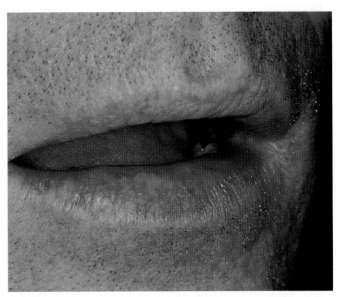

• **Figure 2.37** Solar cheilitis. The color of the vermilion appears mottled and the interface between the vermilion and skin is indistinct.

alveolar ridge. Once the diagnosis of amalgam tattoo has been established, treatment is generally not indicated. Surgical removal of the lesion may be considered if there are esthetic concerns.

Melanosis

Normal physiologic pigmentation of the oral mucosa is common, particularly in dark-skinned individuals (see Figs. 1.18 and 1.50). Melanin pigmentation that occurs after an inflammatory response is called **postinflammatory melanosis** (Fig. 2.36A). The **oral melanotic macule** is a flat, well-circumscribed brown lesion of unknown cause. These are usually small (<1 cm in diameter) and may require biopsy and microscopic examination for diagnosis (Fig. 2.36B). The **labial melanotic macule** on the lower lip vermilion is the most commonly involved site for the melanotic macule. Other sites include the buccal mucosa, gingiva, and palate. The labial melanotic macule characteristically darkens with exposure to sunlight.

Another type of melanosis is called **smoker's melanosis** or **smoking-associated melanosis.** In this type of melanosis the melanin pigmentation is associated with smoking, and the intensity is related to the amount and duration of smoking. Research has suggested that this melanin production in smokers may protect the mucosa from the chemicals in tobacco smoke. The

pigmentation fades when smoking is discontinued. However, this may take months to years. The anterior labial gingiva is the most commonly affected site. Women are affected more frequently than men. A relationship to female hormones and birth control pills has been suggested. Oral mucosal melanin pigmentation may also be associated with genetic, bone, and systemic diseases.

Solar Cheilitis (Actinic Cheilitis)

Sun exposure, particularly in fair-skinned individuals, can result in degeneration of the tissue of the vermilion of the lips, called **solar** or **actinic cheilitis** (Fig. 2.37). The development of this condition is related to the total cumulative exposure to sunlight and the amount of skin pigmentation; it may be seen in individuals of various ages, but usually increases with age. Both the upper and lower lip may be involved; however, the lower lip is usually more severely involved than the upper lip. The ratio of men to women is 10:1, most likely because women protect their lips with lipstick.

The lips appear dry and cracked. The color of the vermilion of the lips appears pale pink and mottled. The interface between the lips and the skin is indistinct, with fissures appearing at right angles to the skin and vermilion junction. Microscopically, the epithelium is thinner than normal and often exhibits abnormal maturational changes that are called *epithelial dysplasia*. Epithelial dysplasia is described in detail in Chapter 7. Degenerative changes are seen in the connective tissue.

No specific treatment is indicated. However, a strong relationship exists between these epithelial and connective tissue changes and the development of squamous cell carcinoma of the vermilion of the lip. The risk is greater for the lower lip than the upper lip. Smoking and alcohol consumption may increase this risk. Biopsy and microscopic examination are indicated for persistent scaling or ulceration. Identification of patients at high risk and those with early indications of sun damage can be helpful in preventing future lesions. Patients at risk should be advised to avoid sun exposure, to use sun-blocking agents for protection, and that they are at increased risk for basal cell carcinoma and squamous cell carcinoma of skin.

Mucous Retention Lesions

Mucous retention lesions include the mucocele, ranula, and mucous cyst.

A **mucocele** is a lesion that forms when a salivary gland duct is severed or ruptured and the mucous salivary gland secretion spills into the adjacent connective tissue. An inflammatory response occurs, granulation tissue forms, and the mucus is walled off to form a cystlike structure lined with compressed granulation tissue. A true cyst is an abnormal sac or cavity lined by epithelium. The mucocele is not a true cyst because the cystic space is not lined with epithelium.

A mucocele presents as a swelling in the tissue that often increases and decreases in size over time. The size of a mucocele may range from a few millimeters to several centimeters. The lower labial mucosa is the most common site of occurrence (Fig. 2.38). However, mucoceles may form in any area of the oral mucosa in which minor salivary glands are found. On the lower labial mucosa, they are usually lateral to the midline. If a mucocele is near the surface, it may appear bluish. The color of the mucosa may appear normal if the mucocele is deeper in the tissue. Most

mucoceles occur in children and adolescents. However, they may occur in adults as well. Some mucoceles resolve spontaneously with no treatment. If they are chronic or persistent, treatment is by surgical excision with removal of the adjacent minor salivary glands. A mucoepidermoid carcinoma may clinically resemble a mucocele and should be considered in the differential diagnosis for lesions that are indurated or persist.

On occasion, an epithelium-lined cystic structure occurs in association with a salivary gland duct. This is also called a **mucocele, mucous cyst,** or **mucous retention cyst.** These occur much less frequently than the type described previously. They are not true cysts, but are dilated salivary gland ducts that are believed to develop as a result of salivary duct obstruction. A ballooning of the duct occurs, which appears microscopically as an epithelium-lined cystlike structure. Mucous cysts usually occur in adults older than 50 years of age. They may occur anywhere in the oral cavity where minor salivary glands are found and are treated by removal of the affected minor salivary glands. Whereas mucoceles are most common on the lower lip, salivary gland tumors are more common on the upper lip.

Ranula is a term used for a larger mucocele-like lesion that forms on the floor of the mouth (Fig. 2.39). The ranula may increase in size during meals. It is associated with the ducts of the sublingual and submandibular glands. The name *ranula* is derived from *rana,* the Latin word for frog (the clinical appearance of the ranula resembles the outpouching that occurs under the jaw of the frog when croaking). The ranula presents as a unilateral, bluish, fluctuant swelling. Obstruction of a salivary duct is considered to be the most likely cause for the development of a ranula. Microscopically, a ranula may resemble either a mucocele or a mucous cyst. Ranulas are treated by surgery, which may include removing part or all of the sublingual or submandibular gland. The cause of obstruction, often a salivary gland stone (sialolith), must be removed.

Sialolith

A **sialolith** is a salivary gland stone. Sialoliths occur in both major and minor salivary glands and form by precipitation of calcium salts around a central core (Fig. 2.40). When they occur in minor glands, a hard, pea-sized nodule may be palpated in soft tissue (Fig. 2.40A). They may cause obstruction of the involved salivary gland. When they occur in the floor of the mouth, they can often

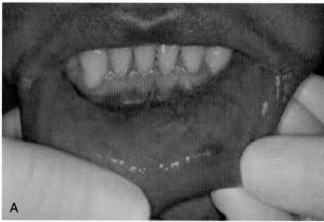

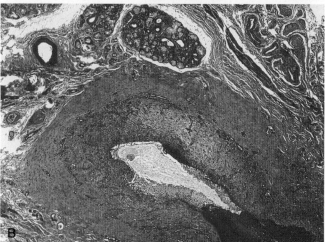

• **Figure 2.38** Mucocele of the lower lip. **A,** Fluid-filled lesion is seen on the lower lip. **B,** Microscopic appearance of a mucocele, showing a cyst-like space lined by granulation tissue (low magnification). (**A** courtesy Dr. A. Ross Kerr.)

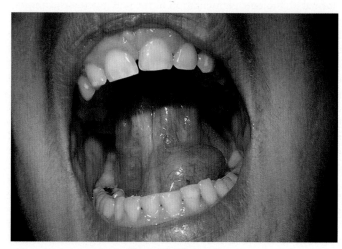

• **Figure 2.39** Ranula.

be seen as a radiopaque structure on an occlusal or panoramic radiograph (Fig. 2.41A-B).

Necrotizing Sialometaplasia

Necrotizing sialometaplasia is a local, painful, benign condition of the salivary glands characterized by moderately painful swelling followed by ulceration in the affected area (Fig. 2.42). It characteristically affects the minor salivary glands located at the junction of the hard and soft palate. It occurs on the hard palate more frequently than the soft palate. It is most common in adults and affects men twice as frequently as women. It is thought to result from blockage of the blood supply to the area of the lesion, resulting in tissue necrosis.

Microscopically, necrosis of the salivary glands is seen. The salivary gland duct epithelium is replaced by squamous epithelium (metaplasia) and appears microscopically as islands of squamous epithelium deep in the connective tissue. The pattern of infiltrating islands may suggest squamous cell carcinoma or mucoepidermoid carcinoma.

If the duration of the ulcer is prolonged, a biopsy and microscopic examination are needed to establish the diagnosis. The ulcer may heal by secondary intention, either spontaneously or following biopsy, usually within a few weeks.

Sialadenitis

Inflammation of salivary gland tissue is called **sialadenitis.** Sialadenitis may be acute or chronic and may be a result of infectious or noninfectious causes. Acute sialadenitis is characterized by an infiltrate of primarily neutrophils, whereas lymphocytes and plasma cells are present in chronic sialadenitis. Several viral infections can cause acute sialadenitis; the most common of these is mumps. Acute bacterial infections result from obstruction of salivary flow due to constriction of a duct or the presence of a sialolith. Decreased salivary flow (xerostomia) may allow bacteria from the

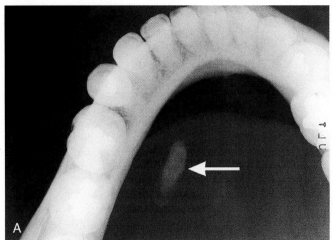

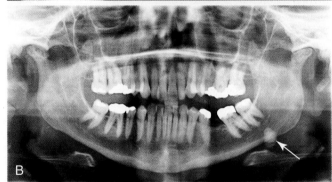

• **Figure 2.41 A,** Occlusal radiograph showing a sialolith (*arrow*) in Wharton's duct. **B,** A panoramic radiograph showing a sialolith (*arrow*). (**A** courtesy Dr. Barry Wolinsky. **B** Courtesy Dr. K.C. Chan.)

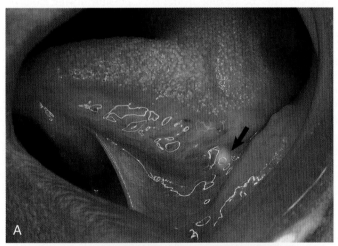

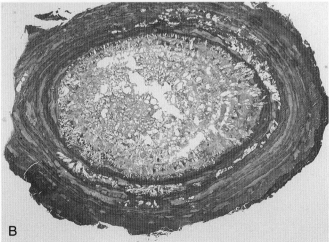

• **Figure 2.40** Sialoliths. **A,** Sialolith (*arrow*) in a minor salivary gland on the floor of the mouth. **B,** Microscopic appearance of a sialolith, showing concentric rings.

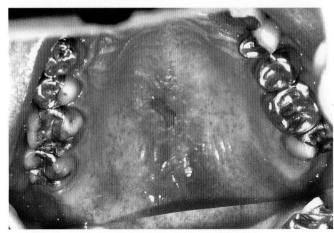

• **Figure 2.42** Necrotizing sialometaplasia.

oral cavity to infect the gland. In some cases the cause cannot be identified. Sialadenitis presents as a painful swelling of the involved salivary gland, usually one of the major glands. Bacterial infection of a major gland may result in a purulent exudate expressed from the ductal opening. Diagnosis may require injection of a radiopaque dye into the gland, followed by taking a radiograph of the gland (a sialogram). Other imaging useful in diagnosis includes magnetic resonance imaging (MRI) and computerized tomography (CT) scans. Microbial culture may be necessary to identify an infectious etiology. Antibiotics may be necessary in cases of bacterial infection.

Acute and chronic sialadenitis may occur in minor salivary glands. This is usually identified microscopically and occurs associated with local trauma or other inflammatory salivary gland conditions.

Reactive Connective Tissue Hyperplasia

Reactive connective tissue hyperplasia consists of proliferating, exuberant granulation tissue and hyperplastic fibrous connective tissue. These lesions result from overzealous repair. They may occur as a response to a single event or as a chronic low-grade injury. The reason for the exuberant overgrowth of reparative tissue is not known.

Pyogenic Granuloma

A **pyogenic granuloma** is a benign, reactive, commonly occurring intraoral lesion that is characterized by a proliferation of connective tissue containing numerous blood vessels and inflammatory cells that resembles granulation tissue. It occurs as a response to injury. The term *pyogenic granuloma* is a misnomer because the lesion does not produce purulent exudate (pyogenic) and is not a true granuloma.

The pyogenic granuloma (Fig. 2.43) is a painless, exophytic mass that usually exhibits an ulcerated surface. It may be either sessile or pedunculated. It is soft to palpation and bleeds easily. The color ranges from pink to deep reddish-purple because of the vascularity of the proliferating tissue. When ulcerated, the fibrin membrane on the surface appears yellowish white. Up to 85% of

intraoral pyogenic granulomas are reported to occur on the gingiva; the maxillary anterior gingiva is a common location. The pyogenic granuloma also occurs in other areas such as the lips, tongue, buccal mucosa, and skin. Pyogenic granulomas may vary considerably in size, from a few millimeters to several centimeters. They usually develop rapidly and then remain static.

Pyogenic granulomas are most common in teenagers and young adults. They may occur at any age and are more common in women than men. Pyogenic granulomas often occur in pregnant women and have been called **pregnancy tumors** (Fig. 2.44). The lesions are microscopically identical to the pyogenic granuloma seen in men and nonpregnant women and may be caused by changing hormonal levels and increased response to oral biofilm. They often regress after delivery, but recur when removed during pregnancy. Similar gingival lesions occur during puberty.

The pyogenic granuloma is treated by surgical excision if it does not resolve spontaneously. On occasion, the lesion may recur if the injurious agent (e.g., calculus) remains.

Peripheral Giant Cell Granuloma

A **giant cell granuloma** is a reactive lesion that is composed of well-vascularized connective tissue with multinucleated giant cells. Red blood cells and chronic inflammatory cells are commonly seen in this lesion. The cause of giant cell granulomas is not clear. They occur only in the jaws, possibly arising from the periodontal ligament or the periosteum, and are thought to be a response to injury. Giant cell granulomas occur both on the gingiva (peripheral giant cell granuloma) and within bone (central giant cell granuloma). The term **peripheral** pertains here to lesions occurring outside the bone, on the gingiva or alveolar mucosa, and the term **central** refers to a lesion occurring within the maxilla and mandible. A description of central giant cell granulomas is included in Chapter 8.

The **peripheral giant cell granuloma** always occurs on the gingiva or alveolar process, usually anterior to the molars. It is considered a reactive lesion, usually occurring as a result of local irritating factors such as dental biofilm or calculus, periodontal disease, fracture restorations, ill-fitting dental appliances, or dental extractions. Peripheral giant cell granulomas associated with

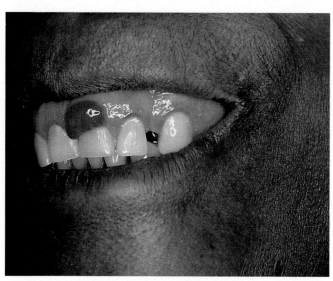

• **Figure 2.43** Pyogenic granuloma.

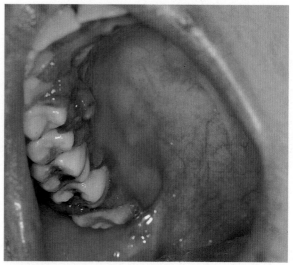

• **Figure 2.44** Pyogenic granuloma of pregnancy (pregnancy tumor).

dental implants have been reported. The peripheral giant cell granuloma may resemble the pyogenic granuloma in clinical appearance (Fig. 2.45 A-C). As with the pyogenic granuloma, surface ulceration may be present. Peripheral giant cell granulomas

may vary in size from 0.5 to 1.5 cm in diameter and are usually dark red to purple because of the numerous blood vessels and extravasated red blood cells present. The peripheral giant cell granuloma may occur at any age, but has been reported to be more frequent in people between 30 and 45 years of age and more common in women than men. Peripheral giant cell granulomas may cause superficial destruction of the alveolar bone, and radiographs may show a cupping or saucerization of bone in the area. They are treated by surgical excision of the lesion and generally do not recur if the source of local irritation is eliminated and the lesion is completely removed.

Peripheral Ossifying Fibroma (Peripheral Fibroma With Calcification)

The peripheral ossifying fibroma is an exophytic, usually well-demarcated sessile or pedunculated gingival lesion (Fig. 2.46A). The pathogenesis of the peripheral ossifying fibroma is uncertain; however, it is considered to be a reactive rather than a neoplastic lesion. Clinically it appears to emanate from the interdental papilla. The lesion is believed to be derived from the cells of the periodontal ligament. It is more common in females than in males

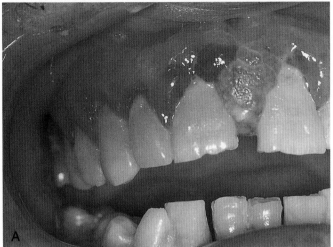

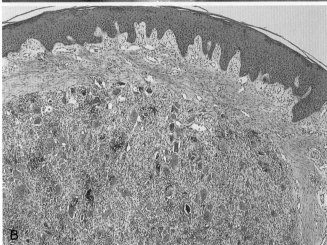

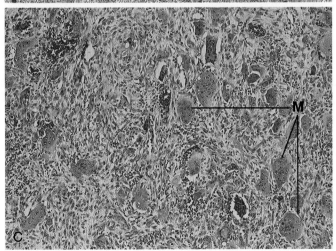

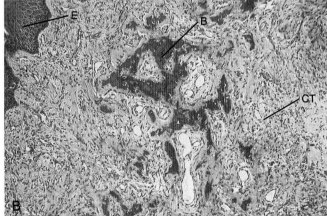

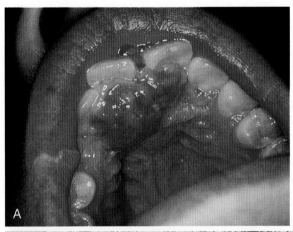

• **Figure 2.45** A, Peripheral giant cell granuloma. B and C, Microscopic appearance of a peripheral giant cell granuloma. Low magnification **(B)** shows the surface epithelium. Higher magnification **(C)** shows multinucleated giant cells (*M*), capillaries, and fibroblasts.

• **Figure 2.46** A, Clinical appearance of a peripheral ossifying fibroma shows an exophytic lesion involving the palatal gingiva of the maxillary anterior teeth. B, Photomicrograph of a peripheral ossifying fibroma shows bonelike calcifications (*B*) in cellular fibrous connective tissue (*CT*). A small amount of surface epithelium (*E*) is also visible.

and most often occurs in young individuals with a peak prevalence in the second decade (ages 10 to 19). It has been reported in both children and adults.

It is composed of cellular fibrous connective tissue interspersed with scattered bone and cementum-like calcifications (Fig. 2.46B). Although the name of this lesion is similar to the central ossifying fibroma, the central ossifying fibroma is a true tumor. The peripheral ossifying fibroma is not a soft tissue counterpart of the central lesion.

Treatment of a peripheral ossifying fibroma consists of complete surgical excision with thorough scaling of the adjacent teeth to remove any irritants that can induce regrowth of the lesion. The recurrence rates for the peripheral ossifying fibroma range from 8% to 16%.

Fibroma, Irritation Fibroma, Traumatic Fibroma, and Focal Fibrous Hyperplasia

The fibroma **(irritation fibroma, traumatic fibroma, focal fibrous hyperplasia)** is a broad-based, persistent exophytic lesion composed of dense, scarlike connective tissue containing few blood vessels (Fig. 2.47). It occurs as a result of chronic trauma or an episode of trauma. Many irritation fibromas likely result from fibrosis of a pyogenic granuloma. As in the normal healing process, the granulation tissue that forms the pyogenic granuloma is replaced by mature fibrous connective tissue. The irritation fibroma is usually a small lesion. Most are less than 1 cm in diameter; fibromas greater than 2 cm in diameter are rare. The fibroma occurs most frequently on the buccal mucosa. It also occurs on the gingiva, tongue, lips, and palate. The color of the irritation fibroma is usually lighter than that of the surrounding mucosa because the connective tissue contains so few blood vessels. The surface is covered by stratified squamous epithelium and may appear opaque and white if it has a thick keratin surface, or it may be ulcerated because of local secondary trauma.

An irritation fibroma is removed surgically. Many benign soft tissue neoplasms resemble the irritation fibroma in clinical appearance. Excision and microscopic examination of the tissue are important to confirm the diagnosis of the lesion. Irritation fibromas usually do not recur at the same site, but additional lesions may occur as a response to additional trauma.

The **frenal tag** is a small fingerlike projection of hyperplastic fibrous tissue attached to the maxillary labial frenum. These are common and do not require removal.

Denture-Induced Fibrous Hyperplasia

Denture-induced fibrous hyperplasia is commonly called **epulis fissuratum**, **denture-associated inflammatory hyperplasia**, or **denture epulis**. This lesion is caused by an ill-fitting full or partial denture and is generally located in the vestibule along the denture flange, most commonly in the anterior maxilla or mandible. The lesion is usually somewhat larger than an irritation fibroma. It is arranged in elongated folds of tissue into which the denture flange fits (Fig. 2.48). It is composed of dense, fibrous connective tissue surfaced by stratified squamous epithelium, the same type of tissue seen in an irritation fibroma. The surface of the lesion is often ulcerated. Because this lesion does not resolve even with prolonged removal of the denture, treatment involves surgical removal of the excess tissue with microscopic examination of the tissue and relining of the prosthesis, or construction of a new denture.

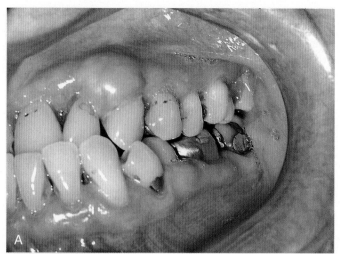
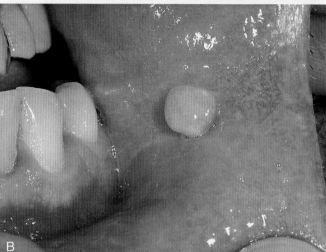
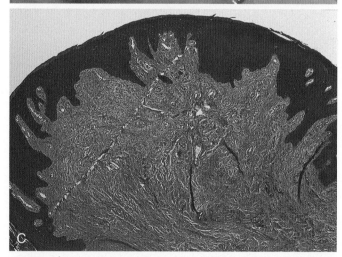

• **Figure 2.47** Irritation fibroma. **A,** Development of fibroma followed by the healing of a periodontal abscess. **B,** Irritation fibroma of the buccal mucosa. **C,** Microscopic appearance of a fibroma. (**A** courtesy Dr. Murray Schwartz.)

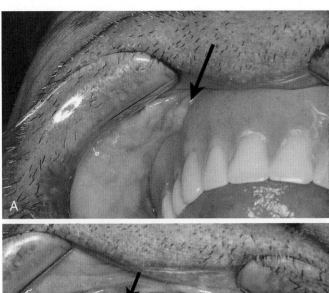

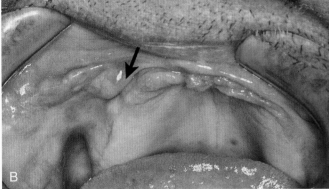

• **Figure 2.48** Denture-induced fibrous hyperplasia (epulis fissuratum; *arrows*). **A,** With denture; **B,** without denture.

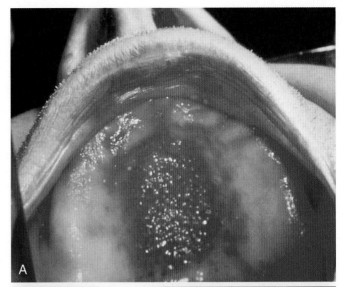

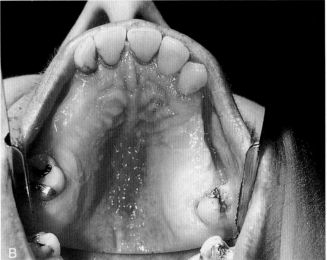

• **Figure 2.49** Papillary hyperplasia of the palate. **A,** Full denture. **B,** Partial denture. (Courtesy Dr. Edward V. Zegarelli.)

Inflammatory Papillary Hyperplasia of the Palate

Papillary hyperplasia of the palate, or **palatal papillomatosis,** is a form of denture-induced hyperplasia. It is also considered a form of denture stomatitis. It is almost always associated with a maxillary removable full or partial denture or an orthodontic appliance. The palatal mucosa, most commonly the vault area, is covered by multiple erythematous papillary projections that give the area a granular or "cobblestone" appearance (Fig. 2.49).

Each of the papillary projections consists of fibrous connective tissue, usually chronically inflamed and surfaced by stratified squamous epithelium. The erythematous appearance is generally due to a superficial infection with the fungus *Candida albicans.* Oral mucosal infections with this fungus are described in Chapter 4. The precise cause of this type of hyperplasia is not known. It is usually related to an ill-fitting upper denture or other removable prosthetic device that is worn continuously, 24 hours a day. Poor denture hygiene can be a contributing factor. Surgical removal of the hyperplastic papillary tissue may be necessary before construction of a new denture.

Gingival Enlargement

Gingival enlargement is characterized by an increase in the size of the marginal and attached gingiva usually involving the interdental papillae (Fig. 2.50). No stippling is seen, and the gingival margins are bulbous and rounded. The tissue consistency may vary from soft to firm, and the appearance may vary from erythematous to a normal pink color, depending on the degree of inflammation and vascularity. Gingival enlargement may be generalized or localized and may vary from mild focal enlargement of interdental papillae to severe generalized gingival enlargement that may cover the crowns of the teeth. Although generally considered to be **gingival hyperplasia,** enlargement of the gingiva may also be the result of hypertrophy.

Many cases are the result of an unusual tissue response to chronic inflammation associated with local irritants such as dental biofilm or calculus. Hormonal changes occurring in pregnancy and puberty and certain drugs such as the anticonvulsive agent phenytoin; calcium channel blockers including nifedipine, verapamil, and amlodipine; oral contraceptive agents; and cyclosporine can increase the tissue response to local factors. Hereditary forms of gingival fibromatosis occur, beginning in early childhood. In some cases the cause of gingival enlargement cannot be identified. Gingival enlargement may occur in some patients with leukemia because of an infiltration of abnormal white blood cells into the gingival tissue. If the tissue is inflamed and bleeds easily, laboratory testing may be appropriate to rule

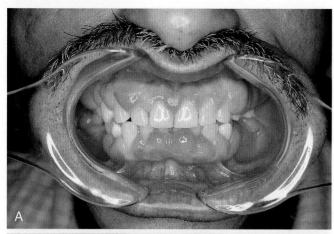

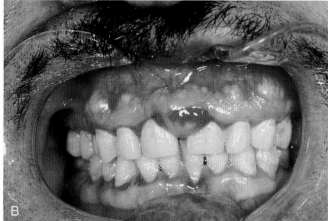

• **Figure 2.50** Gingival enlargement. **A,** Fibrous. **B,** Inflamed.

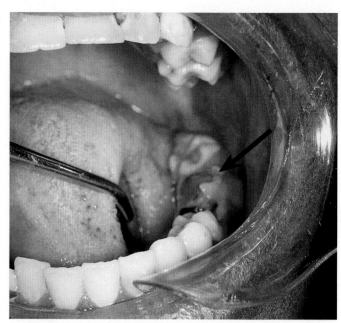

• **Figure 2.51** Chronic hyperplastic pulpitis (pulp polyp) *(arrow)*.

out the gingival enlargement that may occur with leukemia (see Fig. 9.12).

Gingivoplasty (reshaping the gingiva) or *gingivectomy* (removing gingival tissue) may be necessary to recontour the gingival tissue and may have to be done periodically if the cause cannot be eliminated or the medication cannot be changed and gingival enlargement persists. Meticulous oral hygiene and frequent recare appointments may be helpful in reducing enlargement by reducing plaque and calculus.

Chronic Hyperplastic Pulpitis

Chronic hyperplastic pulpitis, or **pulp polyp,** is an excessive proliferation of chronically inflamed dental pulp tissue. In children and young adults it occurs in teeth with large, open carious lesions; both primary and permanent molars may be affected. Chronic hyperplastic pulpitis appears as a red or pink nodule of tissue that often fills the entire cavity in the tooth, with tissue protruding from the pulp chamber (Fig. 2.51). It is usually asymptomatic; because the hyperplastic tissue contains so few nerves, it is usually insensitive to manipulation. The proliferation of pulp tissue rather than pulpal necrosis, which can also result from caries, may be related to the large root opening and blood supply of the tooth involved.

The hyperplastic tissue consists of granulation tissue with inflammatory cells, primarily lymphocytes and plasma cells.

Neutrophils may also be present. The tissue is generally surfaced by stratified squamous epithelium. Because no epithelium exists in normal pulp tissue, this epithelium is thought to result from desquamation of the surface oral mucosa. Chronic hyperplastic pulpitis is treated by either extraction or endodontic treatment of the involved tooth.

Inflammatory Periapical Lesions

Caries or traumatic injury to a tooth may result in a variety of responses: inflammation, infection, chronic hyperplastic pulpitis, and necrosis of the dental pulp. The inflammatory process begins in the dental pulp and then extends into the periapical area, which is the area surrounding the apical portion of the tooth root at the site of the apical foramen. This condition occurs because, once the inflammatory process has been established in the dental pulp, the only route it can follow is through the root canal into the periapical area. The presence of accessory (lateral) canals may lead to areas of inflammation located on the lateral portion of the tooth root.

Periapical Abscess

An acute **periapical abscess** is composed of a purulent exudate (pus or suppuration), surrounded by connective tissue containing neutrophils and lymphocytes located at the apex of a nonvital tooth. The patient complains of severe pain, which is the result of inflammation. The inflammatory exudate puts pressure on nerves, and chemical mediators can also cause pain. The periapical abscess may develop directly from the inflammation in the pulp, or develop in an area of previously existing chronic inflammation. The purulent exudate seeks a path of least resistance and finds either a channel or a fistula (fistulous tract) out of the tissue, or it spreads to contiguous areas through oral and facial tissue spaces (see Fig. 2.3). A **parulis** is a mass of granulation tissue located at the mucosal opening of the fistulous tract. The tooth associated with the abscess is usually quite painful unless a fistulous tract has formed. The tooth may be slightly extruded from its socket. If the acute abscess develops directly from pulpal inflammation, there may initially be no radiographic changes except for a slight thickening of the apical periodontal ligament space. If the abscess develops in a preexisting area of periapical chronic inflammation, a distinct radiolucent area is seen at the apex. The tooth may or may not test positive by electric pulp testing with a vitalometer. The tooth requires treatment even if asymptomatic. If not treated, the infection may spread to surrounding bone (osteomyelitis). If the abscess does not form a fistulous tract, the purulent exudate may spread to the overlying soft tissue (cellulitis). A rare, but very severe, consequence of a dental infection is a rapidly aggressive form of cellulitis called **Ludwig angina.** Ludwig angina involves a massive swelling of the tissue of the floor of the mouth and neck and may be life threatening due to airway obstruction. Pain, dysphasia, fever, chills, and leukocytosis may be present. The swelling is due to edema. Pus is usually not present.

The clinician treats a periapical abscess by establishing drainage, by opening the pulp chamber, or by extracting the tooth. If the abscess has extended into adjacent tissue, an incision may be necessary to establish drainage. In some cases, the tooth is extracted. The patient may also be given antibiotic therapy.

Periapical Granuloma

A **periapical granuloma, dental granuloma,** or **chronic apical periodontitis** is a localized mass of chronically inflamed granulation tissue that forms at the opening of the pulp canal, generally at the apex of a nonvital tooth root (Fig. 2.52). This is a chronic process from the outset, and most cases are completely asymptomatic. In some cases, the tooth is sensitive to pressure and percussion because of the inflammation in the apical area. The tooth may also appear slightly extruded from its socket. The radiographic change may vary from a slight thickening of the periodontal ligament space in the area of inflammation to a diffuse radiolucency to a distinct, well-circumscribed radiolucency surrounding the root apex. Most of these lesions are discovered on radiographic examination.

The periapical granuloma is composed of granulation tissue containing lymphocytes, plasma cells, and macrophages. Neutrophils may also be present, and areas of dense fibrous connective tissue are often seen. The periapical granuloma differs from granulomatous inflammation, which is a distinctive type of inflammation characteristic of certain diseases (e.g., tuberculosis). Epithelial rests of Malassez, which are remnants of tooth-forming tissue of the Hertwig epithelial root sheath, are often present in the periapical granuloma. The periapical granuloma is treated by endodontic therapy (root canal therapy) or extraction of the tooth.

Radicular Cyst (Periapical Cyst)

A **radicular cyst,** or **periapical cyst,** is a true cyst, located at the apex of the root of a nonvital tooth. The radicular cyst consists of a pathologic cavity lined by epithelium. It occurs in association with the root of a nonvital tooth (Fig. 2.53). A true cyst is an abnormal, closed, epithelium-lined cavity in the body. The radicular cyst is the most commonly occurring cyst in the oral region. The epithelial lining of the cyst develops in a periapical granuloma as a result of proliferation of the epithelial rests of Malassez, remnants of the Hertwig epithelial root sheath after tooth development.

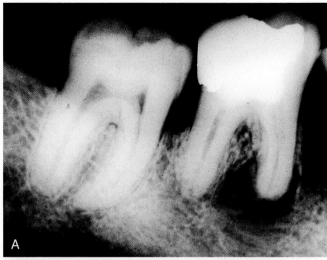

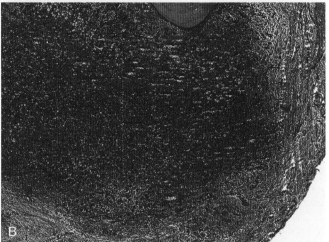

• **Figure 2.52 A,** Radiograph of a periapical granuloma. **B,** Microscopic appearance of a periapical granuloma, showing a collection of inflammatory cells at the apex of a tooth (low magnification). (**A** courtesy Dr. Herbert Frommer.)

A radicular cyst develops when the epithelium within the inflamed connective tissue of the periapical granuloma proliferates, forming an epithelial mass that increases in size through division of the peripheral cells. The peripheral cells are the equivalent of the basal cell layer of the epithelium. As the cells in the central portion of the mass become increasingly separated from the source of nutrition in the connective tissue, they undergo necrosis centrally, forming a cavity that is lined by epithelium and filled with fluid. Microscopically, the tissue surrounding this epithelium-lined cystic cavity is similar to that seen in the periapical granuloma.

Most radicular cysts are asymptomatic and discovered on radiographic examination. The radiographic appearance of the radicular cyst is the same as that of the periapical granuloma. It appears as a radiolucency, usually well circumscribed, that surrounds the apex of a tooth root. It is not possible to differentiate reliably a periapical granuloma from a radicular cyst on the basis of the radiographic appearance alone. A radicular cyst may form in association with any tooth. The cyst may occur lateral to the tooth root rather than at the apex if it is associated with a lateral

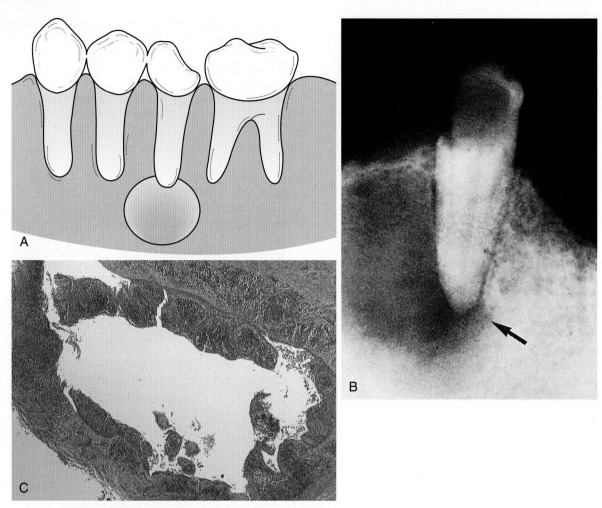

• **Figure 2.53** Radicular cyst. **A,** Diagram of a radicular cyst located around the root of an erupted tooth. **B,** Radiograph showing a well-circumscribed radiolucency (*arrow*) around the root of a tooth. **C,** Microscopic features of a radicular cyst.

pulp canal. *Lateral radicular cyst* may be used to describe this inflammatory cyst when it occurs in this location. Other types of cysts can resemble a radicular cyst radiographically; therefore removal of the cyst and microscopic examination of the tissue are necessary.

The radicular cyst is treated by endodontic therapy (root canal therapy), apicoectomy, or extraction and curettage of the periapical tissue. A **residual cyst** forms when the tooth is removed and all or part of a radicular cyst is left behind (Fig. 2.54). Radiographically, a residual cyst is a well-circumscribed radiolucency located at the site of tooth extraction. It is treated by surgical removal of the cyst.

Tooth Resorption

Tooth structure can be resorbed in the same manner as bone. This occurs normally in the process of exfoliation of deciduous teeth and may also occur in other situations. Resorption of the tooth structure beginning at the outside of the tooth is called *external resorption*. Resorption of the tooth structure from the pulpal aspect of the tooth is called *internal resorption*. External tooth resorption occurs more frequently than internal resorption.

Like bone resorption, tooth resorption can occur when inflammatory tissue is present. External resorption of the root of a tooth can occur when a periapical granuloma is present. Bone resorption as a response to pressure allows orthodontic tooth movement to occur. Pressure can also cause resorption of the tooth structure. This can occur from excessive occlusal or orthodontic forces and with benign and malignant neoplasms. When a tooth that has been avulsed is reimplanted, the root is usually resorbed and then replaced by bone. External root resorption first appears radiographically as a slight raggedness or blunting of the root apex and can proceed to severe loss of tooth substance (Fig. 2.55). The condition is not reversible, but progression of the process can be avoided if the cause can be identified and removed. Resorption of impacted teeth can also occur. Generalized root resorption may also occur after orthodontic tooth movement, and root resorption may be associated with certain neoplasms of the jaws (see Chapter 7). On occasion, resorption may involve the crown of an impacted tooth or the roots of teeth, and the cause cannot be identified. This is called **idiopathic tooth resorption.**

Internal tooth resorption (Fig. 2.56) can occur in any tooth. Usually only a single tooth is involved. In some cases no cause can be identified. However, it is usually associated with an inflammatory response in the pulp. If the process occurs in the coronal part of the tooth, it may be seen clinically as a pinkish area in the crown. The dental hard tissue has resorbed and is thinner than normal, and the pink color results from the vascular, inflamed

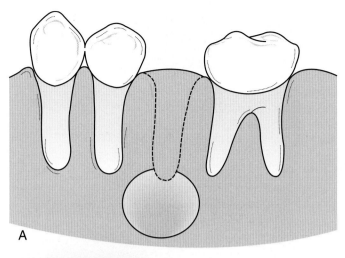

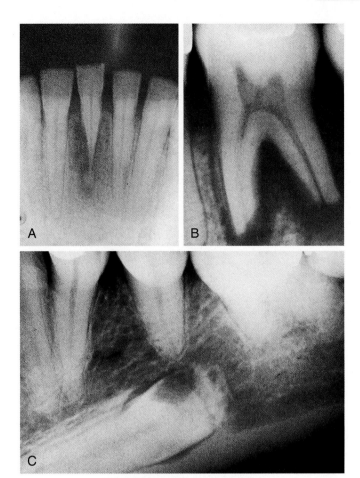

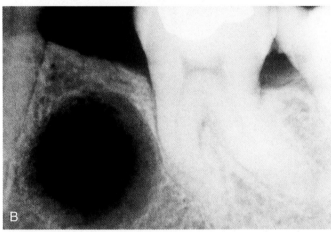

• **Figure 2.54** **A,** Diagram of a residual cyst. **B,** Radiograph of a residual cyst, showing radiolucency at the site of a previously extracted tooth. (Courtesy Drs. Paul Freedman and Stanley Kerpel.)

connective tissue that can be seen through the remaining enamel and dentin, referred to as *pink tooth of Mummery.* When the process involves the root, it can be seen only radiographically. A round-to-ovoid radiolucent area associated with the pulp is seen in the central portion of the tooth.

Endodontic therapy can be performed successfully if internal resorption is discovered early. If not treated, the process can extend through the dental hard tissue and cause a perforation. After this perforation occurs, the tooth must be extracted.

Focal Sclerosing Osteomyelitis

Focal sclerosing osteomyelitis, also called **condensing osteitis,** is a change in bone near the apices of teeth that may be a reaction to low-grade infection. The tooth most commonly associated with focal sclerosing osteomyelitis is the mandibular first molar. On occasion, the mandibular second molar and the mandibular premolars may also be involved.

Radiographically, focal sclerosing osteomyelitis appears as a radiopaque area in the periapical area of teeth (Fig. 2.57). The borders may be diffuse or well defined. On occasion, the periphery of the area is radiolucent; in other cases a central radiolucency surrounded by radiopacity is seen. Microscopically, it is dense bone with little marrow or connective tissue, and little inflammation is

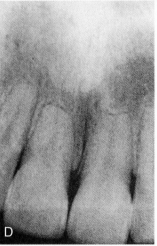

• **Figure 2.55** Tooth resorption. **A,** Root resorption of a mandibular anterior tooth associated with chronic inflammation. **B,** Resorption of tooth structure and bone because of chronic inflammation. **C,** Idiopathic resorption of an impacted tooth. **D,** Generalized root resorption associated with orthodontic tooth movement. (**A** courtesy Dr. Gerald P. Curatola.)

present. Focal sclerosing osteomyelitis is often associated with a carious or restored tooth. It is generally asymptomatic. However, pain may be associated if pulpal inflammatory disease is present. Focal sclerosing osteomyelitis may be present at any age, but it is usually first seen in young adults.

Diagnosis of focal sclerosing osteomyelitis usually can be made on the basis of the characteristic radiographic appearance.

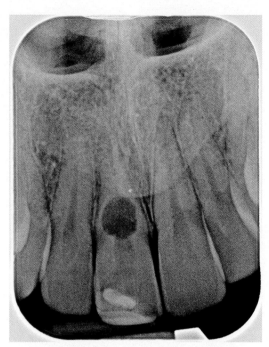

• **Figure 2.56** Internal tooth resorption.

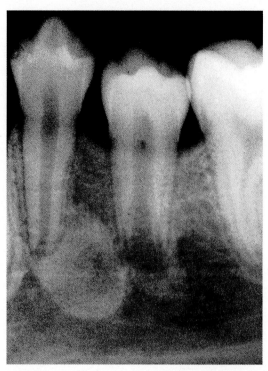

• **Figure 2.57** Focal sclerosing osteomyelitis (condensing osteitis).

Treatment of sclerosing osteomyelitis is not necessary. The sclerotic bone remains even after treatment of the involved tooth. On occasion, biopsy and microscopic examination may be necessary to rule out other radiopaque lesions such as osteoma, complex odontoma, or central ossifying fibroma.

Idiopathic osteosclerosis (dense bone island) can appear radiographically similar to sclerosing osteomyelitis. Unlike sclerosing osteomyelitis, it is not associated with inflammation. The diagnoses of sclerosing osteomyelitis and idiopathic osteosclerosis are made on the basis of their radiographic features. On occasion, biopsy and microscopic examination may be necessary to rule out other radiopaque lesions such as osteoma, complex odontoma, or central ossifying fibroma.

Alveolar Osteitis

Alveolar osteitis, or **"dry socket,"** is a postoperative complication of tooth extraction. The most frequently affected area is the socket of an extracted mandibular third molar. After the extraction of the tooth, the blood clot is lost before healing has taken place. Pain develops several days after the extraction. On examination the tooth socket appears empty, and the bone surfaces are exposed. The patient complains of pain, swelling, bad odor, and bad taste. Because no infection exists, fever is not present. Risk factors for the development of alveolar osteitis include a dissolution of the clot at the surgical site, traumatic extraction, the presence of infection before the extraction, and tobacco smoking after the extraction. There is some evidence that rinsing with chlorhexidine may prevent alveolar osteitis. There is little evidence that supports the effectiveness of any of the interventions to treat alveolar osteitis. Treatment of alveolar osteitis is directed at relief of pain and includes gentle irrigation with chlorhexidine or saline.

Selected References

Books

Fehrenbach MJ, Herring SW: *Illustrated anatomy of the head and neck,* ed 5, St. Louis, 2017, Saunders/Elsevier.

Fehrenbach MJ, Popowics T: *Illustrated dental embryology, histology, and anatomy,* ed 4, St. Louis, 2016, Saunders/Elsevier.

Kumar V, Abbus AK, Aster JC: *Robbins and Cotran pathologic basis of disease,* ed 4, St. Louis, 2015, Saunders/Elsevier.

McCance K, Huether S: *Pathophysiology,* ed 7, St. Louis, 2014, Mosby.

Neville BW, Damm DD, Allen CM, et al: *Oral and maxillofacial pathology,* ed 4, 2016, St. Louis Elsevier.

Regezi JA, Sciubba JJ, Jordan RCK: *Oral pathology: clinical pathologic correlations,* ed 7, St. Louis, 2017, Elsevier.

Journal Articles

Inflammation and Repair

Afsar U, Ahmed AU: An overview of inflammation: mechanism and consequences, *Front Biol* 6(4):274–281, 2011.

Broughton G II, Janis JE, Attinger CE: Wound healing: an overview, *Plast Reconstr Surg* 117(7 Suppl):S1e, 2006.

Buckley CD, Gilroy DW, Serhan CN: Proresolving lipid mediators and mechanisms in the resolution of acute inflammation, *Immunity* 40(3):315–327, 2014.

Eming SA, Krieg T, Davidson JM: Inflammation in wound repair: molecular and cellular mechanisms, *J Invest Dermatol* 127:514, 2007.

Krishnamoorthy S, Honn KV: Inflammation and disease progression, *Cancer Metastasis Rev* 25:481, 2006.

Krishnaswamy G, Ajitawi O, Chi DS: The human mast cell: an overview, *Methods Mol Biol* 315:13, 2006.

Kruger P, et al: Neutrophils: Between host defense, immune modulation, and tissue injury, *PLoS Pathog* 11(3):e1004651, 2015.

Moore K: An anatomy of an infection: overview of the infectious process, *Crit Care Nurs Clin North Am* 19:9, 2007.

Petäjä J: Inflammation and coagulation. An overview, *Thromb Res* 127(Suppl 2):S34–S37, 2011.

Rankin JA: Biological mediators of acute inflammation, *AACN Clin Issues* 15:3, 2004.

Semiali A, Chakir J, Goulet JP, et al: Whole cigarette smoke promotes human gingival epithelial cell apoptosis and inhibits cell repair processes, *J Periodontal Res* 46:533, 2011.

Serhan CN: Controlling the resolution of acute inflammation: a new genus of dual anti-inflammatory and proresolving mediators, *J Periodontol* 79(Suppl 8):1520–1526, 2008.

Lesions from Physical and Chemical Injuries to the Oral Tissue

Bouquot JE, Seime RJ: Bulimia nervosa: dental perspectives, *Pract Periodontics Aesthet Dent* 9:655, 1997.

Ferguson MM, Dunbar RJ, Smith JA, et al: Enamel erosion related to winemaking, *Occup Med* 46:159, 1996.

Gandara BK, Truelove EL: Diagnosis and management of dental erosion, *J Contemp Dent Pract* 1:16, 1999.

Geurtsen W: Rapid general dental erosion by gas-chlorinated swimming pool water: review of the literature and case report, *Am J Dent* 13:291, 2000.

Grippo JO, Simring M, Coleman TA: Abfraction, abrasion, biocorrosion, and the enigma of noncarious cervical lesions: a 20-year perspective, *J Esthet Restor Dent* 24:10, 2012.

Hague AL: Eating disorders: screening in the dental office, *J Am Dent Assoc* 141:675, 2010.

Hanamura H, Houston F, Rylander H, et al: Periodontal status and bruxism: a comparative study of patients with periodontal disease and occlusal parafunctions, *J Periodontol* 58:173, 1987.

Harpenau LA, Noble WH, Kao RT: Diagnosis and management of dental wear, *J Calif Dent Assoc* 39:225, 2011.

Imbery TA, Edwards P: Necrotizing sialometaplasia: literature review and case reports, *J Am Dent Assoc* 127:1087, 1996.

Järvinen V, Meurman JH, Hwärinen H, et al: Dental erosion and upper gastrointestinal disorders, *Oral Surg Oral Med Oral Pathol* 65:298, 1988.

Kapila YL, Kashani H: Cocaine-associated rapid gingival recession and dental erosion: a case report, *J Periodontol* 68:485, 1997.

Lineberry TW, Bostwick JM: Methamphetamine abuse: a perfect storm of complications, *Mayo Clin Proc* 81:77, 2006.

Little JW: Eating disorders: dental implications, *Oral Surg Oral Med Oral Pathol Oral Radiol Endod* 93:138, 2002.

Maron FS: Enamel erosion resulting from hydrochloric acid tablets, *J Am Dent Assoc* 127:781, 1996.

Mitchell-Lewis DA, Phelan JA, Kelly RB, et al: Identifying oral lesions associated with crack cocaine use, *J Am Dent Assoc* 125:1104, 1994.

Owens BM, Johnson WW, Schuman NJ: Oral amalgam pigmentation (tattoos): a retrospective study, *Quintessence Int* 23:805, 1992.

Owens BM, Schuman NJ, Johnson WW: Oral amalgam tattoos: a diagnostic study, *Compendium* 14:210, 1993.

Ozelik O, Haytac MC, Akkaya M: Iatrogenic trauma to oral tissues, *J Periodontol* 76:1793, 2005.

Piotrowski BT, Gillette WB, Handcock EB: Examining the prevalence and characteristics of abfraction-like cervical lesions in a population of US veterans, *J Am Dent Assoc* 132:1694, 2001.

Pullinger AG, Seligman DA: The degree to which attrition characterizes differentiated patient groups of temporomandibular disorders, *J Orofac Pain* 7:196, 1990.

Rawlinson A: Case report: labial cervical abrasion caused by misuse of dental floss, *Dent Health (London)* 26:3, 1987.

Roberts MW, Li SH: Oral findings in anorexia nervosa and bulimia nervosa: a study of 47 cases, *J Am Dent Assoc* 115:497, 1987.

Rossie KM, Guggenheimer J: Thermally induced "nicotine" stomatitis: a case report, *Oral Surg Oral Med Oral Pathol* 70:597, 1990.

Rugh JD, Harlan J: Nocturnal bruxism and temporomandibular disorders, *Adv Neurol* 49:329, 1988.

Rytömaa I, Järvinen V, Kanerva R, et al: Bulimia and tooth erosion, *Acta Odontol Scand* 56:36, 1998.

Silvestre FJ, Perez-Herbera A, Puente-Sandoval A, et al: Hard palate perforation in cocaine abusers: a systematic review, *Clin Oral Investig* 14:621, 2010.

Simmons MS, Thompson DC: Dental erosion secondary to ethanol-induced emesis, *Oral Surg Oral Med Oral Pathol* 64:731, 1987.

Witton R, Brennan PA: Severe tissue damage and neurological deficit following extravasation of sodium hypochlorite solution during routine endodontic treatment, *Br Dent J* 198:749, 2005.

Wray A, McGuirt F: Smokeless tobacco usage associated with oral carcinoma, *Arch Otolaryngol Head Neck Surg* 119:929, 1993.

Zimmers PL, Gobetti JP: Head and neck lesions commonly found in musicians, *J Am Dent Assoc* 125:1487, 1994.

Reactive Connective Tissue Hyperplasia

Bodner L, Peist M, Gatot A, et al: Growth potential of peripheral giant cell granuloma, *Oral Surg Oral Med Oral Pathol Oral Radiol Endod* 83:548, 1997.

Bonetti F, Pelosi G, Martignoni G, et al: Peripheral giant cell granuloma: evidence for osteoclastic differentiation, *Oral Surg Oral Med Oral Pathol* 70:471, 1990.

Brown RS, Sein P, Corio R, et al: Nitrendipine-induced gingival hyperplasia: first case report, *Oral Surg Oral Med Oral Pathol* 70:593, 1990.

Brunet L, Miranda J, Roset P, et al: Prevalence and risk of gingival enlargement in patients treated with anticonvulsant drugs, *Eur J Clin Invest* 31:781, 2001.

Cloutier M, Charles M, Carmichael RP, et al: An analysis of peripheral giant cell granuloma associated with dental implant treatment, *Oral Surg Oral Med Oral Pathol Oral Radiol Endod* 103:618, 2007.

Daley TD, Nartey NO, Wysocki GP: Pregnancy tumor: an analysis, *Oral Surg Oral Med Oral Pathol* 72:196, 1991.

Daley T, Wysocki G, Day C: Clinical and pharmacologic correlations in cyclosporine-induced gingival hyperplasia, *Oral Surg Oral Med Oral Pathol* 62:417, 1986.

Fay AA, Satheesh K, Gapski R: Felodipine-influenced gingival enlargement in an uncontrolled type 2 diabetic patient, *J Periodontol* 76:1217, 2005.

Gould A, Escobar V: Symmetrical gingival fibromatosis, *Oral Surg Oral Med Oral Pathol* 51:62, 1981.

Koutlas IG, Scheithauer BW: Palisaded encapsulated ("solitary circumscribed") neuroma of the oral cavity: a review of 55 cases, *Head Neck Pathol* 4:15, 2010.

Miranda J, Brunet L, Roset P, et al: Prevalence and risk of gingival enlargement in patients treated with nifedipine, *J Periodontol* 72:605, 2001.

Proia NK, Paszkiewicz GM, Nasca MA, et al: Smoking and smokeless tobacco-associated human buccal cell mutations and their association with oral cancer—a review, *Cancer Epidemiol Biomarkers Prev* 15:1061, 2006.

Roberson JB, Crocker DJ, Schiller T: The diagnosis and treatment of central giant cell granuloma, *J Am Dent Assoc* 128:81, 1997.

Silverstein LH, Burton CH Jr, Garnick JJ, et al: The late development of oral pyogenic granuloma as a complication of pregnancy: a case report, *Compendium* 17:192, 1996.

Zain RB, Fei YJ: Fibrous lesions of the gingiva: a histopathologic analysis of 204 cases, *Oral Surg Oral Med Oral Pathol* 70:466, 1990.

Inflammatory Periapical Lesions

Daly B, Sharif MO, Newton T, et al: Local interventions for the management of alveolar osteitis (dry socket), *Cochrane Database Syst Rev* (12):CD006968, 2012.

Gunraj MN: Dental root resorption, *Oral Surg Oral Med Oral Pathol Oral Radiol Endod* 88:647, 1999.

Halabi D, Escobar J, Muñoz C, et al: Logistic regression analysis of risk factors for the development of alveolar osteitis, *J Oral Maxillofac Surg* 70:1040, 2012.

Harris EF, Butler MI: Patterns of incisor root resorption before and after orthodontic correction in cases with anterior open bites, *Am J Orthod Dentofacial Orthop* 101:112, 1992.

Harris EF, Robinson QC, Woods MA: An analysis of causes of apical root resorption in patients not treated orthodontically, *Quintessence Int* 24:417, 1993.

Websites

American Dental Hygienists' Association: Inflammation: the relationship between oral health and systemic disease. Available at http://www.adha.org/CE_courses/course13/indexpg.htm.

Estrela C, Aguirre Guedes O, Almeida Silva J, et al: Diagnostic and clinical factors associated with pulpal and periapical pain (in *Brazilian Dental Journal*). Available at http://www.scielo.br/scielo.php?script=sci_arttext&pid=S0103-64402011000400008&lng=en&nrm=iso&tlng=en.

Kao RT, Harpenau LA: Dental erosion and tooth wear (in *Journal of the California Dental Association*). Available at http://www.cda.org/library/cda_member/pubs/journal/journal_0411.pdf.

Medscape: The biological mechanisms behind injury and inflammation. Available to members at http://www.medscape.com/viewarticle/557490.

Review Questions

1. Which of the following is the body's initial response to injury?
   a. Immune response
   b. Inflammatory response
   c. Repair and regeneration
   d. Hyperplasia and hypertrophy

2. What type of inflammation occurs if the injury is minimal and brief, as well as the source being removed from the tissue?
   a. Fatal
   b. Acute
   c. Chronic
   d. Life-threatening

3. During the inflammatory response, the first microscopic event is:
   a. Dilation of the microcirculation
   b. Increased permeability of the microcirculation
   c. Formation of exudate
   d. Constriction of the microcirculation

4. The directed movement of white blood cells to the area of injury is called:
   a. Pavementing
   b. Margination
   c. Chemotaxis
   d. Hyperemia

5. Which of the following cells are the *most* prevalent cells seen in chronic inflammation?
   a. Neutrophils
   b. Macrophages and lymphocytes
   c. Lymphocytes and plasma cells
   d. Neutrophils and lymphocytes

6. Which of the following is considered a function of the macrophage?
   a. Phagocytosis
   b. Pathologic hyperplasia
   c. Drainage of abscess
   d. Formation of antibodies

7. Which of the following terms is used to describe blood plasma with cells and proteins that leaves the blood vessels and enters the surrounding tissue during inflammation?
   a. Hyperemia
   b. Hypertrophy
   c. Margination
   d. Exudate

8. The process of phagocytosis during inflammation *directly* involves the:
   a. Ingestion of foreign substances by white blood cells
   b. Escape of plasma fluids and proteins from the microcirculation into the surrounding tissue
   c. Displacement of white blood cells to the blood vessel walls
   d. Attachment of white blood cells to the blood vessel walls

9. Which of the following statements is considered *incorrect* concerning the neutrophil?
   a. The neutrophil makes up 30% of white blood cells
   b. The neutrophil contains lysosomal enzymes
   c. The neutrophil is a cell whose main function is phagocytosis
   d. The neutrophil has a multilobed nucleus

10. During the process of inflammation, the second type of white blood cell to emigrate from the blood vessel into the injured tissue is the:
    a. Neutrophil
    b. Red blood cell
    c. Lymphocyte
    d. Macrophage

11. Components of the complement system mediate the inflammatory process by:
    a. Decreasing vascular permeability
    b. Releasing histamine granules from neutrophils
    c. Causing cytolysis of cells
    d. Decreasing phagocytosis

12. Two days after injury, granulation tissue can be described as:
    a. Immature vascular connective tissue
    b. Fluid in the form of exudate
    c. Dense avascular connective tissue
    d. Ulcerated tissue

13. The enlargement of superficial lymph nodes that occurs as a systemic sign of inflammation is:
    a. Called leukocytosis
    b. Regulated by the hypothalamus
    c. Caused by changes in their lymphocytes
    d. A process that involves only the lymph nodes in the submental area

14. Which statement concerning repair in the body is considered *true*?
    a. Repair can be completed with the injurious agents present
    b. Functioning cells and tissue components are always replaced by functioning scar tissue
    c. Repair always results in regeneration
    d. The process of repair is initiated by the inflammatory response

15. The clot that forms during repair after injury:
    a. Consists of fibrous connective tissue
    b. Serves as a guide for migrating epithelial cells
    c. Forms after skin injury, but not after mucosal injury
    d. Occurs only with healing by secondary intention

16. Healing by secondary intention refers to healing of an injury when:
    a. The incision has clean edges joined by sutures
    b. Only a small clot forms
    c. An infection forms in the injured area
    d. There is increased formation of granulation tissue

17. Which of the following is used to describe an increase in the size of an organ or tissue resulting from an increase in the number of its cells?
    a. Hyperemia
    b. Hyperplasia
    c. Inflammation
    d. Hypertrophy

18. Bone tissue repair in the body can be delayed by:
    a. Maintenance of osteoblast-producing tissue
    b. Inadequate movement of bone tissue
    c. Drainage of an area of edema
    d. Reduction in the amount of tissue infection

19. What type of healing is present when there is little loss of the tissue?
    a. Healing by primary intention
    b. Healing by secondary intention
    c. Healing by tertiary intention
    d. Healing does not take place

20. Which of the following cells are similar to smooth muscle cells and help the healing site contract?
    a. Osteoblasts
    b. Myofibroblasts
    c. Macrophages
    d. Neutrophils

21. Which of the following *directly* allows for the presence of fever?
    a. Production of bone tissue
    b. Wound healing
    c. Presence of pyrogens
    d. Production of C-reactive protein

22. Hyperemia is *directly* responsible for which two local clinical signs of inflammation?
    a. Hypertrophy and hyperplasia
    b. Erythema and heat
    c. Abscess and fistula
    d. Necrosis and scarring

23. Which of the following lesions is noted for a microscopic grouping of macrophages usually surrounded by lymphocytes?
    a. Lymphoma
    b. Granuloma
    c. Keloid
    d. Abscess

24. Which one of the following lesions would clinically appear as a pigmented lesion?
    a. Amalgam tattoo
    b. Traumatic ulcer
    c. Frictional keratosis
    d. Aspirin burn

25. Which of the following statements is *false*?
    a. Attrition is the wearing away of tooth structure during mastication
    b. Bruxism is the same process as mastication
    c. Erosion is the loss of tooth structure resulting from chemical action
    d. Abrasion is caused by mechanical, repetitive habits

26. Loss of tooth structure associated with bulimia is caused by:
    a. Attrition
    b. Erosion
    c. Bruxism
    d. Abrasion

27. An aspirin burn in the oral cavity:
    a. Occurs as a result of an overdose of aspirin
    b. Is usually painless
    c. Results from a misuse of aspirin
    d. Can take several weeks to heal

28. A patient has a generalized white appearance of the palate. Tiny erythematous dots can be seen, surrounded by a thickened, raised, white-to-gray area. Overall the palate appears wrinkled. This condition is most likely:
    a. Papillary hyperplasia of the palate
    b. Nicotine stomatitis
    c. An aspirin burn
    d. Necrotizing sialometaplasia

29. Which of the following is the most common cause of a mucocele?
    a. Acute inflammation
    b. Tumor formation
    c. Minor salivary gland duct trauma
    d. A sialolith

30. A ranula is located on the:
    a. Lower lip
    b. Buccal mucosa
    c. Retromolar area
    d. Floor of the mouth

31. Which one of the following lesions would *not* occur on the gingiva?
    a. Irritation fibroma
    b. Pyogenic granuloma
    c. Peripheral giant cell granuloma
    d. Epulis fissuratum

32. Generalized loss of tooth structure primarily on the lingual surfaces of maxillary anterior teeth is associated with:
    a. Erosion
    b. Attrition
    c. Abrasion
    d. Abfraction

33. Which of the following may be a cause of external tooth resorption?
    a. Caries
    b. Salivary gland dysfunction
    c. Chronic inflammation
    d. Medication

34. Which one of the following is considered to be the most likely cause of necrotizing sialometaplasia?
    a. Loss of blood supply
    b. Radiation therapy
    c. Smoking
    d. A sialolith

35. The most common site for a mucocele to occur is the:
    a. Floor of the mouth
    b. Tongue
    c. Buccal mucosa
    d. Lower lip

36. The peripheral giant cell granuloma occurs only on the:
    a. Gingiva or alveolar mucosa
    b. Hard palate
    c. Buccal mucosa
    d. Floor of the mouth

37. A sialolith is:
    a. Chronic inflammation of a salivary gland
    b. Acute inflammation of a salivary gland
    c. A pooling of saliva in the connective tissue
    d. A salivary gland stone

38. Which of the following statements is *false*?
    a. A periapical cyst develops from a periapical granuloma
    b. A periapical abscess always causes radiographic periapical changes
    c. A periapical granuloma is a circumscribed area of chronically inflamed tissue
    d. A periapical cyst is also called a radicular cyst

39. Epulis fissuratum results from irritation caused by:
    a. A denture flange
    b. Denture adhesive
    c. Poor suction from the denture in the palatal vault
    d. An allergic reaction to the acrylic in the denture

40. Which of the following statements is *true*?
    a. A traumatic neuroma is never painful
    b. Necrotizing sialometaplasia is considered a denture-related lesion
    c. Chronic hyperplastic pulpitis is similar to gingival hyperplasia
    d. Gingival enlargement may be caused by medication

41. Loss of tooth structure caused by chemical action describes:
    a. Abrasion
    b. Internal resorption
    c. Erosion
    d. Attrition

42. Which of the following cysts is characteristically associated with a tooth that is nonvital on pulp testing?
    a. Residual
    b. Radicular
    c. Dentigerous
    d. Dermoid

43. Which of the following cysts results when a tooth is extracted without removing the periapical cystic sac?
    a. Radicular
    b. Primordial
    c. Residual
    d. Periodontal

44. The most common cause of a radicular cyst is:
    a. Deep restorations without a base
    b. Caries
    c. Occlusal trauma
    d. Toothbrush abrasion at the cemento-enamel junction

45. The wearing away of tooth structure through an abnormal mechanical action defines:
    a. Attrition
    b. Abrasion
    c. Erosion
    d. Resorption

46. Which one of the following is *not* associated with attrition?
    a. Toothpaste
    b. Bruxism
    c. Mastication
    d. Age

47. Heavy plaque and calculus deposits, mouth breathing, orthodontic appliances, and overhanging restorations best describe some of the causative factors for:
    a. Phenytoin hyperplasia
    b. A reaction from nifedipine
    c. Irritation fibromatosis
    d. Chemical fibromatosis

48. A pink, granular, or "cobblestone-like" appearance of the hard palate under a denture is most likely:
    a. Nicotine stomatitis
    b. Necrotizing sialometaplasia
    c. Papillary hyperplasia of the palate
    d. Multiple fibromas

49. During examination of the dentition, the dental hygienist notes the presence of active wear facets. This indicates that the patient is:
    a. Chewing too vigorously
    b. A bruxer
    c. A vegetarian
    d. Lip biting

50. A patient has a loss of tooth structure on the labial surfaces of the anterior teeth and reports a high intake of citrus fruit juices. The dental hygienist would most likely suspect:
    a. Abrasion
    b. Bulimia
    c. Bruxism
    d. Erosion

51. The amalgam tattoo represents amalgam particles in the tissue and is most commonly observed in the oral cavity on the:
    a. Lateral borders of the tongue
    b. Anterior palate near the rugae
    c. Floor of the mouth
    d. Posterior gingiva and edentulous ridge

52. A pink protruding mass in the occlusal surface of a severely carious mandibular first or second molar is most likely a(n):
    a. Irritation fibroma
    b. Pyogenic granuloma
    c. Pulp polyp
    d. Pulpal granuloma

53. Which of the following drugs does *not* cause gingival enlargement?
    a. Phenytoin (Dilantin)
    b. Cyclosporine
    c. Nifedipine (Procardia)
    d. Tetracycline

54. Traumatic ulcers are usually diagnosed on the basis of:
    a. The patient's medical history
    b. The clinical appearance and history of the ulcers
    c. The results of a biopsy and microscopic examination
    d. A therapeutic diagnosis

55. Which of the following might be identified on a radiograph?
    a. Mucocele
    b. Sialolith
    c. Necrotizing sialometaplasia
    d. Chronic sialadenitis

56. Which of the following is *false* concerning actinic cheilitis?
    a. It affects the vermilion of the lips.
    b. It is caused by sun exposure.
    c. It usually involves the upper lip more severely than the lower lip.
    d. It can be identified by clinical changes in the appearance of the lips.

57. All of the following are systemic manifestations of inflammation *except:*
    a. Leukocytosis
    b. Fever
    c. Hyperemia and erythema
    d. Lymphadenopathy

58. A raised, white line is seen on the buccal mucosa at the level of the occlusal plane. This is best called:
    a. Frictional keratosis
    b. Leukoplakia
    c. Linea alba
    d. A traumatic ulcer

59. Which of the following is *false* concerning a traumatic neuroma? It is:
    a. Caused by an injury to a peripheral nerve
    b. Composed of nerve tissue completely surrounded by a fibrous connective tissue capsule
    c. Composed of a proliferation of small nerves
    d. Often painful

60. Enhancement of phagocytosis is called:
    a. Opsonization
    b. Abfraction
    c. Transudate
    d. Chemotaxis

61. Wedge-shaped defects at the cervical area of teeth define which of the following terms?
    a. Erosion
    b. Abfraction
    c. Attrition
    d. Abrasion

62. Condensing osteitis is diagnosed mainly through which type of diagnostic process?
    a. Clinical
    b. Radiographic
    c. Laboratory
    d. Therapeutic

63. Vomiting after eating is associated with:
    a. Attrition
    b. "Meth mouth"
    c. Bulimia
    d. Anorexia nervosa

64. Which one of the following is used as a cavity sterilization and cauterizing agent?
a. Eugenol
b. Hydrogen peroxide
c. Ferric sulfate
d. Phenol

65. Which one of the following is most commonly seen on the anterior labial gingiva?
a. Smoker's melanosis
b. Amalgam tattoo
c. Melanotic macule
d. Salivary gland tumor

66. Necrotizing sialometaplasia is most commonly found on the:
a. Lower lip
b. Soft palate
c. Hard palate
d. Floor of the mouth

67. The frenal tag is commonly found on the:
a. Floor of the mouth
b. Lingual frenum
c. Maxillary labial frenum
d. Buccal mucosa

68. Candidiasis can be associated with which of the following conditions?
a. Gingival enlargement
b. Papillary hyperplasia
c. Epulis fissuratum
d. Frenal tag

69. You cannot use a radiographic image alone to differentiate a periapical granuloma from which one of the following?
a. Pulp polyp
b. Radicular cyst
c. Abscess
d. Residual cyst

Chapter 2 Synopsis

Condition/Disease	Cause	Age/Race/Sex	Location
Injuries to Teeth			
Attrition *Abrasion* *Abfraction*	Mastication Bruxism	Men are affected more than women	Occlusal/incisal surfaces Proximal
Abrasion *Erosion* *Abfraction*	Repetitive mechanical habit	*	Dependent on cause
Abfraction *Erosion* *Abrasion*	Biomechanical forces on teeth	Adults	Cervical regions of teeth
Erosion *Abfraction* *Attrition* *Enamel hypoplasia*	Chemical action Bulimia	*	Dependent on cause Lingual of maxillary anterior teeth
"Meth mouth" *Rampant caries* *Cocaine use*	Methamphetamine abuse	*	Generalized
Injuries to Soft Tissues			
Chemical burn (e.g., aspirin, phenol)	Caustic chemical in contact with mucosa	*	Site of contact
Electric burn *Herpes simplex*	Live electric cord in contact with mucosa	Infants and young children	Site of contact
Thermal burn *Trauma* *Nicotine stomatitis*	Hot food or liquid	*	Site of contact
Cocaine use *Methamphetamine use*	Crack cocaine Cocaine hydrochloride	*	Midpalate Site of contact
Hematoma *Hemangioma* *Kaposi sarcoma*	Trauma	*	Site of trauma Most common sites are the buccal/labial mucosa

NOTE: Items listed in *italics* under a specific condition/disease should be considered in a differential diagnosis.
N/A, Not applicable.
*No significant information.
†Not covered in this text.

70. In which extraction site is alveolar osteitis usually encountered?
a. Incisor
b. Mandibular third molars
c. Maxillary premolars
d. Maxillary first molar

71. When resorption affects the crown of an unerupted tooth and the cause cannot be identified, it is called:
a. Internal resorption
b. Residual resorption
c. External resorption
d. Idiopathic resorption

72. Which one of the following drug groups is most likely to cause gingival enlargement?
a. Antivirals
b. Diuretics
c. Antibiotics
d. Anticonvulsants

73. Which one of the following periapical conditions is associated with pain?
a. Radicular cyst
b. Periapical abscess
c. Periapical granuloma
d. Residual cyst

74. Which of the following is most likely responsible for internal/external resorption?
a. Inflammatory response
b. Allergic reaction
c. Genetics
d. Systemic disease

75. The most common intraoral site for the pyogenic granuloma is the:
a. Maxillary anterior gingiva
b. Lateral tongue
c. Floor of the mouth
d. Mandibular third molar area

Clinical Features	Radiographic Features	Microscopic Features	Treatment/Management	Diagnostic Process
Flattening of tooth surfaces	N/A	N/A	Prevention Restoration	Clinical
Loss of tooth structure at site of wear	N/A	N/A	Prevention Restoration	Clinical
Wedge-shaped notching at cervical areas of involved teeth	N/A	N/A	Restoration May not require treatment	Clinical
Loss of tooth structure Smooth polished surface	N/A	N/A	Prevention Restoration	Clinical
Generalized extensive destruction of tooth structure	Generalized destruction of teeth	N/A	Restoration Extraction of teeth	Clinical Historical
Painful ulcer with necrotic surface	N/A	†	Palliative	Clinical
Tissue destruction	N/A	†	Tissue repair	Clinical
Painful erythema and superficial ulceration	N/A	†	None/palliative	Clinical
Painful ulceration and erythema Necrotic ulcers	N/A	†	Elimination of cause	Clinical
Red to purple to bluish-black mass lesion Size depends on extent of trauma	N/A	†	None	Clinical

Continued

Chapter 2 Synopsis—cont'd

Condition/Disease	Cause	Age/Race/Sex	Location
Traumatic ulcer 　*Minor aphthous ulcer* 　*Recurrent herpes simplex ulceration*	Trauma to mucosa	*	Site of trauma
Frictional keratosis 　*Lichen planus* 　*Leukoplakia*	Chronic friction against mucosal surface	*	Site of friction
Linea alba 　*Lichen planus*	Teeth clenching/habit	*	Buccal mucosa at occlusal plane
Nicotine stomatitis 　*Papillary hyperplasia* 　*Cocaine use*	Smoking	*	Hard palate
Smokeless tobacco–associated keratosis 　*Frictional keratosis* 　*Leukoplakia*	Chewing tobacco	*	Site where tobacco is habitually placed
Traumatic neuroma 　*Schwannoma*	Injury to a peripheral nerve	*	Site of injured nerve
Amalgam tattoo 　*Melanosis* 　*Oral melanotic macule* 　*Melanotic nevus*	Particles of amalgam in connective tissue	*	Most common on gingiva and edentulous alveolar ridge
Melanosis 　*Amalgam tattoo* 　*Smoker's melanosis*	Smoking (smoker's melanosis), trauma, postinflammatory melanosis, oral and labial melanotic macule, unknown	†	Depends on cause
Solar (actinic) cheilitis 　*Squamous cell carcinoma* 　*Epithelial dysplasia*	Sun exposure	Adults	Vermilion of lips
Mucocele 　*Fibroma*	Severed salivary gland duct	Any age	Most common: lower lip
Ranula 　*Salivary gland tumor* 　*Squamous cell carcinoma*	Obstruction/severing of salivary gland duct	*	Floor of mouth
Sialolith 　*Sialadenitis* 　*Foreign body granuloma*	Precipitation of calcified material around a central core	*	Major and minor salivary glands
Necrotizing sialometaplasia 　*Squamous cell carcinoma* 　*Traumatic ulcer* 　*Aphthous ulcer*	Compromised blood supply to area	*	Most common: junction of the hard and soft palate
Sialadenitis 　*Sialolithiasis*	Infection Obstruction of salivary gland duct	*	Symptomatic when involving major salivary glands
Reactive Connective Tissue Hyperplasia			
Pyogenic granuloma 　*Peripheral giant cell granuloma* 　*Peripheral ossifying fibroma* 　*Fibroma*	Response to injury Puberty Pregnancy	*	Most common: gingiva Also other areas

NOTE: Items listed in *italics* under a specific condition/disease should be considered in a differential diagnosis.
N/A, Not applicable.
*No significant information.
†Not covered in this text.

Clinical Features	Radiographic Features	Microscopic Features	Treatment/Management	Diagnostic Process
Painful, mucosal ulceration	N/A	Ulcer with eosinophils present in inflammatory infiltrate	Elimination of cause	Clinical
White mucosal surface	N/A	Hyperkeratosis	Elimination of cause	Clinical
Anterior-to-posterior white line	N/A	Epithelial hyperplasia and hyperkeratosis	None	Clinical
White, opacification of the palatal mucosa with raised red dots	N/A	Hyperkeratosis with inflamed minor salivary glands	Elimination of cause	Clinical
Granular to white, wrinkled appearance	N/A	Hyperkeratosis and epithelial hyperplasia Can have epithelial atypia	Elimination of cause	Clinical Microscopic
Painful, submucosal nodule	N/A	Mass of nerve cells	Surgical excision	Microscopic
Bluish-gray macule	Fine opaque granules	Black granular material in connective tissue	No treatment after identification	Clinical Microscopic Radiographic
Diffuse grayish-brown color of areas on the gingiva; localized macular pigmentation	N/A	Melanin pigment in basal layer of epithelium and in underlying connective tissue	Fades with decreased smoking None	Clinical Microscopic
Indistinct, fissured skin–mucosal interface	N/A	Degenerative changes in connective tissue	Protect lips and skin from sun exposure	Clinical
Localized tissue swelling that increases/decreases in size	N/A	Extravasated mucus in tissue surrounded by granulation tissue	Excision May spontaneously resolve	Clinical Microscopic
Fluid-filled swelling that increases/decreases in size	N/A	Resembles mucocele or mucous cyst	Surgery	Clinical
Obstruction of the gland Hard nodule in soft tissue	Floor of the mouth: radiopaque structure (seen in occlusal or panoramic radiograph)	Calcified structure arranged in concentric rings	Surgical removal of stone	Clinical Radiographic Microscopic
Moderately painful swelling and ulceration Acute onset	N/A	Necrosis of the salivary glands Replacement of salivary duct epithelium with squamous epithelium	Spontaneous resolution	Microscopic
Painful swelling of gland	N/A	Acute or chronic inflammatory infiltrate in salivary gland	Antibiotic if infection	Clinical Laboratory Microscopic
Deep red-purple exophytic lesion, usually ulcerated	N/A	Ulcerated granulation tissue	Surgical excision	Microscopic

Continued

Chapter 2 Synopsis—cont'd

Condition/Disease	Cause	Age/Race/Sex	Location
Peripheral giant cell granuloma *Pyogenic granuloma* *Peripheral ossifying fibroma* *Fibroma*	Unknown	Any age More frequent between 40 and 60 yr of age More common in women than men	Gingiva
Irritation fibroma *Benign soft tissue tumor*	Trauma	*	Common on the gingiva Many other oral locations
Denture-induced fibrous hyperplasia (epulis fissuratum) *Fibroma* *Squamous cell carcinoma*	Ill-fitting denture Continuous wearing of denture	*	Vestibule along a denture border
Papillary hyperplasia of the palate *Nicotine stomatitis*	Constant wearing of maxillary removable prosthesis	*	Hard palate
Gingival enlargement *Medication related* *Chronic inflammation* *Genetic* *Leukemic infiltrate*	Response to chronic inflammation Idiopathic Drug reaction Hormonal changes Genetic	*	Gingiva: generalized or localized
Chronic hyperplastic pulpitis	Caries	Children and young adults	Primary or permanent molars
Inflammatory Periapical Lesions			
Periapical abscess *Periapical granuloma* *Radicular cyst*	Inflammation of the dental pulp Preexisting periapical chronic inflammation	*	Roots of primary or permanent teeth
Periapical granuloma *Radicular cyst* *Periapical abscess*	Pulpal inflammation and necrosis	*	Roots of primary or permanent teeth
Radicular cyst (periapical cyst) *Periapical granuloma*	Nonvital tooth	*	Roots of primary or permanent teeth
Residual cyst *Keratocystic odontogenic tumor (odontogenic keratocyst)*	Radicular cyst not removed with extracted tooth		Site of tooth extraction
Resorption of teeth (external resorption, internal resorption) *Caries*	Chronic inflammation Chronic pulpal inflammation		Roots of primary or permanent teeth Dental hard tissue within root or crowns
Focal sclerosing osteomyelitis *Idiopathic osteosclerosis* *Periapical cemento-osseous dysplasia*	Low-grade chronic infection	*	Bone adjacent to any tooth Mandibular first molar most common
Alveolar osteitis ("dry socket")	Postoperative complication of tooth extraction	*	Extraction site

NOTE: Items listed in *italics* under a specific condition/disease should be considered in a differential diagnosis.
N/A, Not applicable.
*No significant information.
†Not covered in this text.

Clinical Features	Radiographic Features	Microscopic Features	Treatment/Management	Diagnostic Process
Deep red exophytic lesion	N/A	Many multinucleated giant cells in well-vascularized connective tissue	Surgical excision	Microscopic
Broad-based, pink exophytic lesion	N/A	Dense fibrous connective tissue usually surfaced by normal epithelium	Surgical excision	Microscopic
Elongated folds of exophytic tissue surrounding denture flange	N/A	Dense fibrous connective tissue surfaced by epithelium that may be hyperplastic and ulcerated	Surgical excision Fabrication of new denture	Clinical Microscopic
Mucosa surfaced by multiple, erythematous papillary projections	N/A	Papillary projections composed of fibrous connective tissue (usually inflamed) surfaced by squamous epithelium	Surgical removal of papillary tissue Fabrication of new denture	Clinical
Increase in the bulk of the free and attached gingiva No stippling Erythematous to normal color	N/A	Connective tissue (usually inflamed) surfaced by squamous epithelium	Gingivectomy Meticulous oral hygiene	Clinical Microscopic
Red or pink nodule protruding from the pulp chamber of a tooth with a large, open carious lesion	N/A	Granulation tissue surfaced by squamous epithelium	Extraction of tooth or endodontic treatment	Clinical
Pain, swelling, fistula, slight extrusion of tooth	None Thickening of periodontal ligament space Periapical radiolucency	Acute inflammatory infiltrate	Establish drainage	Clinical
Asymptomatic Tooth sensitive to percussion Slight extrusion of tooth	Slight thickening of periodontal ligament space Periodontal radiolucency	Chronic inflammatory infiltrate	Endodontic therapy Extraction	Radiographic Microscopic
Most are asymptomatic	Radiolucency associated with the root of a nonvital tooth	Space lined by epithelium surrounded by an infiltrate of chronic inflammatory cells	Endodontic therapy Apicoectomy Extraction and curettage of the extraction site	Radiographic Microscopic
	Radiolucency at the site of tooth extraction		Surgical removal	
Asymptomatic May see pinkish color if crown involved	Blunting of root apex to severe loss of root substance Round to ovoid radiolucency in the central part of the tooth	N/A	Identify and remove cause Root canal therapy Extraction	Radiographic
Asymptomatic	Radiopaque area below roots of the tooth	Dense bone	None	Radiographic
Pain develops several days after extraction	N/A	N/A	Gentle irrigation Insertion of medicated dressing	Clinical

3

Immunity and Immunologic Oral Lesions

MARGARET J. FEHRENBACH, JOAN ANDERSEN PHELAN, AND OLGA A.C. IBSEN

OBJECTIVES

After studying this chapter, the student will be able to:

1. Define each of the words in the vocabulary list for this chapter.
2. Describe the differences between an immune response and an inflammatory response.
3. Do the following related to cellular involvement in the immune response:
   - List the three main types of lymphocytes and their origins.
   - Describe the involvement of B-cell lymphocytes and plasma cells in the production of antibodies.
   - List and describe the different types of T-cell lymphocytes and their functions.
   - Describe the functions of natural killer cells.
4. Describe the origin of macrophages and dendritic cells and list their activities in the immune response.
5. Describe where cytokines are produced and the roles they play in the immune response.
6. Describe the differences between humoral immunity and cell-mediated immunity and include the cells involved in each.
7. Describe the differences between passive and active immunity and give an example for each type of immunity.
8. List and describe four types of hypersensitivity reactions and give an example for each type of hypersensitivity.
9. Define autoimmunity and describe how it results in disease.
10. Define immunodeficiency and describe how it results in disease.
11. Do the following related to aphthous ulcers:
    - Describe and contrast the clinical features of each of the three types of aphthous ulcers.
    - Describe the diagnosis, treatment, and prognosis of aphthous ulcers.
    - List systemic diseases associated with aphthous ulcers.
12. Describe and compare the clinical features of urticaria, angioedema, contact mucositis, and fixed drug eruption.
13. Describe the clinical features of erythema multiforme and Stevens-Johnson syndrome.
14. Do the following related to lichen planus:
    - Describe the clinical and microscopic features of lichen planus.
    - Name and describe the types of lichen planus.
    - Discuss the diagnosis, treatment, and prognosis of lichen planus.
15. List the triad of systemic signs that comprise reactive arthritis (Reiter syndrome) and describe the oral lesions that occur in this condition.
16. Name the two cells that characterize Langerhans cell histiocytosis microscopically and describe the radiographic appearance of jaw lesions in Langerhans cell histiocytosis.
17. Do the following related to autoimmune diseases with oral manifestations:
    - Describe the oral manifestations, diagnosis, treatment, and prognosis of each of the following autoimmune diseases: Sjögren syndrome, lupus erythematosus, pemphigus vulgaris, mucous membrane pemphigoid, bullous pemphigoid, and Behçet syndrome.
    - Define desquamative gingivitis, describe the clinical features, and list three diseases in which desquamative gingivitis may occur.
    - Describe the clinical features of Behçet syndrome.
18. Do the following related to immunodeficiency:
    - Describe the difference between primary and secondary immunodeficiency.
    - List and describe three examples of primary immunodeficiency.
    - List four causes of secondary immunodeficiency.

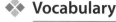 Vocabulary

Acantholysis (akan″-thol′ĭ-sis) Dissolution of the intercellular bridges of the prickle cell layer of the epithelium.

Acquired immune response An immune response to a foreign substance based on the specific memory of a past exposure to that same foreign substance.

Active immunity A type of immunity based on antibodies developed in response to an antigen, which includes both natural and acquired types.

Adjuvants (ajə′-vənts) The agents that can be added to a vaccine to modify the immune response.

Allergen (al′ər-jen) An antigen that produces a hypersensitivity or allergic reaction.

Allergy (al′ər-je) Hypersensitivity acquired through exposure to a particular allergen that elicits an exaggerated reaction on reexposure to the same allergen.

Anaphylaxis (an″ə-fə-lak′sis) A severe immediate type of hypersensitivity in which an exaggerated immunologic reaction occurs on reexposure to a foreign protein or other substance after sensitization, resulting in not only hives, itching, and swelling, but also vascular collapse and shock, as well as death.

Antibody (an′tĭ-bod″e) A protein molecule or immunoglobulin that is secreted by plasma cells and reacts with a specific antigen; includes five classes: IgA, IgD, IgE, IgG, and IgM.

Antibody titer (an′tĭ-bod″e ti′tər) The level of antibody in the blood that can be measured by a diagnostic laboratory test.

Antigen (an′tĭ-jən) Any substance able to induce a specific immune response.

Attenuated (ə-ten′u-āt) The ability to reduce the virulence of a pathogenic microorganism but still keep it viable, as is done in the development of certain vaccines.

Autoantibody (aw″to-an′tĭ-bod″e) An antibody that reacts against a tissue constituent of one's own body.

Autoimmune disease An immunopathologic condition characterized by tissue trauma caused by an immune response against tissue constituents of one's own body.

B-cell lymphocyte A type of lymphocyte that develops in lymphoid tissue other than the thymus and that can later differentiate into a plasma cell that produces antibody, the main initiator of humoral immunity.

Cell-mediated immunity A type of immunity in which the major role is played by T-cell lymphocytes.

Connective tissue diseases A category of autoimmune diseases with connective tissue as the primary target of the pathology.

Cytokines (si″to-kĭns) The proteins produced by various cell types for the purpose of intercellular communication or signaling; immunologic cytokines are involved as biochemical mediators in the immune response.

Delayed hypersensitivity (hi″pər-sen″sĭ-tiv′ĭ-te) A type of hypersensitivity reaction that takes time to develop after T-cell lymphocytes are previously introduced to an antigen to either directly cause damage to the tissue cells or recruit other cells that cause the damage.

Dendritic cell (den′dritik) A type of white blood cell that acts as an antigen-presenting cell in the skin and mucosa.

Dysgeusia (dis-gu′ze-ah) An alteration in taste.

Humoral immunity (hyoo′mərəl imyoo′nĭ-te) A type of immunity in which both the B-cell lymphocytes and the antibodies they produce as plasma cells play a predominant role.

Hypersensitivity (hi″pər-sen″sĭ-tiv′ĭ-te) An altered state of reactivity in which the body reacts to a foreign agent such as an allergen with an exaggerated immune response; includes the four types, types I through IV.

Hyposalivation (hi″po-sal″ĭ-va′shən) Decreased salivary flow that may result in xerostomia (dry mouth).

Immune complex (im′u-n) The combination of an antibody and antigen, producing a complex that can initiate a hypersensitivity or allergic reaction.

Immunization (im″u-nĭ-za′shən) An induction of active immunity, such as when the pathogenic microorganism used to induce active immunity is encountered after vaccination.

Immunodeficiency (im″u-no-də-fish′ən-se) A type of immunopathologic condition that involves a compromised or entirely absent immune system involving its white blood cells and their products.

Immunoglobulins (im″u-no-glob′u-lins) The proteins that, when secreted by plasma cells, serve as antibodies designed to respond to a specific antigen.

Immunomodulator (im″u-no-mod′u-la″tor) A substance that alters the immune response by augmenting or reducing the ability of the immune system to produce antibodies or sensitized cells that recognize and react with the antigen that initiated their production.

Interferon (in″ter-fēr′on) A family of glycoproteins that have immunoregulatory, antineoplastic, and antiviral activity; it is one of the cytokines.

Langerhans cell (lahng′ər-hahnz) A specialized dendritic cell found in the skin and mucosa that is involved in the immune response.

LE cell Mature neutrophil with a phagocytized spherical inclusion derived from another neutrophil; it is used as a marker of autoimmune diseases.

Lymphocytes (lim′fo-sīts) The white blood cells involved in the immune response that have three major subsets: the B-cell lymphocyte, T-cell lymphocyte, and natural killer cell.

Lymphoid tissue (lim′foid) Tissue composed of lymphocytes supported by a meshwork of connective tissue; includes tonsillar tissue, lymph nodes, and lymphatic organs.

Lymphokines (lim′fo-kīns) The subset of cytokines produced by B-cell or T-cell lymphocytes in contact with antigens that serve as biochemical mediators in an immune response.

Macrophage (mak′ro-fāj) A large tissue-bound mononuclear phagocyte derived from monocytes circulating in the blood, which can become mobile when stimulated by inflammation and interact with lymphocytes in an immune response as well as during inflammation.

Monokines (mon′o-kīns) The subset of cytokines primarily produced by monocytes or macrophages that serve as biochemical mediators in an immune response.

Mucositis (mu″ko-si′tis) The inflammation of a mucosal tissue due to a disease process.

Natural killer cell Type of lymphocyte that is part of the initial innate immune response, which by unknown mechanisms is able to directly destroy cells recognized as foreign.

Nikolsky sign (nikol′ske) Diagnostic sign whereby the superficial epithelium separates easily from the basal layer on exertion of firm, sliding manual pressure with the fingers or a tongue blade.

Passive immunity Type of immunity that uses antibodies produced by another person to protect an individual against infectious disease, which includes both natural and acquired.

Plasma cell (plæzmə) The cell derived from B-cell lymphocytes that produces antibodies in response to the presence of antigen.

Pruritus (proo-ri′təs) The symptom of severe itching due to a disease process, possibly a hypersensitivity reaction or allergy.

Rheumatoid factor (roo′mə-toid) Antibody that binds to certain antibodies found in the serum of patients with rheumatoid arthritis and connective tissue diseases such as Sjögren syndrome. Current assays test for IgM-class rheumatoid factor.

Schirmer test (shər′mər) A test that measures lacrimal gland flow by placing special filter paper strips inside the lower eyelid for 5 minutes.

Serum sickness (sir′əm) A classic example of type III hypersensitivity that involves a drug allergy to antitoxin serum from horses.

Syndrome (sin′drōm) A group of signs and symptoms that occur together.

Symblepharon (sim-blef′ă-ron) Fibrous adhesion between the eyeball and conjunctiva.

T-cell lymphocyte A lymphocyte that matures in the thymus and is mainly responsible for initiating cell-mediated immunity as well as modulating humoral immunity.

Thymus (thi′məs) Organ consisting of lymphoid tissue located high in the chest, which is large in an infant and gradually shrinks in size in adulthood; site of T-cell lymphocyte maturation.

Xerostomia (zēr″o-sto′me-ə) Dryness of the mucous membranes, including the oral cavity; usually caused by hyposalivation or decreased salivary flow.

The inflammatory response, as described in Chapter 2, is a rapid first line of defense against injury. The immune response, which is described in this chapter, follows the inflammatory response as the second line of defense that is necessary for complete recovery. This chapter begins with a description of the acquired immune response and then includes a discussion of the most commonly encountered oral diseases that may result from harmful effects of such a response. Surveillance against neoplastic cells also involves the immune response and is described, along with the neoplastic process and neoplastic oral lesions, in Chapter 7. In contrast, using the immune response against cancer by way of immunotherapy marks an entirely different way of treating not only infection, as discussed later in this chapter, but also cancer—by targeting the immune system, not the tumor itself.

Immune Response

The immune response can either be innate in its origin or can be acquired. The innate immune response does not involve memory and is described, along with inflammation, in Chapter 2. In contrast, the acquired immune response involves a complex network of white blood cells, all involved with memory. Similar to the inflammatory response, the immune response may also result in an increased level of tissue damage and disease as it fights against what it considers to be foreign.

Like the inflammatory response, the **acquired immune response** defends the body against injury, particularly from foreign substances such as microorganisms (Fig. 3.1). The immune response differs from the inflammatory response in that it has the capacity for memory and responds more quickly to a foreign

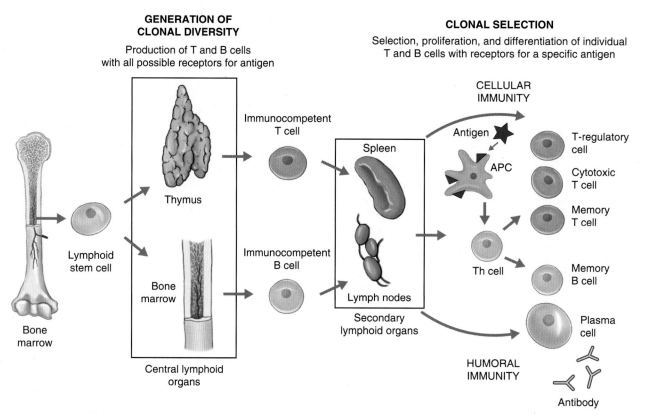

GENERATION OF CLONAL DIVERSITY
Production of T and B cells with all possible receptors for antigen

CLONAL SELECTION
Selection, proliferation, and differentiation of individual T and B cells with receptors for a specific antigen

• **Figure 3.1** Overview of immune response. (From McCance K, Huether S: *Pathophysiology*, ed 7, St. Louis, 2014, Mosby.)

substance if encountered again. It works amid the background of an already activated inflammatory response and innate immune response, as well as a working repair process.

Immunity is the increased responsiveness that results from the retained memory of an already encountered antigen. Thus memory is a characteristic function of the acquired immune response. This contrasts with the inflammatory response, which is not capable of memory. Certain lymphocytes—B-memory and T-memory lymphocytes—retain the memory of an antigen after an initial encounter. For this reason, the immune response to that antigen is much more rapid and stronger the next time it is encountered.

Antigens in the Immune Response

Antigens, or *immunogens,* are foreign substances against which the immune system defends the body. These substances are mainly proteins and are often microorganisms and their toxins. The immune system tolerates the components of the body, or *self,* with their various types of diversity. In contrast, antigens are substances that the immune system recognizes as foreign or *nonself.* Transformed human cells such as neoplasm cells or cells infected with viruses can become antigens. Human tissue, as in the case of an organ transplant, tissue graft, or incompatible blood transfusion, can also become an antigen.

The body reacts to the introduction of an antigen in various ways. In one type of disease, an autoimmune disease, parts of an individual's own body become antigens. In another type of disease, an immunodeficiency, the body no longer recognizes certain antigens as foreign. In another type of reaction involving hypersensitivity, the body overreacts to what it sees as foreign, creating a multitude of complications. Thus disease can occur when the immune response identifies components of self as antigen, does not recognize foreign material as antigen, or overreacts to antigens.

Cellular Involvement in the Immune Response

The white blood cells, or *leukocytes,* were introduced in Chapter 2. A more complex network of white blood cells is involved in the immune response than in the inflammatory response. These cells can produce cell products or cytokines that are active during the immune response.

The primary white blood cells involved in the immune response are **lymphocytes.** These cells are able to recognize and respond to an antigen when it is in contact with receptor sites located on the cell surface. Lymphocytes, like other white blood cells, are derived from hematopoietic stem cells in the bone marrow (see Fig. 2.8). Lymphocytes constitute 20% to 25% of the white blood cell population. They are mobile antigen-sensitive cells with a long life. They have a round nucleus and only a small amount of cytoplasm. Different types of lymphocytes have differing functions.

The three main types of lymphocytes are the B-cell lymphocyte, the T-cell lymphocyte, and the natural killer cell. The macrophage and the dendritic cell are also part of the immune response. The three main types of lymphocytes cannot be distinguished morphologically by light or electron microscopy. Subtle differences between the lymphocytes can be recognized by immunocytochemical techniques designed to identify unique marker molecules

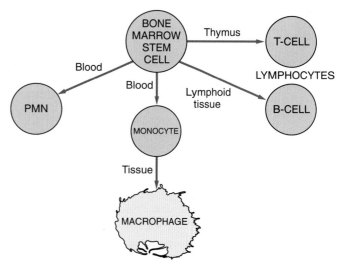

• **Figure 3.2** Primary cells of the immune response include the lymphocytes, both B-cell lymphocytes and T-cell lymphocytes. Lymphocytes, polymorphonuclear neutrophils *(PMN),* and, macrophages are derived from stem cells in the bone marrow.

on the surface of these cells. In practice, this can be done by immunohistochemical staining of tissue sections or cytologic smear preparations with specific, color-coded antibodies.

B-Cell Lymphocytes

The **B-cell lymphocyte,** or *B cell,* develops from a hematopoietic stem cell in the bone marrow and then resides and matures in **lymphoid tissue** such as spleen, lymph nodes, and tonsillar tissue (Fig. 3.1 and Fig. 3.2). The location of cervical lymph nodes is shown in Fig. 2.14; tonsillar tissue is located nearby in the oropharynx as well as in the oral cavity. When antigen stimulates a B cell, the B cell travels to the site of the injury. The two main types of B cells that develop when stimulated by an antigen are the B-memory cell and the plasma cell.

The *B-memory cell* retains a memory of the antigen. In the presence of an antigen recognized by the B-memory cell, this cell reacts by duplicating itself many times over in a process called *clonal selection.* All of these newly formed B cells retain the capacity to recognize the previously encountered antigen. Thus B cells can internalize the antigens and thereafter function as *antigen-presenting cells,* or APCs, by presenting the internalized antigens to T cells.

The **plasma cell** is a fully differentiated descendant of B-cell lymphocytes. The plasma cell produces and releases many copies of a particular protein that is now considered an **antibody** in response to the presence of antigen. The plasma cell has a round, pinwheel-shaped nucleus and visible cytoplasm. The newly produced antibodies circulating within the blood serum are called **immunoglobulins.** Five different general types of immunoglobulins exist: (1) IgA, (2) IgD, (3) IgE, (4) IgG, and (5) IgM (Table 3.1). They all are variations of the same basic structure (Figs. 3.3 and 3.4). The level of antibody in the blood is called the **antibody titer.** This can be measured by a diagnostic laboratory test and is useful in the diagnosis and evaluation of infectious disease.

Each immune response involves specific antibodies produced in response to a specific antigen by a specific plasma cell. This specificity is a characteristic function of the immune response. The

TABLE 3.1	Antibodies or Immunoglobulins
Immunoglobulin (Ig)	**Description**
IgA	Has two subgroups: serous in the blood and secretory in the saliva and other secretions such as tears and breast milk; aids in defense against proliferation of microorganisms in body fluids as well as protecting mucosal sites such as gastrointestinal and genitourinary tracts
IgD	Functions in the activation of B-cell lymphocytes and is only found on their surface; thus is not released separately into serum or body fluids
IgE	Involved in hypersensitivity or allergic reactions because it can bind to mast cells and basophils to bring about the release of biochemical mediators such as histamine; and it also attacks parasites
IgG	Major antibody in blood serum at about 75% and as the smallest it can pass the placental barrier; produced in large amounts in secondary immune response and serves as the first passive immunity for the newborn
IgM	Involved in early immune responses because of its involvement with IgD in the activation of B-cell lymphocytes; activates complement and reacts to blood group antigens as well as to neutralize microorganisms

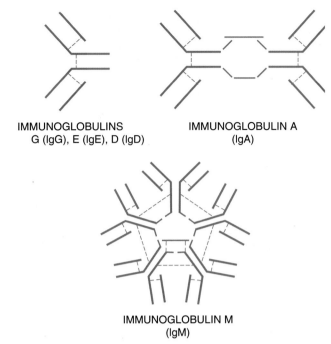

IMMUNOGLOBULINS
G (IgG), E (IgE), D (IgD)

IMMUNOGLOBULIN A
(IgA)

IMMUNOGLOBULIN M
(IgM)

• **Figure 3.4** Five general types of antibodies or immunoglobulins (Ig) in serum include the same basic structure arranged differently. This variation in structure allows them to function differently.

T-Cell Lymphocytes

After it develops from a hematopoietic stem cell in the bone marrow, the **T-cell lymphocyte**, or *T cell*, travels to the **thymus**, a lymphoid organ located in the chest, and is processed into a mature cell and then can reside in lymphoid tissue such as the spleen (see Figs. 3.1 and 3.2). The thymus is a primary lymphoid organ located high in the upper chest or thorax; it is quite large in infants and shrinks as an individual matures. The spleen is in the abdomen; it is involved in production and removal of blood cells.

The T cell can be distinguished from other lymphocytes, such as B cells and natural killer cells, by the presence of a special receptor on its cell surface that is called the *T-cell receptor* (TCR). The T cells use TCR to recognize antigens. Other receptors are also present on the surface of the T cell and can interact with each other. The TCR is linked to a membrane protein of the CD3 cell receptor, and a TCR-CD3 complex is considered essential for the activity of T cells. Different types of T cells have different functions in the immune response. The different types of T cells include the T-helper cell, the T-suppressor cell, the T-cytotoxic cell, and the T-memory cell (Fig. 3.5).

The *T-helper cell* (Th cell) increases the functioning of the B cell, enhancing the antibody response produced by the plasma cell. The T-helper cell is easily identifiable by the CD4 cell receptor on its surface. The *T-suppressor cell* (T-regulatory cell) carries the CD8 cell receptor as well as other markers on its surface and suppresses the functioning of the B cell. The *T-cytotoxic cell* also carries the CD8 cell receptor, but it is active in surveillance against virally infected cells and neoplastic cells, directly attacking these cells. Both CD4 and CD8 cell receptors serve as markers for determining the amount of T-helper, T-suppressor, or T-cytotoxic cells in blood. Thus T cells within cell-mediated immunity also begin and regulate as well as coordinate the overall immune response.

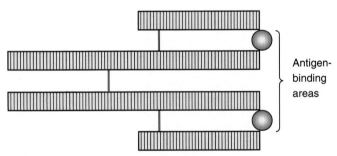

Antigen-binding areas

• **Figure 3.3** Antibody or immunoglobulin (Ig) basic structure, with four protein chains with two identical heavy polypeptide chains and two identical light chains, forming a Y-shape. The tips of the arms are called the *variable region* because they vary greatly, creating a pocket uniquely shaped to enfold, or "bind," a specific antigen (Fab). The stem or base, called the *constant region*, is identical in all antibodies of the same class and serves to link the antibody to other cells and products in the immune response (Fc).

combination of a specific antibody with a specific antigen is called an **immune complex.** The formation of an immune complex usually renders the antigen inactive. Immune complexes may also be involved in certain disease states. Some of these are discussed later in this chapter.

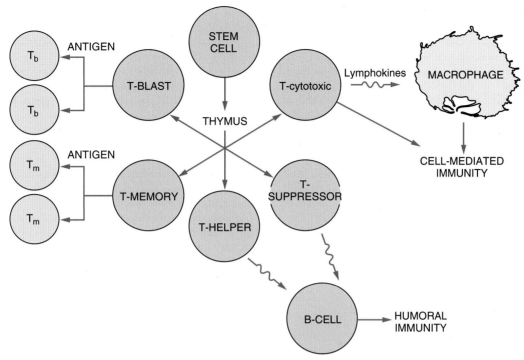

• **Figure 3.5** Various types of T-cell lymphocytes and their involvement in the immune response.

Similarly to B-memory cells, the *T-memory cell* retains a memory of the antigen. In the presence of an antigen recognized by the T-memory cell, this cell reacts by duplicating itself many times over in a process called *clonal selection* similar to the B-cell lymphocyte. All of these newly formed T cells retain the capacity to recognize the previously encountered antigen and serve, as in many cases, as potentially cancer- or infection-fighting T cells.

All processed antigens are presented to T cells in the context of the *major histocompatibility complex* (MHC) proteins expressed on the surface of B-cell APCs. These MHC proteins, first identified on white blood cells, are also known as *human leukocyte antigens* (HLAs), although they are also expressed on other cells in the body. A unique set of MHC antigens determines the individuality of each person; only identical twins have the same MHC antigens. In immune reactions, as discussed later in the chapter, the MHC antigens regulate the cell-to-cell contact during antigen presentation. The MHC is also important for organ transplantation, and most transplant rejection reactions result from the HLA incompatibility of the host and the donor.

Natural Killer Cells

The **natural killer cell,** or *NK cell,* is a large lymphocyte that plays a part in the innate immune response of the body and also develops from a bone marrow stem cell. NK cells have the ability to destroy foreign cells soon after their appearance because they recognize them as foreign without first having to recognize them as specific antigens and go through any system checks. These cells are usually located only within the microcirculation and not in the outlying tissue.

The NK cell type seems to be active against viruses and cancer cells because it contains granules with enzymes that kill these invaders. However, in some situations, such as human immunodeficiency virus (HIV) infection, NK cell function is compromised and the virus is able to evade the NK cell response.

Macrophages

As discussed in Chapter 2, the **macrophage** is a large tissue-bound mononuclear phagocyte derived from monocytes circulating in the blood, which can become mobile when stimulated by inflammation. The macrophage is not only present in the connective tissue during inflammation, but it is also involved as an accessory cell in the evolving immune response to an antigen (see Fig. 3.2). Within this added role, the macrophage is active in phagocytosis of foreign substances and assists both the B cell and T cell during the immune response.

Along with phagocytosis, the macrophage acts to process and present antigen material on its surface to the T-helper cell as APCs. This stimulates both types of lymphocytes to travel from the lymphoid tissue or surrounding blood vessels to the injury site. Thus the macrophage functions as an APC, acting as a messenger between both the inflammatory response and immune response.

The macrophage carries receptors for lymphokines produced by the lymphocytes, as discussed earlier, which allow it to be activated into a single-minded pursuit of specific foreign material such as microorganisms or neoplastic cells. When activated, the macrophage can function in many other different ways, always amplifying the immune response. Unlike lymphocytes, the macrophage does not retain memory of an encountered antigen and needs to be reactivated during each encounter.

Dendritic Cells

The **dendritic cell** (DC) is a white blood cell whose main function is to process antigenic material and present it on its surface to other cells of the immune system. The DC functions as an APC, acting as a link between innate immunity and acquired immunity. It is similar in function to a B-cell lymphocyte and macrophage.

The DC is present in tissue that is in contact with the external environment, such as the skin and mucosa. It can also be found in an immature state in the blood. At certain developmental stages, it grows branched projections or dendrites. Thus although similar in appearance, these are structures distinct from the dendrites of neurons. Once activated, it migrates to the lymph nodes or other lymphoid tissue, where it interacts with T cells and B cells to initiate and shape the acquired immune response.

In the skin and mucosal tissue such as the oral mucosa, there is a specialized dendritic cell type, a **Langerhans cell** (LC), which contains large cell organelles called *Birbeck granules*. Langerhans cells in the genital mucosa may be the initial cellular targets of infection with HIV. Because the epithelium of the sublingual oral mucosa is particularly thin with the microcirculation nearby, it provides a useful route of entry for drugs and allergens during desensitization therapy by way of the numerous Langerhans cells.

Cytokines in the Immune Response

Cytokines are produced by the cells of the immune system and play a prominent role in the activation of the immune response. Cytokines are signaling proteins that are able to affect the behavior of other cells; thus they are considered immunomodulating agents. Immunomodulating agents, or **immunomodulators,** alter the immune response by either adding to or reducing the functions of the response.

Cytokines are one way that lymphocytes communicate with each other and with other immune system cells, thus the designation of cytokines as a type of signaling protein. B cells and T cells produce their own cytokines, a subset called **lymphokines** (Fig. 3.5). Monocytes or macrophages produce their own cytokines, a subset called **monokines**. Dendritic cells, such as the Langerhans cells, also produce and react to cytokines.

Different cytokines have differing functions within the immune response (Table 3.2). They can activate macrophages and enhance the ability of macrophages to destroy foreign cells. These types of killer cytokines may also be involved in various other functions concerning white blood cells, fibroblasts, and endothelial cells. They are also responsible for the systemic effects of inflammation such as loss of appetite and increased heart rate.

One of the first cytokines to be discovered within the body was **interferon**. Produced by T cells and macrophages (as well as by cells outside the immune system), interferons are a group of proteins with antiviral properties. Discovered more recently,

chemokines are a group of cytokines that are named for their ability to induce chemotaxis in nearby responsive cells. These signaling proteins may be involved in controlling infection as part of the immune response, as well as being involved in several developmental processes during embryogenesis.

Major Divisions of the Immune Response

The two major divisions of the immune response are humoral immunity and cell-mediated immunity (Fig. 3.6). These two divisions differ in their reaction to an antigen. However, these divisions are interrelated, and present understanding of the immune response recognizes that these divisions do not function as distinctly separate mechanisms.

Humoral immunity, or *antibody-mediated immunity,* involves the production of antibodies, with the B-cell lymphocytes as the primary cells. Humoral immunity is responsible for protection against many pathogenic microorganisms such as bacteria and viruses.

The other division of the immune system is **cell-mediated immunity,** or *cellular immunity;* it involves lymphocytes, usually T cells, working alone or assisted by macrophages. The cell-mediated division regulates both major divisions of the immune system.

TABLE 3.2	Cytokines
Cytokine	**Function**
Interferons	Various functions involving white blood cells, fibroblasts, and endothelial cells
Interleukins	Stimulate white blood cell proliferation and other functions
Lymphotoxin	Destroys fibroblasts
Macrophage-activating factor	Activates macrophages to produce and secrete lysosomal enzymes
Macrophage chemotactic factor	Stimulates macrophage emigration
Migration inhibitory factor	Inhibits macrophage activity
Tumor necrosis factor	Various functions involving white blood cells and fibroblasts

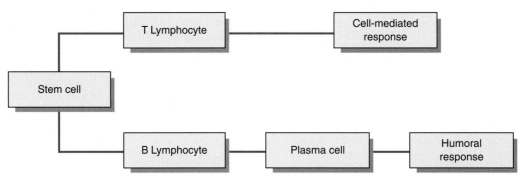

• **Figure 3.6** The two major divisions of the immune response: humoral immunity and cell-mediated immunity.

Types of Immunity

The two types of immunity that can occur are passive and active. **Passive immunity** refers to the use of antibodies produced by another person to protect an individual against infectious disease. This type of immunity can occur naturally or it can be acquired.

The process of *natural passive immunity* occurs when antibodies from a mother pass through the placenta to the developing fetus. These antibodies protect a newborn infant from disease while the infant's own immune system matures.

Passive immunity can also be acquired by injecting a person with antibodies against a microorganism to which the person has not previously been exposed. This is done to confer immediate protection against the disease caused by that microorganism. These antibodies are collected from individuals who have already had the disease and have naturally produced antibodies to the pathogenic microorganism. This process of *acquired passive immunity* is short lived but can act immediately. This type of immune therapy is used because the unprepared immune system of an individual takes longer to produce antibodies, and in the meantime the disease may develop. Acquired passive immunity may be provided to dental personnel who do not have immunity to hepatitis B after needlestick or other occupational exposure incidents, using hepatitis B immunoglobulin.

Active immunity uses antibodies produced by one's own body to protect against infectious disease, and it can occur naturally or be acquired. It occurs naturally when a pathogenic microorganism causes disease. Protection against further attack by that microorganism is conferred to the individual if the body recovers from the disease.

A less risky way of achieving active immunity is by an acquired or artificial means. This production of acquired active immunity is called **immunization.** A person is injected with or ingests either altered pathogenic microorganisms or products of those microorganisms. The altered microorganism or products of the microorganisms cannot produce infection but are able to act as an antigen. This is called a *vaccine,* and the process is called *vaccination.* When the pathogenic microorganism is encountered after vaccination, the immune system produces a stronger, faster response and prevents development of the disease.

Immunization lowers the risk of a microorganism causing disease because it safely prepares the immune system to fight future attacks by the disease-causing microorganism. In some cases more than one exposure to the antigen is needed to ensure adequate immunity; a repeated exposure by way of a vaccination is called a *booster.* Immunization by vaccination is used to protect children and adults against many diseases. Dental personnel should be vaccinated against the hepatitis B virus because of their high risk of occupational exposure to that virus.

Killed-type vaccines consist of heat- or chemical-treated microorganisms or toxins; these treatments make killed-type vaccines safe, but in some cases they may be less effective than vaccines that have been attenuated. An **attenuated** vaccine consists of genetically altered pathogenic microorganisms that have reduced virulence but are still viable (or live) so as to undergo limited replication. **Molecular vaccines** are composed of critical antigenic determinants from cloned bacteria, yeast, or synthetic peptides that are developed with the aid of recombinant DNA techniques.

In some cases, **adjuvants** may be added to the vaccine. This addition can modify the immune response by boosting it so that it gives a higher level of antibody production and longer-lasting immunity, thus minimizing the amount of injected foreign substance.

An alternative approach to vaccination that is being studied is known as *DNA vaccination* and involves genetically engineering a vaccine from an infectious agent's DNA. This new approach has a number of potential advantages over conventional vaccines, including the ability to induce a wider range of immune response types.

Immunopathology

The immune response helps defend the body against disease-producing antigens, but it can also malfunction and cause tissue damage, resulting in the production of lesions. **Immunopathology** is the study of diseases caused by the malfunctioning of the immune system. These immunopathologic conditions include hypersensitivity, autoimmune disease, and immunodeficiency. Examples of each of these immunopathologic conditions, in which damage is directly caused by the immune response, are discussed next. Some of these conditions fall into the category of a **syndrome,** which is a group of signs and symptoms that occur together to define the disease state. Many different syndromes are described in various chapters in this text.

Hypersensitivity

Hypersensitivity, or **allergy,** comprises the same basic types of reactions that occur when the immune response is fighting microorganisms and protecting the body against disease. However, these hypersensitivity or allergenic reactions are exaggerated immune responses to an antigen or *immunogen* causing an immunopathologic condition, along with tissue destruction.

Antigens that induce a hypersensitivity or allergic response are also called **allergens.** Many small molecules can function as *haptens:* antigens that are too small to be immunogens by themselves but become immunogenic in combination with larger molecules that function as *carriers* for the hapten. For example, the antigens of penicillin and poison ivy are haptens, but they initiate allergic responses only after binding to large-molecular-weight proteins in the allergic individual's blood or skin.

Four main types of hypersensitivity reactions can occur; they are classified by the nature of the immune response that causes the disease (Table 3.3).

Type I Hypersensitivity

Type I hypersensitivity, or *anaphylactic type hypersensitivity,* is a reaction that occurs immediately—within minutes—after

TABLE 3.3   Hypersensitivity or Allergy Reactions

Type of Reaction	Example(s)
Type I or anaphylactic type	Hay fever, asthma, anaphylaxis
Type II or cytotoxic type	Autoimmune hemolytic anemia
Type III or immune complex type	Autoimmune diseases such as systemic lupus erythematosus
Type IV or cell-mediated type	Granulomatous diseases such as tuberculosis as well as graft and organ transplant rejection

exposure to a previously encountered allergen in this case, such as pollen, latex, or penicillin. With type I hypersensitivity, plasma cells produce IgE as a response to the allergen. The newly produced IgE binds to mast cells located in tissue, causing them to release their granules containing histamine, a well-known potent biochemical mediator of inflammation. This results in edema caused by increased dilation and permeability of blood vessels and in constriction of smooth muscle in the bronchioles of the lungs.

This type of hypersensitivity includes hay fever and urticaria or hives, as well as more serious conditions, including asthma and anaphylaxis. **Anaphylaxis** is a type of hypersensitivity that can be life threatening because the individual may not be able to breathe as a result of the oropharyngeal tissue swelling and constriction of the bronchioles, which requires immediate treatment with epinephrine. Drugs that suppress inflammation, such as antihistamines and corticosteroids, may be helpful in reducing symptoms of some forms of type I hypersensitivity.

Type II Hypersensitivity

With type II hypersensitivity, or *cytotoxic type hypersensitivity,* antibody combines with an antigen that is bound to the surface of tissue cells, usually a circulating red blood cell. Activated complement components, as well as both IgG and IgM antibodies in blood, participate in this type of hypersensitivity reaction. The result is the destruction of the tissue that has the antigen on the surface of its cells. A type II reaction occurs in incompatible blood transfusions and in rhesus (Rh) incompatibility. In the latter case, the mother's antibodies cross the placenta and destroy the newborn's red blood cells, resulting in possibly fatal hemolytic anemia.

Type III Hypersensitivity

Type III hypersensitivity, or *immune complex type hypersensitivity,* is marked by the formation of immune complexes between microorganisms and antibody in the circulating blood. The complexes leave the blood and are deposited in various types of tissue or even in a localized area in an organ. In either case the deposition results in the initiation of an acute inflammatory response. Neutrophils are attracted to the tissue in which the complexes have been deposited. As a result of phagocytosis and death of the neutrophils, lysosomal enzymes are released, causing tissue destruction.

Type IV Hypersensitivity

Type IV hypersensitivity, or *cell-mediated type hypersensitivity,* involves a cell-mediated immune response rather than a humoral response that produces antibodies. T-cell lymphocytes that have been introduced to an antigen previously either directly cause damage to the tissue cells or recruit other cells that cause the damage. This type of hypersensitivity reaction is also called **delayed hypersensitivity** because the reaction takes 2 to 3 days to develop.

This process by T cells is used when diagnosing tuberculosis. During the tuberculin skin test, a visible skin reaction occurs if the individual tested has previously been exposed to the microorganism that causes tuberculosis. This process is also how an infection by tuberculosis can be controlled in the body under the right circumstances.

This type of hypersensitivity is also responsible for the rejection of tissue grafts and transplanted organs, as well as an allergy to nickel found in some jewelry and older dental restorations. New strategies for prevention of rejection, such as synthetic production of therapeutic antibodies against specific T-cell receptors, may

produce fewer long-term side effects than the chemotherapies now routinely used.

Drug Hypersensitivity

Drugs can act as allergens and cause a hypersensitivity or allergic reaction. Many factors influence the risk of a hypersensitivity or allergic reaction to a drug. The route of administration influences how the reaction will be manifested and its severity. Topical administration of drugs (via the skin or mucous membranes) may cause a greater number of reactions than the oral (or swallowed) or parenteral (or administered by injection) route of administration; however, the reaction that occurs after parenteral administration may be more widespread and severe because the allergen can be carried quickly to many parts of the body by the circulating blood.

Patients with multiple allergies are more likely to also have allergic reactions to drugs. For this reason, in addition to the specific allergy involved, a complete allergy history is an important component of a patient's medical history. Patients with autoimmune diseases such as systemic lupus erythematosus (SLE) commonly have adverse reactions to medications. Children, with their newer and less strong levels of immunity, are less likely than adults to have an allergic reaction to a drug.

Drugs can be involved in any of the previously described hypersensitivity reactions. Type I hypersensitivity to a drug can include anaphylaxis, urticaria (or hives), and angioedema (or localized swelling). A systemic anaphylactic reaction is more likely to occur with an injected drug, but can also occur with a drug administered orally, and can be fatal. For example, the drug penicillin may cause a systemic anaphylactic reaction in approximately 1 in 10,000 patients and causes about 300 deaths per year in the United States.

The classic example of type III hypersensitivity is **serum sickness,** which involves a drug allergy. This name was given to a reaction that occurred frequently when patients were given large amounts of antitoxin serum from horses to provide passive immunity in the treatment of diphtheria and tetanus. However, this risky method is no longer the way by which passive immunity to these diseases is provided.

The drug penicillin is the single most common cause of serum sickness today; other drugs such as barbiturates can also cause this reaction. The signs and symptoms of serum sickness include rash or urticaria, fever, painful swelling of the joints as in arthritis, renal disturbance or failure, edema around the eyes, and cardiac inflammation.

Drugs can also be involved in a type IV hypersensitivity reaction. This T-cell–mediated allergic reaction can occur in response to topically applied substances and can produce contact dermatitis, a type of skin inflammation, as well as contact **mucositis,** which is an inflammation of the mucosal tissue.

Autoimmune Diseases

The immune system learns to differentiate between one's own cells or tissue and foreign substances early in embryologic development. This recognition and the nonresponsiveness of the immune system to one's own cells or tissue usually produce a type of *immunologic tolerance.*

In an **autoimmune disease,** the recognition mechanism breaks down and certain body cells are no longer tolerated. The immune system now treats body cells as antigens, creating an immunopathologic condition. An autoimmune disease may involve a single cell type or a single organ or may be even more extensive, involving multiple organs. Certain types of tissue and even entire organs may be damaged. Genetic factors may play a role in the predisposition of an individual to autoimmune disease, and viral infection may also be involved.

Certain autoimmune diseases are also called **connective tissue diseases** because connective tissue is the primary target of the pathology. Several autoimmune diseases have oral manifestations and are described later in this chapter.

Immunodeficiency

Immunodeficiency is a type of immunopathologic condition that involves a compromised or entirely absent immune system involving white blood cells and their products in number, function, or interrelationships. This condition may be congenital (present at birth) or acquired (developed after birth). Immunodeficiency may be inherited genetically, or it can be caused by numerous other environmental factors.

When a person's immune system is not functioning adequately, infections and neoplasms may develop undeterred by any defense mechanisms. In addition, research has shown that stress and depression may be associated with decreased levels of immune function. This could be an important factor in increasing the risk of disease. Acquired immunodeficiency syndrome (AIDS) from HIV infection is an example of an immunodeficiency that has numerous oral manifestations.

Oral Immunologic Lesions and Diseases

Aphthous Ulcers and Recurrent Aphthous Stomatitis

Recurrent aphthous ulcers, also known as *canker sores* or *aphthous stomatitis,* are a painful type of oral ulcers for which the cause remains unclear. Aphthous ulcers are one of the most common oral lesions. Reported incidence ranges from 5% to 56%. The highest incidence was found in professional school students and the lowest in male hospitalized patients. They frequently occur in episodes. The first episode of these ulcers usually occurs in childhood and adolescence, and they are somewhat more common in females than in males. The clinical appearance, history, and location of the ulcers are important in establishing the diagnosis.

Trauma is the most commonly reported precipitating factor in the development of aphthous ulcers. They are often reported to occur after trauma to the oral mucosa during dental procedures (e.g., in the area of film or sensor placement or at the injection site for local anesthetics) or with the manipulation of oral tissue during dental hygiene treatment. Some patients associate the initiation of aphthous ulcers with eating certain foods such as citrus fruits. However, it is possible that patients perceive these foods as causative because of the sensitivity of the ulcers to foods with a high acid content, or the foods themselves may have caused trauma to the oral mucosa. The recurrence of aphthous ulcers has been associated with menstruation, whereas pregnancy has been found to produce a decrease in the episodes. Studies have found that iron, folic acid, and vitamin B_{12} deficiencies are more common in individuals with recurrent aphthous stomatitis. These ulcers also occur in association with certain systemic diseases, as well as with tobacco cessation. Emotional stress has also been suggested as a contributing factor.

A genetic predisposition is supported by family history and the frequency of certain genetic markers. Substantial evidence indicates that aphthous ulcers have an immunologic pathogenesis. Patients in whom aphthous ulcers develop have slightly elevated levels of antibodies to oral mucous membranes. Microscopically, an infiltrate of lymphocytes is present in the lesion, suggesting that cell-mediated immunity may be important in development of the ulcers. The infiltrate contains mainly T-helper cells in the prodromal stage and T-cytotoxic cells in the ulcerative phase; T-helper cells return in the healing stage. The T-cytotoxic cells are probably responsible for the ulceration. However, the specific antigen to which they are responding has not yet been identified. Studies have suggested that sodium lauryl sulfate in some oral health care products may give rise to oral ulceration that resembles aphthous ulcers. Medications, including nonsteroidal antiinflammatory drugs (NSAIDs), beta-blockers, and microbial agents, have been implicated in the pathogenesis of aphthous ulcers. Other possible antigens include dairy products, fruits, coffee, dyes, and preservatives. Aphthous ulcers are oral manifestations of many systemic disorders. Once the systemic disease is under control, the episodes of oral aphthous ulcers decrease. Research has not identified a link between microbes and aphthous ulcers. However, the potential role of microbes in the pathogenesis of aphthous ulcers is an area that is still being explored.

Types of Aphthous Ulcers

There are three forms of recurrent aphthous ulceration: (1) minor, (2) major, and (3) herpetiform, with the three forms differing in the size and duration of the ulcers.

Minor aphthous ulcers are the most commonly occurring type affecting about 80% of patients with recurrent aphthous ulcers. They appear as discrete, "punched-out," round-to-oval ulcers that can be as large as 1 cm in diameter and exhibit a yellowish-white fibrin center (pseudomembrane) surrounded by a halo of erythema (Fig. 3.7). Minor aphthous ulcers are more common in the anterior than the posterior part of the mouth. The ulcers often have a prodromal period of 1 to 2 days, which is characterized by a burning or tingling sensation or soreness in the area in which the ulcer will eventually form. Although they are small, these ulcers can be exquisitely painful, and single or multiple lesions may be present. They heal spontaneously in 7 to 10 days.

Major aphthous ulcers, also known as *Sutton disease* and *periadenitis mucosa necrotica recurrens* are larger than 1 cm in diameter and are deeper and last longer than minor aphthous ulcers (Fig. 3.8). In addition, they can be more painful, often occur in the posterior part of the mouth, and are less common compared with minor aphthous ulcers. They can take several weeks to heal and frequently result in scarring. Ulcers that resemble major aphthous ulcers have been reported to occur in patients with HIV infection, Behçet syndrome, Crohn disease, and reactive arthritis

Herpetiform aphthous ulcers are the smallest, at 1 to 2 mm, and the least common type (Fig. 3.9). They are mistakenly called *herpetiform* because they resemble ulcers caused by the herpes simplex virus, but like the other types of aphthous ulcers they do not have a known cause. They are painful and may develop anywhere in the oral cavity.

Diagnosis

The diagnosis of the type of aphthous ulcers is made on the basis of their distinctive clinical appearance, the location of the lesions,

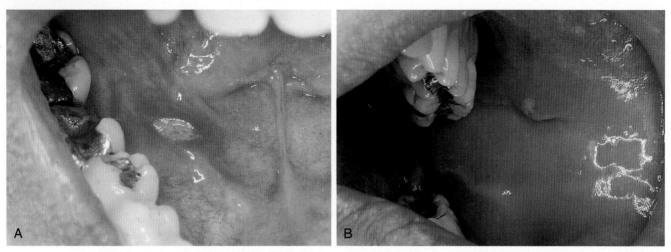

• **Figure 3.7** Minor aphthous ulcers. **A,** On the floor of the mouth. **B,** On the buccal mucosa, on the papilla of the Stenson duct.

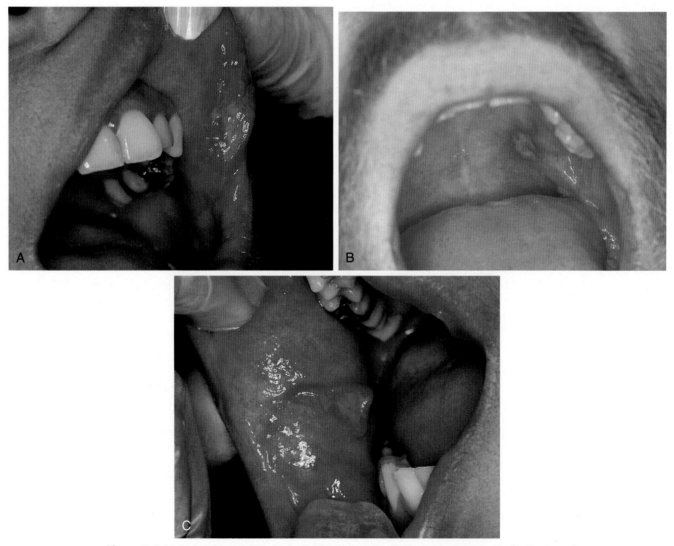

• **Figure 3.8** Major aphthous ulcers. **A,** On the labial mucosa. **B,** On the soft palate. **C,** On the buccal mucosa.

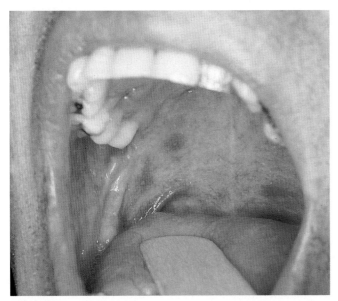

• **Figure 3.9** Herpetiform aphthous ulcers on the palate. These are the smallest of the aphthous ulcers.

TABLE 3.4	**Clinical Features of the Three Types of Recurrent Aphthous Ulcers**		
	TYPE OF RECURRENT APHTHOUS ULCER		
Feature	Minor	Major	Herpetiform
Size	Small, 3–5 mm	Large, 5–10 mm	Smallest, 1–2 mm
Location on nonkeratinized mucosa	More anterior	More posterior	Anywhere
Number	1–5	1–10	1–100
Appearance	Shallow	Deep	Shallow
Scarring	No	Yes	No
Pain	Yes	Yes	Yes

and a complete patient history (Table 3.4). It is important to note that laboratory results are not specific for any form of aphthous ulcer.

The location of the ulcers is important in differentiating between recurrent aphthous ulcers and recurrent intraoral ulceration caused by the herpes simplex virus. The differentiation between aphthous ulcers and herpes simplex ulcers is described in Chapter 4 (see Table 4.2). Aphthous ulcers appear on nonkeratinized oral mucosa that is nonattached, that is, not fixed to bone, such as the buccal and labial mucosa, vestibular tissue, and the floor of the mouth, as well as the lateral and ventral surfaces of the tongue. In contrast, ulcers resulting from recurrence of the herpes simplex virus, when they occur intraorally, appear on keratinized mucosa such as the oral mucosa of the palate and gingival tissue (i.e., the mucosa fixed to bone). Because major aphthous ulcers may clinically resemble squamous cell carcinoma or deep fungal infections, a biopsy may be necessary to rule out these conditions. However, as with minor aphthous ulcers, biopsy

and microscopic features are nonspecific and not diagnostic for major aphthous ulcers.

Herpetiform aphthous ulcers may also be difficult to distinguish clinically from primary herpetic gingivostomatitis. However, no systemic signs or symptoms exist as in primary herpes simplex infection. Herpetiform aphthous ulcers have been reported to respond to topical application of liquid tetracycline, which may be helpful in confirming the diagnosis of herpetiform aphthous ulcers.

When a patient develops multiple aphthous ulcers, it is important to consider that they might be associated with a systemic disease. Other signs and symptoms that may suggest systemic disease should be considered when reviewing the patient's medical history. These include the presence of chronic gastrointestinal symptoms such as diarrhea and discomfort (Crohn disease, gluten-sensitive enteropathy/celiac disease, inflammatory bowel syndrome, intestinal lymphoma, ulcerative colitis), arthritis and skin lesions (Behçet syndrome), and childhood periodic fevers (cyclic neutropenia and PFAFA [periodic fever, aphthous stomatitis, pharyngitis, and adenitis] syndrome).

Treatment and Prognosis

The local application of topical corticosteroids and topical nonsteroidal antiinflammatory agents is helpful in the management of aphthous ulcers, and topical anesthetics such as lidocaine and benzocaine can help decrease the pain. Topical corticosteroids and nonsteroidal antiinflammatory agents are most effective when applied very early in the development of the ulcer, during the prodromal or preulcerative period; systemic steroids may be necessary for managing patients with major aphthous ulcers. Differentiating recurrent aphthous ulcers from recurrent herpes simplex virus ulceration is important because topical steroid application can exacerbate herpes simplex virus infection. The clinical presentation and diagnosis of recurrent herpes simplex infection is described in Chapter 4, and Table 4.2 summarizes the differences between these two types of recurrent ulceration.

Nicotine replacement therapy has been suggested to be helpful when aphthous ulcers occur in association with tobacco cessation.

Urticaria and Angioedema

Urticaria and angioedema have a similar causal background in that they are skin and oral mucosal hypersensitivity reactions. The lesions are caused by localized areas of increased vascular permeability in the superficial connective tissue beneath the epithelium.

Urticaria, also called *hives,* appears as multiple areas of well-demarcated edema and erythema of the skin, usually accompanied by itching **(pruritus)** (Fig. 3.10A-B). **Angioedema** appears as a diffuse edema (swelling) of tissue caused by permeability of deeper blood vessels (Fig. 3.11). The skin covering the swelling appears normal, and angioedema is usually not accompanied by itching. Urticaria and angioedema both may occur in acute self-limited episodes. On occasion, chronic or recurrent forms may occur each time the patient comes in contact with the allergen.

In many cases of urticaria and angioedema the cause cannot be identified. Infection, trauma, emotional stress, and certain systemic diseases have been reported to cause these lesions, and ingested allergens are frequent causes of urticaria.

Several mechanisms are capable of causing the increased vascular permeability that results in both urticaria and angioedema,

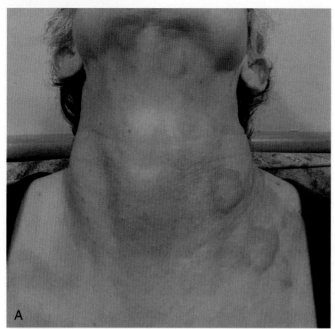

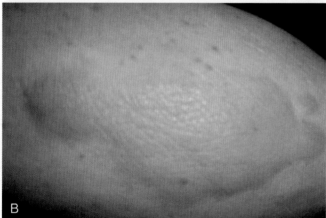

• **Figure 3.10** **A** and **B,** Two examples of urticaria (hives). (**A** courtesy Denise Cuttita.)

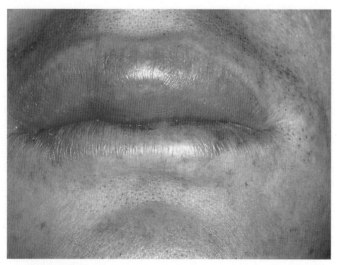

• **Figure 3.11** Angioedema. (Courtesy Dr. Edward V. Zegarelli.)

including the release of the chemical mediator histamine from mast cells stimulated by IgE antibodies (type I hypersensitivity) and the activation of IgG or IgM antibodies along with trauma, causing vascular permeability. Acetylsalicylic acid (aspirin) and nonsteroidal antiinflammatory drugs (NSAIDs), such as ibuprofen, can produce a nonspecific effect that can cause vascular permeability. A rare hereditary form of angioedema exists in which uncontrolled activation of the complement cascade occurs, resulting in prolonged vascular permeability.

Diagnosis

The diagnoses for both urticaria and angioedema are based on the clinical appearance of the lesions, the patient's history, and the history of the lesion. Avoidance of the causative agent, if identified, is important in managing patients with recurring urticaria and angioedema.

Treatment and Prognosis

Antihistaminic drugs (e.g., diphenhydramine [Benadryl]) are the standard drugs used to treat urticaria and angioedema. Immediate treatment is important. Angioedema involving the larynx and pharynx can cause asphyxiation and therefore may be fatal. Immediate treatment with epinephrine is necessary in these cases.

Allergic Contact Mucositis and Dermatitis

Allergic contact mucositis and allergic **contact dermatitis** are lesions that result from the direct contact of an allergen with the oral mucosa and the skin, respectively. The development of these conditions involves a T cell within a cell-mediated immune response and is an example of type IV hypersensitivity. The exact underlying immunologic basis is not always clear.

In contact mucositis the mucosa becomes erythematous and edematous, often accompanied by burning and pruritus (Fig. 3.12A). The mucositis occurs where the offending agent has contacted the mucosa, giving it a smooth, shiny appearance that is firm to palpation. Small vesicles and ulcers may appear in the affected areas. In contact dermatitis the initial lesion may be erythematous, with swelling and vesicles. Later the area becomes crusted, scaly, and white (Fig. 3.12B).

Preservatives in local anesthetics and components of topical medication are common causes of allergic reactions. Acrylics, metal-based alloys, epoxy resins, and the flavoring agents in chewing gum and dentifrices and mouthwashes all have been reported to cause contact mucositis. Tartar control toothpastes may have high concentrations of cinnamon-containing flavoring agents. Cinnamon oil as a flavoring agent is responsible for multiple abnormal oral mucosal responses. Patients may be unaware that products they are using contain cinnamon oil.

Contact dermatitis, particularly affecting the hands, may occur in response to the materials used in dentistry. The routine use of gloves in dental care has decreased the incidence of this type of dermatitis; however, latex gloves and glove powder have also been responsible for contact dermatitis in some individuals (see Fig. 3.12B). Due to the high prevalence of latex allergies, latex is disappearing from the dental environment.

Diagnosis

When the cause of the contact mucositis or dermatitis is suspected, skin testing for sensitivity to the particular substance can help confirm the agent that has caused the lesion.

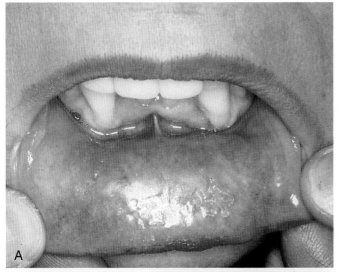

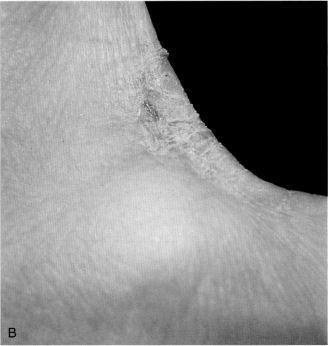

• **Figure 3.12** A, Contact mucositis on the labial mucosa, from acrylic. B, Contact dermatitis on the skin between the thumb and index finger, from latex gloves. (**A** courtesy Dr. Edward V. Zegarelli.)

Treatment and Prognosis

Topical and systemic corticosteroids may be used in the management of these lesions in some patients.

Fixed Drug Eruptions

Fixed drug eruptions are lesions that appear in the same site each time a drug is introduced. The lesions generally appear suddenly after a latent period of several days and subside when the drug is discontinued. They appear again when the drug is reintroduced, usually with greater intensity. Clinically there may be single or multiple slightly raised, reddish patches or clusters of macules on the skin or rarely the mucous membranes in the oral cavity. Pain and pruritus may be associated with these lesions.

The fixed drug eruption is a type III hypersensitivity reaction in which immune complexes are deposited along the endothelial wall of blood vessels. The ensuing inflammatory reaction causes vasculitis and subsequent damage to the vessel wall, giving rise to erythema and edema of the superficial layers of the skin or mucosa. If possible, the drug causing the reaction should be identified and its use discontinued. Some medications associated with fixed drug eruptions are barbiturates, chlorhexidine, lidocaine, penicillamine, sulfonamides, and tetracycline.

Erythema Multiforme

Erythema multiforme (EM) is an acute, self-limited disease that affects the skin and mucous membranes. The cause is not clear, but some evidence exists that it is a hypersensitivity reaction; however, the type has not been determined.

Erythema multiforme most commonly occurs in young adults under 30 years old. Studies differ as to whether there is a male or female predominance. It includes a wide range of clinical disease. Erythema multiforme involving oral mucosa and some skin sites is called **erythema multiforme minor**. Involvement of two or more mucosal sites with widespread skin involvement is called **erythema multiforme major**. In approximately 50% of cases of erythema multiforme minor, a triggering event can be identified. These include herpes simplex infection, *Mycoplasma pneumoniae* infection, and drug exposure, particularly antibiotics and analgesics. Erythema multiforme major is usually triggered by drug exposure rather than infection.

Both erythema multiforme minor and major may affect the oral mucosa. They usually have an explosive onset of lesions on the oral mucosa, lips, and skin. Prodromal symptoms include fever, malaise, headache, cough, and sore throat. It may be chronic on occasion, or there may be recurrent acute episodes because it seems to be related to persistent antigenic stimulus.

The oral lesions are usually ulcers (Fig. 3.13A-B). Diffuse, large, superficial erythematous areas may also occur. The ulcers frequently form on the lateral borders of the tongue. Crusted and bleeding lips are frequently seen in erythema multiforme, and gingival and palatal mucosal involvement is rare. However, gingival involvement in erythema multiforme has been reported.

The characteristic skin lesion is called a *target* or *bull's-eye* lesion, which consists of concentric rings of erythema alternating with normal skin color, with the darkest color at the center of the lesion. The term *erythema multiforme* refers to the variety of skin lesions that can occur, which range from target lesion macules to plaques to bullae (Fig. 3.13C-D). Erythema multiforme can affect the oral mucosa either alone or in association with skin lesions. Skin lesions can occur without the presence of any oral lesions.

Diagnosis

The diagnosis of erythema multiforme is made on the basis of the clinical features and the exclusion of other diseases; the microscopic appearance is nonspecific. Biopsy and microscopic examinations are helpful in some cases for excluding other diseases with similar clinical features but more distinctive microscopic features.

Treatment and Prognosis

If a cause can be identified, first remove the cause if possible. Topical corticosteroids may be helpful in mild cases of erythema multiforme, but systemic corticosteroid treatment is usually needed. Long-term systemic antiviral medication is used in some cases to attempt to decrease recurrent episodes that are suspected of being stimulated by a herpes simplex virus infection.

Stevens-Johnson Syndrome

In the past a condition known as *Stevens-Johnson syndrome* was considered a very severe form of erythema multiforme. More recently, Stevens-Johnson syndrome has been separated from the erythema multiforme spectrum and classified as a variant of toxic epidermal necrolysis (TEN) (Fig. 3.14), a rare and usually severe adverse reaction to certain drugs. Stevens-Johnson syndrome presents with mucosal lesions that are more extensive and painful than erythema multiforme. The lips are generally more extensively encrusted and bloody than in erythema multiforme. These conditions tend to occur in older individuals and affect females more than males. Lesions involving the genital mucosa and the mucosa

of the eyes may also be involved. Skin involvement in Stevens-Johnson syndrome involves less than 10% of the body, whereas skin involvement in toxic epidermal necrolysis involves greater than 30%.

Treatment of Stevens-Johnson syndrome and toxic epidermal necrolysis involves removing the causative drug, intravenous hydration, and corticosteroid therapy. Mortality resulting from Stevens-Johnson syndrome is reported to be up to 5%; mortality for toxic epidermal necrolysis is reported to be up to 30%.

Lichen Planus

Lichen planus is a benign, chronic disease affecting the skin and oral mucosa. In some patients this disease may affect both the skin and the oral mucosa; in others either oral mucosa or skin alone may be affected.

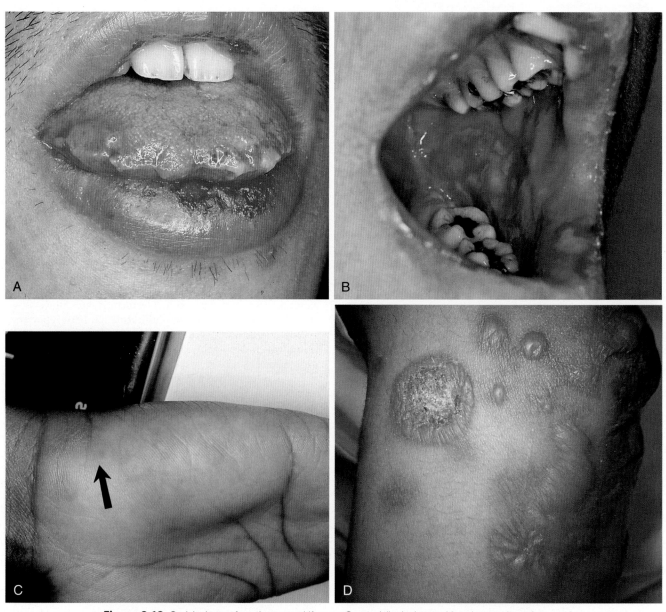

• **Figure 3.13** Oral lesions of erythema multiforme: Crusted lip lesions with edema, ulceration, and erythema **(A)** and erythematous and ulcerated lesions of the lips and buccal mucosa **(B)**. Skin lesions of erythema multiforme: Target lesion (*arrow*) **(C)** and bullae **(D)**. (**C** courtesy Dr. Edward V. Zegarelli.)

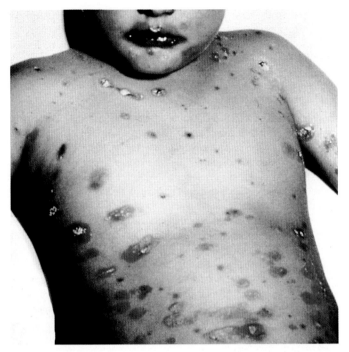

• **Figure 3.14** Stevens-Johnson syndrome. (Courtesy Dr. Sidney Eisig.)

The classic appearance of lichen planus affecting the oral mucosa is an arrangement of interconnecting white lines and circles (sometimes referred to as a *lacelike pattern*) (Fig. 3.15A). The slender white lines are called *Wickham striae*. The fundamental lesion is a small, papular, pinhead-sized, domed or hemispheric, glistening white nodule on the mucosa. The clinical appearance depends on the arrangement of these minute papules and striae. The most common location is the buccal mucosa. However, lichen planus also occurs on the tongue, lips, floor of the mouth, and gingiva. Lesions of lichen planus are frequently distributed symmetrically in the oral cavity.

The prevalence of lichen planus in the general population of the United States has been reported to be about 1%, with individuals ranging in age from 13 to 78 years. The disease is most common in middle age and has a slight female predilection. Most cases are asymptomatic, discovered on routine oral examination. There are also skin lesions.

Many factors have been implicated in lichen planus; however, the cause remains unknown. Erosive lesions tend to worsen with emotional stress. Many drugs and chemicals have been shown to produce lichenoid lesions (lesions that resemble lichen planus), but these have a different microscopic appearance from true lichen planus.

Types of Lichen Planus

Several forms of lichen planus have been described. The most common form is **reticular lichen planus.** In this form oral lesions are composed of Wickham striae along with slightly raised

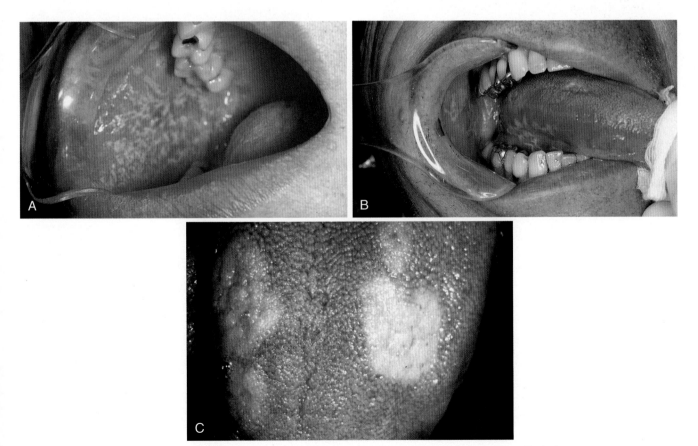

• **Figure 3.15** **A and B,** Two examples of the oral lesions of lichen planus. **C,** The plaquelike lesions on the tongue of a patient with lichen planus. (**A** courtesy Dr. Edward V. Zegarelli.)

white plaquelike areas that do not rub off. The raised lines of Wickham striae are composed of 2- to 4-mm papules that, strung together, form the raised lines of Wickham striae that are often arranged in a "lacelike" pattern (Fig. 3.15A-B). These are often found bilaterally on the posterior buccal mucosa. The tongue, palate, and gingiva may also be involved. Plaquelike lesions are sometimes seen on the tongue of patients with lichen planus (see Fig. 3.15C).

Erosive lichen planus and **bullous lichen planus** are those forms in which the epithelium separates from the connective tissue, resulting in erosions, bullae, or ulcers. These forms are less common (Fig. 3.16). The striated lesions commonly occur on the buccal mucosa and may also occur on other mucosal tissue and the lips. Lichen planus can also present with gingival lesions that are clinically described as **desquamative gingivitis** (Fig. 3.17). Bullous lichen planus is a severe form of erosive lichen planus that involves the formation of large blisters (bullae) that occur when the epithelium separates from the connective tissue.

With the skin lesions of lichen planus, itching or pruritus may be present. Skin lesions of lichen planus are described as purple, pruritic papules (Fig. 3.18). Scaly purplish lesions can occur anywhere on the skin, but the most common sites are the lumbar region, the flexor surfaces of the wrist and elbow, and the anterior surface of the ankles. Some patients with lichen planus have only skin lesions, some have only oral lesions, and others have both skin and oral lesions.

Diagnosis

The diagnosis of lichen planus is made on the basis of both the distinctive clinical features and the microscopic appearance of the tissue obtained through scalpel biopsy (Fig. 3.19). The epithelium is generally parakeratotic and may be either hyperplastic or atrophic. The characteristic microscopic features include degeneration of the basal cell layer of the epithelium in small-to-extensive areas (described as hydropic degeneration because the basal cells appear clear and fluid filled), sawtooth-shaped rete ridges, and a broad band of lymphocytes in the connective tissue immediately subjacent to the degenerated basal cell layer epithelium.

In erosive areas the separation of the epithelium from the connective tissue occurs at the interface of the epithelium and connective tissue. Epithelial atypia and dysplasia may also occur in lesions that appear clinically as lichen planus, and it has been suggested that these lesions may be premalignant.

Treatment and Prognosis

Lichen planus is a chronic disease. Treatment is indicated only when lesions are symptomatic. Erosive lesions usually respond quickly when topical corticosteroid medication is applied. The

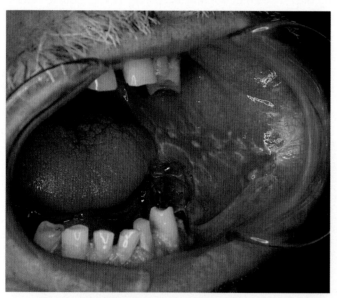

• **Figure 3.16** Erosive lichen planus on the buccal mucosa.

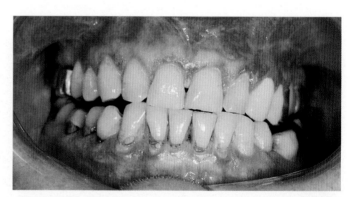

• **Figure 3.17** Desquamative gingivitis seen in lichen planus. (Courtesy Dr. Edward V. Zegarelli.)

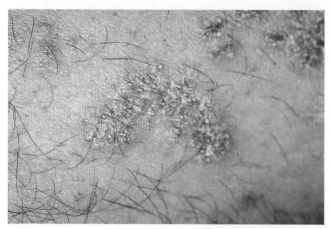

• **Figure 3.18** Skin lesions of lichen planus presenting as scaly purplish lesions.

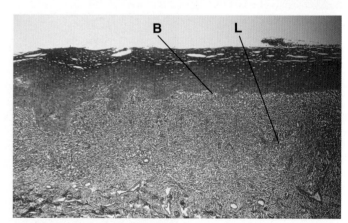

• **Figure 3.19** Microscopic appearance of lichen planus. Degeneration of the basal cell layer of the epithelium (B) and the bandlike infiltrate of lymphocytes (L).

most commonly prescribed are triamcinolone, fluocinonide, betamethasone, clobetasol, and dexamethasone. Oral candidiasis may be an adverse effect of treatment of erosive lichen planus with corticosteroid medication. The patient complains of a burning sensation, and mucosal lesions consistent with candidiasis are present. Antifungal medication is introduced when this occurs. Improvement of gingival lesions with meticulous oral hygiene has been reported.

The possibility of an increased risk of the development of squamous cell carcinoma in patients with lichen planus remains controversial. Erosive lesions have been suggested to be associated with this increased risk. A recent study has suggested that the risk is associated with lichenoid mucositis and not lichen planus.

Lichenoid mucositis has been described by the World Health Organization as a condition in which lesions clinically and histopathologically resemble lichen planus but do not fully meet either the characteristic clinical or histopathologic features. Lichenoid mucositis is composed of a mixed inflammatory infiltrate rather than only lymphocytes and may extend deeper into the connective tissue. Oral lesions diagnosed as lichenoid mucositis may be a response to a topical agent (i.e., amalgam, nickel, cinnamon) or many systemic medications. If a drug can be identified as the causative agent of lichenoid-appearing lesions, discontinuation of the drug should cause the lesions to disappear. However, at times it is not possible to discontinue the drug. Because of the concern about development of malignancy in erosive lichenoid lesions, regular follow-up of patients with erosive lichen planus or lichenoid mucositis is recommended with biopsy of any suspicious lesions. Suggested follow-up intervals range from 3 to 6 months.

Reactive Arthritis (Reiter Syndrome)

Reactive arthritis, or Reiter syndrome, is a chronic disease that classically comprises the triad of three features: (1) arthritis, (2) urethritis, and (3) conjunctivitis. All the components of the syndrome may be present with a case of reactive arthritis, but polyarthritis is generally the most prominent component of this syndrome.

Reactive arthritis characteristically develops 1 to 6 weeks after a sexually transmitted or gastrointestinal infection: *Chlamydia, Salmonella, Shigella,* and *Yersinia* are most common. Reactive arthritis is also associated with HIV infection. The pathogenesis of this syndrome is not clear; an abnormal immune response to a microbial antigen is considered the most likely mechanism. Diagnostic tests for the initiating infection are generally negative by the time signs and symptoms appear. An antigenic marker called *HLA-B27* is present in most patients with reactive arthritis, suggesting a strong genetic influence. Reactive arthritis is far more prevalent in men than in women (9:1).

Urethritis and conjunctivitis are often early clinical signs. The conjunctivitis is usually mild, but some individuals experience iritis (inflammation of the iris). Fever, malaise, and weight loss may be associated with this condition. The arthritis usually involves the joints of the lower extremities such as the knees and ankles and may be asymmetric and migratory, acute, chronic, or recurrent. Temporomandibular joint involvement has been reported. The condition is usually benign and self-limited. Radiographically, a periosteal proliferation can be detected on the heels, ankles, metatarsals, phalanges, knees, and elbows.

Skin and mucous membrane lesions are seen in many patients with reactive arthritis. Oral lesions occur almost anywhere in the oral cavity (Fig. 3.20). Aphthous-like ulcers, erythematous lesions, and areas of depapillation of the dorsal surface of the tongue that mimic erythema migrans have been described in patients with reactive arthritis.

Diagnosis

The diagnosis of reactive arthritis is made on the basis of the clinical signs and symptoms along with identification of the HLA-B27 antigenic marker.

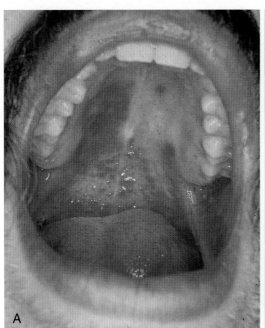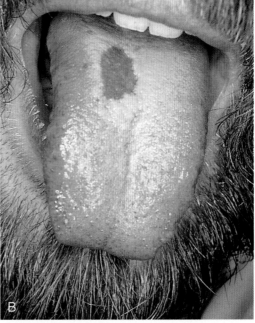

• **Figure 3.20** Reactive arthritis. **A,** Ulcerative lesions on the palate. **B,** Lesion on the tongue.

Treatment and Prognosis

Reactive arthritis lasts from 3 months to a year. About 50% of patients with reactive arthritis will be free of symptoms by 6 months; but about 20% may proceed to chronic disease. During that time, the patient may experience spontaneous remission, but recurrent attacks are common. Aspirin or other NSAIDs are generally used for treatment, as well as antibiotics for possible coexistent infection. Systemic corticosteroid therapy may be needed in severe cases. Physical therapy may help reduce the arthritis.

Langerhans Cell Histiocytosis (Langerhans Cell Disease)

Langerhans cell histiocytosis (LCH), also called *Langerhans cell disease*, is a group of rare disorders characterized by the presence of histiocytes-like cells and eosinophils. The histiocytes-like cells, called *Langerhans cells,* are not histiocytes or macrophages. Recent studies suggest that these cells are most likely derived from myeloid dendritic cells rather than the Langerhans cells of the skin and mucosa. The cause and pathogenesis of Langerhans cell histiocytosis remains unclear; a reactive process, a primary immunodeficiency disease, and a neoplastic process have all been suggested. Recent evidence supports a neoplastic process.

This group of diseases was formerly called *histiocytosis X* and included three main forms: (1) acute disseminated form (Letterer-Siwe disease), (2) chronic disseminated or multifocal form (Hand-Schüller-Christian disease with its triad of punched-out radiolucent lesions of the skull, exophthalmos, and diabetes insipidus), and (3) solitary eosinophilic granuloma. There is much overlap in the clinical presentation of Langerhans cell histiocytosis. These traditional categories did not match the clinical presentation and prognosis of most patients with a diagnosis of Langerhans cell histiocytosis; therefore the spectrum of the cell has been stratified into two basic categories: (1) single-system disease with unifocal and multifocal involvement and (2) multisystem disease with or without organ dysfunction. Bone is the most common site of involvement in single-system disease followed by skin, lymph node, and lung. Sites involved in multisystem disease include bone, skin, liver, spleen, and bone marrow. Involvement of liver, spleen, and bone marrow place patients at higher risk of death from the disease.

Biopsy and histopathologic examination is necessary for a diagnosis of Langerhans cell histiocytosis. Lesions are characterized by a diffuse infiltrate of large histiocyte-like cells accompanied by a prominent infiltrate of eosinophils (Fig. 3.21). Lymphocytes and neutrophils may also be present. The presence of eosinophils is thought to result from the production of an eosinophilic chemotactic factor produced by Langerhans cells. Langerhans cells can be distinguished from other cells that look microscopically similar by immunohistochemical staining. A structure called a **Birbeck granule** can be identified in the cytoplasm of Langerhans cells by electron microscopy.

Langerhans cell histiocytosis occurs most often in children and in white individuals of Northern European ancestry. Although cases may present over a wide age range, 50% of cases are diagnosed in children less than 15 years of age. Single or solitary bone lesions are the most common presentation. The involved sites differ in relationship to the patient's age. Younger children tend to have lesions in the skull and femur; patients over 20 years of age tend to have bone lesions in the ribs, shoulder girdle, and

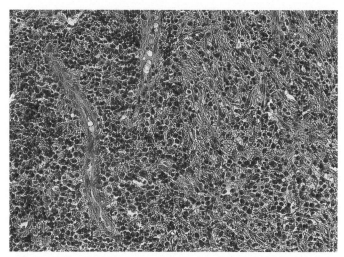

• **Figure 3.21** Langerhans cell histiocytosis (Langerhans cell disease) microscopic appearance (high magnification) with a combination of Langerhans cells and eosinophils.

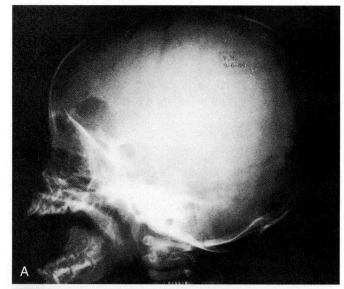

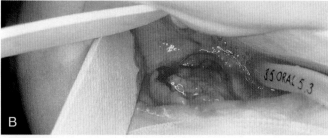

• **Figure 3.22** Langerhans cell histiocytosis (Langerhans cell disease): **A,** Skull radiograph. **B,** Ulcerated lesion of the mandible. (Courtesy Dr. Sidney Eisig.)

mandible (Fig. 3.22A). Children are more likely to have visceral involvement (i.e., liver, spleen).

Jaw lesions are seen in 10% to 20% of all cases of Langerhans cell histiocytosis. Radiographically these appear as punched-out radiolucencies because they do not have a sclerotic border. A scooped-out appearance may be seen when the alveolar bone is destroyed that may be suggestive of periodontal disease. Bone destruction may result in loose teeth. Dull pain may accompany bone lesions. Proliferative or ulcerating lesions may develop if the disease perforates the bone (Fig. 3.22B).

Treatment of Langerhans cell histiocytosis depends on the site and extent of disease and ranges from excision of single lesions to radiation therapy for persistent lesions and chemotherapy for more widespread disease

The **eosinophilic granuloma of bone** is the name traditionally used for the solitary or chronic localized form. The eosinophilic granuloma occurs mainly in older children and young adults. The skull and its mandible are typically involved with eosinophilic granuloma (Fig. 3.23). Cases of multifocal eosinophilic granuloma have also been reported. Eosinophilic granuloma is treated by conservative surgical excision; recurrence is rare. Low-dose radiation therapy may also be used for treatment of more severe or persistent cases.

Autoimmune Diseases With Oral Manifestations

Several autoimmune diseases affect the oral cavity (Table 3.5). In this type of disease tissue damage occurs because the immune system treats the person's own cells and tissue types as antigens. It is important to note that an individual with one autoimmune disease has an increased risk of developing another, so dental personnel must keep a patient's medical history current and ask for a medical consultation if warranted.

Sjögren Syndrome

Sjögren syndrome is a chronic, systemic, autoimmune disease that affects the salivary and lacrimal glands, resulting in a decrease in saliva and tears. This combination of dry mouth (**xerostomia**) and dry eyes (**xerophthalmia**) with Sjögren syndrome is also called **sicca syndrome** (*sicca*, dry). Decreased salivary flow, or **hyposalivation,** results in dry mouth, or xerostomia; decreased lacrimal flow results in dry eyes (**xerophthalmia**) with resultant damage to the eyes (**keratoconjunctivitis sicca**). The specific cause of Sjögren syndrome is not known. There is evidence for a genetic influence, and certain viruses have been implicated. Both cellular and humoral immunity are involved in the pathogenesis.

In some patients only the mouth and eyes are involved. In others the autoimmune process can be more extensive. Salivary and lacrimal gland involvement without the presence of another autoimmune disease is considered **primary Sjögren syndrome.** When another autoimmune disease accompanies salivary and lacrimal gland involvement, the combination is considered **secondary Sjögren syndrome.** About 50% of individuals with Sjögren syndrome have another autoimmune disease. As with most autoimmune diseases, Sjögren syndrome is much more common in women than in men (9:1).

The oral manifestation of Sjögren syndrome is xerostomia (dry mouth), which occurs as a result of hyposalivation (decreased salivary flow) and causes the mucosa to become erythematous. Patients have oral discomfort, and lack of saliva causes the mouth to feel sticky. Lips are cracked and dry and may have angular cheilitis. Intraoral examination reveals very dry mucosa and a generalized loss of both filiform and fungiform papillae (atrophy) on the dorsal surface of the tongue (Fig. 3.24). Patients with xerostomia have difficulty eating and swallowing and often

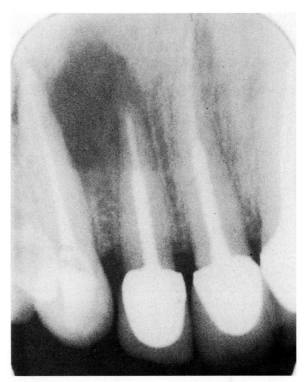

• **Figure 3.23** Langerhans cell histiocytosis (Langerhans cell disease) in the solitary or chronic localized form of an eosinophilic granuloma, showing a well-circumscribed radiolucency. (Courtesy Drs. Paul Freedman and Stanley Kerpel.)

TABLE 3.5	Autoimmune Diseases With Oral Manifestations
Disease	**Oral Manifestation**
Sjögren syndrome	Xerostomia and parotid gland enlargement
Systemic lupus erythematosus	White erosive oral lesions
Pemphigus vulgaris	Mucosal ulceration with bullae
Benign mucous membrane pemphigoid	Mucosal ulceration and desquamative gingivitis
Behçet syndrome	Aphthous-like ulcers
Pernicious anemia*	Mucosal atrophy and ulceration with loss of both filiform and fungiform lingual papillae

*Described in Chapter 9.

complain of taste distortion (**dysgeusia**). They are at high risk for the development of caries, periodontal disease, and oral candidiasis.

Both major and minor salivary glands are affected. Parotid salivary gland enlargement, usually bilateral and symmetric, occurs in about 50% of patients (Fig. 3.25). The characteristic microscopic appearance of these enlarged parotid glands consists of replacement of the glands by lymphocytes and changes in the epithelium of the ducts that appear as islands of epithelium (epimyoepithelial islands). Biopsy of the minor salivary glands is sometimes performed to assist in the diagnosis of Sjögren syn-

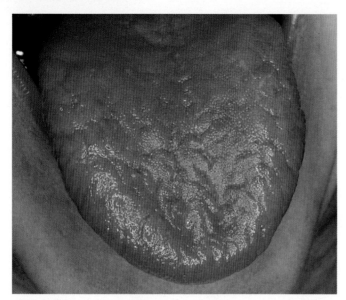

• **Figure 3.24** Sjögren syndrome with severe xerostomia and a lack of papillae on the dorsal tongue.

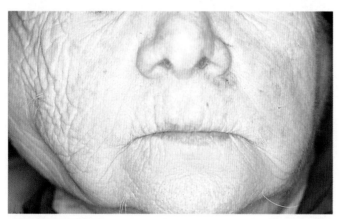

• **Figure 3.25** Bilateral parotid gland enlargement seen in Sjögren syndrome. (Courtesy Dr. Louis Mandel.)

drome. The minor glands show aggregates of lymphocytes surrounding the salivary gland ducts (Fig. 3.26).

In addition to the oral findings, patients with decreased lacrimal flow experience xerophthalmia causing burning and itching of the eyes and photophobia (abnormal visual intolerance of light). Severe ocular involvement may lead to keratoconjunctivitis sicca with ulceration and opacification of the cornea.

In some patients with Sjögren syndrome, the **Raynaud phenomenon,** a circulatory disorder affecting the fingers and toes, may also occur. Both cold and emotional stress tend to trigger the reaction, which is characterized by an initial pallor of the skin that results from vasoconstriction and reduced blood flow. The initial pallor is followed by cyanosis, which occurs because of the decreased blood flow. When the skin is rewarmed, the blood vessels dilate, and the hyperemia results in a reddening of the skin. Finally, in minutes to hours the color returns to normal. The Raynaud phenomenon can occur alone or in association with autoimmune diseases other than Sjögren syndrome. Patients with Sjögren syndrome may also have myalgia (muscle pain or tenderness), arthralgia (joint pain), and chronic fatigue.

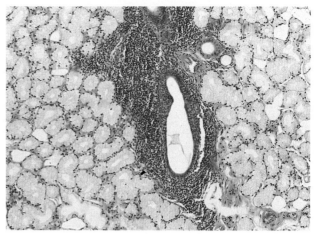

• **Figure 3.26** Microscopic appearance (high magnification) of a minor salivary gland in Sjögren syndrome, showing aggregates of lymphocytes surrounding the salivary gland ducts. (Courtesy Dr. Harry Lumerman.)

Laboratory abnormalities are important in the diagnosis of Sjögren syndrome. A positive result for **rheumatoid factor (RF),** a serum antibody to IgG (i.e., an antibody to an antibody), is found in 90% of patients with Sjögren syndrome. Rheumatoid factor is also found in patients with other autoimmune diseases such as rheumatoid arthritis. **Autoantibodies,** called *anti–Sjögren syndrome A* and *anti–Sjögren syndrome B,* are also found in patients with Sjögren syndrome. Other laboratory abnormalities include mild anemia, a decreased white blood cell count, an elevated erythrocyte sedimentation rate, and a diffuse elevation of serum immunoglobulins.

Diagnosis

The diagnosis of Sjögren syndrome is made when at least two of its three components are present: (1) xerostomia, (2) keratoconjunctivitis sicca, and (3) rheumatoid arthritis or another autoimmune disease. Laboratory findings supporting the diagnosis include positive Sjögren syndrome antibodies (SS-A, SS-B), positive rheumatoid factor (RF), or positive antinuclear antibodies (ANAs). Rheumatoid factor is present in up to 55% of patients with Sjögren syndrome, although they may not have rheumatoid arthritis. Xerostomia can result from conditions other than autoimmune disease, such as with many prescribed and over-the-counter medications. Measurement of stimulated and unstimulated salivary flow and biopsy of minor salivary glands of the lower lip can be helpful in the diagnosis of Sjögren syndrome. In addition, a characteristic pattern is seen in a parotid gland sialogram, with its pattern reflecting a lack of functioning glandular elements (Fig. 3.27).

Keratoconjunctivitis is confirmed by eye examination. Lacrimal flow is measured using filter paper (**Schirmer test**), but special examination techniques are necessary to demonstrate the corneal erosions.

Treatment and Prognosis

Sjögren syndrome is usually treated symptomatically. Nonsteroidal antiinflammatory agents are used for the arthritis; in severe cases corticosteroids and other immunosuppressive drugs may be necessary. Saliva substitutes are helpful, and for some patients the use of a humidifier at night makes the xerostomia more tolerable. Pilocarpine has been used to attempt to increase salivary flow in some patients. Sugarless gum or lozenges may be used to

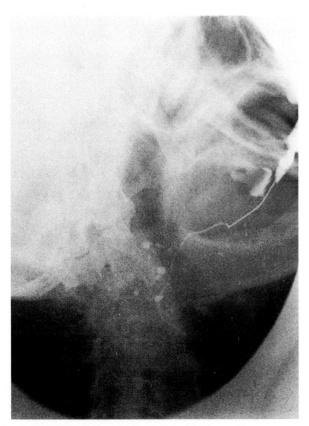

• **Figure 3.27** Sialogram of the parotid gland in Sjögren syndrome. (Courtesy Dr. Louis Mandel.)

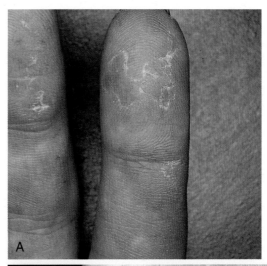

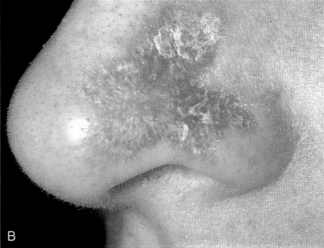

• **Figure 3.28** A and B, Skin lesions of systemic lupus erythematosus. (**B** courtesy Dr. Edward V. Zegarelli.)

stimulate saliva production. However, the greater the destruction of salivary gland tissue, the less saliva will be stimulated. An "artificial tears" formula containing methylcellulose helps to protect the eye from the drying effects of the disease. Glasses provide shielding and are helpful to minimize the drying effects of wind and air-conditioning.

Maintaining good oral hygiene and using oral lubricants and rinses can minimize the effects of xerostomia, as does the use of xylitol and remineralizing compounds such as MI paste™ (Recaldent), a paste with bioavailable calcium and phosphate. Fluoride rinses and toothpastes containing fluoride may help prevent caries. An electric toothbrush may help patients to more easily maintain optimum oral health care. The interval between recall appointments should be sufficiently short to ensure early detection and treatment of root caries.

For most patients the course of the disease is chronic and benign. However, patients are at risk for the development of other, more serious autoimmune diseases, such as lupus erythematosus, and for lymphoma and Waldenström macroglobulinemia, a disorder characterized by a high concentration of IgM in serum. Therefore patients with Sjögren syndrome should be closely monitored by a physician.

Systemic Lupus Erythematosus

Systemic lupus erythematosus is an acute and chronic inflammatory autoimmune disease of unknown cause. Genetics and environmental influences have been implicated in the pathogenesis of this disease.

Systemic lupus erythematosus affects women eight times more frequently than men, predominantly during the childbearing years. It occurs three times more frequently in black women than in white women. It is usually chronic and progressive, with periods of remission and exacerbation, and it is a syndrome rather than a specific disease entity. Systemic lupus erythematosus includes a wide spectrum of disease activity and signs and symptoms that range from lesions confined to the skin (discoid lupus erythematosus) to a widespread, debilitating, life-threatening disease with multiple organ involvement. Up to 50% of patients have kidney involvement, which can lead to kidney failure. Cardiac involvement includes pericarditis and valvular disease.

Both cellular and humoral immunity are impaired in systemic lupus erythematosus. The effect on cellular immunity results in the deregulation of humoral immunity. Antigen–antibody complexes are deposited in various organs and stimulate an inflammatory response, which may be responsible for the tissue damage that occurs in systemic lupus erythematosus. **Antiuclear antibodies (ANAs)**, which are autoantibodies to the patient's DNA, are present in serum. These circulating antibodies are responsible for the positive ANA test result. Production of these antibodies is enhanced by estrogen. Antibodies to lymphocytes are present in some patients. Skin lesions are among the most common signs of the disease (Fig. 3.28). The most common skin lesion is an erythematous rash involving areas of the body exposed to sunlight; the classic "butterfly" rash occurs over the bridge of the nose, and there may be erythematous lesions on the fingertips. The lesions can heal with scarring in the center as they continue to spread at the periphery. They tend to worsen when exposed to sunlight. Atrophy and hypopigmentation or hyperpigmentation can follow these lesions. Other skin lesions such as bullae, purpura, a discoid rash, vitiligo, or subcutaneous nodules can also occur.

Arthritis and arthralgia are common manifestations of systemic lupus erythematosus. Any joint can be involved. Symptoms resemble rheumatoid arthritis but without severe deformities. The Raynaud phenomenon occurs in 15% of patients. Myalgia and myositis (inflammation of muscle) also occur. A retinal vasculitis causes degeneration of the nerve fiber layer of the retina and can cause loss of vision. Psychoses and depression are signs of central nervous system (CNS) involvement, and seizures can be present. Involvement of the pleura may cause shortness of breath and chest pain. Pericarditis, cardiac arrhythmias, and endocarditis may be seen late in the disease. Kidney involvement is common. Thrombocytopenia may also occur in patients with systemic lupus erythematosus.

Oral lesions appear as erythematous plaques or erosions most commonly involving the buccal mucosa, palate, and gingiva. White striae radiating from the center of the lesion are usually present. The lesions may resemble lichen planus but are less symmetric in their distribution. The involvement of the oral mucosa in this disease is usually mild (Fig. 3.29). Petechiae and gingival bleeding may be present in patients with severe thrombocytopenia. Patients with systemic lupus erythematosus may develop other autoimmune diseases such as Sjögren syndrome and rheumatoid arthritis.

Diagnosis

The diagnosis of systemic lupus erythematosus is usually based on the classic multiorgan involvement and the presence of circulating antinuclear antibodies (ANAs) in serum. **LE cells,** mature neutrophils that have phagocytized spherical inclusions derived from other neutrophils, may be identified in circulating blood. However, the diagnosis of systemic lupus erythematosus is difficult if the onset is slow and insidious.

The microscopic appearance of oral lesions resembles that of lichen planus because it also involves destruction of the basal cells. However, the inflammatory infiltrate is distributed around blood vessels in the connective tissue rather than in a subepithelial band. Direct immunofluorescence and immunohistochemical testing of skin and mucosal lesions shows granular and linear deposits of immunoglobulins along the basement membrane area.

Treatment and Prognosis

Once the diagnosis of systemic lupus erythematosus is made, the decision as to whether treatment is indicated depends on the degree of disease activity. This once-fatal disease is now managed with several drugs. Aspirin and nonsteroidal antiinflammatory agents are used for mild signs and symptoms. Hydroxychloroquine, an antimalarial agent, and systemic corticosteroids combined with other immunosuppressive agents such as azathioprine and cyclophosphamide are also used. Topical corticosteroids may be used to treat oral lesions.

If the course of the disease is mild and only a few organs are involved, the prognosis is good; however, the disease can also be fatal. Kidney involvement can be associated with severe hypertension and rapid onset of renal failure, which is a cause of death in patients with systemic lupus erythematosus. Other common causes of death include hemorrhage secondary to thrombocytopenia, nervous system involvement, and infection.

Systemic lupus erythematosus is an extremely complex disease. A medical consultation may be needed before dental treatment to identify the extent of systemic involvement and to clarify which drugs may be used in dental treatment.

Pemphigus Vulgaris

Pemphigus vulgaris is a severe, progressive autoimmune disease that affects both the skin and mucous membranes. Pemphigus

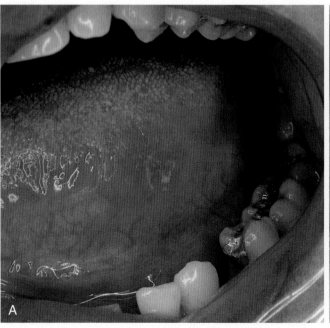
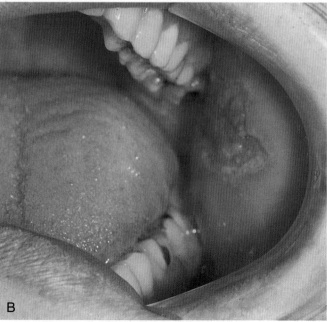

• **Figure 3.29** **A** and **B,** Oral lesions of systemic lupus erythematosus.

vulgaris is characterized by intraepithelial vesicle formation that results from breakdown of the cellular adhesion between epithelial cells. This type of epithelial cell separation is called **acantholysis.** The patient with pemphigus vulgaris has circulating autoantibodies that are reactive against components of the epithelial cell attachment mechanism. The higher the titer of circulating antibodies, the greater the epithelial destruction. These autoantibodies are also found in surrounding epithelial cells. *Pemphigus vulgaris* is the most common form of pemphigus. *Vulgaris* is Latin for "common" and when used in the name of a disease indicates the most common form. Three other forms of pemphigus are *pemphigus vegetans, pemphigus foliaceus,* and *pemphigus erythematosus.* These are much rarer conditions overall, but all are characterized by epithelial acantholysis (breakdown of cellular adhesion within the prickle cell layer of the epithelium). Only pemphigus vulgaris and pemphigus vegetans affect the oral mucosa; pemphigus vegetans is thought to be a variant of pemphigus vulgaris.

No gender predilection exists. A broad age range has been reported, including both children and elderly individuals, with most cases occurring after 50 years of age. The estimated prevalence of pemphigus vulgaris in the general population is 1 in 5 million. Genetic and ethnic factors have been reported; it is reported to be more prevalent among South Asian, Ashkenazi Jewish, and Mediterranean populations.

In more than 50% of cases of pemphigus vulgaris the first signs of disease occur in the oral cavity; oral lesions can precede cutaneous lesions by up to a year. The appearance of oral lesions ranges from shallow ulcers to fragile vesicles or bullae. Because the bullae are so fragile, they rupture soon after they form; the detached epithelium remains as a gray membrane (Fig. 3.30). The ulcers are painful and range in size from small to very large. Gentle finger pressure with movement on clinically normal mucosa or skin can produce a cleavage in the epithelium and result in the formation of a bulla. This is called the **Nikolsky sign.**

Skin lesions in pemphigus vulgaris include erythema, vesicles, bullae, erosions, and ulcers. Ocular involvement is rare. Microscopically, the tissue shows an intact basal layer of epithelium attached to the underlying connective tissue (Fig. 3.31). The loss of desmosomal attachments between the epithelial cells results in detached cells that appear rounded. These loose, rounded, acantholytic cells are **Tzanck cells** and are present in the area of

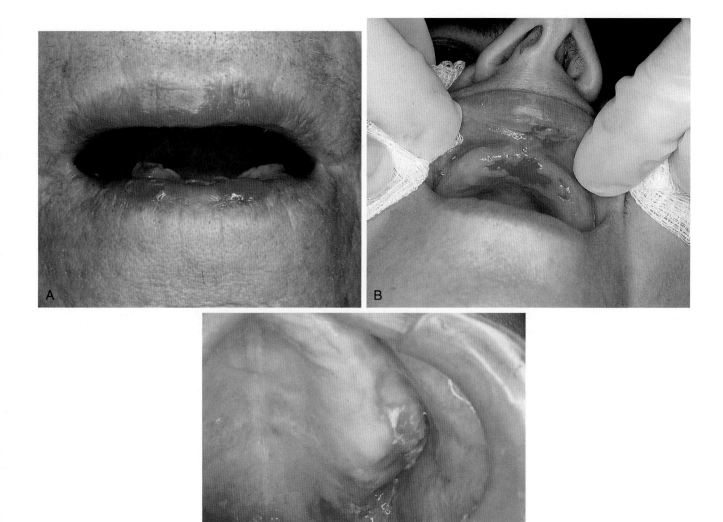

• **Figure 3.30** A to C, Oral lesions in pemphigus vulgaris. (**B** courtesy Dr. Fariba Younai; **C,** courtesy Dr. Sidney Eisig.)

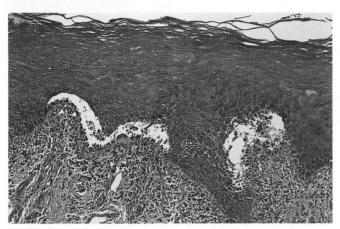

• **Figure 3.31** Microscopic appearance of pemphigus vulgaris (low magnification), showing acantholysis of the epithelium and the intact basal layer attached to the connective tissue.

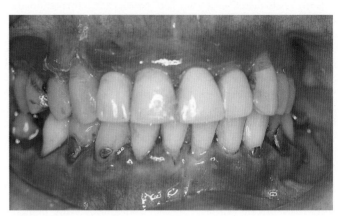

• **Figure 3.32** Desquamative gingivitis in mucous membrane pemphigoid. (Courtesy Dr. Victor M. Sternberg.)

separation. Tzanck cells may also be seen on cytologic smear, but the diagnosis must be confirmed by biopsy.

Diagnosis

The diagnosis of pemphigus vulgaris is made by biopsy and microscopic examinations. Direct or indirect immunofluorescence is also used in the diagnosis. Direct immunofluorescence is performed on biopsy tissue obtained from perilesional, normal-appearing mucosa and identifies autoantibodies present in the tissue. The tissue is viewed through a special microscope, with fluorescence seen surrounding the cells in the prickle cell layer. The tissue must be placed in a different fixative solution than tissue submitted for routine microscopic examination, and is usually sent to a specialized laboratory. In indirect immunofluorescence the patient's serum is used to detect the presence of circulating autoantibodies. These circulating autoantibodies are present in 80% of patients with pemphigus vulgaris, and therefore this is a very useful diagnostic test for this disease.

Treatment and Prognosis

The treatment of pemphigus vulgaris generally involves high doses of systemic corticosteroids, often in combination with other immunosuppressive drugs such as azathioprine and methotrexate. The amount of autoantibodies present in the patient's serum correlates with the severity of lesions; therefore the concentration (titer) of autoantibodies is used to determine disease activity and response to the drug therapy.

Pemphigus vulgaris was at one time a life-threatening disease. The mortality rate is now about 8% to 10% within the first 5 years and is related to the complications of corticosteroid treatment rather than to the disease itself. Long-term adverse effects of systemic corticosteroid treatment include adrenal suppression, peptic ulcers, susceptibility to infection, osteoporosis, and kidney disease. As with other autoimmune diseases, patients with pemphigus vulgaris may develop another autoimmune disease. Patients with pemphigus vulgaris should be under the care of a physician who specializes in immunosuppressive therapy.

Mucous Membrane Pemphigoid

Mucous membrane pemphigoid, also known as **cicatricial pemphigoid** and **benign mucous membrane pemphigoid,** is a chronic autoimmune disease that affects the oral mucosa, conjunctiva, genital mucosa, and skin. Mucous membrane pemphigoid is twice as common in women compared with men, is most frequently diagnosed in women over 50 years of age, and is not as severe a disease as pemphigus vulgaris. The name *cicatricial pemphigoid* refers to healing of the lesions with scarring. The most significant complication of mucous membrane pemphigoid is eye involvement. Scarring of lesions involving the conjunctiva result in adhesions between the lining of the globe of the eye and the conjunctiva. These adhesions are called **symblepharons**. Oral lesions rarely result in scarring. Autoantibodies and complement components have been identified in mucous membrane pemphigoid at the basement membrane of the epithelium; lesions occur as a result of cleavage of the epithelium from the underlying connective tissue.

Oral mucosal lesions in mucous membrane pemphigoid appear as vesicles or bullae that, unlike the lesions of pemphigus vulgaris, may be intact because the epithelium is not as friable as in pemphigus vulgaris. Oral lesions of mucous membrane pemphigoid are frequently limited to the gingiva. The gingival lesions have been called *desquamative gingivitis* (Fig. 3.32). The appearance ranges from erythema to ulceration and involves both the marginal and attached gingiva. *Desquamative gingivitis* is a clinical and descriptive term, and similar lesions can be seen in lichen planus and pemphigus vulgaris. In this disease, as in pemphigus vulgaris, a Nikolsky sign can be produced on normal-appearing tissue by gentle friction. Bullae, erosions, and ulcers can also occur in other locations in the oral cavity. The bullae of mucous membrane pemphigoid are thick walled, much less fragile, and persist longer than those of pemphigus vulgaris.

Diagnosis

The diagnosis of mucous membrane pemphigoid is made by biopsy and microscopic examination. On microscopic examination the epithelium appears to separate from the connective tissue at the basement membrane, with no degeneration of the basal cells of the epithelium as in lichen planus or acantholysis as in pemphigus vulgaris (Fig. 3.33). An inflammatory infiltrate, usually including prominent plasma cells and eosinophils, is seen in the connective tissue. In mucous membrane pemphigoid, direct immunofluorescence shows a linear pattern of fluorescence at the basement membrane. Indirect immunofluorescence, identifying

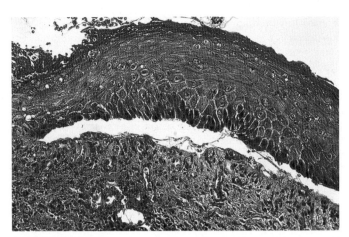

• **Figure 3.33** Microscopic appearance of mucous membrane pemphigoid (low magnification), showing a separation of the epithelium from the connective tissue at the basement membrane area.

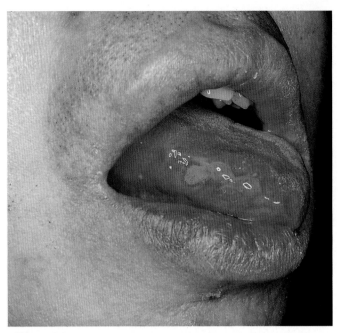

• **Figure 3.34** Aphthous-like ulcer on the tongue in Behçet syndrome.

autoantibodies in serum, is usually not helpful in the diagnosis of mucous membrane pemphigoid.

Treatment and Prognosis

Mucous membrane pemphigoid is a chronic disease that follows a benign course. Topical corticosteroid application is helpful in the management of mild cases. Trays can be fabricated to carry the corticosteroid medication in order to treat gingival lesions. Systemic medications include dapsone and combinations of tetracyclines (minocyline, doxycycline) and niacinamide. In more severe cases, high doses of systemic corticosteroids (e.g., prednisone) and other immunosuppressive agents may be needed. The disease may be difficult to control and slow to respond to therapy. Patients may experience episodes of exacerbation followed by periods of remission.

Bullous Pemphigoid

Some investigators have suggested that bullous and mucous membrane pemphigoid are variants of a single disease. However, differences exist between the two diseases that make this inference questionable.

Most patients with bullous pemphigoid are older than age 70, and no gender predilection exists. Oral lesions are less common in bullous pemphigoid than in mucous membrane pemphigoid, occurring in only about one third of patients. When they occur, the gingival lesions are very similar to those of mucous membrane pemphigoid, and other mucosal lesions are more extensive and painful.

Diagnosis

As in mucous membrane pemphigoid, the microscopic appearance of bullous pemphigoid shows a cleavage of the epithelium from the connective tissue at the basement membrane. Unlike mucous membrane pemphigoid, in bullous pemphigoid circulating autoantibodies are usually detectable; and unlike pemphigus vulgaris, the circulating autoantibodies do not correlate with disease activity.

Treatment and Prognosis

High doses of systemic corticosteroids and NSAIDs are used in the management of bullous pemphigoid. The disease is chronic, with periods of remission, unlike mucous membrane pemphigoid in which the lesions are more chronic and progressive. The disease is usually not life threatening. The risk of serious problems is generally related to the immunosuppressive medications.

Behçet Syndrome (Behçet Disease)

Behçet syndrome (**Behçet disease**) is a chronic, recurrent, and multisystem autoimmune disease. The manifestations of the syndrome are due to systemic vasculitis. The pathogenesis is unclear, but the disease is thought to represent an abnormal immune response that is triggered by an infectious or environmental antigen. Oral ulcers, genital ulcers, and ocular inflammation are common manifestations of the syndrome, which also includes skin lesions, gastrointestinal and genitourinary disease, arthritis, and central nervous system involvement. Evidence for an immunologic pathogenesis includes the identification of antibodies to human mucosa in patients with Behçet syndrome and the association between Behçet syndrome and HLA-B51.

Behçet syndrome emerges in patients between 30 and 40 years of age. There is an increased prevalence of this syndrome in individuals from the Middle Eastern and Mediterranean countries and Asia. Large epidemiologic studies suggest that the sex distribution is about equal. However, a male predominance is reported in Middle Eastern and Mediterranean countries and a female predominance in Japan and Korea. Behçet syndrome is rare in the United States.

Mucocutaneous lesions are the hallmark of the syndrome. Oral ulcers are present in almost all patients with Behçet syndrome (91% to 100%). The oral ulcers that occur in Behçet syndrome are painful and recurrent and very similar in appearance to minor aphthous ulcers (Fig. 3.34). They are surrounded by a larger area of erythema than classic aphthous ulcers. Ulcers resembling major and herpetiform aphthous ulcers have also been reported. Genital ulcers occur in 57% to 93% of patients. They are usually small and do not recur as often as oral ulcers. In males the scrotum is most commonly affected; the vulva and vagina in females. Ocular lesions usually begin with photophobia and can develop into conjunctivitis and uveitis. The skin lesions show a papular pattern of pustules and are most common on the trunk, genitals, and limbs.

Diagnosis

There is no laboratory finding that is diagnostic of Behçet syndrome. Criteria for diagnosis include recurrent oral ulceration plus two of the following: recurrent genital ulceration, eye lesions, skin lesions, or a positive pathergy test. The **pathergy test** is most useful in Middle Eastern patients. The test involves inserting a sterile needle under the skin. A raised erythematous area or a pustule develops within 1 to 2 days.

Treatment and Prognosis

Systemic and topical corticosteroids, as well as immunosuppressive drugs, are used in the management of Behçet syndrome. Chlorambucil is used for the ocular lesions; occasionally other immunosuppressive drugs are needed. Behçet disease is a lifelong disorder with a series of remissions and exacerbations. CNS involvement may result in paralysis or dementia. The prognosis is poor for patients with CNS involvement.

Immunodeficiency

Immunodeficiency can involve various components of the immune system, either alone or together. It can involve the cell-mediated (T-cell) response or the humoral (B-cell or antibody) response. Deficiencies in phagocytosis are also considered deficiencies in immunity. Immunodeficiency diseases are divided into primary and secondary immunodeficiencies. Primary immunodeficiencies are those of genetic origin; secondary immunodeficiencies result from an underlying disorder. The signs and symptoms that occur in a person with immunodeficiency depend on the degree of the deficiency and the type of immune response involved. The most common complication arising in persons with either primary or secondary immunodeficiency is infection. The type of infection is related to the type of immunodeficiency. Individuals with deficiency in humoral immunity are more likely to develop bacterial infections; those with deficiency in cell-mediated immunity are more likely to develop viral infections, fungal infections, and infections by intracellular bacteria such as tuberculosis. Autoimmune diseases such as autoimmune-type thrombocytopenia and neoplasms such as lymphoma may also be associated with certain immunodeficiencies.

Primary Immunodeficiencies

Primary immunodeficiencies are immunodeficiencies of genetic or developmental origin and can involve B cells, T cells, or both. These primary immunodeficiencies have provided much information about the functions of the different immunologic responses and are extremely rare. The following are several examples of primary immunodeficiencies.

Isolated IgA deficiency is the most common primary immunodeficiency. It affects about 1/500 individuals, primarily of European ancestry. It is much rarer among individuals of African or Asian ancestry. It is characterized by low levels of both serum and secretory IgA. There is impaired differentiation of B lymphocytes to IgA-producing plasma cells. As a result individuals with this deficiency are susceptible to respiratory, gastrointestinal, and genitourinary infection. They have an increased risk of respiratory allergy, systemic lupus erythematosus, and RA.

X-linked congenital agammaglobulinemia, also called **Bruton disease,** is a disorder in which B-cell precursors stop maturing before they complete immunoglobulin gene development. B-cell lymphocyte precursors in bone marrow are normal, but plasma cells are deficient throughout the body. As a result there is a lack of immunoglobulins produced; T cells are normal. This immunodeficiency occurs almost entirely in males, and the signs of the deficiency become evident at about 6 months of age. Babies with this immunodeficiency develop bacterial infections and gastrointestinal viral infections.

Thymic hypoplasia, also called **DiGeorge syndrome,** is a disorder in which the thymus is deficient or lacking; therefore T lymphocytes do not mature. There is a low number of T-cell lymphocytes circulating in blood, and T-cell areas of lymph nodes and the spleen are depleted. B-cell lymphocytes and their ability to mature to plasma cells and produce immunoglobulins are not affected; however, the T-helper cell increases the functioning of the B cell, enhancing the antibody response produced by the plasma cell. Infants and children with this syndrome are extremely susceptible to fungal and viral infections and bacterial infections that require T-cell and B-cell cooperation.

Severe combined immunodeficiency is a group of genetically inherited syndromes that have defects in both humoral (B-cell) and cell-mediated (T-cell) immune responses. Infants with these syndromes present with recurrent, severe infections by a wide range of pathogens. In the past, most infants with this type of immunodeficiency died within the first year of life. Bone marrow transplant has dramatically improved survival.

Leukocyte adhesion deficiency is a primary immunodeficiency characterized by defects in function of neutrophils. The neutrophils are not able to migrate (chemotaxis) and are not able to phagocytose and destroy bacteria. This results in persistent bacterial infections, including gingival and periodontal infection.

Secondary Immunodeficiencies

Secondary immunodeficiencies are those that occur as a result of an underlying disorder. They are much more common than the primary immunodeficiency disorders. Immunodeficiencies occur with the use of **immunosuppressive drugs,** including corticosteroids; drugs that are used, along with radiation, to suppress the immune system in organ and bone marrow transplantation; drugs that are used to treat autoimmune diseases; and drugs used for cancer chemotherapy. Table 3.6 lists some of the most common drugs that can cause immunodeficiency and the reasons they are generally used. Disorders that can have accompanying immunodeficiency include **malnutrition,** which can lead to inadequate synthesis of antibodies; **renal diseases** in which antibodies are excreted abnormally; and **HIV infection** (described in detail in Chapter 4), which affects the number and function of T-helper (CD4) lymphocytes, DCs, and macrophages. In patients with **diabetes mellitus** (described in detail in Chapter 9), T-cell lymphocyte function and neutrophil function are depressed. Taking a patient's medical history is important in identifying potential secondary immunodeficiencies.

TABLE 3.6   Examples of Drugs That Can Cause Immunosuppression

Name	Use
Azathioprine	Prevention of rejection of renal transplants Treatment of rheumatoid arthritis
Cyclosporine	Prevention of rejection of renal transplants
Cyclophosphamide	Cancer chemotherapy
Methotrexate	Cancer chemotherapy
Prednisone	Treatment of allergic diseases, inflammatory diseases (arthritis), autoimmune diseases (such as rheumatoid arthritis, pemphigus vulgaris, Behçet syndrome, lupus erythematosus); also used as a component of cancer chemotherapy

Selected References

Books

Fehrenbach MJ, Herring SW: *Illustrated anatomy of the head and neck*, ed 5, St. Louis, 2017, Elsevier.

Fehrenbach MJ, Popowics T: *Illustrated dental embryology, histology, and anatomy*, ed 4, St. Louis, 2016, Elsevier.

Fehrenbach MJ, Weiner J: *Saunders review of dental hygiene*, ed 2, St. Louis, 2009, Saunders.

Kumar V, Abbus AK, Aster JC: *Robbins and Cotran pathologic basis of disease*, ed 4, St. Louis, 2015, Saunders.

Kumar V, Cotran RS, Robbins SL: *Robbins basic pathology*, ed 9, Philadelphia, 2013, Saunders.

McCance K, Huether S: *Pathophysiology*, ed 6, St. Louis, 2010, Mosby.

McCance K, Huether S: *Pathophysiology*, ed 7, St. Louis, 2014, Mosby.

Neville BW, Damm DD, Allen CM, et al: *Oral and maxillofacial pathology*, ed 4, St. Louis, 2016, Elsevier.

Regezi JA, Sciubba JJ, Jordan RCK: *Oral pathology: clinical pathologic correlations*, ed 7, St. Louis, 2017, Elsevier.

Parham P: *The immune system*, ed 4, New York, 2015, Garland Science.

Journal Articles

Immunity

Chaplin DD: Overview of the human immune response, *J Allergy Clin Immunol* 125(2 Suppl 2):S3, 2010.

Grivennikov SI, Greten FR, Karin M: Immunity, inflammation, and cancer, *Cell* 140:883, 2010.

Hovav A-H: Dendritic cells of the oral mucosa, *Mucosal Immunol* 7(1):27, 2014.

Ledford H: Cancer treatment: The killer within, *Nature* 508(7494):24–26, 2014.

Pradeu T, Jaeger S, Vivier E: The speed of change: towards a discontinuity theory of immunity?, *Nat Rev Immunol* 13(10):764, 2013.

Immunologic Oral Lesions

Adizie T, Moots B, Hodkinson B, et al: Inflammatory arthritis in HIV positive patients: a practical guide, *BMC Infect Dis* 16:100, 2016.

Al-Johani KA, Fedele S, Porter SR: Erythema multiforme and related disorders, *Oral Surg Oral Med Oral Pathol Oral Radiol Endod* 103:642, 2007.

Belenguer-Guallar I, Jiménez-Soriano Y, Claramunt-Lozano A: Treatment of recurrent aphthous stomatitis. A literature review, *J Clin Exp Dent* 6:168, 2014.

Bosch X: Systemic lupus erythematosus and the neutrophil, *N Engl J Med* 365:758, 2011.

Calapai G, Miroddi M, Mannucci C, et al: Oral adverse reactions due to cinnamon-flavoured chewing gums consumption, *Oral Dis* 20:637, 2014.

Celenano A, Tovaro S, Yap T, et al: Oral erythema multiforme: trends and clinical findings of a large retrospective European case series, *Oral Surg Oral Med Oral Pathol Oral Radiol* 120:707, 2015.

Chavan M, Jain H, Diwan N, et al: Recurrent aphthous stomatitis: a review, *J Oral Pathol Med* 418:577, 2012.

Epstein JB, Wan LS, Gorsky M, et al: Oral lichen planus: progress in understanding its malignant potential and the implications for clinical management, *Oral Surg Oral Med Oral Pathol Oral Radiol Endod* 96:32, 2003.

Iwai S, Sueki H, Watanabe H, et al: Distinguishing between erythema multiforme major and Stevens-Johnson syndrome/toxic epidermal necrolysis immunopathologically, *J Dermatol* 39:1, 2012.

Jurge S, Kuffer R, Scully C, et al: Recurrent aphthous stomatitis, *Oral Dis* 12:1, 2006.

Mockenhaupt M: The current understanding of Stevens-Johnson syndrome and toxic epidermal necrolysis, *Expert Rev Clin Immunol* 7:803, 2011.

Rohekar S, Pope J: Epidemiologic approaches to infection and immunity: the case of reactive arthritis, *Curr Opin Rheumatol* 21:14, 2009.

Tasher D, Somekh E, Dalal I: PFAPA syndrome: new clinical aspects disclosed, *Arch Dis Child* 91:981, 2006.

van der Meij EH, Mast H, van der Waal I: The possible premalignant character of oral lichen planus and oral lichnoid lesions: a prospective five-year follow-up study of 192 patients, *Oral Oncol* 43(8):742, 2007.

Wolf R, Lipozencic J: Shape and configuration of skin lesions: targetoid lesions, *Clin Dermatol* 29:504, 2011.

Websites

Centers for Disease Control and Prevention: Frequently asked questions about multiple vaccinations and the immune system. Available at http://www.cdc.gov/vaccinesafety/Vaccines/multiplevaccines.html.

Review Questions

1. The immune system usually defends the body against foreign substances that are called:
   a. Plasma cells
   b. Antibodies
   c. Antigens
   d. Lymphocytes

2. Memory is an important function of the immune system because it:
   a. Retains the memory of the antibody
   b. Allows faster future immune responses
   c. Allows faster inflammatory responses
   d. Weakens future immune responses

3. Immunization with a vaccine works by:
   a. Increasing the risk of an antigen-causing disease
   b. Using antibodies produced by another person
   c. Passing antibodies from the mother to the fetus
   d. Producing active acquired immunity

4. Which of the following statements is an important fact concerning the B-cell lymphocyte?
   a. It has CD4 receptors on its surface.
   b. It matures and resides in the thymus.
   c. It is produced from plasma cells.
   d. It is derived from a hematopoietic stem cell.

5. A macrophage is a cell of the immune system that:
   a. Retains a memory of an encountered antigen
   b. Produces antibodies
   c. Undergoes   B-cell   phagocytosis   initially   during inflammation
   d. Can be activated by lymphokines

6. Which statement is *correct* when applied to natural killer cells?
   a. They do not circulate within the body.
   b. They secrete antibodies.
   c. They are part of the body's innate immunity.
   d. They are a type of T-cell lymphocyte.

7. In which type of immunopathology are the cells of the body *no* longer tolerated and treated by the immune system as antigens?
   a. Hypersensitivity
   b. Immunodeficiency
   c. Hyperplasia
   d. Autoimmune disease

8. During the anaphylactic type of hypersensitivity reaction, the plasma cells:
   a. Produce antibody called IgE
   b. React with lymphocytes
   c. Combine with antigen
   d. Form immune complexes with antigen

9. Which type of hypersensitivity reaction involves activated complement?
   a. Type I
   b. Cytotoxic
   c. Type III
   d. Anaphylactic

10. What type of lymphocyte matures in the thymus, produces lymphokines, and can increase or suppress humoral immunity?
    a. T-cell lymphocyte
    b. Plasma cell
    c. Natural killer cell
    d. Macrophage

11. In the immune system, antibodies are:
    a. Also called immunoglobulins
    b. Also called cytokines
    c. Directly produced by lymphocytes
    d. Directly produced from mast cells

12. Which of the following types of immunologic disease involve either a decreased number or activity of lymphoid cells?
    a. Autoimmune
    b. Hypersensitivity
    c. Immunodeficiency
    d. Reactive hyperplasia

13. Humoral immunity involves the production of:
    a. Antigens
    b. Antibodies
    c. Autoimmune cells
    d. Toxins

14. The diagnostic laboratory measurement of antibody level in the blood is called:
    a. Phagocytosis
    b. Immunization
    c. Titer
    d. Pavementing

15. Which type of immunity may be provided immediately to dental personnel after needlestick accidents?
    a. Natural passive immunity
    b. Acquired passive immunity
    c. Natural active immunity
    d. Acquired active immunity

16. Which of the following situations would result in the *least* risk of drug allergy?
    a. Application of topical medication
    b. Presence of infection
    c. Presence of multiple allergies
    d. Use with children

17. Which of the following is involved in the regulation of *both* humoral and cell-mediated immunity?
    a. Humoral immunity
    b. Cell-mediated immunity
    c. Innate immunity
    d. Bone marrow cells

18. Which of the following is involved in the communication between lymphocytes within the immune system?
    a. Histamine
    b. Complement
    c. Bradykinin
    d. Cytokines

19. Which one of the following types of hypersensitivity reactions can also be referred to as *delayed hypersensitivity*?
    a. Type I
    b. Type II
    c. Type III
    d. Type IV

20. Which of the following statements concerning the dendritic cell is considered correct?
    a. It is found in an immature state within tears.
    b. It is a specialized type in oral mucosa called a Langerhans cell.
    c. It is similar to lymphocytes in morphology and function.
    d. It interacts only with macrophages during the immune response.

21. What marker does the T-cytotoxic cell carry?
    a. CD4
    b. CD8
    c. C-reactive protein
    d. IgG

22. Which of the general types of immunoglobulin is a *major* antibody found in blood serum and serves as the first passive immunity for the newborn?
    a. IgA
    b. IgD
    c. IgG
    d. IgM

23. Which one of the following is the *most* common cause of serum sickness?
    a. Aspirin
    b. Antihistamines
    c. Corticosteroids
    d. Penicillin

24. Which type of IgA is present in *both* tears and saliva?
    a. Purulent
    b. Serous
    c. Secretory
    d. Reactive

25. What type of hypersensitivity reaction is involved in a fixed drug eruption when it occurs in the oral cavity?
    a. Type I
    b. Type II
    c. Type III
    d. Type IV

26. Which is one of the important factors for safety when using a live vaccine?
    a. Heat stable
    b. Attenuated
    c. Virulence
    d. Synthetic peptides

27. Which of the following descriptions is *correct* when used to describe cytokines?
    a. Affect only nephrons within the kidneys
    b. Include both lymphokines and monokines
    c. Administered parenterally with asthma attacks
    d. Produced in the liver in response to low serum levels

28. Which of the following cells is *not* known to function as an antigen-presenting cell within the immune system?
    a. T-cell lymphocytes
    b. B-cell lymphocytes
    c. Macrophages
    d. Dendritic cells

29. Which of the following can be considered *correct* when discussing interferon?
    a. Was only recently discovered by researchers
    b. Falls under the category of cytokines
    c. Can be produced by B-cell lymphocytes and macrophages
    d. As a protein has potent antibacterial properties

30. Many small molecules can function as haptens, which can be immunogenic in combination with larger molecules that function as:
    a. Boosters
    b. Monokines
    c. Immunoglobulins
    d. Carriers

31. All of the following are examples of hypersensitivity reactions *except:*
    a. Major aphthous ulcers
    b. Urticaria
    c. Angioedema
    d. Contact dermatitis and mucositis

32. Reactive arthritis is known for being:
    a. An infectious disease
    b. An immunodeficiency disease
    c. An immunologic disorder
    d. More common in women than in men

33. A target lesion on the skin is associated with which of the following diseases?
    a. Behçet syndrome
    b. Systemic lupus erythematosus
    c. Lichen planus
    d. Erythema multiforme

34. Tzanck cells are seen in which of the following conditions?
    a. Pemphigus vulgaris
    b. Erythema multiforme
    c. Systemic lupus erythematosus
    d. Behçet syndrome

35. The oral lesions in Reiter syndrome may resemble:
    a. Pemphigus vulgaris
    b. Lichen planus
    c. Angioedema
    d. Erythema migrans

36. Aphthous ulcers are seen in all of the following systemic diseases *except:*
    a. Behçet syndrome
    b. Langerhans cell histiocytosis
    c. Ulcerative colitis
    d. Cyclic neutropenia

37. The two cell types that microscopically characterize Langerhans cell histiocytosis are:
    a. Lymphocytes and plasma cells
    b. Fibroblasts and lymphocytes
    c. Eosinophils and mononuclear cells
    d. Neutrophils and lymphocytes

38. Which one of the following is the name of the solitary bone lesion of Langerhans cell histiocytosis that may occur in the mandible?
    a. Pyogenic granuloma
    b. Eosinophilic granuloma
    c. Periapical granuloma
    d. Traumatic granuloma

39. All of the following are traditional categories of Langerhans cell histiocytosis except one. Which one is the exception?
    a. Hand-Schüller-Christian disease
    b. Chronic disseminated reticulosis
    c. Letterer-Siwe disease
    d. Eosinophilic granuloma

40. The *most* characteristic oral manifestation of Sjögren syndrome is:
    a. Xerostomia
    b. Erythema migrans
    c. Erythema multiforme
    d. Acute disseminated reticulosis

41. Which of the following statements about autoimmune disease with oral manifestations is *false?*
    a. The bullae in pemphigus vulgaris are more fragile than those in bullous pemphigoid.
    b. Acantholysis of the epithelium is seen in pemphigus vulgaris.
    c. In pemphigoid the separation of the epithelium from the connective tissue occurs at the basement membrane.
    d. Skin lesions are common in mucous membrane pemphigoid.

42. Which is the *most* distinct and definitive characteristic that distinguishes pemphigus from pemphigoid?
    a. Size of the ulcerations
    b. Age and gender of the patient
    c. The histopathologic findings
    d. Nikolsky sign

43. Desquamative gingivitis may be present in all of the following *except:*
    a. Cicatricial pemphigoid
    b. Pemphigus vulgaris
    c. Lichen planus
    d. Aggressive periodontal disease

44. Which of the following orofacial structures could create a life-threatening situation for the patient from angioedema involvement?
    a. Lips
    b. Mucosa
    c. Eyelids
    d. Epiglottis

45. Which of the following is a pathologic condition producing a characteristic butterfly-shaped lesion on the face and oral ulcers, occurs more frequently in females than males, and for which the result of a blood test is important in its diagnosis?
    a. Pemphigus
    b. Erosive lichen planus
    c. Desquamative gingivitis
    d. Lupus erythematosus

46. Which one of the following is involved in the Raynaud phenomenon?
    a. Kidney tissue
    b. Ocular components
    c. Fingers and toes
    d. Joints

47. Which of the following can be used in the management of herpetiform ulcerations?
    a. Laser nephelometer
    b. Topical tetracycline
    c. Rheumatoid factor
    d. Rh incompatibility

48. What is the *most* common location for Wickham striae in the intraoral region?
    a. Dorsal surface of tongue
    b. Floor of mouth
    c. Buccal mucosa
    d. Vermilion border

49. Which of the following statements is *false?*
    a. All primary immunodeficiencies are combined B-lymphocyte and T-lymphocyte deficiencies.
    b. Primary immunodeficiencies are less common than secondary immunodeficiencies.
    c. Persons with T-lymphocyte deficiencies are susceptible to viral and fungal infections.
    d. Secondary immunodeficiency can result from corticosteroid medication.

50. Which of the following conditions is very serious and can be life threatening if untreated?
    a. Pemphigus vulgaris
    b. Contact dermatitis
    c. Necrotizing sialometaplasia
    d. Eosinophilic granuloma

51. Sawtooth-shaped epithelial rete ridges, degeneration of the basal cells of the epithelium, and a bandlike infiltrate of lymphocytes in the connective tissue subjacent to the epithelium are classic histopathologic features of:
    a. Erythema multiforme minor
    b. Benign mucous membrane pemphigoid
    c. Pemphigus vulgaris
    d. Lichen planus

52. Acantholysis and Tzanck cells are associated with which condition?
    a. Pemphigus vulgaris
    b. Aphthous ulcers
    c. Erythema multiforme
    d. Mucous membrane pemphigoid

Chapter 3 Synopsis

Condition/Disease	Cause	Age/Race/Gender	Location
Minor aphthous ulcers *Major aphthous* *Herpetiform aphthous ulcers*	Unclear immunologic pathogenesis involving cell-mediated immunity Trauma is most common precipitating factor	More common in younger than older individuals Affects women more than men	Oral mucosa not covering bone Anterior more than posterior
Major aphthous ulcers (Sutton disease) *Erythema multiforme* *Pemhigus vulgaris*	Unclear immunologic pathogenesis involving cell-mediated immunity	*	Oral mucosa not covering bone Often occur in the posterior oral cavity
Herpetiform aphthous ulcers *Herpes simplex ulcers* *Minor aphthous ulcers*	Unclear immunologic pathogenesis involving cell-mediated immunity	*	Anywhere in the oral cavity
Urticaria (hives) *Angioedema* *Contact dermatitis*	Type I hypersensitivity Release of IgG, IgM—often in response to ingested allergen Infection, trauma, and emotional stress are also associated with urticaria Localized vascular permeability in superficial connective tissue	*	Skin
Angioedema *Urticaria*	Type I hypersensitivity Trauma, release of IgG or IgM Permeability of deeper blood vessels	*	Skin or mucosa
Contact mucositis *Urticaria* *Aphthous ulcers*	Direct contact of allergen with mucosa	*	Mucosa in contact with allergen
Contact dermatitis	Direct contact of allergen with skin	*	Skin in contact with allergen
Fixed drug eruptions *Contact dermatitis*	Type III hypersensitivity	*	Same site each episode Usually skin Occasionally oral mucosa
Erythema multiforme *Aphthous ulcers* *Primary herpes simplex infection*	Unclear: evidence for hypersensitivity reaction that in some cases may be associated with infectious agents, such as a herpesvirus infection	Most frequent in young adults Affects men more than women	Skin and mucous membranes
Stevens-Johnson syndrome (a variant of toxic epidermal necrolysis)	Drug exposure from multiple medications	Younger adults	Primarily skin; mucous membranes

NOTE: Items listed in *italics* under a specific condition/disease should be considered in a differential diagnosis.
ASA, Acetylsalicylic acid (aspirin); N/A, not applicable.
*No significant information.
†See reference materials.

Clinical Features	Radiographic Features	Microscopic Features	Treatment	Diagnostic Process
Painful, discrete, round to oval, yellowish-white ulcers Halo of erythema Up to 1 cm in diameter Spontaneous healing in 7-10 d	N/A	Ulcer with lymphocytic infiltrate	Topical corticosteroids	Clinical
Painful Greater than 1 cm in diameter Often deeper than minor aphthous ulcers May last several weeks Often heal with scarring	N/A	May require biopsy for diagnosis to rule out other causes of ulceration	Topical or systematic corticosteroids Biopsy to rule out ulceration from other cause	Clinical Microscopic
Painful, small 1- to 2-mm ulcers Often occur in groups Resolve spontaneously	N/A	Unclear	Topical corticosteroids Topical tetracycline	Clinical
Multiple areas of well-demarcated swelling accompanied by itching (pruritus) Self-limiting episodes	N/A	†	Identification and avoidance of causative agent Antihistaminic drugs	Clinical
Diffuse swelling of tissue Usually no itching Self-limiting episodes	N/A	†	Identification of causative agent Antihistaminic drugs	Clinical
Smooth, shiny, firm mucosa with erythema and edema May form vesicles Often an itching or burning sensation is present	N/A	†	Identification of causative agent Topical and systemic corticosteroids	Clinical
Erythema Swelling vesicles to encrusted, scaly, white appearance	N/A	†	Identification of causative agent Topical and systemic corticosteroids	Clinical
Lesions appear when drug is introduced and subside when drug is discontinued with increasing intensity Single- to-multiple raised, reddish patches or clusters of macules Pain/pruritus may be present	N/A	†	Identification and discontinuation of causative drug	Clinical
Skin: characteristic target lesions; also macules, plaques, bullae Mucosa: erythema; ulcers; crusted, bleeding lips Explosive onset Minor and major types depending on degree of tissue and skin involvement	N/A	Nonspecific	Identification of causative agent if possible Topical/systemic corticosteroids	Clinical
Skin: Less than 10% of body affected with lesions; erythematous macules on trunk of body Flu-like prodromal symptoms	N/A	Subepithelial blisters; necrosis of basal keratinocytes; few inflammatory cells in connective tissue	Discontinue the drug that was most likely the cause	Clinical Microscopic

Continued

Chapter 3 Synopsis—cont'd

Condition/Disease	Cause	Age/Race/Gender	Location
Lichen planus	Unknown	Broad age range Increased prevalence in middle age Male/Female predominance not consistent among different studies	Skin and oral mucosal lesions Oral mucosa: buccal mucosa, tongue, labial mucosa, floor of mouth, gingiva
Reactive arthritis (Reiter syndrome) *Erythema migrans* *Erythema multiforme*	Abnormal immunologic response to infectious agent Genetic influence: presence of HLA-B27	Affects men much more than women (10 to 15:1)	Conjunctiva Urethra Oral mucosa Skin Knee and ankle joints
Langerhans cell histiocytosis (Langerhans cell disease) *Chronic periodontitis*	Unclear: suggestive reactive process, immunologic disease, neoplastic process		
Acute disseminated form (Letterer-Siwe disease)		Affects children under 3 years of age	Disseminated disease
Chronic disseminated multifocal form (Hand-Schüller-Christian disease)		Affects children under 5 years of age	Multiple locations
Solitary (chronic) localized form (eosinophilic granuloma)	Unclear: suggested reactive process, immunologic disease, neoplastic process	Affects older children and young adults Affects males more than females (2:1)	Bone: skull and mandible are commonly involved
Sjögren syndrome *Drug-related xerostomia*	Autoimmune disease Decreased lacrimal flow Decreased salivary flow	*	Eyes Oral cavity
Systemic lupus erythematosus *Lichen planus* *Minor aphthous ulcers*	Autoimmune disease	Affects women more than men (8:1), blacks more than whites (3:1)	Multiple sites Skin Mucous membranes Joints Eyes Central nervous system Kidneys, heart, and other organs

NOTE: Items listed in *italics* under a specific condition/disease should be considered in a differential diagnosis.
ASA, Acetylsalicylic acid (aspirin); N/A, not applicable.
*No significant information.
†See reference materials.

Clinical Features	Radiographic Features	Microscopic Features	Treatment	Diagnostic Process
Oral lesions Wickham striae Erosive and plaquelike lesions may occur Gingival lesions: desquamative gingivitis	N/A	Degeneration of the basal layer of the epithelium Broad band of lymphocytes in the connective tissue subjacent to the epithelium	None if asymptomatic Topical corticosteroids if symptomatic Follow-up evaluation	Clinical Microscopic
Syndrome triad: arthritis, urethritis, conjunctivitis Skin lesions Oral lesions Aphthous-like ulcers Lesions resembling erythema migrans Erythematous lesions	N/A	†	ASA and nonsteroidal antiinflammatory drugs	Clinical
†	N/A	†	Chemotherapy Poor prognosis	Chemotherapy Poor prognosis
Classic triad: skull radiolucencies, exophthalmos, diabetes insipidus Oral: sore mouth with or without ulceration; halitosis; gingivitis; unpleasant taste; loose, sore teeth; early exfoliation of teeth	Radiolucencies ("punched-out" areas) of skull Maxilla/mandible radiolucencies, including alveolar bone	Infiltrate of Langerhans cells and eosinophils	†	Clinical Microscopic
N/A	Radiolucency may resemble periodontal disease or may be well-circumscribed radiolucency May be multifocal	Infiltrate of Langerhans cells and eosinophils	Conservative surgical excision Low-dose radiation treatment	Microscopic
Primary Sjögren syndrome: dry eyes (xerophthalmia), dry mouth (xerostomia) Secondary Sjögren syndrome: dry eyes (xerophthalmia), dry mouth (xerostomia) Along with another autoimmune disease	Sialogram shows characteristic features (see text)	Salivary gland changes: lymphocytic infiltration and epimyoepithelial islands	Xerostomia: saliva substitutes Saliva stimulation: pilocarpine	Clinical Radiographic Microscopic Laboratory
Oral lesions Erythematous plaques or erosions White striations radiating from center of lesion	N/A	Destruction of the basal layer of the epithelium with inflammatory infiltrate around blood vessels Immunohistochemical testing Granular and linear deposits of immunoglobulins along basement membrane zone	Antiinflammatory and immunosuppressive agents	Laboratory Microscopic Clinical

Continued

Chapter 3 Synopsis—cont'd

Condition/Disease	Cause	Age/Race/Gender	Location
Pemphigus vulgaris *Mucous membrane pemphigoid*	Autoimmune disease	Affects children and adults Most common in fourth to fifth decade More common in Ashkenazi Jews	Mucous membranes Skin
Mucous membrane pemphigoid (cicatricial pemphigoid, benign mucous membrane pemphigoid) *Lichen planus* *Pemphigus vulgaris*	Autoimmune disease	Adults	Mucous membranes Most common: gingival May affect eyes
Bullous pemphigoid *Pemphigus vulgaris*	Autoimmune disease	80% affected are over 60 yr	Mucous membranes Skin
Behçet syndrome *Minor aphthous ulcers*	Autoimmune disease	Mean age of onset, 30 yr	Mucous membranes Oral Genital Ocular
Primary Immunodeficiencies			
Isolated IgA deficiency	Developmental/low levels of serum and secretory IgA	Children/adults Primarily European ancestry	Systemic
X-linked congenital agammaglobulinemia (Bruton disease)	Developmental/congenital/B-cell precursors stop maturing	Infants/males	Systemic
Thymic hypoplasia (DiGeorge syndrome)	Developmental – Thymus is absent	Infants	Systemic
Severe combined immunodeficiency	Defects in both B-cell and T-cell immune responses	Infants	Systemic
Leukocyte adhesion deficiency	Defects in functions of neutrophils	Adults/children	Systemic
Secondary Immunodeficiencies			
HIV infection/AIDS	See Chapter 4		
Diabetes mellitus	See Chapter 9		
Immunosuppressive drugs	See Chapter 9		

NOTE: Items listed in *italics* under a specific condition/disease should be considered in a differential diagnosis.
ASA, Acetylsalicylic acid (aspirin); *N/A,* not applicable.
*No significant information.
†See reference materials.

Clinical Features	Radiographic Features	Microscopic Features	Treatment	Diagnostic Process
Progressive involvement of mucous membranes and skin Oral lesions Painful, erythema, vesicles, bullae, erosions Positive Nikolsky sign	N/A	Intact basal layer attached to the underlying connective tissue Acantholysis of the prickle cell layer Tzanck cells	Corticosteroids and other immunosuppressive agents	Laboratory Microscopic
Oral lesions Desquamative gingivitis Bullae, erosions, ulcers Lesions heal with scarring	N/A	Epithelium detaches from the connective tissue at the basement membrane	Topical/systemic corticosteroids	Microscopic
Oral lesions as in cicatricial pemphigoid but less common	N/A	Epithelium detaches from the connective tissue at the basement membrane	Systemic corticosteroids and other antiinflammatory agents	Microscopic
Oral lesions: aphthous-like ulcers	N/A	†	Corticosteroids and other immunosuppressive agents	Clinical
Respiratory, gastrointestinal, genitourinary infection	N/A	N/A	Not covered	Clinical Laboratory
Bacterial and gastrointestinal viral infections	N/A	N/A	Not covered	Clinical Laboratory
Fungal/viral infections Bacterial infections that require T/B cell cooperation	N/A	N/A	Not covered	Clinical Laboratory
Severe recurrent infections	N/A	N/A	Bone marrow transplant	Clinical Laboratory
Persistent bacterial infections, gingival and periodontal infection	Not covered	Not covered	Not covered	Clinical Laboratory

4

Infectious Diseases

JOAN ANDERSEN PHELAN

OBJECTIVES

After studying this chapter, the student will be able to:

1. Define each of the words in the vocabulary list for this chapter.
2. Describe the factors that allow opportunistic infections to develop, state the difference between an inflammatory and an immune response to infection, and list two examples of opportunistic infections that can occur in the oral cavity.
3. Do the following related to bacterial infections:
   - For each of the following infectious diseases, name the organism causing it, list the route or routes of transmission of the organism and the oral manifestations of the disease, and describe how the diagnosis is made: impetigo, tuberculosis, actinomycosis, syphilis (primary, secondary, tertiary), necrotizing ulcerative gingivitis, pericoronitis, and osteomyelitis (acute and chronic).
   - Describe the relationship between streptococcal tonsillitis, pharyngitis, scarlet fever, and rheumatic fever.
4. Do the following related to fungal infections:
   - List and describe four forms of oral candidiasis.
   - Discuss deep fungal infections.
   - Describe mucormycosis.
5. Do the following related to viral infections:
   - Discuss how a human papillomavirus (HPV) infection occurs.
   - List and describe the three benign lesions caused by HPV infections in the oral cavity: verruca vulgaris, condyloma acuminatum, and focal epithelial hyperplasia.

- Discuss the two major types of the herpes simplex virus.
- Describe the clinical features of herpes labialis.
- Describe the clinical features of recurrent intraoral herpes simplex infection and compare them with the clinical features of minor aphthous ulcers.
- Describe the clinical characteristics of herpes zoster when it affects the skin of the face and oral mucosa.
- List and describe four diseases associated with the Epstein-Barr virus.
- List and describe two diseases caused by coxsackieviruses that have oral manifestations, and state the routes of transmission of coxsackieviruses.
- Describe measles and mumps.
6. Do the following related to human immunodeficiency virus (HIV) and acquired immunodeficiency syndrome (AIDS):
   - Describe how HIV infection is diagnosed.
   - Describe the spectrum of HIV disease, including initial infection, latent infection, and the development and diagnosis of AIDS.
   - List and describe the clinical appearance of five oral manifestations of HIV infection.

❖ Vocabulary

Granuloma (gran″u-lo′mə) A tumorlike mass of inflammatory tissue consisting of a central collection of macrophages, often including multinucleated giant cells, surrounded by lymphocytes.

Granulomatous disease (gran″u-lom′ə-təs dĭ-zēz′) A disease characterized by the formation of granulomas.

Herpetic whitlow (hər-pe′tik hwit′lo) An infection caused by herpes simplex virus infection that involves the distal phalanx of a finger.

Incubation period (in″ku-ba′shən pe′re-od) The period between the infection of an individual by a pathogen and the manifestation of the disease it causes.

Malaise (mah-lāz′) A vague, indefinite feeling of discomfort, debilitation, or lack of health.

Nonpathogenic microorganisms (non-path-o-jen′ik mi″kro-or′gən-iz-əm) Microorganisms that do not cause disease.

Opportunistic infection (op″ər-too-nis′tik in-fek′shən) A disease caused by a microorganism that does not ordinarily cause disease but becomes pathogenic under certain circumstances.

Paresthesia (par″əs-the′zhə) An abnormal sensation such as burning, prickling, or tingling.

Pathogenic microorganism (path-o-jen′ik mi″kro-or′gən-iz-əm) A microorganism that causes disease.

Pruritus (proo-ri′təs) Itching.

Subclinical infection (səb-klin′i-kəl in-fek′shən) An infectious disease not detectable by the usual clinical signs.

Humans are surrounded and inhabited by an enormous number of microorganisms. The ability of these organisms to cause disease depends on both the microorganism and the state of the body's defenses. The organism must be capable of causing disease, and the individual must be susceptible to the disease. Microorganisms are traditionally divided into those that produce disease (**pathogenic microorganisms**) and those that do not (**nonpathogenic microorganisms**). To cause disease the organism must gain access to the body, accommodate to growth in the human environment, and avoid multiple host defenses. These defense mechanisms include intact skin and mucosal surfaces, antimicrobial secretory and excretory products on the skin and mucosa, saliva, the competition among the components of the normal microflora, the inflammatory response, and the immune response.

Numerous infectious diseases can affect the tissues of the oral cavity. Bacterial, fungal, and viral infections are the most common, but even protozoan and helminthic infections, although extremely rare, have been reported.

The oral cavity can be the primary site of involvement of an infectious disease, or a systemic infection can have oral manifestations. These infections are transmitted from one individual to another by several different routes. Organisms can be transferred through the air on dust particles or water droplets. Some organisms require intimate and direct contact to be transferred. Some can be transferred on hands and objects, and others such as hepatitis B must be transferred from one person to another in blood or other body fluids. Microorganisms that initially invade the oral tissues can cause a local infection, systemic infection, or both. Microorganisms circulating in the bloodstream can cause lesions in the oral cavity, and microorganisms causing infection in the lungs can be transferred to oral tissues when they are present in sputum. The oral cavity contains numerous microorganisms that make up the normal oral microflora. Changes such as a decrease in salivary flow, antibiotic administration, and immune system alterations affect the oral microflora so that organisms that are usually nonpathogenic are able to cause disease. This type of infection is called an **opportunistic infection.**

Microorganisms penetrating epithelial surfaces act as foreign material and stimulate the inflammatory and immune responses. The inflammatory response, including the cells of innate immunity (primarily neutrophils and macrophages) is nonspecific, resulting in edema and the accumulation of a large number of white blood cells at the site (see Chapter 2). The responses of the immune system, both humoral and cell mediated, are highly specific; microorganisms are antigens, and specific antibodies are formed in response to specific antigens (see Chapter 3).

Humoral immunity (immunity that is mediated by antibodies) is an effective defense against some microorganisms, and cell-mediated immunity (immunity in which T lymphocytes are responsible for the response) is the primary defense against others, such as intracellular bacteria (tuberculosis), viruses, and fungi. Microbial infections are responsible for many more diseases than those included in this chapter. The diseases discussed here are common, cause specific oral lesions, and help illustrate principles of infectious disease. Dental caries and periodontal disease clearly are infectious diseases that are important to dental hygienists. However, they are not included in this text because they are usually studied in courses other than oral pathology. The dental hygienist frequently encounters oral infectious diseases and must be able to recognize their clinical features and significance.

Bacterial Infections

Impetigo

Impetigo is a bacterial skin infection caused primarily by *Staphylococcus aureus,* often in combination with *Streptococcus pyogenes.* Impetigo most commonly involves the skin of the face or extremities and is usually seen in young children. The organisms are present on skin. Nonintact skin is necessary for infection; areas of trauma such as cuts and abrasions and areas of dermatitis are likely sites of this infection. The lesions of impetigo are infectious. Direct contact is required for transmission. Impetigo presents as either vesicles that rupture, resulting in thick, amber-colored crusts, or as longer-lasting bullae. The lesions may follow a pattern that corresponds to fingernail scratches or areas of perioral irritation. Lesions may itch (**pruritus),** and regional lymphadenopathy may be present. Systemic manifestations such as fever and **malaise** generally do not occur with this infection. When impetigo affects the perioral skin, the lesions may resemble recurrent herpes simplex infection (herpes simplex infection is discussed later in this chapter). However, recurrent herpes simplex infection (herpes labialis) is much less common than impetigo in small children. The diagnosis of impetigo is made on the basis of the clinical presentation or by identification of the bacteria from cultures of the lesions. Topical or systemic antibiotics are used for treatment.

Tonsillitis and Pharyngitis

Tonsillitis and **pharyngitis** are inflammatory conditions of the tonsils and pharyngeal mucosa. Many different organisms cause them, including streptococci, adenoviruses, influenza viruses, and Epstein-Barr virus (EBV). The clinical features include sore throat, fever, tonsillar hyperplasia, and erythema of the oropharyngeal mucosa and tonsils.

Streptococcal tonsillitis and pharyngitis are common bacterial infections that are spread by contact with infectious nasal or oral secretions. The appearance of streptococcal tonsillitis and pharyngitis (i.e., "strep throat") closely resembles tonsillitis and pharyngitis caused by other infections, such as viral infections. Specific laboratory tests, including a rapid antigen detection test, are available for diagnostic confirmation of streptococcal infection. Antibiotics are used to treat streptococcal infection.

Tonsillitis and pharyngitis caused by group A β-hemolytic streptococci are significant because of their relationship to scarlet fever and rheumatic fever. **Scarlet fever** usually occurs in children. In addition to fever, patients with scarlet fever develop a generalized red skin rash that is caused by a toxin released by the bacteria. In addition to streptococcal tonsillitis and pharyngitis, oral manifestations of scarlet fever include petechiae on the soft palate and an appearance of the tongue that has been called **strawberry tongue.** The fungiform papillae are red and prominent, with the dorsal surface of the tongue exhibiting either a white coating or erythema. Throat culture is helpful in confirming the diagnosis of streptococcal pharyngitis in a patient with scarlet fever.

Rheumatic fever is a childhood disease that follows a group A β-hemolytic streptococcal infection, usually tonsillitis and pharyngitis. Antibodies are made to the cell wall of the bacteria, and these antibodies react with many different tissues. As a result, rheumatic fever is characterized by an inflammation involving the heart, joints, and central nervous system. Rheumatic fever may result in permanent damage to heart valves. Rheumatic fever is rare in developed countries because of rapid diagnostic tests for streptococcal sore throat and subsequent antibiotic treatment.

Tuberculosis

Tuberculosis is an infectious chronic **granulomatous disease** usually caused by the organism *Mycobacterium tuberculosis.* The chief form of the disease is a primary infection of the lung. Inhaled droplets containing the bacteria lodge in the alveoli of the lungs. After undergoing phagocytosis by macrophages, the organisms are resistant to destruction and multiply in the macrophages. They then disseminate in the bloodstream. After a few weeks, dissemination ceases. The signs and symptoms of this lung infection include fever, chills, fatigue and malaise, weight loss, and persistent cough. The bacteria can be carried to widespread areas of the body and cause involvement of organs such as the kidneys and liver. This is called **miliary tuberculosis.** Involvement of the submandibular and cervical lymph nodes (usually as a result of ingesting the organism in nonpasteurized milk) causes enlargement of those nodes and is called **scrofula** or **tuberculous lymphadenitis.** The lung infection can occur at any age. Most commonly, foci of infection in the lungs become completely walled off and heal by fibrosis and calcification. A reactivation of the primary lesion can occur years after the initial infection. This reactivation is usually the result of a compromised immune response.

Oral lesions associated with tuberculosis occur but are rare. They most likely appear when organisms are carried from the lungs in sputum and transmitted to the oral mucosa (Fig. 4.1). The tongue and palate are the most common sites for oral lesions of tuberculosis, but they may occur anywhere in the oral cavity, even in bone. Oral lesions appear as painful, nonhealing, slowly enlarging ulcers that can be either superficial or deep.

Diagnosis

Oral lesions of tuberculosis are identified by biopsy and microscopic examination of the tissue. The characteristic histopathologic lesions of tuberculosis are **granulomas.** The granulomas are composed of areas of necrosis surrounded by macrophages,

multinucleated giant cells, and lymphocytes. Similar lesions occur in deep fungal infections and foreign-body reactions. Staining the tissue to be examined microscopically with a special stain may reveal the organisms. Tissue culture to diagnose tuberculosis requires a specialized laboratory.

A skin test is used to determine whether an individual has been exposed and infected with *M. tuberculosis.* An antigen called **purified protein derivative** (PPD) is injected under the top layer of the skin. If the individual's immune system has previously encountered the antigen (*M. tuberculosis*), a positive inflammatory skin reaction occurs (a type IV delayed-hypersensitivity reaction). This skin reaction indicates previous infection with the bacteria but not necessarily active disease. When a skin test result is positive, chest radiographs are taken to determine whether active tuberculosis disease is present. Once the skin test result is positive, it will always test positive.

Effective drug treatment for tuberculosis became available in the 1940s. In the United States most tuberculosis treatment centers had closed by the mid-1970s. State health departments reported a dramatic increase in new cases in the mid-1980s, particularly in densely populated urban areas. The increase in new cases of tuberculosis was suggested to be related to HIV infection and to noncompliance of patients with therapy. Recent public health efforts have focused on ensuring compliance with antituberculosis drug treatment; as a result the number of new cases reported has decreased.

Tuberculosis is an infectious disease that could potentially be transmitted occupationally to dental health care personnel. Routine use of universal precautions, including eye protection, mask, or facial shield, is important in preventing the transmission of airborne droplet infections such as tuberculosis. However, for patients with active tuberculosis, routine dental treatment is deferred. When emergency dental treatment is needed for patients with active tuberculosis, the use of a special mask is recommended to ensure prevention of transmission of the tuberculosis organism.

Treatment and Prognosis

Oral lesions resolve with treatment of the patient's primary (usually pulmonary) disease. Combinations of several different medications, including isoniazid, rifampin, and rifapentine, are used to treat tuberculosis. Treatment continues for many months and may continue for as long as 2 years. Patients usually become noninfectious shortly after treatment begins. Consultation with the patient's physician should confirm that treatment is ongoing and that the patient is no longer infectious.

Actinomycosis

Actinomycosis is an infection caused by a filamentous bacterium called *Actinomyces israelii.* These organisms were at one time thought to be fungi; therefore the name ends in the suffix "mycosis," which usually indicates a fungal infection.

The most characteristic form of the disease is the formation of abscesses that tend to drain by the formation of sinus tracts (Fig. 4.2). The colonies or organisms appear in the pus as tiny, bright-yellow grains and are called *sulfur granules* because of their yellow color. The organisms can also be identified by microscopic examination. These organisms are common inhabitants of the oral cavity. It is not clear why they only occasionally cause disease. Predisposing factors have not been identified. The infection is often preceded by tooth extraction or an abrasion of the mucosa.

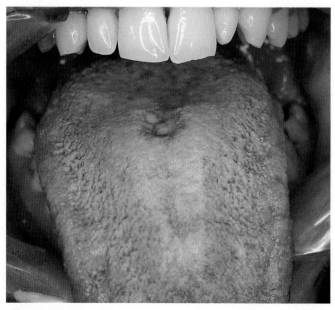

• **Figure 4.1** This ulcer on the tongue tested positive for tuberculosis organisms.

In general, the clinician makes a diagnosis of actinomycosis by identifying the colonies in the tissue from the lesion. Actinomycosis is treated with long-term high doses of antibiotics.

Syphilis

Syphilis is a disease caused by the spirochete *Treponema pallidum.* The organism is transmitted from one person to another by direct contact. The spirochete, a corkscrewlike bacterium, can penetrate mucous membranes, but requires a break in the continuity of the skin surface to invade through the skin. The organisms die quickly when exposed to air and changes in temperature. Syphilis is usually transmitted through sexual contact with a partner who has active lesions. It can also be transmitted by transfusion of infected blood or by transplacental inoculation of a fetus from an infected mother.

The disease occurs in three stages: (1) primary, (2) secondary, and (3) tertiary (Table 4.1). The lesion of the primary stage, called the **chancre**, is highly infectious and forms at the site at which the spirochete enters the body (Fig. 4.3). Regional lymphadenopathy accompanies the chancre. The lesion heals spontaneously after several weeks without treatment, and the disease enters a latent period.

The secondary stage occurs about 6 weeks after the primary lesion appears. In the secondary stage diffuse eruptions of the skin and mucous membranes occur. The skin lesions have many forms. The oral lesions are called **mucous patches** and appear as multiple painless, grayish-white plaques covering ulcerated mucosa. The lesions of secondary syphilis are the most infectious. They undergo spontaneous remission, but can recur for months or years. After remission the disease may remain latent for many years.

The tertiary lesions occur years after the initial infection if the infection has not been treated. They chiefly involve the cardiovascular system and the central nervous system. The localized tertiary lesion is called a **gumma** and is noninfectious. A gumma can occur in the oral cavity; the most common sites are the tongue and palate. The lesion appears as a firm mass that eventually becomes an ulcer. The gumma is a destructive lesion and can lead to perforation of the palatal bone.

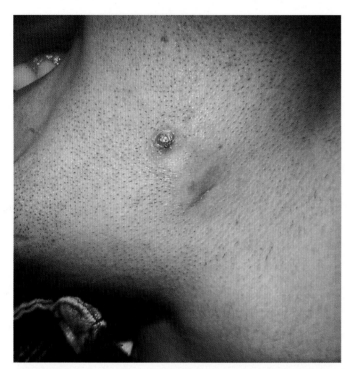

• **Figure 4.2** Actinomycosis. The skin lesion is over the mandible, and the incision and drainage site is seen below the lesion. "Sulfur granules" were noted in the exudate draining from the site, and the condition was treated with long-term antibiotic therapy.

TABLE 4.1	Stages of Syphilis	
Stage	**Oral Lesion**
Primary	Chancre
Secondary	Mucous patch
Latent	None
Tertiary	Gumma

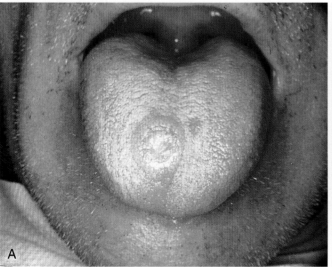
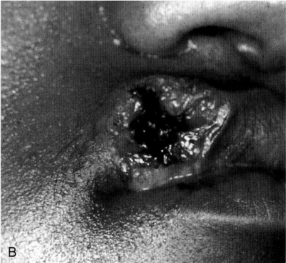

• **Figure 4.3 A,** Chancre on tongue seen in primary syphilis. **B,** Chancre on lip. (**A** courtesy Dr. Norman Trieger; **B** courtesy Dr. Edward V. Zegarelli.)

Congenital Syphilis

Syphilis can be transmitted from an infected mother to the fetus because the organism can cross the placenta and enter the fetal circulation. **Congenital syphilis** often causes serious and irreversible damage to the child, including facial and dental abnormalities. The developmental disorders that result from fetal and neonatal syphilis are described in Chapter 5.

Diagnosis and Treatment

The diagnosis of syphilitic lesions occurring on skin can be made by a special microscopic technique called a **dark-field examination** to identify the spirochetes. However, other spirochetes are present in the oral cavity; therefore this examination is not reliable for oral lesions. Two of the serologic (blood) tests that are commonly used to confirm the diagnosis of syphilis include (1) the Venereal Disease Research Laboratory (VDRL) test, and (2) the fluorescent treponemal antibody absorption (FTA-ABS) test. These tests may produce negative results in primary syphilis because sufficient antibodies may not have formed for the test result to be positive. It may take 4 weeks to 6 months for sufficient antibodies to develop for the test to become positive. If syphilis continues to be suspected, retesting is done. A rapid finger prick-screening test for syphilis was approved by the Food and Drug Administration (FDA) in 2014. This test allows a diagnosis within 15 minutes and immediate treatment, but it still requires sufficient antibodies for a positive result. As with the routine test, a negative test requires retesting if syphilis continues to be suspected.

Syphilis is generally treated with penicillin. The VDRL test is used again to evaluate the success of treatment. The antibody titer decreases if treatment has been successful. The FTA-ABS test remains positive after treatment.

Necrotizing Ulcerative Gingivitis

Necrotizing ulcerative gingivitis (NUG) was formerly called **acute necrotizing ulcerative gingivitis**. This condition is more chronic than acute and is therefore most appropriately called necrotizing ulcerative gingivitis. It is a painful erythematous gingivitis with necrosis of the interdental papillae (Fig. 4.4). Necrotizing ulcerative gingivitis is usually caused by a combination of a fusiform bacillus and a spirochete (*Borrelia vincentii*) and is associated with decreased resistance to infection.

The gingiva is painful and erythematous, with necrosis of the interdental papillae generally accompanied by a foul odor and metallic taste. The necrosis results in cratering of the interdental papillae area. Sloughing of the necrotic tissue presents as a pseudomembrane over the tissues. Systemic manifestations of infection such as fever and cervical lymphadenopathy may be present. Clinical features distinguish necrotizing ulcerative gingivitis from acute marginal gingivitis and the gingival component of acute primary herpes simplex infection (see Fig. 4.20B).

Treatment of necrotizing ulcerative gingivitis includes tissue debridement with topical or local anesthetic, rinsing with chlorhexidine or diluted hydrogen peroxide, and systemic antibiotic therapy with metronidazole or penicillin. The dental hygienist plays an important role in the treatment of necrotizing ulcerative gingivitis.

Pericoronitis

Pericoronitis is an inflammation of the mucosa around the crown of a partially erupted, impacted tooth (Fig. 4.5). The soft tissue around the mandibular third molar is the most common location for pericoronitis. The inflammation is usually the result of infection by bacteria that are part of the normal oral microflora, which proliferate in the pocket between the soft tissue and the crown of the tooth. Compromised host defenses, ranging from minor illnesses to immunodeficiency, are associated with an increased risk of pericoronitis. Trauma from an opposing molar and impaction of food under the soft tissue flap (operculum) covering the distal portion of the third molar may also precipitate pericoronitis.

Diagnosis

The diagnosis of pericoronitis is made on the basis of the clinical presentation. The tissue around the crown of a partially erupted tooth is swollen, erythematous, and painful.

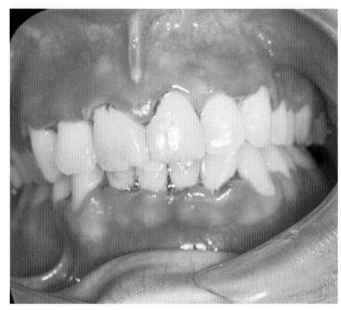

• **Figure 4.4** Necrotizing ulcerative gingivitis.

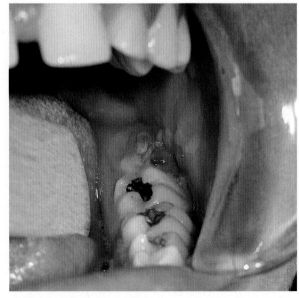

• **Figure 4.5** Pericoronitis. (Courtesy Dr. Kenneth Fleisher.)

Treatment and Prognosis

Treatment of pericoronitis includes mechanical debridement and irrigation of the pocket and systemic antibiotics. Extraction of the impacted molar is usually necessary to prevent recurrence.

Acute Osteomyelitis

Acute osteomyelitis involves acute inflammation of the bone and bone marrow (Fig. 4.6A). Acute osteomyelitis of the jaws is most commonly a result of the extension of a periapical abscess. It may follow fracture of the bone or surgery and may also result from bacteremia. Pain and lymphadenopathy are significant features.

Diagnosis

The diagnosis of the specific organism causing acute osteomyelitis is based on culture results, and treatment is based on antibiotic sensitivity testing. In acute osteomyelitis bone loss is rapid. Early radiographic changes are evident in 2 to 3 weeks. Microscopic examination shows nonviable bone, necrotic debris, acute inflammation, and bacterial colonies in the marrow spaces.

Treatment and Prognosis

The treatment of acute osteomyelitis involves drainage of the purulent exudate from the area and the use of appropriate

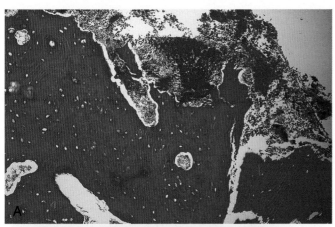
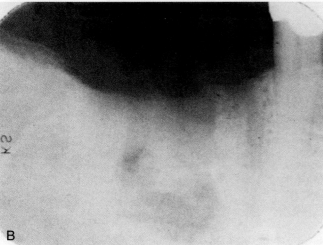

• **Figure 4.6** A, Low-power microscopy of acute osteomyelitis, showing nonviable bone. Bacterial colonies and inflammatory cells are seen between trabeculae of bone. **B,** Diffuse, irregular radiographic changes seen in chronic osteomyelitis.

antibiotics. Surgical debridement of necrotic tissue may also be needed. Once successfully treated, prognosis is good.

Chronic Osteomyelitis

Chronic osteomyelitis is a long-standing inflammation of bone. It may occur in inadequately treated acute osteomyelitis, long-term inflammation of bone with no recognized acute phase, Paget disease of bone, sickle cell disease, or bone irradiation that results in decreased vascularity. The involved bone is painful and swollen, and radiographic examination reveals a diffuse and irregular radiolucency that can eventually become radiopaque as bone forms within the chronically inflamed tissue (Fig. 4.6B). When radiopacity develops, the condition is called **chronic sclerosing osteomyelitis.** Recently cases of osteonecrosis of the mandible and maxilla have been reported in patients taking bisphosphonate medication. This may appear clinically similar to chronic osteomyelitis. Bisphosphonate-associated osteonecrosis is described in Chapter 9.

Diagnosis

The diagnosis of chronic osteomyelitis is based on duration, biopsy results, and the microscopic examination, which shows chronic inflammation of bone and marrow. Bacterial culture may be helpful, but the bacteria may be difficult to identify.

Treatment

Treatment of chronic osteomyelitis involves debridement and administration of systemic antibiotics. In some patients the use of hyperbaric oxygen may be needed to successfully treat this condition.

Fungal Infections

Candidiasis

Candidiasis, also called **candidosis, moniliasis,** and **thrush,** occurs as a result of an overgrowth of the yeastlike fungus *Candida albicans.* It is the most common oral fungal infection. This fungus is part of the normal oral microflora in many individuals, particularly those individuals with diabetes mellitus and those who wear dentures. Overgrowth of *C. albicans* is associated with many different conditions (Box 4.1).

Newborn infants are particularly susceptible to an overgrowth of this fungus because they do not have either an established oral microflora or a fully developed immune system. Pregnant women

---

• **BOX 4.1** **Conditions Associated With Overgrowth of *Candida albicans***

- Antibiotic therapy
- Cancer chemotherapy
- Corticosteroid therapy
- Dentures
- Diabetes mellitus
- Human immunodeficiency virus infection
- Hypoparathyroidism
- Infancy (newborn)
- Malignancies involving bone marrow
- Primary T-lymphocyte deficiency
- Xerostomia

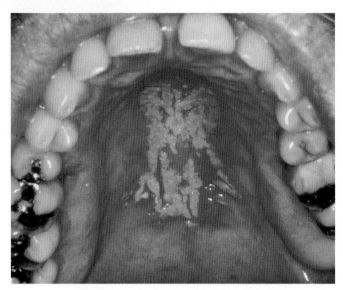

• **Figure 4.7** Pseudomembranous candidiasis.

often have *Candida* vaginitis because they are somewhat immunosuppressed in order to maintain the fetus. The organism is transmitted to the infant while it passes through the birth canal. Antibiotics can alter the bacteria of the oral microflora, which can allow the overgrowth of *C. albicans*. Systemic and topical corticosteroids, diabetes, and cell-mediated immune system deficiency are other factors that allow the overgrowth of this fungus. Candidiasis is one of the most common oral lesions that occur in association with immunodeficiency. Candidiasis generally affects the superficial layers of the epithelium; therefore when it is present, the proliferating organisms are easily identified in a mucosal smear (cytologic preparation) prepared from a sample obtained by scraping the surface of the lesion.

Types of Oral Candidiasis

Several forms of oral candidiasis exist; recognition of their clinical features is important so that candidiasis is appropriately included in the differential diagnosis of a variety of clinical presentations. The types of oral candidiasis are as follows:

• Pseudomembranous
• Erythematous
• Denture stomatitis (chronic atrophic candidiasis)
• Chronic hyperplastic (*Candida* leukoplakia)
• Angular cheilitis

Pseudomembranous Candidiasis

A white curdlike material is present on the mucosal surface in **pseudomembranous candidiasis** (Fig. 4.7). The underlying mucosa is erythematous. On occasion, a burning sensation is felt, and the patient may complain of a metallic taste.

Erythematous Candidiasis

An erythematous, often painful, mucosa is the presenting complaint in **erythematous candidiasis** (Fig. 4.8). This type of candidiasis may be localized to one area of the oral mucosa or be more generalized. Irregular, patchy depapillation of the tongue is often seen in this type of candidiasis.

Denture Stomatitis

Denture stomatitis is the most common type of candidiasis affecting the oral mucosa. It is also called **chronic atrophic**

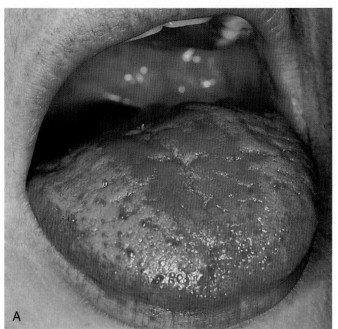

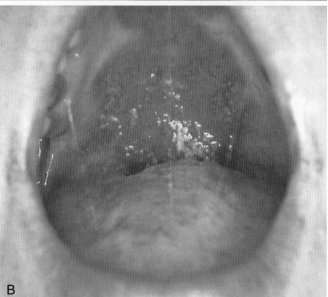

• **Figure 4.8** Erythematous candidiasis. **A,** Recent-onset and erythematous lesions elsewhere in the oral cavity differentiate this from median rhomboid glossitis. **B,** Response to antifungal treatment confirmed the diagnosis of oral candidiasis in this patient.

candidiasis (Fig. 4.9). This type of candidiasis also presents as erythematous mucosa, but the erythematous change is limited to the mucosa covered by a full or partial denture. The lesions may vary from petechiae-like to more generalized and granular. It is most common on the palate and maxillary alveolar ridge. Denture stomatitis is asymptomatic and is usually discovered by the dentist or dental hygienist during a routine oral examination.

Chronic Hyperplastic Candidiasis

Chronic hyperplastic candidiasis (Fig. 4.10) appears as a white lesion that does not wipe off the mucosa. **Candidal leukoplakia** and **hypertrophic candidiasis** are other names for this type of oral candidiasis. An important diagnostic feature of this type of

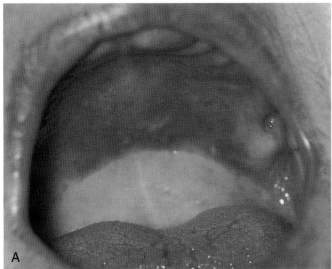
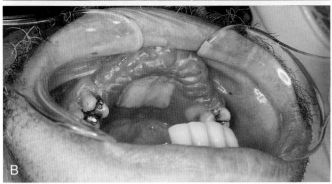

• **Figure 4.9** Chronic atrophic candidiasis (denture stomatitis). **A,** Full denture. **B,** Partial denture.

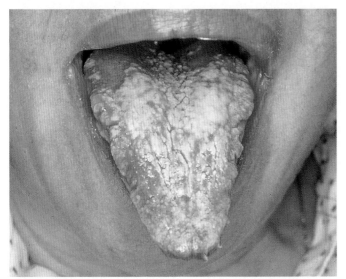

• **Figure 4.10** Chronic hyperplastic candidiasis. The white appearance of the tongue did not wipe off, and it disappeared with antifungal treatment.

candidiasis is its response to antifungal medication: when leuko-plakia is caused by candidiasis, it disappears when treated with antifungal medication (therapeutic diagnosis). If the lesion does not respond to antifungal therapy, biopsy should be considered to establish the diagnosis of the lesion.

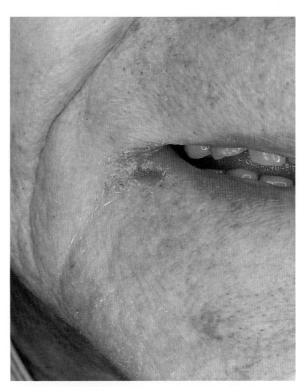

• **Figure 4.11** Angular cheilitis.

Angular Cheilitis
Angular cheilitis is an inflammatory condition characterized by erythema and fissuring at the labial commissures (Fig. 4.11). It may be unilateral or bilateral. Angular cheilitis is most commonly caused by *Candida* organisms and often accompanies intraoral candidiasis. Angular cheilitis may be caused by other factors such as nutritional deficiencies or a combination of *Candida* and bacteria. However, it most commonly results from a *Candida* infection.

Chronic Mucocutaneous Candidiasis
A severe form of candidiasis that usually occurs in patients who are severely immunocompromised is called **chronic mucocutaneous candidiasis.** The patient has skin lesions as well as chronic oral and genital mucosal candidiasis. Oral involvement may appear as pseudomembranous, erythematous, or hyperplastic candidiasis, and angular cheilitis is common. The skin lesions usually involve the nails and skinfolds.

Median Rhomboid Glossitis (Central Papillary Atrophy)
Several studies have reported an association between **median rhomboid glossitis** (Fig. 4.12, see also Fig. 1.55), also called *central papillary atrophy,* and candidiasis. It appears as an erythematous, often rhombus-shaped, flat-to-raised area on the midline of the posterior dorsal tongue. *Candida* organisms have been identified in some lesions, and some lesions disappear with antifungal treatment. However, the response to antifungal treatment is not consistent; therefore although this lesion has been associated with candidiasis, the cause is not yet clear.

Diagnosis and Treatment
Because *Candida* is part of the oral microflora in many individuals, a culture is not useful for diagnosis. A positive culture result indicates that the organisms are present but not that they are causing infection. Clinical features and the use of the mucosal

smear (cytologic preparation) (Fig. 4.13) are usually more helpful. A sample from the surface of the lesion is obtained by scraping vigorously with a tongue blade, wooden spatula, cotton applicator, or specially designed brush, and the scrapings are spread on a glass slide and fixed with alcohol. The slide is then sent to an oral pathology laboratory for staining and examination. In addition to the smear, the response of the lesion to antifungal treatment is important in confirming the diagnosis of candidiasis. Lesions caused by *Candida* should resolve with antifungal treatment. Both topical and systemic medications are used for candidiasis. However, in some patients, particularly those who are immunocompromised, candidiasis is persistent and recurrent.

Although the final diagnosis and management of a patient with oral candidiasis is the responsibility of the dentist, dental hygienists are often the first to recognize the oral changes characteristic of this condition. Recurrent oral candidiasis may be an early sign of a severe underlying medical problem.

Deep Fungal Infections

Oral lesions occur in some deep fungal infections (e.g., *histoplasmosis, coccidioidomycosis, blastomycosis,* and *cryptococcosis*). They are all characterized by primary involvement of the lungs. Oral lesions are caused by implantation of the organism carried by sputum from the lungs to the oral mucosa.

Infections caused by these organisms are more common in certain areas of the United States than in others. Histoplasmosis is widespread in the midwestern United States, and coccidioidomycosis is more prevalent in parts of the western United States, particularly the San Joaquin Valley of California. Blastomycosis is common in the Ohio and Mississippi River basin areas. Therefore oral lesions caused by these organisms are most likely seen in areas of the country in which the infection is most common.

Cryptococcosis is transmitted through inhalation of organisms contained in dust from bird droppings, particularly from pigeons. In addition to the regional distribution of these infections, reactivation, including the development of oral lesions, can occur in patients who are immunocompromised.

Diagnosis

The initial signs and symptoms of these deep fungal infections are usually related to the primary lung infection. Oral lesions are preceded by pulmonary involvement. These oral lesions are chronic, nonhealing ulcers that can resemble squamous cell carcinoma (Fig. 4.14). Diagnosis is made by biopsy and microscopic examination. Special staining of the tissue reveals the organisms, which can be identified by their microscopic appearance. The tissue can also be cultured; this is useful in establishing the diagnosis.

Treatment

Systemic antifungal medications such as amphotericin B or ketoconazole or itraconazole are used to treat these infections. However, latent infections may remain even after treatment and may reappear if the individual's immune system becomes deficient.

Mucormycosis

Mucormycosis, also called **phycomycosis,** is a rare fungal infection. The organisms are a common inhabitant of soil and are usually nonpathogenic. However, infection with this organism occurs in diabetic and severely debilitated patients. The disease often involves the nasal cavity, maxillary sinus, and hard palate and can present as a proliferating or destructive mass in the maxilla. The diagnosis is made by biopsy and identification of the organisms in the tissue.

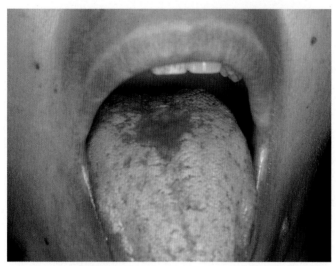

• **Figure 4.12** Median rhomboid glossitis.

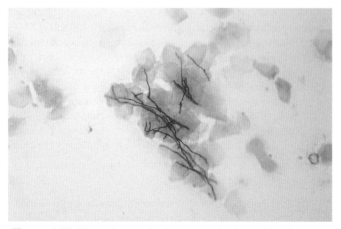

• **Figure 4.13** Photomicrograph of a smear showing epithelial cells and *Candida* organisms.

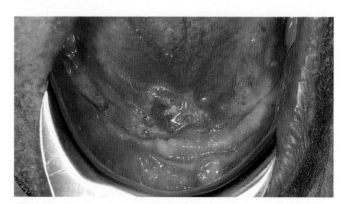

• **Figure 4.14** Oral lesions of histoplasmosis in this patient clinically resemble squamous cell carcinoma. (Courtesy Dr. A. Ross Kerr.)

Viral Infections

Human Papillomavirus Infection

Human papillomavirus (HPV) selectively infects skin and oral mucosa. Infection occurs by direct contact. More than 130 different types of human papillomavirus have been identified; some of these types have been found to cause neoplasia and therefore are called *high-risk types*. Others that cause benign lesions or are not associated with lesions are called *low-risk types*. About 35 different types of human papillomavirus have been identified in oral mucosa. A recent study that examined both high-risk and low-risk types of human papillomavirus in the oral cavity found the overall prevalence of human papillomavirus in the oral cavity to be 6.9%. This included both high-risk and low-risk types. High-risk types that have been associated with oral squamous cell carcinoma include HPV types 16 and 18. Human papilloma virus has been clearly associated with carcinoma of the vaginal cervix (cervical cancer). High-risk types have been identified and associated with squamous cell carcinomas that form in the oropharyngeal region (see Chapter 7). Evidence of their role in the pathogenesis of these cancers is emerging, but is not yet completely clear.

For human papillomavirus to infect skin and oral mucosa, it must infect the basal cells of the epithelium. This usually requires a break in the surface of these tissues. Human papillomavirus matures in the spinous layer and then the virus is released on the surface of the tissue. Proliferation of the basal cells of the infected epithelium is a characteristic of benign lesions that are caused by human papillomavirus infection.

Like other viruses, human papillomavirus incorporates itself into the nuclear material of infected cells. Human papillomavirus–infected cells, called *koilocytes,* are characterized microscopically by an irregular nucleus surrounded by clear cytoplasm (Fig. 4.15).

Three benign lesions caused by human papillomavirus infection are seen in the oral cavity. These include the verruca vulgaris, condyloma acuminatum, and focal epithelial hyperplasia. Examples of low-risk types associated with these lesions include HPV types 2, 6, 11, 13, 27, 32, and 57. These are described in this chapter. The benign squamous papilloma, described in Chapter 7, is also most likely caused by human papillomavirus infection.

The relationship between human papillomavirus and oral cancer is further described in Chapter 7.

Verruca Vulgaris

The **verruca vulgaris,** or common wart, is a papillary oral lesion caused by several different types of human papilloma virus. HPV type 2 is the type most commonly found in verruca vulgaris. It is a common skin lesion. Oral lesions are less common than skin lesions, but they do occur. The virus is inoculated by direct contact and may be transmitted from skin to oral mucosa. The lips are one of the most common intraoral sites for this lesion. Autoinoculation occurs through finger sucking or fingernail biting in patients with verrucae on the hands or fingers (Fig. 4.16). The verruca vulgaris is usually a white, papillary, exophytic lesion (Fig. 4.17) that closely resembles and is related to the benign tumor of squamous epithelium called the **papilloma** (see Chapter 7).

Microscopically, the verruca vulgaris consists of fingerlike projections of markedly keratotic, stratified squamous epithelium

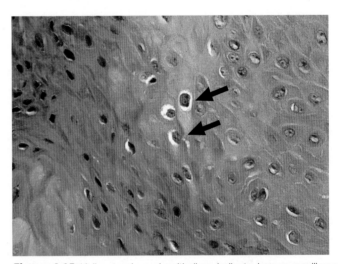

• **Figure 4.15** Koilocytes in oral epithelium indicate human papilloma virus infection. Cells with irregular nuclei are surrounded by clear cytoplasm *(arrows)*.

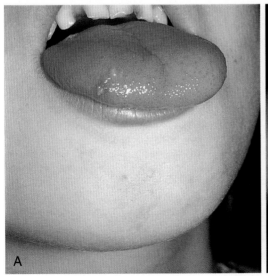
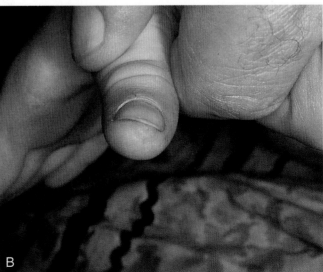

• **Figure 4.16** A and B, Verruca vulgaris on the tongue of a child with a similar lesion on the thumb. (Courtesy Dr. Edward V. Zegarelli.)

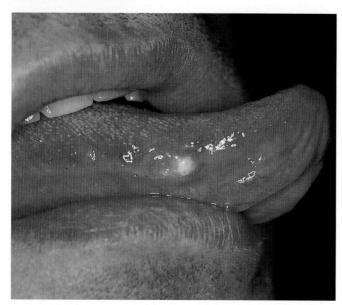

• **Figure 4.17** Verruca vulgaris on the lateral aspect of the tongue in an adult.

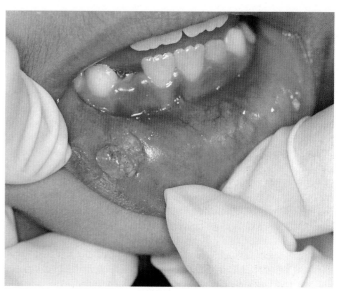

• **Figure 4.18** Condyloma acuminatum. The presence of condyloma acuminatum in a child is strongly suggestive of sexual abuse. (Courtesy Dr. Sidney Eisig.)

that exhibits a prominent granular cell layer; numerous cells with clear cytoplasm, called *koilocytes,* are present in the upper spinous layer of the epithelium. These cells contain viral particles that are visible by electron microscopic examination. Each of the projections contains a central core of fibrous connective tissue containing many blood vessels. The vacuolated cells in the epithelium contain the viral particles.

Diagnosis
Biopsy and microscopic examination reveal the light microscopic features of this lesion. Immunologic staining is also useful in identifying these viruses.

Treatment and Prognosis
Conservative surgical excision is the treatment of choice for verruca vulgaris. These lesions may recur. In addition, patients with skin lesions should be instructed to refrain from finger sucking or fingernail biting to prevent reinoculation and development of new lesions.

Condyloma Acuminatum

The **condyloma acuminatum** is a benign papillary lesion caused by other types of human papilloma virus. The virus is generally transmitted by sexual contact and is most commonly found in the anogenital region. It is transmitted to the oral cavity through oral-genital contact or self-inoculation. HPV types 6 and 11 are the most common types associated with condyloma acuminatum.

Oral condylomas appear as papillary, bulbous masses and can occur anywhere in the oral mucosa (Fig. 4.18). Multiple lesions may be present. They have been reported to occur on the tongue, buccal mucosa, palate, gingiva, and alveolar ridge. The oral condyloma tends to be more diffuse than the papilloma or verruca vulgaris and is generally not as well keratinized as the verruca vulgaris. The condyloma is pink, whereas the verruca vulgaris is usually white.

Microscopically, the condyloma acuminatum is composed of fingerlike (papillary) projections of epithelium covering cores of

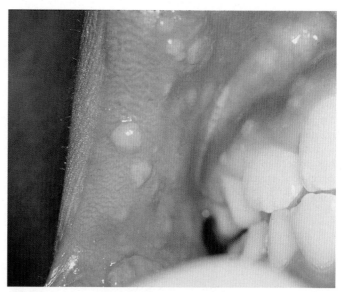

• **Figure 4.19** Multifocal epithelial hyperplasia. (Courtesy Dr. Stanley Kerpel.)

connective tissue. The epithelium is thickened, and cells with clear cytoplasm are seen throughout the epithelium. These clear cells contain viral particles that can be identified through immunologic staining.

When the condyloma acuminatum occurs in the oral cavity, it is generally treated by conservative surgical excision. However, recurrence is common, and multiple lesions make management difficult. Patients should be instructed to avoid oral-genital contact with an infected partner to prevent reinoculation.

Multifocal Epithelial Hyperplasia

Multifocal epithelial hyperplasia, also called *Heck disease,* is characterized by the presence of multiple whitish to pale pink nodules distributed throughout the oral mucosa (Fig. 4.19). The disease is most common in children and was first described in

Native Americans, but it has since been described in many different areas of the world. Low-risk HPV types 13 and 32 have been identified in epithelium of multifocal epithelial hyperplasia. The lesions are generally asymptomatic and do not require treatment. They resolve spontaneously weeks to months after onset. Microscopically, the lesions show thickened epithelium with broad, connected rete ridges. Cells in the epithelium that have clear cytoplasm, consistent with koilocytes, may also be seen in the lesions of multifocal epithelial hyperplasia.

Herpes Simplex Infection

Two major forms of the herpes simplex virus exist: type 1 and type 2. Oral infections are generally caused by type 1, and genital infections are most commonly caused by type 2. Oral infection with the herpes simplex virus occurs in an initial (primary) form and a recurrent (secondary) form. The herpes simplex virus is one of a group of viruses called human herpesviruses (HHVs). Other herpesviruses include varicella-zoster virus (VZV), Epstein-Barr virus (EBV), cytomegalovirus (CMV), and Kaposi sarcoma–associated herpesvirus (KSHV; human herpesvirus 8). Herpes simplex viruses have the ability to persist in an individual in a clinically quiescent or latent state. For many individuals, the primary infection undergoes remission without the virus being completely eliminated.

Primary Herpetic Gingivostomatitis

The oral disease caused by initial infection with the herpes simplex virus is called **primary herpetic gingivostomatitis** (Fig. 4.20). Painful, erythematous, and swollen gingivae and multiple tiny vesicles on the perioral skin, vermilion border of the lips, and oral mucosa characterize the disease. These vesicles progress to form ulcers. Systemic symptoms such as fever, malaise, and cervical lymphadenopathy generally occur first, followed by gingival involvement and the appearance of mucosal vesicles and ulcers. The disease most commonly occurs in children between the ages of 6 months and 6 years. However, it may occur at any age if an individual who has not been previously exposed to the virus comes into contact with it or if a sufficient level of antibodies has not developed to confer protection against reinfection. Because many more individuals have antibodies to herpes simplex than have a history of the disease, the majority are thought to be **subclinical infections.** The disease is usually self-limited. The lesions heal spontaneously in 1 to 2 weeks.

Recurrent Herpes Simplex Infection

In many individuals, after the primary infection, the herpes simplex virus tends to persist in a latent state, usually in the nerve tissue of the trigeminal ganglion, and causes localized recurrent infections. It has been estimated that one third to one half of the population of the United States experience **recurrent herpes simplex infection.** The most common type of recurrent oral herpes simplex infection occurs on the vermilion border of the lips and is called **herpes labialis** (Fig. 4.21), which is also called a **cold sore** or **fever blister.** Recurrent infections are often produced by certain stimuli such as sunlight, menstruation, fatigue, fever, and emotional stress. These stimuli are thought to trigger viral replication and immunologic changes that result in clinical lesions.

Recurrent herpes simplex infection can also occur intraorally (Fig. 4.22). The appearance and location of these lesions are important to distinguish them from aphthous ulcers (Table 4.2).

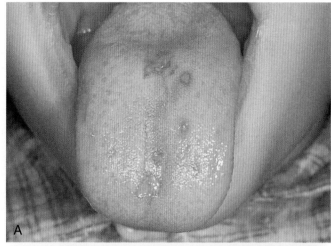

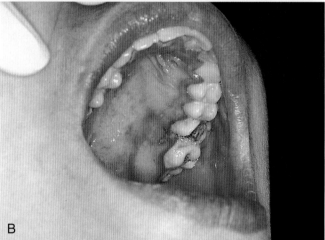

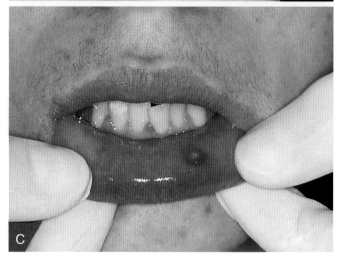

• **Figure 4.20 A,** Primary herpetic gingivostomatitis in a child. **B** and **C,** Primary herpetic gingivostomatitis in an adolescent. (**A** courtesy Dr. Edward V. Zegarelli.)

Recurrent intraoral herpes simplex occurs on keratinized mucosa that is fixed to bone, most commonly the hard palate and gingiva. The lesions appear as painful clusters of tiny vesicles or ulcers that can coalesce to form a single ulcer with an irregular border. Usually patients experience prodromal symptoms such as pain, burning, or tingling in the area in which the vesicles develop. The

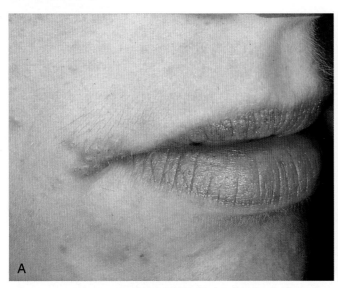
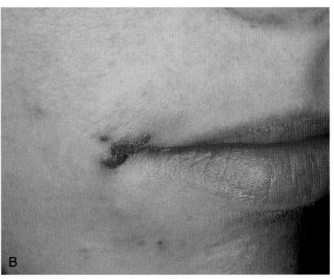

• **Figure 4.21** Herpes labialis. **A,** Twelve hours after onset. **B,** Forty-eight hours after onset.

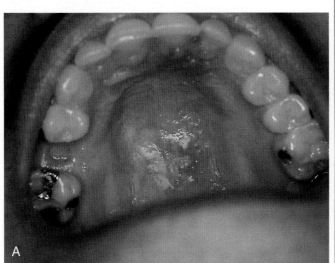
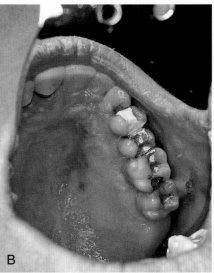

• **Figure 4.22 A** and **B,** Recurrent intraoral herpes simplex.

TABLE 4.2	Comparison of the Clinical Features of Recurrent Minor Aphthous Ulcers and Recurrent Herpes Simplex Ulceration	
Feature	**Recurrent Minor Aphthous Ulcers**	**Recurrent Herpes Simplex Ulceration**
Location	Nonkeratinized mucosa	Keratinized mucosa
Number	One to several	Multiple (crops)
Vesicle precedes ulcer	No	Yes
Pain	Yes	Yes
Size	<1 cm	1–2 mm
Borders	Round to oval	Clusters of ulcers coalesce to form a large irregular ulcer
Recurrent	Yes	Yes

lesions heal without scarring in 1 to 2 weeks. Episodes of recurrence vary from once a month in some individuals to once a year in others. Activation of latent herpes simplex infection has been identified as an initiator of recurrent erythema multiforme (see Chapter 3).

Herpes simplex virus is transmitted by direct contact with an infected individual, and the lesions of the primary infection occur at the site of inoculation. The herpes simplex virus can be isolated from both primary and recurrent lesions. The amount of virus present is highest in the vesicle stage. In some individuals the virus is present in the oral cavity, even when no lesions are present. Herpes simplex virus can cause a painful infection of the fingers called a **herpetic whitlow.** Before the routine use of gloves during dental treatment, this was an occupational hazard for dentists and dental hygienists (Fig. 4.23). Herpetic whitlow can be either a primary or a recurrent infection. Herpes simplex virus can also cause eye infection (Fig. 4.24). Routine barrier infection control procedures (mask, eye protection, and gloves) are important in preventing the transmission of the herpes simplex virus to dental health care providers.

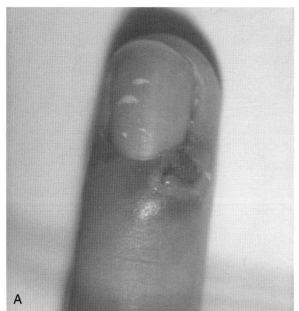

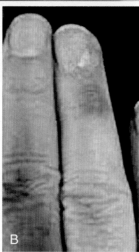

• **Figure 4.23 A,** Herpetic whitlow in a dental hygienist (initial lesion).
B, Recurrent lesion occurred many, many years later. (Courtesy Susan
Rod Graham.)

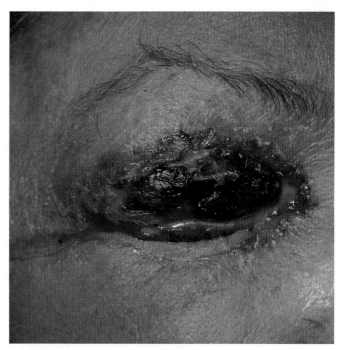

• **Figure 4.24** Herpetic eye infection. (Courtesy Dr. Sidney Eisig.)

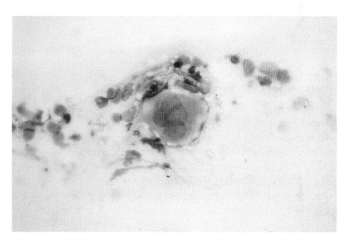

• **Figure 4.25** Cytologic smear preparation showing a virally altered cell
(Tzanck cell) resulting from herpes simplex infection. (Courtesy Dr. Harry
Lumerman.)

Diagnosis

The diagnosis of herpes simplex infection, both primary and
recurrent, is generally based on the clinical characteristics of the
disease (see Table 4.2). In immunocompromised patients the
characteristic clinical features may be lacking. A viral culture can
be performed to confirm the diagnosis. This procedure requires a
special culture medium and at least 2 days before results are
available.

Herpes simplex virus causes changes in epithelial cells that can
be seen microscopically. These virally altered cells can be seen in
tissue obtained by biopsy or on a smear taken by scraping the
basal cells of the lesion and spreading them on a glass slide, fixing
them with alcohol, and submitting them to an oral pathology
laboratory for staining and examination (Fig. 4.25). The virally
altered epithelial cells that are seen on a cytologic preparation
(smear) from patients with herpes simplex infection are called
Tzanck cells. These are different from the Tzanck cells that are
seen in pemphigus vulgaris (see Chapter 3) but have the same
name. Smears of herpes simplex ulceration have been reported to
be positive for virally altered cells only about 50% of the time.

Treatment

Antiviral drugs such as acyclovir are available for the treatment of
herpes simplex infection and are used for treating genital herpes
simplex infection. Antiviral drugs have not been shown to be
consistently effective in treating the intraoral lesions of herpes
simplex infection except in immunocompromised patients. The
use of sunscreens may prevent the development of herpes labialis.
Systemic antiviral medication has been approved by the FDA for
treating and preventing herpes labialis. Topical application of
antiviral drugs may prevent or decrease the duration of herpes
labialis when they are administered very early in the development
of the lesion (prodromal period), before epithelial damage has
occurred.

Varicella-Zoster Virus

The **varicella-zoster virus** (VZV) causes both chickenpox (varicella) and shingles (herpes zoster). Respiratory aerosols and

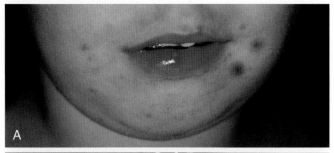

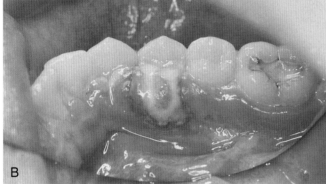

• **Figure 4.26** Chickenpox. **A,** Skin lesions. **B,** Gingival lesion. (Courtesy Dr. Roger S. Kitzis.)

contact with secretions from skin lesions transmit the virus. Both chickenpox and herpes zoster are contagious.

Chickenpox

Chickenpox is a highly contagious disease that causes vesicular and pustular eruptions of the skin and mucous membranes, along with systemic symptoms such as headache, fever, and malaise (Fig. 4.26). The **incubation period** is about 2 weeks. Chickenpox usually occurs in children; although oral lesions occur, they generally do not cause severe discomfort. Usually an individual has only a single episode of chickenpox, but second, milder forms have also been described. Recovery generally occurs in 2 to 3 weeks.

Herpes Zoster

Although chickenpox has been described in adults, the virus usually causes a different form of disease in this population. The form that usually occurs in adults is called **herpes zoster** or **shingles.** It is characterized by a unilateral, painful eruption of vesicles along the distribution of a sensory nerve (Fig. 4.27). Whether or not the varicella-zoster virus is harbored in the sensory ganglia during the interval between chickenpox and herpes zoster in a manner similar to that of the herpes simplex virus is not clear. However, herpes zoster often occurs in association with immunodeficiency or certain malignancies such as Hodgkin disease and leukemia. A vaccine is available to prevent varicella-zoster infections. It is given to children to prevent chickenpox and to older adults to prevent the recurrence of the infection as herpes zoster.

The depression of cell-mediated immunity appears to be important in the development of herpes zoster. Any of the three branches of the trigeminal nerve may be affected: (1) the ophthalmic branch, (2) the maxillary branch, or (3) the mandibular branch (Fig. 4.28). Oral lesions occur when the maxillary and/or mandibular branches are affected. Skin lesions on the forehead and around the eye occur when the ophthalmic branch is involved. The oral lesions, like the skin lesions, are characterized by their

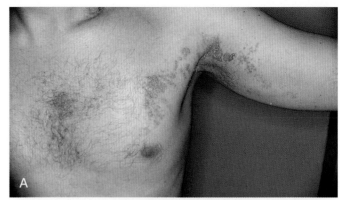

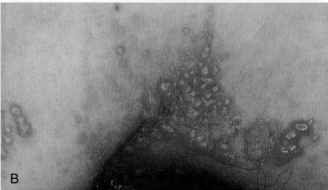

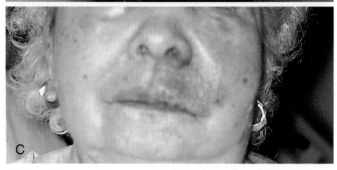

• **Figure 4.27** Herpes zoster. **A,** Unilateral distribution of vesicles along the distribution of a sensory nerve. **B,** Same patient as **A** showing many vesicles coalescing to form large lesions. **C,** Unilateral facial lesions occurring along the distribution of the maxillary branch of the trigeminal nerve. This patient also had intraoral lesions on the same side.

unilateral distribution. Prodromal symptoms of pain, burning, or both, called **paresthesia,** often precede the development of vesicles. Oral lesions are painful and begin as vesicles that progress to ulcers. The disease usually lasts for several weeks, and in some patients, neuralgia, which takes months to resolve, may follow the resolution of the lesions.

Diagnosis

The diagnosis of varicella (chickenpox) and herpes zoster is generally made on the basis of the clinical features. Biopsy or a cytologic mucosal smear (cytologic preparation) of the lesion may show the same type of virally altered epithelial cells that are seen in herpes simplex infection (Tzanck cells). Laboratory identification of varicella-zoster virus is also helpful.

Treatment

Varicella generally requires only supportive treatment. Antiviral drugs are used for immunocompromised patients and for patients

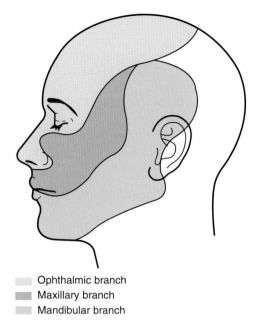

Ophthalmic branch
Maxillary branch
Mandibular branch

• **Figure 4.28** Diagram of the branches of the trigeminal nerve.

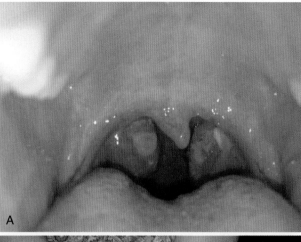

• **Figure 4.29** Infectious mononucleosis. **A,** Intraoral lesions. **B,** Skin rash on hands. (Courtesy Laura J. Greco, RDH, MSEd.)

with herpes zoster. In some patients corticosteroids have been used in an attempt to prevent the pain of postherpetic neuralgia.

Epstein-Barr Virus Infection

The **Epstein-Barr virus** (EBV) has been implicated in several diseases that occur in the oral region, including infectious mononucleosis, nasopharyngeal carcinoma, Burkitt lymphoma, and hairy leukoplakia. Nasopharyngeal carcinoma and Burkitt lymphoma are rare malignant neoplasms. Infectious mononucleosis and hairy leukoplakia are discussed here.

Infectious Mononucleosis

Infectious mononucleosis is an infectious disease caused by the Epstein-Barr virus. It is characterized by sore throat, fever, generalized lymphadenopathy, enlarged spleen, malaise, and fatigue. Palatal petechiae occur in infectious mononucleosis, usually appearing early in the course of the disease (Fig. 4.29). The mechanism for the development of these petechiae is unclear. The diagnosis is confirmed by the identification in the blood of mononucleosis cells, which are atypical activated T lymphocytes. A skin rash may appear briefly during early onset of this condition. Severe complications such as hepatitis occur in some patients. In developed countries infectious mononucleosis occurs principally in late adolescence among young adults in the upper socioeconomic classes. The virus is transmitted by close contact. Contact with saliva during kissing is a frequent route of transmission of Epstein-Barr virus. In most patients infectious mononucleosis is a benign, self-limited disease that resolves within 4 to 6 weeks. In some patients fatigue lasts much longer. Multiple recurrences occur in some patients.

Hairy Leukoplakia

Hairy leukoplakia is characterized by an irregular, corrugated white lesion most commonly occurring on the lateral border of

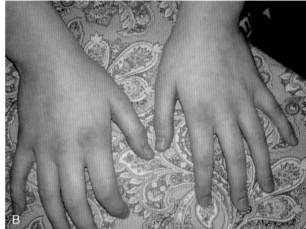

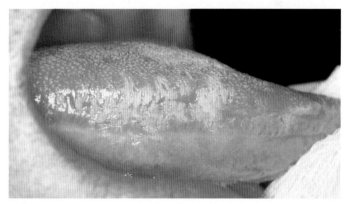

• **Figure 4.30** Hairy leukoplakia seen here in an HIV-infected patient is an oral epithelial lesion caused by the Epstein-Barr virus.

the tongue (Fig. 4.30). Epstein-Barr virus has been identified in the epithelial cells of hairy leukoplakia and is considered to be the cause of the lesion. Hairy leukoplakia was first identified in patients infected with human immunodeficiency virus (HIV) and occurs most commonly in these patients; it has also been reported in immunocompromised patients not infected with human immunodeficiency virus (i.e., organ transplant patients). Hairy leukoplakia is discussed later in this chapter as an oral manifestation of human immunodeficiency virus infection.

Coxsackievirus Infections

The **coxsackieviruses,** named for the town in New York State where the virus was first discovered, cause several different infectious diseases. Three of these have distinctive oral lesions and are discussed here. Fecal-oral contamination, saliva, and respiratory droplets can all be the means of transmission.

Herpangina

Herpangina characteristically includes vesicles on the soft palate (Fig. 4.31A), along with fever, malaise, sore throat, and difficulty swallowing (dysphagia). An erythematous pharyngitis is also present. The disease is usually mild to moderate and resolves in less than 1 week without treatment.

Hand-Foot-and-Mouth Disease

Hand-foot-and-mouth disease usually occurs in epidemics in children younger than 5 years of age. Oral lesions are generally painful vesicles and ulcers that can occur anywhere in the mouth. Multiple macules or papules occur on the skin, typically on the feet, toes, hands, and fingers (Fig. 4.31B-C). Lesions resolve spontaneously within 2 weeks.

Diagnosis

Although the oral lesions may resemble herpes simplex infection, the distribution of the skin lesions and the mild systemic symptoms usually help to differentiate the two conditions. Viral culture and measurement of circulating antibodies to the type of coxsackievirus that causes hand-foot-and-mouth disease may help to confirm the diagnosis but generally are not necessary.

Treatment

The disease is generally mild and of short duration. Treatment usually is not required.

Acute Lymphonodular Pharyngitis

Acute lymphonodular pharyngitis is another coxsackievirus infection that is characterized by fever, sore throat, and mild headache. Hyperplastic lymphoid tissue of the soft palate or tonsillar pillars appears as yellowish or dark pink nodules. The disease generally lasts several days to 2 weeks and does not usually require treatment.

Other Viral Infections That May Have Oral Manifestations

Measles

Measles is a highly contagious disease causing systemic symptoms and a skin rash that results from a type of virus called a **paramyxovirus.** The disease most commonly occurs in childhood. Early in the disease, **Koplik spots,** which are small erythematous macules with white necrotic centers, may occur in the oral cavity.

Mumps

Mumps, or **epidemic parotitis,** is a viral infection of the salivary glands that is also caused by a paramyxovirus. The disease most commonly occurs in children and is characterized by painful

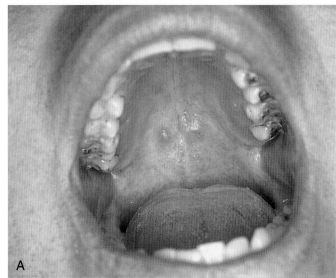
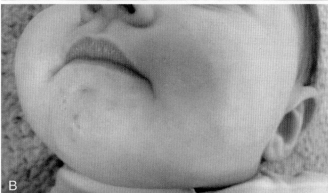
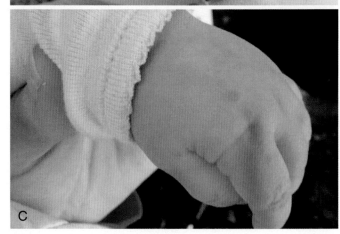

• **Figure 4.31** A, Herpangina. **B** and **C,** Hand-Foot-and-Mouth Disease in a 9-month-old infant. Papules on skin. (**B** and **C** courtesy Jill Lanzilotta.)

swelling of the salivary glands, most commonly bilateral swelling of the parotid glands.

Human Immunodeficiency Virus and Acquired Immunodeficiency Syndrome

The virus associated with **acquired immunodeficiency syndrome (AIDS)** was identified in 1983; in 1986 it was designated as **human immunodeficiency virus (HIV).** HIV is transmitted by

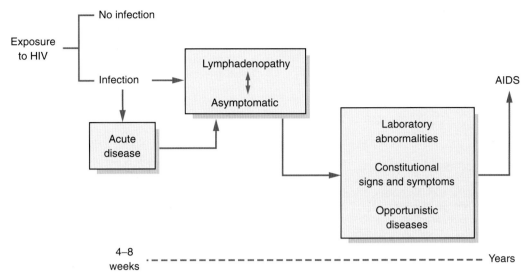

• **Figure 4.32** Spectrum of human immunodeficiency virus *(HIV)* disease. *AIDS,* acquired immunodeficiency syndrome.

sexual contact with infected persons, by contact with infected blood and blood products, and to infants of infected mothers. HIV infects cells of the immune system. The HIV virus infects cells that have the CD4 receptor on their cell surfaces. The most important of the cells of the immune system that the virus infects is the CD4⁺ T-helper lymphocyte. This lymphocyte is important both in cell-mediated immunity and in regulating the immune response. As the disease progresses, this lymphocyte becomes depleted. Other cells that may be infected with HIV include macrophages, Langerhans cells, dendritic cells, and cells of the nervous system.

The Spectrum of Human Immunodeficiency Virus

Many individuals experience an acute disease that occurs shortly after infection with human immunodeficiency virus, whereas other individuals remain asymptomatic. The acute disease resolves, and infected individuals may have no signs or symptoms of disease for some time. In most patients infected with human immunodeficiency virus, a progressive immunodeficiency eventually develops. As the immune system begins to fail, the number of CD4⁺ lymphocytes decreases; nonspecific problems such as fatigue and opportunistic infections such as oral candidiasis may develop. As the immune system becomes profoundly deficient, life-threatening opportunistic infections and cancers occur. The most severe result of infection with human immunodeficiency virus is acquired immunodeficiency syndrome (Fig. 4.32).

Diagnosing Acquired Immunodeficiency Syndrome

The diagnosis of AIDS is well defined. The definition of AIDS has been established by the Centers for Disease Control and Prevention (CDC) and revised several times since the disease was first identified in the early 1980s as the disease has become better understood and new laboratory tests allow more accurate measurement of antibodies and virus. The most recent definition was published by the CDC in 2014. In the most recent definition, AIDS is designated as Stage 3 HIV infection, whereas early

infection is designated as Stage 0. The most recent definition of AIDS in adults and adolescents includes HIV infection with severe CD4⁺ lymphocyte depletion (less than 200 CD4⁺ lymphocytes per microliter [μL] of blood). The normal CD4⁺ lymphocyte count is between about 550 and 1000 lymphocytes/μL blood. The revised definition continues to include a number of opportunistic diseases such as *Pneumocystis carinii* pneumonia, esophageal candidiasis, and Kaposi sarcoma (Box 4.2). Also included is HIV-related wasting syndrome, pulmonary tuberculosis, recurrent pneumonia, and invasive cervical cancer.

Human Immunodeficiency Virus Testing

Tests that identify antibodies to human immunodeficiency syndrome are the tests generally used to determine whether a person has been infected with human immunodeficiency virus. Recently, a rapid HIV test has been approved. This test identifies antibodies to human immunodeficiency virus either in oral fluid or in blood. The oral test uses a collector specially designed to obtain a sample of transudate through the oral mucosa. Oral fluid testing has been approved as a test that can be done by people at home. A positive oral fluid test is confirmed by a blood test using a more specific test called a **Western blot test.** A negative test does not require confirmation. Routine HIV testing of blood generally uses a blood test called an **enzyme-linked immunosorbent assay (ELISA).** When this test is positive twice, it is also followed by the more specific **Western blot test.** To be considered seropositive for human immunodeficiency virus, a person must have two positive ELISA results followed by a positive Western blot test result. Other tests such as the polymerase chain reaction (PCR) and a nucleic acid test identify virus rather than antibody. These are not generally used as screening tests. They are used to measure the amount of virus circulating in blood (viral load) and to assess the effectiveness of treatment. HIV testing is now becoming a component of the laboratory tests that accompany routine physical examinations. In the United States different states have different laws concerning HIV testing. In some states informed consent by the patient and pretest counseling may be required before HIV testing can be done. In other states an individual must specifically opt out of HIV testing or it will be included in routine laboratory testing. HIV testing is an important means of controlling human immunodeficiency virus infection by allowing infected individuals to be treated, and as a result, their viral load and potential infectivity are decreased.

Clinical Manifestations

The initial infection with human immunodeficiency virus may be completely asymptomatic. However, early in human immunodeficiency virus infection the amount of circulating virus is very high, and the risk of transmission to others may be very high. In some individuals lymphadenopathy may develop; in still others an acute illness resembling infectious mononucleosis and lasting 8 to 14 days can occur. When this acute illness develops, the patient may have sore throat, general malaise, myalgia and arthralgia, lymphadenopathy, and fever. Patients with acute infection can also have oral candidiasis, skin rash, nausea, and diarrhea. After this acute illness, some individuals have persistent lymphadenopathy, but many become completely asymptomatic.

The virus infects cells of the immune system; as a result this system stops protecting the individual against certain infections and tumors. In time, as the immune system becomes deficient, a variety of signs and symptoms can develop, signaling changes in the immune system. Several of these signs and symptoms occurring together are sometimes called *AIDS-related complex*. They

include oral candidiasis, fatigue, weight loss, and lymphadenopathy. Human immunodeficiency virus can also infect cells of the nervous system, resulting in dementia in some patients.

Antibodies to human immunodeficiency virus generally begin to be detectable in blood about 6 weeks after the initial infection. However, in some individuals antibodies may not be detectable for 6 months and occasionally for up to 1 year or more.

The spectrum of HIV infection includes the full range of problems that result from infection with this virus, from asymptomatic infection to AIDS. AIDS represents terminal HIV infection in this spectrum. It is not yet known how many of the persons who become infected with the human immunodeficiency virus go on to experience immunodeficiency, opportunistic diseases, or dementia. Some patients who are human immunodeficiency virus seropositive appear to remain immunocompetent for many years. Cofactors that can contribute to the development of the immunodeficiency are being studied. The results of natural history studies have shown that without treatment most HIV-infected individuals will develop AIDS.

Medical Management

Tests such as the polymerase chain reaction (PCR) are used to measure the amount of human immunodeficiency virus circulating in serum. This is called the *viral load*. Measurement of viral load along with the CD4+ lymphocyte count is used to assess HIV infection. Patients with HIV infection are managed with combinations of different types of antiretroviral (anti-HIV) drugs and drugs that prevent and treat opportunistic diseases. The combination of drugs is called *highly active antiretroviral therapy* (HAART or ART). Measurement of viral load is used to evaluate the effectiveness of antiretroviral therapy. Management of HIV infection is continually changing in response to the results of ongoing clinical drug trials. With antiretroviral treatment, many individuals infected with human immunodeficiency virus may live long and relatively healthy lives.

Oral Manifestations

Oral lesions were prominent features of acquired immune disease syndrome and human immunodeficiency virus infection before HAART/ART therapy was available (Box 4.3). Some of these lesions are known to be indicators of developing immunodeficiency and predictors of the development of acquired immune disease syndrome in individuals who are human immunodeficiency virus seropositive. The oral lesions that occur develop because of the deficiency in cell-mediated immunity and the deregulation of immunologic responses that occurs when the T-helper cells (CD4+ lymphocytes) become depleted. Oral lesions include opportunistic infections, tumors, and autoimmune-like diseases. As a result of management of human immunodeficiency virus infection with antiviral therapy, oral manifestations of HIV infection are much less common than earlier in the history of this disease.

Oral Candidiasis

Oral candidiasis occurs frequently in individuals with cell-mediated immunodeficiency and is one of the most common oral lesions seen in persons with HIV infection (Fig. 4.33). It is also called *thrush*. All of the different types of oral candidiasis described earlier in this chapter, including mucocutaneous candidiasis, can occur. It is important to remember that candidiasis can be associated with a variety of conditions other than HIV infection, such

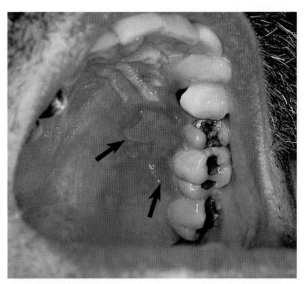

• **Figure 4.34** Herpes simplex ulceration of the hard palate in a patient with human immunodeficiency virus infection. *Arrows* point to the periphery of the ulcer.

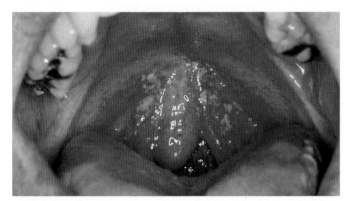

• **Figure 4.33** Candidiasis in a patient with human immunodeficiency virus infection. Removable white plaques are present on the mucosa of the soft palate.

as uncontrolled diabetes, other immunodeficiency diseases, antibiotic treatment, and xerostomia. Both topical and systemic antifungal treatment can be used to control oral candidiasis in the patient with immunodeficiency caused by HIV infection. Recurrence is common.

In persons who are known to be infected with human immunodeficiency virus, the development of oral candidiasis is worrisome because it generally signals the beginning of a progressively severe immunodeficiency. It may also be a sign of acute HIV infection. Persons with unexplained oral candidiasis should be referred to a physician for evaluation if the cause of the candidiasis cannot be determined. Studies have shown oral candidiasis to be a very early sign of developing immunodeficiency and predictive of the development of AIDS in a person who is infected with human immunodeficiency virus. Oral lesions caused by other fungal infections such as histoplasmosis and coccidioidomycosis have also been reported in persons with human immunodeficiency virus infection, but they are rare.

Herpes Simplex Infection

Ulcers caused by the herpes simplex virus occur in persons with HIV infection (Fig. 4.34). Herpes labialis and lesions consistent with intraoral recurrent herpes simplex infection can also develop in persons with HIV infection. The clinical characteristics of these lesions are the same as those occurring in immunocompetent individuals. However, when the immune system, particularly cell-mediated immunity, becomes deficient, HIV-infected individuals are at risk for the development of ulcers caused by the herpes simplex virus that do not have the same clinical characteristics as those seen in immunocompetent persons. These appear as persistent, superficial, painful ulcers that can be located anywhere in the oral cavity. Small, characteristic herpes simplex–like ulcers can be seen surrounding larger ulcers, but their presence cannot be depended on for diagnosis. The diagnosis of these ulcers is made by several methods, including viral culture, cytologic smear, biopsy, and response to the antiviral medication acyclovir.

Ulceration of the oral mucosa from herpes simplex infection that has been present for more than 1 month is an oral lesion that meets the criteria for the diagnosis of AIDS. This can occur only when a person has profound immunodeficiency. Oral ulcers caused by cytomegalovirus may also occur in HIV-infected individuals who are severely immunodeficient. These ulcers are much rarer than those caused by herpes simplex virus.

Herpes Zoster

Herpes zoster is caused by the VZV and is described earlier in this chapter. When herpes zoster occurs in a person with HIV infection, it generally follows the usual pattern (see Figs. 4.27 and 4.28). Although the infection can disseminate, most cases are self-limited. In the facial and oral area the lesions appear as distinctly unilateral ones following the distribution of one or more branches of the trigeminal nerve. The development of herpes zoster in a person infected with human immunodeficiency virus is a sign of developing immunodeficiency.

Hairy Leukoplakia

Hairy leukoplakia is caused by the Epstein-Barr virus and is discussed earlier in this chapter. It was first described in individuals with HIV infection; although it has been reported in HIV-negative individuals, most cases are an oral manifestation of HIV infection.

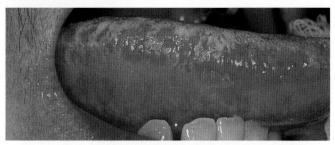

• **Figure 4.35** Hairy leukoplakia.

It almost always occurs on the lateral borders of the tongue and may extend onto the dorsal and ventral tongue (Fig. 4.35; and see Fig. 4.30). On the lateral tongue it appears as an irregular white lesion that has a corrugated surface. The corrugations may not be present when the lesions extend onto the dorsal or ventral tongue. Microscopically, this lesion shows hyperkeratosis (often with hair-like projections), epithelial hyperplasia, vacuolated epithelial cells, and little or no inflammatory infiltrate in the underlying connective tissue.

Other white lesions, such as those resulting from chronic tongue chewing and hyperplastic candidiasis, can resemble hairy leukoplakia clinically. Biopsy of the lesions can reveal a microscopic appearance that is consistent with hairy leukoplakia. However, the most reliable method of diagnosis is identification of the Epstein-Barr virus in the lesion.

In general, hairy leukoplakia is not treated. Lesions may respond to antiviral medication such as acyclovir or zidovudine but recur when treatment is discontinued. Studies have shown hairy leukoplakia to be predictive of the development of AIDS in HIV-infected persons.

Human Papillomavirus Infections

Lesions caused by human papillomaviruses are described earlier in this chapter. Papillary oral lesions resulting from several different papillomaviruses have been described in persons with human immunodeficiency virus infection. They are either normal in color or have a slightly erythematous mucosa (Fig. 4.36). These lesions may be persistent and may occur in multiple oral mucosal locations. Results of studies have suggested that the prevalence of these human papillomavirus lesions has not decreased with antiretroviral therapy as has the prevalence of most other HIV-associated oral lesions. Diagnosis of these lesions is made by biopsy and microscopic examination, with special tests to identify papillomavirus. Human papillomavirus lesions in patients with HIV infection are difficult to control, and recurrence and proliferation are common.

Kaposi Sarcoma

Kaposi sarcoma is one of the opportunistic neoplasms that occur in patients with human immunodeficiency virus infection. Human herpesvirus type 8 (HHV-8), or KSHV, has been associated with this neoplasm. Oral lesions appear as reddish-purple, flat or raised lesions and are seen anywhere in the oral cavity. The most common locations are the palate and gingiva (Fig. 4.37). This lesion was common before antiretroviral therapy was available, but is now seen much less frequently.

The diagnosis is made by biopsy. However, the clinical appearance of the lesion can be used when it is characteristic and the diagnosis of Kaposi sarcoma has been made at another site. At present no effective treatment for Kaposi sarcoma exists. Surgical excision to decrease the size of the lesion is sometimes attempted,

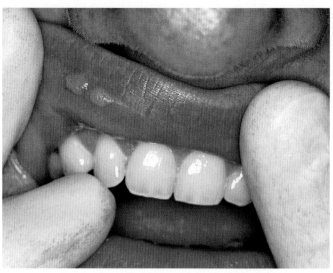

• **Figure 4.36** Papillary lesion of the upper lip caused by human papillomavirus in a patient with human immunodeficiency virus infection.

as are radiation treatment and chemotherapy. Kaposi sarcoma is one of the intraoral lesions that may fulfill the criteria for the diagnosis of AIDS.

Lymphoma

Non-Hodgkin lymphoma is another of the malignant tumors that occur in association with HIV infection. It occasionally occurs in the oral cavity. Epstein-Barr virus has been associated with this neoplasm. These tumors have appeared as nonulcerated, necrotic, or ulcerated masses and have been surfaced by either ulcerated or normal-colored erythematous mucosa (Fig. 4.38).

The diagnosis is made by biopsy and microscopic examination. Treatment involves several different chemotherapeutic drugs. Oral lymphoma is another oral lesion that may meet the criteria for the diagnosis of AIDS.

Gingival and Periodontal Disease

In patients with human immunodeficiency virus infection, unusual forms of gingival and periodontal disease can develop. These occur in HIV-infected individuals whose immune system has become deficient, and have been called **linear gingival erythema** and **necrotizing ulcerative periodontitis.** A condition resembling necrotizing ulcerative gingivitis also occurs in individuals with HIV infection.

Linear gingival erythema has three characteristic features: (1) spontaneous bleeding, (2) punctate or petechiae-like lesions on the attached gingiva and alveolar mucosa, and (3) a bandlike erythema of the gingiva that does not respond to therapy. Linear gingival erythema is different from typical gingivitis in that gingivitis is generally not characterized by spontaneous bleeding, and the erythema of typical gingivitis responds within a few days to 1 week to scaling, root planing, and improvement of oral hygiene. Linear gingival erythema occurs independently of oral hygiene status.

Some patients experience gingivitis that resembles necrotizing ulcerative gingivitis, and it can be either generalized or localized to specific areas. Necrotizing ulcerative periodontitis resembles necrotizing ulcerative gingivitis in that patients experience pain, spontaneous gingival bleeding, interproximal necrosis, and interproximal cratering (Fig. 4.39). Patients also experience intense erythema and, most characteristically, extremely rapid bone loss.

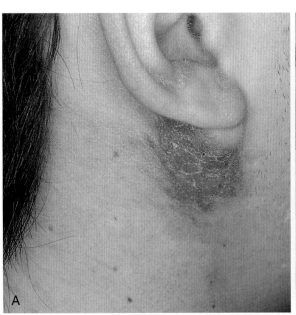
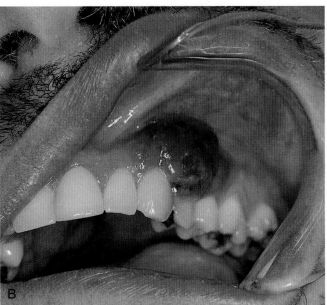

• **Figure 4.37** Kaposi sarcoma in a patient with acquired immunodeficiency syndrome. **A,** Skin. **B,** Gingiva. (Courtesy Dr. Fariba Younai.)

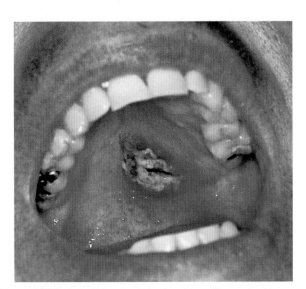

• **Figure 4.38** Intraoral lymphoma in a patient with acquired immunodeficiency syndrome.

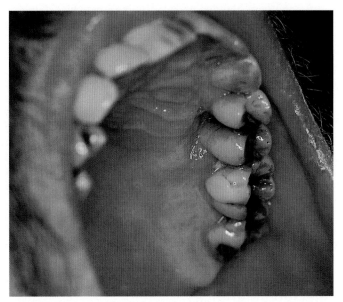

• **Figure 4.39** Atypical periodontal disease in a patient with human immunodeficiency virus infection.

Necrotizing stomatitis is characterized by extensive focal areas of bone loss along with the features of necrotizing ulcerative periodontitis.

The specific causes of these atypical gingival and periodontal diseases remain unclear. The microbiota associated with these diseases is being studied and has not been found to be distinctly different from that of inflammatory periodontal disease. These atypical gingival and periodontal conditions are not common in HIV-infected individuals and appear to occur in patients whose immune systems have become severely compromised.

Treatment of HIV gingivitis and periodontitis involves scaling, root planing, and soft tissue curettage. In addition, intrasulcular lavage with povidone-iodine, use of a chlorhexidine mouth rinse, and short-term systemic metronidazole administration have been

helpful in the treatment of these conditions. Good oral hygiene, including the use of smaller toothbrushes and interproximal cleaning devices, has been a component of management.

Most HIV-infected patients do not have HIV-associated gingival and periodontal problems. However, recognition of early lesions is essential to prevent extensive bone loss, and frequent recall is helpful in early identification of gingival and periodontal disease. Lack of response to periodontal treatment is a clue to the recognition of HIV-associated gingivitis and periodontitis.

Spontaneous Gingival Bleeding

A decrease in the number of platelets resulting from an autoimmune type of thrombocytopenic purpura is occasionally seen in patients with human immunodeficiency virus infection. These

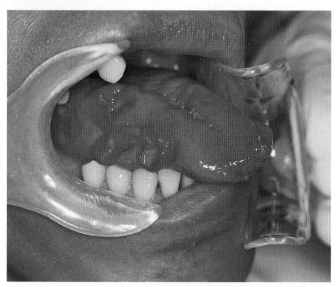

• **Figure 4.40** Persistent, nonspecific (major aphthouslike) ulcers in a patient with human immunodeficiency virus infection. (Courtesy Dr. Sidney Eisig.)

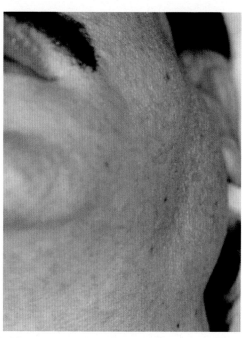

• **Figure 4.41** Salivary gland enlargement was bilateral in this patient with human immunodeficiency virus infection.

patients can have bleeding gums or mucosal petechiae. Gingival bleeding not related to thrombocytopenia has also been described in linear gingival erythema and necrotizing ulcerative periodontitis. A platelet count should be considered before deep scaling procedures are performed.

Aphthous Ulcers

Characteristic minor aphthous ulcers occur in patients with human immunodeficiency virus infection and AIDS. Studies have suggested that an increase in the incidence of these ulcers occurs in patients with HIV infection. The clinical appearance and behavior of minor aphthous ulcers in HIV-infected patients are the same as in other individuals (see Chapter 3). Minor aphthous ulcers are diagnosed on the basis of their clinical appearance.

Ulcers that resemble major aphthous ulcers also occur in patients with HIV infection (Fig. 4.40). They appear as deep, persistent, painful ulcers and must be differentiated from infectious ulcers. Biopsy and microscopic examination of these ulcers do not show any evidence of an infectious cause. These ulcers respond to topical and systemic corticosteroid therapy. Topical application of tetracycline and thalidomide has also been used in the management of these ulcers. Similar ulcers have been reported in the esophagus of patients with HIV infection.

Salivary Gland Disease

Bilateral parotid gland enlargement has been reported to occur in patients who are HIV-positive (Fig. 4.41). The microscopic appearance is reported to be that of a benign lymphoepithelial lesion, often with a prominent cystic component. Xerostomia has been reported to be associated with HIV infection. The cause is not clear. It may be related to medication administration or salivary gland disease.

Selected References

Books

Kumar V, Abbas AK, Fausto N, et al: *Robbins basic pathology*, ed 9, Philadelphia, 2013, Saunders.

Langlais RP, Miller CS, Gehrig JS: *Color atlas of common oral diseases*, ed 5, Philadelphia, 2017, Lippincott Williams and Wilkins.

Neville BW, Damm DD, Allen CM, et al: *Oral and maxillofacial pathology*, ed 4, St. Louis, 2016, Elsevier.

Regezi JA, Sciubba JJ, Jordan RCK: *Oral pathology: clinical-pathologic correlations*, ed 7, Philadelphia, 2017, Elsevier.

Journal Articles

Alves M, Mulligan R, Passaro D, et al: Longitudinal evaluation of loss of attachment in HIV-infected women compared to HIV-uninfected women, *J Periodontol* 77:773, 2006.

Centers for Disease Control and Prevention: 1993 revised classification system for HIV infection and expanded surveillance case definition for AIDS among adolescents and adults, *MMWR Recomm Rep* 41(RR–17):1, 1992.

Cleveland JL, Junger ML, Saraiya M, et al: The connection between human papillomavirus and oropharyngeal squamous cell carcinomas in the United States: implications for dentistry, *J Am Dent Assoc* 142:915, 2011.

Depaola LG: Human immunodeficiency virus disease: natural history and management, *Oral Surg Oral Med Oral Pathol Oral Radiol Endod* 90:266, 2000.

Eisen D: The clinical characteristics of intraoral herpes simplex virus infection in 52 immunocompetent patients, *Oral Surg Oral Med Oral Pathol Oral Radiol Endod* 86:432, 1998.

Gillison ML, Broutian T, Pickard RK, et al: The prevalence of oral HPV infection in the United States, 2009-2010, *JAMA* 307:693, 2012.

Greenspan D, Gange SJ, Phelan JA, et al: Incidence of oral lesions in HIV-1–infected women: reduction with HAART, *J Dent Res* 83:145, 2004.

Harris AM, Van Wyk CW: Heck's disease (focal epithelial hyperplasia): a longitudinal study, *Community Dent Oral Epidemiol* 21:82, 1993.

Hodgson TA, Greenspan D, Greenspan JS: Oral lesions of HIV disease and HAART in industrialized countries, *Adv Dent Res* 19:57, 2006.

Holbrook WP, Gunnlaugur TG, Ragnarsson KT: Herpetic gingivostomatitis in otherwise healthy adolescents and young adults, *Acta Odontol Scand* 59:113, 2001.

Iacopino AM, Wathen WF: Oral candidal infection and denture stomatitis: a comprehensive review, *J Am Dent Assoc* 123:46, 1992.

Jones AC, Gulley ML, Freedman PD: Necrotizing ulcerative stomatitis in human immunodeficiency virus–seropositive individuals: a review of the histopathologic, immunohistochemical, and virologic characteristics of 18 cases, *Oral Surg Oral Med Oral Pathol Oral Radiol Endod* 89:323, 2000.

Koorbusch GF, Fotos P, Terhark K: Retrospective assessment of osteomyelitis, *Oral Surg Oral Med Oral Pathol* 74:149, 1992.

Kulak-Ozkan Y, Kazazoglu E, Arikan A: Oral hygiene habits, denture cleanliness, presence of yeasts and stomatitis in elderly people, *J Oral Rehabil* 29:300, 2002.

Leggott PJ: Oral manifestations of HIV infection in children, *Oral Surg Oral Med Oral Pathol* 73:187, 1992.

Leigh JE, Kishore S, Fidel PL Jr: Oral opportunistic infections in HIV-positive individuals: review and role of mucosal immunity, *AIDS Patient Care* 18:443, 2004.

MacPhail LA, Komaroff E, Alves ME, et al: Differences in risk factors among clinical types of oral candidiasis in the Women's Interagency HIV Study, *Oral Surg Oral Med Oral Pathol Oral Radiol Endod* 93:45, 2002.

Morrow DJ, Sandhu HS, Daley TD: Focal epithelial hyperplasia (Heck's disease) with generalized lesions of the gingiva: a case report, *J Periodontol* 64:63, 1993.

Narana N, Epstein JB: Classifications of oral lesions in HIV infection, *J Clin Periodontol* 28:137, 2001.

Pankhurst CL: Candidiasis (oropharyngeal), *Clin Evid* 15:1849, 2006.

Patton LL, Ranganathan K, Naidoo S, et al: Oral lesions, HIV phenotypes, and management of HIV-related disease: Workshop 4A, *Adv Dent Res* 23:112, 2011.

Peterman TA, Heffelfinger JD, Swint EB, et al: The changing epidemiology of syphilis, *Sex Transm Dis* 32(10 Suppl):S4, 2005.

Rautava J, Syrjänen S: Human papillomavirus infections in the oral mucosa, *J Am Dent Assoc* 142:905, 2011.

Robinson JL, Vaudry WL, Dobrovolsky W: Actinomycosis presenting as osteomyelitis in the pediatric population, *Pediatr Infect Dis J* 24:365, 2005.

Ryder MI: An update on HIV and periodontal disease, *J Periodontol* 73:1071, 2002.

Shirlaw PJ, Chikte U, MacPhail L, et al: Oral and dental care and treatment protocols for the management of HIV-infected patients, *Oral Dis* 8(Suppl 2):136, 2002.

Siegel MA: Diagnosis and management of recurrent herpes simplex infections, *J Am Dent Assoc* 133:1245, 2002.

Soysa NS, Samaranayake LP, Ellepola AN: Diabetes mellitus as a contributory factor in oral candidosis, *Diabet Med* 23:455, 2006.

Watkins P: Impetigo: aetiology, complications and treatment options, *Diabet Med* 19:51, 2005.

Websites

New York State Department of Health AIDS Institute: HIV clinical resource [clinical guidelines]. Available at http://www.hivguidelines.org.

Centers for Disease Control and Prevention: Hand, foot, and mouth disease. Available at http://www.cdc.gov/hand-foot-mouth/index.html.

Review Questions

1. The most specific of the body's defense mechanisms against infection is:
   a. Intact skin
   b. The immune response
   c. Skin secretions
   d. The inflammatory response

2. Which statement is *false?*
   a. The primary lesion of syphilis is called a chancre.
   b. The secondary lesion of syphilis occurs at the site of inoculation with the organism.
   c. The tertiary lesion of syphilis is called a gumma.
   d. Syphilis is caused by the spirochete *Treponema pallidum.*

3. Perioral lesions of impetigo may resemble:
   a. Syphilis
   b. Herpes labialis
   c. Herpes zoster
   d. Actinomycosis

4. Which of the following is *not* associated with group A, β-hemolytic streptococcal infection?
   a. Tonsillitis
   b. Syphilis
   c. Scarlet fever
   d. Rheumatic fever

5. Oral candidiasis is caused by a:
   a. Bacterium
   b. Yeastlike fungus
   c. Spirochete
   d. Protozoan

6. Which statement is *false?*
   a. Angular cheilitis may be caused by *Candida albicans.*
   b. White lesions resulting from candidiasis may not rub off the mucosal surface.
   c. Erythematous candidiasis is usually completely asymptomatic.
   d. Denture stomatitis may be a form of oral candidiasis.

7. Which type of infection is involved when normal components of the oral microflora can cause disease?
   a. Chronic inflammatory
   b. Opportunistic
   c. Hyperplastic
   d. Granulomatous

8. The most characteristic clinical feature of herpes zoster is:
   a. Ulcer formation
   b. Pain
   c. Unilateral distribution of lesions
   d. Abscesses that drain through fistulas

9. A cytologic smear may be helpful in the diagnosis of:
   a. Coxsackievirus infection
   b. Human papillomavirus infection
   c. Tuberculosis
   d. Candidiasis

10. Which condition is *not* associated with the Epstein-Barr virus?
    a. Hairy leukoplakia
    b. Herpangina
    c. Nasopharyngeal carcinoma
    d. Infectious mononucleosis

11. Which of the following stages of syphilis is *not* infectious?
    a. Primary
    b. Secondary
    c. Tertiary
    d. All stages are equally infectious

12. Which of the following is *not* associated with syphilis?
    a. Mucous patch
    b. Venereal Disease Research Laboratories and fluorescent treponemal antibody
    c. Dark-field microscopy
    d. Hypodontia

13. Which of the following microorganisms causes tuberculosis?
    a. Mycobacterium israelii
    b. Actinomycosis israelii
    c. Mycobacterium tuberculosis
    d. Treponema pallidum

14. A positive skin reaction to PPD indicates:
    a. Active tuberculosis
    b. Contagious tuberculosis
    c. If a person has ever been infected with the tuberculosis bacteria
    d. Need for antibiotic therapy

15. A specific clinical characteristic found in actinomycosis is:
    a. Periapical radiolucency
    b. Filamentous bacteria
    c. Fungal infection
    d. Sulfur granules present in exudate

16. Which of the following is *not* a clinical characteristic of necrotizing ulcerative gingivitis?
    a. Painful gingiva
    b. Xerostomia
    c. Foul odor
    d. Metallic taste

17. Which of the following is associated with chronic osteomyelitis?
    a. Sickle cell anemia
    b. Paget disease of bone
    c. Radiation treatment involving bone
    d. All of the above

18. Which of the following is *not* associated with the development of oral candidiasis?
    a. Antibiotic therapy
    b. HIV infection
    c. Xerostomia
    d. Herpangina

19. Verruca vulgaris:
    a. Clinically resembles an irritative fibroma
    b. Is caused by a human papillomavirus
    c. Is most commonly seen on the buccal mucosa
    d. Clinically resembles a pyogenic granuloma

20. Another name for a common wart is:
    a. Papilloma
    b. Verruca vulgaris
    c. Condyloma acuminatum
    d. Fibroma

21. Which of the following is caused by a papillomavirus and is considered a sexually transmitted disease?
    a. Actinomycosis
    b. Syphilis
    c. Condyloma acuminatum
    d. Infectious mononucleosis

22. Painful oral ulcers, gingivitis, fever, malaise, and cervical lymphadenopathy in a child younger than 6 years old would cause the hygienist to suspect which of the following diseases?
    a. Herpangina
    b. Heck disease
    c. Primary herpes simplex infection
    d. Herpetic whitlow

23. The most common form of recurrent herpes simplex infection is:
    a. Herpes zoster
    b. Herpetic whitlow
    c. Herpangina
    d. Herpes labialis

24. The primary infection with the varicella-zoster virus is called:
    a. Primary herpetic gingivostomatitis
    b. Chickenpox
    c. Shingles
    d. Measles

25. Herpangina is caused by:
    a. Coxsackievirus
    b. Herpes simplex virus
    c. Varicella-zoster virus
    d. Epstein-Barr virus

26. Antibody testing to determine whether a person has been infected with human immunodeficiency virus includes which of the following tests?
    a. Schilling
    b. Schirmer
    c. Prothrombin time and partial thromboplastin time
    d. Enzyme-linked immunosorbent assay and Western blot

27. Which one of the following oral conditions is an early sign of a deficiency in the immune system and is commonly found in patients with HIV infection?
    a. Erythema migrans
    b. Advanced periodontitis
    c. Candidiasis
    d. Histoplasmosis

28. Hairy leukoplakia most commonly occurs on the:
    a. Buccal mucosa
    b. Dorsal tongue
    c. Lateral tongue
    d. Soft palate

29. Which one of the following oral conditions is *not* a lesion associated with HIV or AIDS?
    a. Candidiasis
    b. Hairy leukoplakia
    c. Kaposi sarcoma
    d. Leukoedema

30. Linear gingival erythema has specific characteristics that include spontaneous bleeding, petechiae on the attached gingiva and alveolar mucosa, and a band of erythema at the gingival margin. Which one of the following statements is *true?*
    a. These tissues respond well to scaling and root planing.
    b. Excellent oral hygiene and home care techniques will eliminate these gingival conditions.
    c. This condition will automatically develop into advanced periodontal disease in all patients infected with human immunodeficiency virus.
    d. Patients with linear gingival erythema do not respond to scaling or oral hygiene techniques; the gingival condition exists independently of the patient's oral hygiene status.

31. Which of the following statements is *false* concerning primary herpetic gingivostomatitis?
    a. After primary herpes simplex infection, the latent infection is usually in the trigeminal ganglion.
    b. The virus is able to survive outside the body and is therefore easily transmitted by fomites.
    c. The initial oral infection is usually due to HSV type 1.
    d. The HSV altered epithelial cell is called a Tsanck cell.

32. Which of the following clinical features would help differentiate between recurrent oral mucosal simplex infection and recurrent aphthous stomatitis?
    a. The location of the ulcers; herpes simplex ulceration occur on keratinized epithelium and aphthous ulcers occur on nonkeratinized epithelium.
    b. Systemic signs and symptoms accompany recurrent herpes simplex infection, but do not accompany recurrent aphthous ulcers.
    c. Recurrent herpes simplex ulceration is painful; recurrent aphthous ulcers are usually asymptomatic.
    d. Recurrent aphthous ulcers take much longer to heal than recurrent herpes simplex ulceration.

33. Which of the following statements is false concerning oral human papilloma virus (HPV) infection?
    a. HPV may be present in the oral mucosa without any signs or symptoms.
    b. HPV causes papillary oral mucosal lesions.
    c. HPV is transmitted by droplet infection.
    d. Microscopically, HPV-infected epithelial cells are called koilocytes.

34. Which of the following is the best diagnostic test for oral candidiasis?
    a. A mucosal smear (cytologic preparation) showing fungal hyphae
    b. A mucosal smear (cytologic preparation) showing Tzanck cells
    c. A positive culture for *Candida albicans*
    d. A blood test for *Candida* antibodies

35. Which of the following is the name of the oral lesions of primary syphilis?
    a. Gumma
    b. Mucous patch
    c. Chancre
    d. Verruca vulgaris

36. All of the following statements are correct statements concerning HIV infection except one. Which one is the exception?
    a. Two positive Elisa tests followed by a positive Western blot test confirms HIV infection.
    b. Initial infection with HIV can be asymptomatic.
    c. Antibodies to HIV are usually detectable in the blood by 2 weeks after infection.
    d. PCR is a test that measures viral load.

37. All of the following are characteristic features of hand-foot-and-mouth disease except one. Which one is the exception?
    a. Occurs in epidemics in children younger than 5 years.
    b. Is caused by Epstein-Barr virus.
    c. Is characterized by painful oral vesicles.
    d. Is characterized by multiple papules on the skin.

38. "Strawberry tongue" is associated with which condition?
    a. Herpangina
    b. Scarlet fever
    c. Rheumatic fever
    d. Tuberculosis

39. Which one of the following is considered a deep fungal infection?
    a. Median rhomboid glossitis
    b. Angular cheilitis
    c. Histoplasmosis
    d. Herpangina

Chapter 4 Synopsis

Condition/Disease	Cause	Age/Race/Sex	Location
Bacterial Infections			
Impetigo *Herpes labialis*	*Staphylococcus aureus* or occasionally *Streptococcus pyogenes*	Most commonly seen in children	Skin, most commonly on face and extremities
Tonsillitis and pharyngitis *Bacterial vs. viral infection*	*Streptococcus pyogenes* Other bacteria and viruses	Children and adults	Posterior oral cavity Tonsils Oropharynx
Tuberculosis *Deep fungal infections, i.e., histoplasmosis*	*Mycobacterium tuberculosis*	*	Primary infection of lung Bacteria can spread to other areas of the body
Actinomycosis *Other bacterial infections*	*Actinomyces israelii*	*	Skin/oral mucosa

Syphilis
Primary:
  Nonspecific oral ulcer
  Traumatic ulcer
Secondary:
  Hyperplastic candidiasis
Tertiary:
  Phycomycosis/mucormycosis
	Treponema pallidum	Usually seen in sexually active adults
		Congenital: infected mother to fetus
			Primary: site of inoculation
			Secondary: diffuse lesions of skin and mucous membranes
			Tertiary: cardiovascular system
			Central nervous system: oral lesions may occur

Necrotizing ulcerative gingivitis (NUG) *Primary herpetic gingivo-stomatitis*	*Borrelia vincentii* plus fusiform bacillus	Adolescents and adults	Gingiva
Pericoronitis	Inflammatory process, usually bacterial infection	More common in adolescents and young adults at the eruption of third molars	Tissue around the crown of a partially erupted impacted tooth
Acute osteomyelitis *Osteonecrosis*	Bacterial infection	*	Bone
Chronic osteomyelitis *Osteonecrosis*	Bacterial infection	*	Bone
Fungal Infections			
Oral candidiasis *Erythematous candidiasis* *Allergic mucositis*	Opportunistic infectious disease *Candida albicans*	Children and adults	Oral mucosa

NOTE: Items listed in *italics* under a specific condition/disease should be considered in a differential diagnosis.
N/A, Not applicable.
*No significant information.
†Not covered in this text.

Clinical Features	Radiographic Features	Microscopic Features	Treatment	Diagnostic Process
Vesicles or crusted lesions	N/A	N/A	Topical or systemic antibiotics	Clinical Laboratory
Enlarged tonsils Mucosal erythema	N/A	N/A	Systemic antibiotic if bacterial	Clinical Laboratory
Oral lesions: rare Painful, nonhealing, slowly enlarging, deep or superficial ulcers Most common locations are tongue and palate	N/A	Granulomas containing the causative organism	Combination antituberculosis agents	Laboratory Microscopic
Draining abscesses "Sulfur granules" in pus draining from abscess	N/A	Bacterial colonies in tissue from the lesion	Long-term, high-dose antibiotic therapy	Clinical Microscopic
Oral lesions Primary: chancre Secondary: mucous patches Tertiary: gumma	N/A	Skin: dark-field identification of spirochetes	Antibiotic agents (usually penicillin)	Clinical Laboratory
Painful, erythematous gingivitis with necrosis and cratering of the interdental papillae, foul odor, metallic taste Fever, cervical lymphadenopathy	N/A	N/A	Antibiotic agents Debridement of necrotic tissue Oral hygiene care	Clinical
Erythematous, painful, swollen tissue around the crown of the partially erupted tooth	Impacted tooth can be seen on radiograph	N/A	Debridement and irrigation Antibiotic therapy Extraction of impacted tooth	Clinical
	No radiographic change unless present for more than 1 wk	Nonviable bone Necrotic debris Acute inflammation Bacterial colonies	Antibiotic therapy Drainage of area	Clinical Laboratory
Involved bone is painful with swelling	Irregular radiolucency	Chronic inflammation of bone and bone marrow	Debridement Antibiotic therapy Hyperbaric oxygen	Clinical Radiographic Laboratory
Appearance depends on type Pseudomembranous Erythematous Chronic atrophic (denture stomatitis) Chronic hyperplastic Angular cheilitis Chronic mucocutaneous	N/A	*Candida* hyphae present on mucosal smear (cytologic preparation) *Candida* hyphae in biopsy tissue	Antifungal therapy	Clinical Microscopic Therapeutic

Continued

Chapter 4 Synopsis—cont'd

Condition/Disease	Cause	Age/Race/Sex	Location
Deep Fungal Infections			
Histoplasmosis	*Histoplasma capsulatum*	*	Primary: lung infection
Coccidioidomycosis	*Coccidioides immitis*		Secondary: oral mucosal involvement
Blastomycosis	*Blastomyces dermatitidis*		
Cryptococcosis	*Cryptococcus neoformans*		
Squamous cell carcinoma (a differential diagnosis of any of the four deep fungal infections listed above)			
Mucormycosis	†	*	Nasal cavity
			Maxillary sinus
			Hard palate
Viral Infections			
Verruca vulgaris	A human papillomavirus	Children and adults	Skin
Papilloma			Lips: most common oral location
Condyloma acuminatum	A human papillomavirus	Usually adults	Oral mucosa: any location
Other viral papillomas			
Multifocal epithelial hyperplasia	A human papillomavirus	Occurs in children	Oral mucosa
Coxsackievirus infections			
Primary herpetic gingivostomatitis	Herpes simplex virus	Generally in children	Lips, gingival and oral mucosa
Erythema multiforme	Most oral infections are type 1; some are type 2	Less common in adolescents and adults	
Recurrent herpes simplex infection	Herpes simplex virus	Usually seen in adolescents and adults	Herpes labialis: vermilion of lips
Traumatic ulcer			Recurrent intraoral form: keratinized mucosa (hard palate and gingiva)
Aphthous ulcer			
Chickenpox	Varicella-zoster virus	Usually seen in children	Skin
		Less common in adolescents and adults	Mucous membranes

NOTE: Items listed in *italics* under a specific condition/disease should be considered in a differential diagnosis.

N/A, Not applicable.

*No significant information.

†Not covered in this text.

Clinical Features	Radiographic Features	Microscopic Features	Treatment	Diagnostic Process
Chronic nonhealing ulcers	Irregular radiolucency if bone involvement	Causative organism identified in biopsy tissue	Appropriate antifungal agents	Microscopic
Proliferating mass with destruction of bone	Irregular radiolucency if bone involvement	Causative organism identified in biopsy tissue	Appropriate antifungal agent Management of underlying disease	Microscopic
White, papillary exophytic lesion resembling a papilloma	N/A	Fingerlike projection of keratotic squamous epithelium with central cores of well-vascularized fibrous connective tissue Cells with clear cytoplasm in the upper spinous layer	Surgical excision Immunologic staining to identify presence of papillomavirus May recur	Microscopic
Pink, papillary lesion usually more diffuse than papilloma or verruca vulgaris There may be multiple lesions	N/A	Thickened epithelium with fingerlike projections covering cores of connective tissue Cells with clear cytoplasm seen throughout the epithelium	Surgical excision Recurrence is common	Microscopic
Multiple whitish to pale pink nodules distributed throughout the oral mucosa	N/A	Thickened epithelium with broad, connected rete bridges Cells with clear cytoplasm seen in the epithelium	Self-limited disease	Clinical Microscopic
Multiple tiny vesicles that progress to form painful ulcers Painful, erythematous, swollen gingival Fever, malaise, cervical lymphadenopathy	N/A	Virally altered epithelial cells in mucosal smear or biopsy tissue (Tzanck cells)	Self-limited disease	Clinical Microscopic
Focal crops of tiny vesicles that coalesce to form a single ulcer Prodromal symptoms	N/A	Virally altered epithelial cells in mucosal smear (cytologic preparation) or biopsy tissue (Tzanck cells)	Self-limited disease	Clinical
Vesicular and pustular eruptions Oral lesions usually do not cause severe discomfort	N/A	Virally altered epithelial cells in mucosal smear (cytologic preparation) or biopsy tissue (Tzanck cells)	Self-limited disease	Clinical

Continued

Chapter 4 Synopsis—cont'd

Condition/Disease	Cause	Age/Race/Sex	Location
Herpes zoster *Recurrent herpes simplex infection*	Varicella-zoster virus	Occurs in adults	Skin Mucous membranes
Infectious mononucleosis *Lymphadenopathy* *Lymphoma*	Epstein-Barr virus	Usually occurs in adolescents and young adults	Systemic disease
Herpangina *Other coxsackievirus infections* *Primary herpes simplex infections*	A coxsackievirus	Usually young children and adults	Soft palate
Hand-foot-and-mouth-disease *Other coxsackievirus infections*	A coxsackievirus	Affects children under 5 yr	Oral mucosa Skin: feet, hands, fingers
Acute lymphonodular pharyngitis *Other coxsackievirus infections* *Streptococcal pharyngitis*	A coxsackievirus	Children	Nodular lesions on the soft palate and tonsillar area
Measles *Rubella*	A paramyxovirus	Most commonly occurs in children	Primarily skin Oral mucosa: early lesions
Mumps *Sialadenoses* *Lymphadenopathy*	A paramyxovirus	Most commonly occurs in children	Salivary glands
HIV infection/AIDS	Immune deficiency resulting from infection with the human immunodeficiency virus	Newborn infants to adults	Systemic disease

NOTE: Items listed in *italics* under a specific condition/disease should be considered in a differential diagnosis.
N/A, Not applicable.
*No significant information.
†Not covered in this text.

Clinical Features	Radiographic Features	Microscopic Features	Treatment	Diagnostic Process
Unilateral distribution of painful vesicles along a sensory nerve Prodromal symptoms	N/A	Virally altered epithelial cells in mucosal smear (cytologic preparation (cytologic preparation) or biopsy tissue (Tzanck cells)	Antiviral agents Corticosteroids	Clinical
Palatal petechiae Sore throat Fever Generalized lymphadenopathy Enlarged spleen Malaise Fatigue	N/A	Atypical white blood cells in blood	Usually self-limited disease	Laboratory
Fever Malaise Vesicles on the soft palate	N/A	N/A	Self-limited disease	Clinical
Oral lesions: vesicles anywhere in the mouth	N/A	N/A	Self-limited disease	Clinical
Sore throat Fever Mild headache Oral lesions in the posterior oral cavity	N/A	*	Self-limited disease	Clinical
Oral mucosa: Koplik spots—erythematous macules with white necrotic centers	N/A	N/A	Self-limited disease	Clinical
Painful, usually bilateral enlargement of salivary glands	N/A	N/A	Self-limited disease	Clinical
Opportunistic diseases Oral manifestations include oral candidiasis, herpes simplex infection, herpes zoster, hairy leukoplakia, papillomavirus lesions, Kaposi sarcoma, lymphoma, atypical periodontal disease, major aphthouslike ulcers, salivary gland disease, xerostomia, and mucosal pigmentation Autoimmune-type thrombocytopenia may result in spontaneous gingival bleeding	Severe and rapid bone loss seen in atypical periodontal disease	Dependent on opportunistic disease	Combination antiretroviral agents Management of specific opportunistic disease	Laboratory Microscopic

5

Developmental Disorders

OLGA A.C. IBSEN

OBJECTIVES

After studying this chapter, the student will be able to:

1. Define each of the words in the vocabulary list for this chapter.
2. Compare and contrast developmental disorders, inherited disorders, and congenital disorders.
3. Describe the embryonic development of the face, oral cavity, and teeth.
4. Discuss developmental soft tissue abnormalities such as ankyloglossia, commissural lip pits, and a lingual thyroid.
5. Do the following related to developmental cysts:
   - Describe the differences between odontogenic and nonodontogenic cysts.
   - Distinguish between intraosseous cysts and extraosseous cysts.
   - Name four odontogenic cysts that are intraosseous.
   - Name two odontogenic cysts that are extraosseous.
   - Name four nonodontogenic cysts that are intraosseous.
   - Name four nonodontogenic cysts that are found in the soft tissues of the head, neck, and oral region.

6. Do the following related to developmental abnormalities of teeth:
   - List, define, and discuss three abnormalities that affect the number of teeth.
   - List, define, and discuss two abnormalities that affect the size of teeth.
   - List, define, and discuss five abnormalities that affect the shape of teeth.
   - List, define, and discuss four abnormalities that affect the structure of teeth.
   - Define, identify, and discuss each of the following abnormalities that affect the eruption of teeth: impacted teeth, embedded teeth, and ankylosed teeth.
7. Identify the diagnostic process that contributes most significantly to the final diagnosis for each developmental anomaly discussed in this chapter.

❖ Vocabulary

Ankyloglossia (ang″kə-lo-glos′e-ə) Extensive adhesion of the tongue to the floor of the mouth or the lingual aspect of the anterior portion of the mandible.

Ankylosed teeth (ang′kə-lōzd tēth) Teeth that are fused to the alveolar bone; a condition especially common with retained deciduous teeth.

Anodontia (an″o-don′shə) Congenital lack of teeth.

Anomaly (ə-nom′ə-le) Marked deviation from normal, especially as a result of congenital or hereditary defects.

Commissure (kom′i-sūr) The site of union of corresponding parts (e.g., the corners of the lips) (labial commissure, commissural lip pits).

Concrescence (kən-kres′əns) In dentistry, a condition in which two adjacent teeth become united by cementum.

Congenital disorder (kən-jen′ĭ-təl dis-or′dər) A disorder that is present at and existing from the time of birth.

Cyst (sist) An abnormal sac or cavity lined by epithelium and surrounded by fibrous connective tissue.

Dens in dente (dens in den′te) "A tooth within a tooth"; a developmental anomaly that results when the enamel organ invaginates into the crown of a tooth before mineralization.

Dentinogenesis (den″tĭ-no-jen′ə-sis) The formation of dentin.

Differentiation (dif″ər-en″she-a′shən) The distinguishing of one tissue from another.

Dilaceration (di-las″ər-a′shən) An abnormal bend or curve, as in the root of a tooth.

Fusion (fu′zhən) The union of two adjacent tooth germs.

Gemination (jem″ĭ-na′shən) "Twinning"; when a single tooth germ attempts to divide, resulting in the incomplete formation of two teeth; the tooth usually has a single root and root canal.

Hypodontia (hi″po-don′shə) Partial anodontia; the lack of one or more teeth.

Hypercementosis (hi′pĕr-sē′men-tō′sis) Excessive cementum on the roots of teeth.

Impacted teeth (im-pak′təd tēth) Teeth that cannot erupt into the oral cavity because of a physical obstruction.

Macrodontia (mak″ro-don′shə) Abnormally large teeth.

Macrognathia (mak″ro-nath′e-ah) Enlarged jaw.

Microdontia (mi″kro-don′shə) Abnormally small teeth.

Multilocular (mul″tĭ-lok′ū-lər) A radiographic appearance in which many circular radiolucencies exist; these can appear "soap bubble–like" or "honeycomb-like."

Nodule (nod′ūl) A small solid mass that can be detected through touch.

Oligodontia (ol″ĭ-go-don′she-ə) A subcategory of hypodontia in which six or more teeth are missing.

Predilection (prĕd-ĭ-lĕk′shən) A disposition in favor of something; preference.

Proliferation (pro-lif″ə-ra′shən) The multiplication of cells.

Stomodeum (sto″mo-de′əm) The embryonic invagination that becomes the oral cavity.

Supernumerary (soo″per-noo′mər-ar″e) In excess of the normal or regular number, as in teeth.

The development of the human body is an extremely complex process that begins when an egg is fertilized by a sperm. It continues with a series of cell divisions, multiplications, and **differentiation** into various tissues and structures. A failure or disturbance that occurs during these processes may result in a lack, excess, or deformity of a body part. These disorders are called **developmental disorders** or **developmental anomalies.**

Inherited disorders are different from developmental disorders in that they are caused by an abnormality in the genetic makeup (genes and chromosomes) of an individual and transmitted from parent to offspring through the egg or sperm. Inherited disorders are discussed in Chapter 6.

A **congenital disorder** is one that is present at birth. It can be either inherited or developmental; however, the cause of most congenital abnormalities is unknown.

The complex process of **proliferation** and differentiation that takes place in the human body provides numerous possibilities for errors or defects in development. The head and neck region is a common location for such errors because of its intricate sequence and pattern of development. This chapter includes descriptions of developmental disorders of the face, oral cavity, and teeth with which the dental hygienist should be familiar.

Some of the developmental disturbances discussed in this chapter can be identified clinically, whereas others are identified by radiographic examination; still others require biopsy and microscopic examinations. A thorough clinical examination, including examination of extraoral and intraoral structures, is an essential component. Dental radiographs are an important part of the examination. Any developmental anomalies observed either clinically or radiographically are documented in the patient's record even if no treatment is indicated. The patient is informed of all dental anomalies, their possible implications, and the treatment necessary, if any. In some instances referral to a specialist is indicated. To better understand these developmental disorders, a brief review of the embryonic development of the face, oral cavity, and teeth is included in this chapter.

Embryonic Development of the Face, Oral Cavity, and Teeth

Face

Development of the face is a process of selective growth, or proliferation and differentiation (Figs. 5.1 and 5.2). During the third week of embryonic life, an **invagination,** or infolding, of the ectoderm forms the primitive oral cavity, which is called the **stomodeum.** Just above the stomodeum is a process called the **frontal process,** and just below it is a structure called the first **branchial arch.** Additional branchial arches form below the first branchial arch. All of the face and most of the structures of the oral cavity develop from either the frontal process or the first branchial arch. The first branchial arch divides into two **maxillary processes** and the **mandibular process.** The maxillary processes give rise to the upper part of the cheeks, the lateral portions of the upper lip, and part of the palate. The mandibular arch forms the lower part of the cheeks, the mandible, and part of the tongue.

As development continues, two pits (called **olfactory pits**) mark the future openings of the nose that develop on the surface of the frontal process. They divide the frontal process into three parts: (1) the **median nasal process,** (2) the **right lateral nasal process,** and (3) the **left lateral nasal process.** The lateral nasal processes form the sides of the nose, whereas the median nasal process forms the center and tip of the nose. Later, the median nasal process grows downward between the maxillary processes to

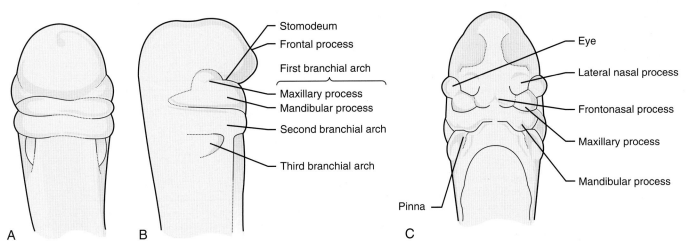

• **Figure 5.1** In the third week of embryonic life, an invagination, or infolding, of the ectoderm forms the primitive oral cavity, called the *stomodeum.* **A and B,** As facial development continues, the first branchial arch divides into two maxillary processes. **C,** The fourth week of development.

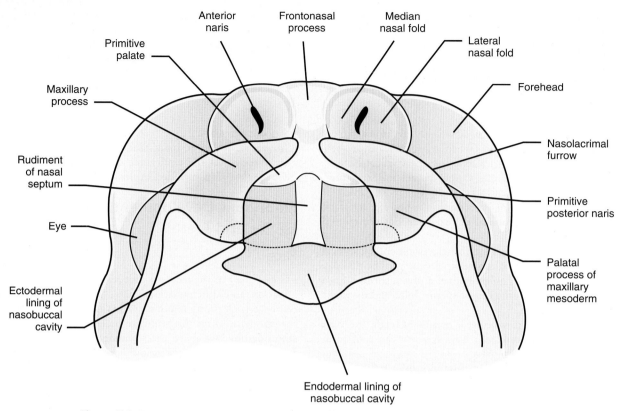

• **Figure 5.2** The right and left palatine processes fuse to form the maxilla and premaxilla. A Y-shaped pattern results.

form a pair of bulges called the **globular process.** This continues to grow downward, forming the portion of the upper lip called the **philtrum.** Most of these developments are completed by the end of the eighth week of embryonic life.

Oral and Nasal Cavities

The area of the palate called the **premaxilla** develops from the globular process. The lateral **palatine processes** (left and right) are formed from the maxillary processes. These lateral palatine processes then fuse with the premaxilla. The fusion creates a Y-shaped pattern (see Fig. 5.2). The nasal septum arises from the median nasal process. The right and left maxillary processes fuse together with the nasal septum at the center of the palate.

The tongue develops from the first three branchial arches. The second and third branchial arches are located just below the first branchial arch (Fig. 5.1B). The body of the tongue forms from the first branchial arch, and the base of the tongue forms from the second and third branchial arches.

Teeth

Tooth development, or **odontogenesis,** in the human embryo begins at about the fifth week of embryonic life and involves both ectoderm and ectomesenchyme. The ectomesenchyme is derived from neural crest cells.

Odontogenesis begins with the formation of a band of ectoderm in each jaw called the **primary dental lamina.** Ten small knoblike proliferations of epithelial cells develop on the primary dental lamina in each jaw (Fig. 5.3A). Each of these proliferations

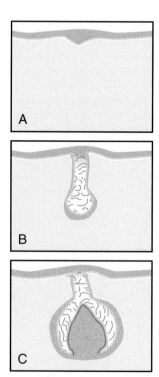

• **Figure 5.3** Development of a tooth germ, showing initiation of dental lamina **(A),** proliferation of dental lamina **(B),** and differentiation of the components of the tooth germ **(C).** (From Bath-Balogh M, Fehrenbach MF: *Illustrated dental embryology, histology, and anatomy,* ed 3, St. Louis, Saunders, 2012.)

extends into the underlying mesenchyme, becoming the early enamel organ for each of the primary teeth (Fig. 5.3B).

The tooth germ is composed of three parts: (1) the enamel organ, (2) the dental papilla, and (3) the dental sac, or *follicle* (Fig. 5.3C). The enamel organ develops from ectoderm, and the dental papilla and dental sac or follicle develop from mesoderm. Cell differentiation in the enamel organ progresses to produce ameloblasts, which form enamel. In the dental papilla odontoblasts are produced to form dentin. The permanent, or **succedaneous,** enamel organs form at the same time.

Formation of dental hard tissues occurs during the fifth month of gestation (Fig. 5.4). **Dentinogenesis** is the formation of **dentin.** Dentin is the first mineralized tooth tissue to appear. When it begins to form, the mesenchymal tissue within the tooth germ is called the **dental papilla.** After dentin is produced, the dental papilla is called the *dental pulp.* **Enamel** is the product of the enamel organ. Enamel matrix begins to form shortly after dentin, and mineralization and maturation of enamel follow the formation of the matrix. **Amelogenesis** refers to the formation of enamel. The enamel is highly mineralized epithelial tissue, and 90% of its volume is occupied by hydroxyapatite crystals.

The dental sac, or follicle, that surrounds the developing tooth germ provides cells that form cementum, the periodontal ligament, and alveolar bone. **Cementogenesis** (the formation of **cementum**) occurs after crown formation is complete. An epithelial structure called the **Hertwig epithelial root sheath** proliferates to shape the root of the tooth and induces the formation of the root dentin. Cells of the Hertwig epithelial root sheath must break up and pull away from the root surface before cementum can be produced. Very little cementum is produced until the tooth has erupted and is in occlusion and functioning. Root length is not completed until 1 to 4 years after the tooth erupts into the oral cavity.

Developmental Soft Tissue Abnormalities

Ankyloglossia

Ankyloglossia is a developmental anomaly of the tongue. It is an extensive adhesion of the tongue to the floor of the mouth, caused by a complete or partial fusion of the lingual frenum to the floor of the mouth. The condition is often referred to as "tongue-tied." Ankyloglossia is derived from the Greek words *ankylos,* meaning adhesion, and *glossa,* meaning tongue. It is four times more common in boys than in girls.

Complete ankyloglossia is rare and seen in 3 out of 10,000 adults. Partial ankyloglossia appears clinically as a very short lingual frenum connecting the anteroventral portion of the tongue to the floor of the mouth (Fig. 5.5). Patients with a short lingual frenum may exhibit no adverse effects, but some may have problems with speech. Gingival recession and bone loss can occur if the frenum is attached high on the lingual alveolar ridge. Treatment may not be necessary. Surgical removal of a portion of the lingual frenum, known as **frenectomy,** is the usual treatment for ankyloglossia. Some infants with breastfeeding problems are successfully treated with a frenectomy.

Commissural Lip Pits

Commissural lip pits are epithelium-lined blind tracts located at the corners of the mouth on the vermilion border **(commissures)** (Fig. 5.6). These tracts may be shallow, or they may be several millimeters deep. They are a relatively common developmental **anomaly** that can be unilateral or bilateral. The cause of commissural lip pits has been linked to family history. They are more often seen in adult males. The commissural lip pit may be observed during clinical examination. Because they are asymptomatic, no treatment is needed.

Another lip pit that occasionally may be seen is the **paramedian lip pit (congenital lip pit)**. It occurs near the midline of the vermilion border of the lower lip and may appear as either a unilateral or bilateral depression. They are referred to as *congenital fistulas of the lower lip* because they may contain salivary secretions and can be seen in patients with cleft lip or cleft palate. They are inherited as an autosomal-dominant trait. No treatment is indicated for paramedian lip pits.

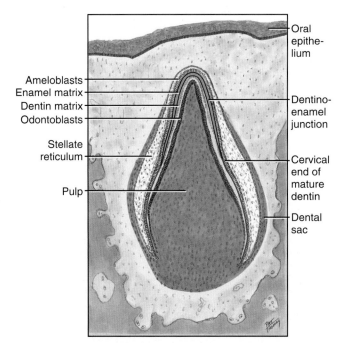

• **Figure 5.4** Deposition of enamel and dentin. (From Bath-Balogh M, Fehrenbach MF: *Illustrated dental embryology, histology, and anatomy,* ed 3, St. Louis, Saunders, 2012.)

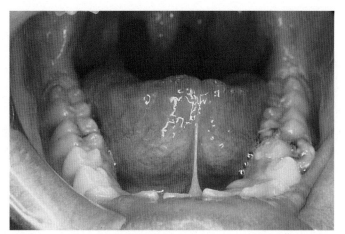

• **Figure 5.5** Ankyloglossia. The short lingual frenum is attached near the tip of the tongue. (Courtesy Dr. George Blozis.)

Lingual Thyroid

A **lingual thyroid,** or **ectopic lingual thyroid,** is a mass of thyroid tissue located between the foramen cecum on the tongue and the epiglottis, away from the normal anatomic location of the thyroid gland. It is an uncommon developmental anomaly that results from the failure of the primitive thyroid tissue to migrate from its developmental location in the area of the foramen cecum on the posterior portion of the tongue to its normal position in the neck.

Clinically, the lingual thyroid nodule appears as a smooth nodular mass at the base of the tongue posterior to the circumvallate papillae at the midline. It can be asymptomatic or can cause a feeling of fullness in the throat and difficulty in swallowing, speaking, or breathing. Microscopically, the lingual thyroid is composed of immature or mature thyroid tissue.

On occasion, the size of the lingual thyroid necessitates its removal. However, this nodule may be the patient's only functioning thyroid tissue. A thyroid scan should be performed to determine the presence of functioning thyroid tissue. If a normally located thyroid gland is lacking or nonfunctional, the lingual thyroid is not removed.

Developmental Cysts

A **cyst** is an abnormal, pathologic sac or cavity lined by epithelium and surrounded by fibrous connective tissue. Cysts occur throughout the body, including the oral region.

The cysts discussed in this chapter are all related to the development of the face, jaws, and teeth. Some have a distinctive microscopic appearance, and a definitive diagnosis is based on microscopic examination of the tissue. Other cysts are lined by less distinctive epithelium. The diagnosis of these cysts is based on both the microscopic appearance of the tissue and the location of the cyst.

The most common cyst observed in the oral cavity is caused by pulpal inflammation and is called a **radicular cyst (periapical cyst).** This cyst is described in Chapter 2. It develops from a preexisting periapical granuloma found at the apex of a nonvital tooth. The radicular cyst is always associated with a nonvital tooth, and diagnosis can be made only through microscopic examination because the radiographic appearance can be similar to other lesions. A **residual cyst** is a radicular cyst that remains after extraction of the offending tooth. Again, these two cysts are inflammatory reactions. Because cysts are commonly observed in the jaws and surrounding soft tissues, the dental hygienist should understand their diagnostic criteria, pathogenesis, and prognosis. The preliminary identification of a cystic lesion is within the scope of dental hygiene practice.

Developmental cysts are classified as **odontogenic** (related to tooth development) and **nonodontogenic** (not related to tooth development). Cysts are also classified according to location, cause, origin of the epithelial cells, and microscopic appearance (Table 5.1). Developmental cysts can vary in size from small, asymptomatic lesions to large lesions that can cause expansion of bone. Very large and long-standing lesions can resorb tooth structure or move teeth. Oral cysts that occur within bone are called **intraosseous cysts,** and cysts that occur in soft tissue are called **extraosseous cysts.**

Radiographically, cysts within bone generally appear as well-circumscribed radiolucencies. All cysts may appear **unilocular,** but some are more likely to appear as **multilocular** radiolucencies. When a cyst is found within soft tissue, there is no radiographic feature.

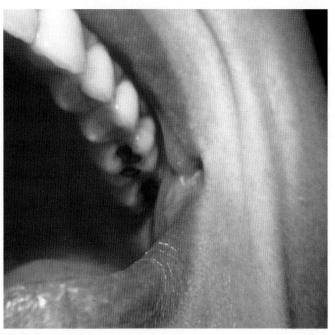

• **Figure 5.6** Commissural lip pit. A deep depression is seen at the labial commissure.

TABLE 5.1	**Classification of Developmental Cysts**			

ODONTOGENIC		NONODONTOGENIC	
Intraosseous	**Extraosseous**	**Intraosseous**	**Extraosseous**
Dentigerous cyst	Eruption cyst	Nasopalatine duct cyst	Nasolabial cyst
Primordial cyst		Median palatal cyst	Branchial cleft cyst (cervical lymphoepithelial cyst and intraoral lymphoepithelial cyst)
Odontogenic keratocyst (keratocystic odontogenic tumor)		Globulomaxillary cyst	Epidermal cyst
Lateral periodontal cyst	Gingival cyst	Median mandibular cyst	Thyroglossal tract cyst

Odontogenic Cysts

Dentigerous Cyst

A **dentigerous cyst,** also called a **follicular cyst,** forms around the crown of an unerupted or developing tooth (Fig. 5.7). It is the most commonly occurring type of developmental odontogenic cyst. The radicular cyst is the most common odontogenic cyst, but it is an inflammatory, not developmental, cyst. The epithelial lining originates from the reduced enamel epithelium after the crown has completely formed and calcified. Fluid accumulates between the crown and the reduced enamel epithelium. The reduced enamel epithelium results from remnants of the enamel organ. The most common location for the dentigerous cyst is around the crown of an unerupted or impacted mandibular third molar. However, a dentigerous cyst may also form around the crowns of other unerupted or **impacted teeth** such as the maxillary cuspid or a supernumerary tooth. The cyst may develop in both males and females. However, there is a higher incidence in males, and this cyst is most often seen in young adults from 15 to 30 years of age with a higher **predilection** for whites than blacks. The size of these cysts can range from small and asymptomatic to very large. When large, it is capable of displacing teeth or causing a fracture of the mandible. Ameloblastoma or odontogenic keratocyst (OKC; keratocystic odontogenic tumor) should be considered in the differential diagnosis of these very large cysts.

Radiographically, the dentigerous cyst appears as a well-defined, unilocular radiolucency around the crown of an unerupted or impacted tooth attached at the cemento-enamel junction (Fig. 5.8A-B). Microscopically, the dentigerous cyst is a true cyst because the lumen is lined by epithelium, most characteristically cuboidal epithelium, surrounded by a wall of connective tissue (Fig. 5.8C). It may also be lined with stratified squamous epithelium. The lumen may be filled with a watery or serous fluid. Radiographically, research studies have shown that a dentigerous

cyst should be suspected when the radiolucency is at least 4 mm in size.

Treatment of a dentigerous cyst involves the complete removal of the cystic lesion and usually the tooth involved. If it is not removed, the cyst wall continues to enlarge. In addition, a risk exists that a neoplasm (i.e., ameloblastoma, intraosseous mucoepidermoid carcinoma, intraosseous squamous cell carcinoma) may develop (see Chapter 7).

Eruption Cyst

An **eruption cyst** is similar to a dentigerous cyst, but it is found in the soft tissue around the crown of an erupting tooth. Clinically, it presents as a swelling of the gingival mucosa over the crown of an erupting tooth. If there is blood in the fluid, there is a purplish color to the tissue at the eruption site and the term *eruption hematoma* is used. It can sometimes be seen radiographically along with the clinical lesion.

The eruption cyst can be seen in deciduous and permanent teeth, but it is most commonly associated with the deciduous mandibular central incisors and the maxillary first permanent molars.

Because the tooth erupts through the cyst, this condition usually does not require treatment. On occasion, the dome of the eruption cyst is removed to expose the crown. The tooth is then allowed to erupt naturally and more quickly.

Primordial Cyst

A **primordial cyst** develops in place of a tooth and is most commonly found in place of the third molar or posterior to an erupted third molar (Fig. 5.9). It originates from remnants and degeneration of the enamel organ. A history that the tooth was never present is an essential component of the diagnostic process. Microscopically, primordial cysts often turn out to be odontogenic keratocysts (OKC).

Primordial cysts are most often seen in the young adult; no sex **predilection** has been reported. Clinically, the cyst usually is asymptomatic and is discovered on radiographic examination. Radiographically, it is a well-defined, radiolucent lesion that can be either unilocular or multilocular. The microscopic appearance and diagnosis of the primordial cyst may vary. Microscopically, the lumen is lined by stratified squamous epithelium surrounded by parallel bundles of collagen fibers. A layer of orthokeratin or parakeratin can cover the epithelium. The term *primordial cyst* simply refers to its development in place of a tooth. For this reason, biopsy and microscopic examination of primordial cysts are essential. Microscopically, a primordial cyst can be an odontogenic keratocyst or a lateral periodontal cyst.

Treatment of a primordial cyst involves surgical removal of the entire lesion. The prognosis depends on the histology; the risk of recurrence depends on the microscopic diagnosis. For example, if the cyst is microscopically an odontogenic keratocyst, the risk of recurrence is greater than if the cyst is lined by nonkeratinized stratified squamous epithelium.

Odontogenic Keratocyst

An **odontogenic keratocyst** (OKC) is an odontogenic developmental cystic lesion that is characterized by its unique microscopic appearance and frequent recurrence. The diagnosis is based on its histopathologic findings. The lumen is lined by epithelium that is 8 to 10 cell layers thick and surfaced by parakeratin. The basal cell layer is palisaded and prominent; the

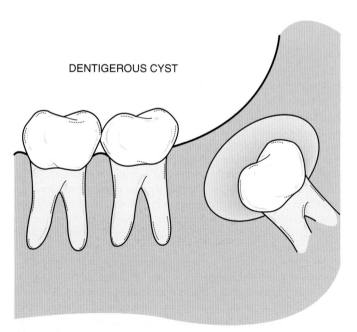

DENTIGEROUS CYST

• **Figure 5.7** Schematic of a dentigerous cyst located around the crown of an unerupted or impacted tooth.

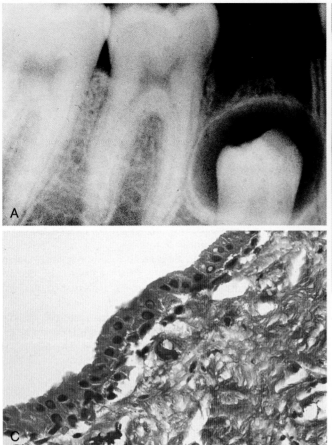

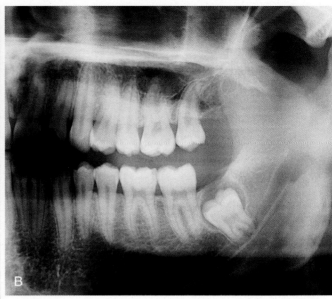

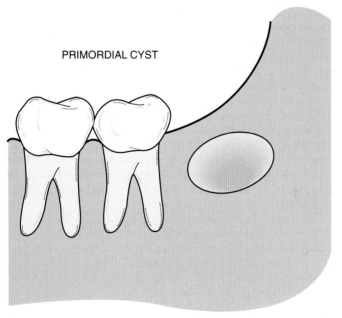

• **Figure 5.8** Radiographs of dentigerous cysts around the crown of an unerupted bicuspid **(A)** and an impacted third molar **(B)**. **C,** Microscopic appearance of a dentigerous cyst. (**B** courtesy Laura J. Greco.)

PRIMORDIAL CYST

• **Figure 5.9** Primordial cyst occurring in place of a tooth: the third molar, in this instance.

interface between the epithelium and the connective tissue is flat (Fig. 5.10).

In 2005 the World Health Organization reclassified the odontogenic keratocyst as **keratocystic odontogenic tumor** on the basis of its aggressive behavior, unique histopathology, and specific genes identified in the epithelial cells. These genetic alterations have been identified in neoplasms. The diagnosis of odontogenic keratocyst is still frequently used, and often both diagnoses are used together.

These cysts are most often seen in the mandibular third-molar region and can involve a slight predilection for males; most are diagnosed between 10 and 50 years of age. Radiographically, the odontogenic keratocyst frequently appears as a well-defined, multilocular, radiolucent lesion (Fig. 5.10C). Unilocular lesions may also occur, and the radiographic appearance can be identical to that of an odontogenic tumor. The odontogenic keratocyst can move teeth and resorb tooth structure, but does not usually cause expansion of bone. Bony expansion can be seen in the dentigerous cysts of equal size. The odontogenic keratocyst is also associated with nevoid basal cell carcinoma syndrome (Gorlin syndrome) (see Chapter 6).

Treatment of an odontogenic keratocyst is rather aggressive because of the high recurrence rate (Fig. 5.10D-E). The cyst generally extends beyond the borders that are seen on the radiograph because it extends between the trabeculae of bone. Therefore thorough surgical excision and osseous curettage are essential. Careful follow-up and evaluation are necessary because up to 25% recurrence is reported.

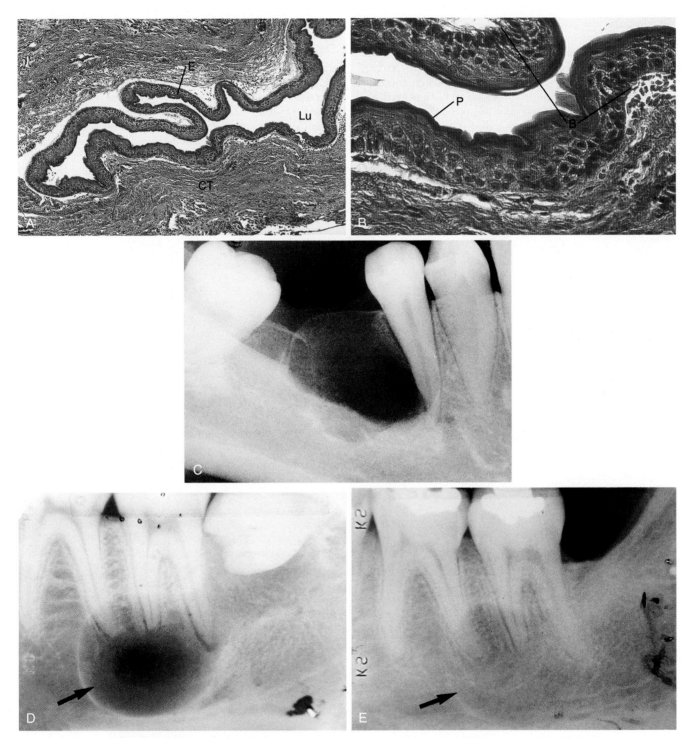

• **Figure 5.10 A,** Microscopic appearance of an odontogenic keratocyst (OKC), showing a thin uniform epithelial lining (low power). Lu, Lumen; E, epithelium; CT, connective tissue. **B,** Microscopic appearance of an OKC, showing a corrugated parakeratotic surface (P) and a prominent basal cell layer (B) (high power). **C,** Radiograph of an OKC, showing a multilocular radiolucency. **D,** Radiograph of an OKC extending to the third molar. **E,** Same patient in **(D),** 2 years later, showing recurrence of OKC. The reader should note that the third molar has been removed.

An **orthokeratotic odontogenic cyst** is an odontogenic cyst that is lined by orthokeratin rather than parakeratin. It does not have the characteristic histopathologic appearance of the keratocystic odontogenic tumor/odontogenic keratocyst and has a much lower rate of recurrence.

Calcifying Odontogenic Cyst

The **calcifying odontogenic cyst,** also referred to as a **Gorlin cyst**, is a developmental nonaggressive cystic lesion lined by odontogenic epithelium that closely resembles the epithelium of the odontogenic tumor called an **ameloblastoma.** Microscopically, it has an additional characteristic feature called **ghost cells.** Radiographically, the calcifying odontogenic cyst usually appears as a well-defined radiolucency. In up to 50% of cases there are radiopaque structures identified within the radiolucency. The average age at diagnosis is 30. The calcifying odontogenic cyst is usually found in the incisor or canine area of either arch. In general, the cyst is treated conservatively and does not recur. A solid variant of the calcifying odontogenic cyst is called the *odontogenic ghost cell tumor;* it has been suggested that this solid variant represents a neoplasm rather than a cyst. Because of its microscopic resemblance to the ameloblastoma and the solid variant of this odontogenic cystic lesion, the calcifying odontogenic cyst is described in detail in Chapter 7.

Lateral Periodontal Cyst, Gingival Cyst, and Botryoid Odontogenic Cyst

The **lateral periodontal cyst** is a developmental odontogenic cyst that occurs on the lateral root surface of mandibular canine and premolar teeth and can be seen in the same area in the maxilla. It presents as an asymptomatic, unilocular or multilocular radiolucent lesion that is most often seen in adults between 50 and 70 years of age.(Fig. 5.11A). The botryoid odontogenic cyst is considered a variant of the lateral periodontal cyst. The botryoid cyst is usually multilocular, but may also be unilocular (Fig. 5.11B). The microscopic appearance is the same for both (Fig. 5.11C). The diagnosis botryoid odontogenic cyst is used for multicystic

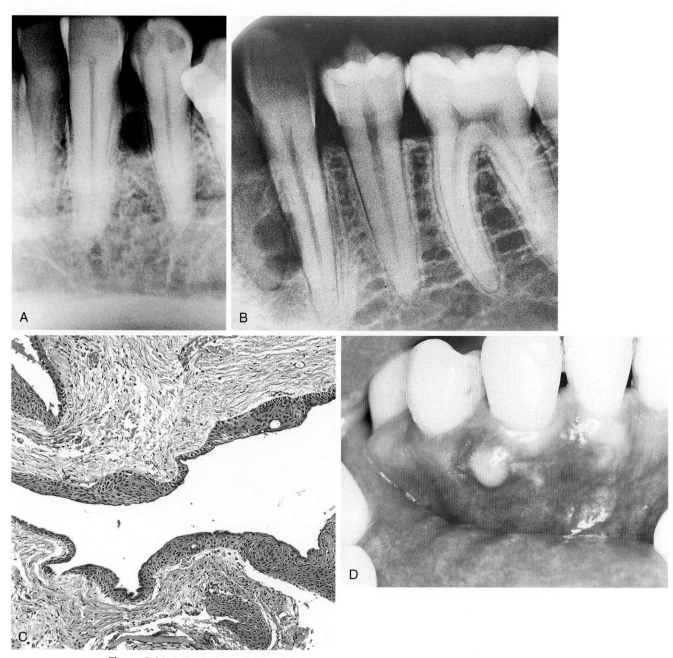

• **Figure 5.11** **A,** Radiograph of a lateral periodontal cyst. This well-defined radiolucency is located lateral to the tooth root. **B,** Radiograph of a botryoid cyst showing the biloculated radiolucency lateral to the tooth root. **C,** Microscopic appearance of a lateral periodontal cyst, showing a thin epithelial lining with focal epithelial thickenings. **D,** Gingival cyst. (**D** courtesy Drs. Paul Freedman and Stanley Kerpel.)

and multilocular variants. The botryoid odontogenic cyst is also most common in the mandibular cuspid and premolar area of the mandible and is reported to have a greater recurrence potential than the lateral periodontal cyst. These are also generally treated by conservative enucleation of the cyst. Microscopically, the lateral periodontal cyst and the botryoid cyst show a thin epithelial lining with focal epithelial thickenings. The **gingival cyst** exhibits the same type of epithelial lining as the lateral periodontal cyst and is located in the soft tissue of the same area. The gingival cyst appears as a small bulge or swelling of the attached gingiva or interdental papillae (Fig. 5.11D).

The lateral periodontal cyst is found most often in males. No sex predilection has been reported for gingival cysts. Both the lateral periodontal cyst and the gingival are treated by surgical excision.

A few cases of recurrence of lateral periodontal cysts have been reported. Some of these have been multilocular variants and were probably better classified as botryoid odontogenic cysts. The prognosis is excellent.

Glandular Odontogenic Cyst

The **glandular odontogenic cyst** is a rare developmental odontogenic cyst. It was initially identified as a separate entity in 1988 and was called a *sialo-odontogenic cyst*. The name *glandular odontogenic cyst* was adopted by the World Health Organization in 1992, and this has become the preferred name for this cyst.

Glandular odontogenic cysts exhibit a distinctive microscopic appearance. They are usually multicystic lesions. The epithelial lining of this cyst varies from cuboidal to columnar cells, and mucous cells are frequently also present. Intraepithelial microcysts, or ductlike spaces, are seen within the epithelium and clear epi-

thelial cells and mucous cells are also noted. Epithelial thickenings showing whorls of cells similar to those in the lateral periodontal cyst and botryoid cyst are also often seen.

The glandular odontogenic cyst often presents as an enlargement of the bone; the anterior and posterior mandible and anterior maxilla are the most commonly reported locations. About 75% of cases have been reported in the mandible. Both men and women may develop this cyst, and there is a peak incidence in the fifth decade. The radiographic appearance may be unilocular but is often multilocular, appearing similar to that of an ameloblastoma or odontogenic keratocyst. When not completely surgically removed, these cysts have a high recurrence rate. A recurrence rate of up to 30% has been reported.

Nonodontogenic Cysts

Nasopalatine Canal Cyst

A **nasopalatine canal cyst (incisive canal cyst)** is a developmental cyst located within the nasopalatine canal or the incisive papilla. When found in the papilla, it is referred to as a **cyst of the palatine papilla.** This cyst arises from epithelial remnants of the embryonal nasopalatine ducts. The lesion is most commonly seen in adults between 40 and 60 years of age, and a strong predilection exists for males. The cyst is usually asymptomatic. Clinically, there may be a small pink bulge near the apices and between the roots of the maxillary central incisors on the lingual surface. The adjacent teeth are usually vital.

Radiographically, the nasopalatine canal cyst is a well-defined, radiolucent lesion that is often heart shaped (Fig. 5.12A), resulting from the anatomic Y shape of the canal. When it is heart shaped, it is evenly distributed to the right and left of the midline. The

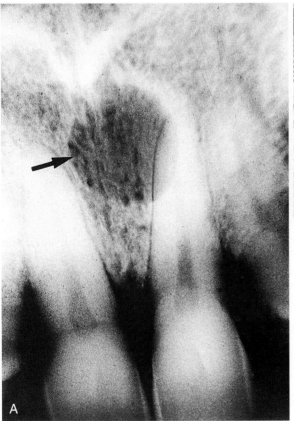

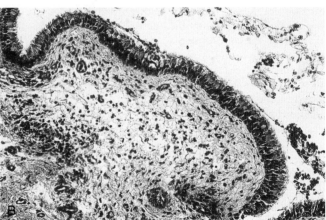

• **Figure 5.12** **A,** An incisive canal cyst may be located in the anterior maxilla in either bone or soft tissue or both. This radiograph of an incisive canal cyst shows a well-circumscribed radiolucency between the maxillary central incisors. **B,** Microscopic appearance of an incisive canal cyst, showing a pseudostratified, ciliated, columnar epithelial lining.

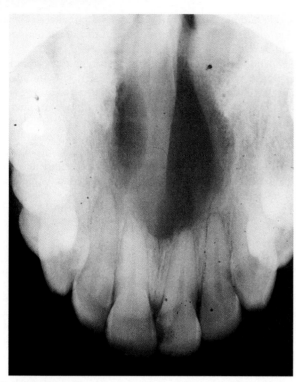

• **Figure 5.13** Radiograph of a median palatine cyst, showing a well-defined radiolucency located in the midline of the maxilla.

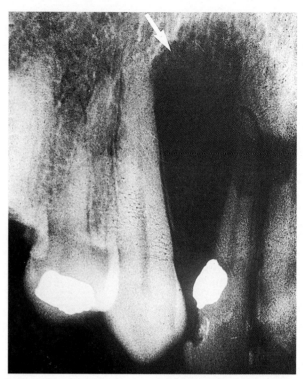

• **Figure 5.14** Radiograph of a globulomaxillary cyst, showing the characteristic pear-shaped radiolucency (*arrow*) between the roots of the maxillary lateral incisor and cuspid.

average size is 1 to 2 cm in diameter. If the nasopalatine canal cyst develops in the soft tissue of the incisive papilla without any bone involvement, it is called a *cyst of the incisive papilla.*

Microscopically, the cyst is lined by epithelium that varies from stratified squamous to pseudostratified ciliated columnar epithelium (Fig. 5.12B). The connective tissue wall contains nerves and blood vessels that are normally found in the area and may also contain inflammatory cells.

Treatment of a nasopalatine canal cyst is surgical enucleation. It is especially important that surgery take place in the edentulous patient before the fabrication of a prosthesis. Recurrence is rare.

Median Palatine Cyst

A **median palatine cyst** is a rare fissural cyst that appears as a well-defined unilocular radiolucency and is located in the midline of the hard palate (Fig. 5.13). The cyst is thought to be a more posterior form of a nasopalatine canal cyst. Clinically, it is a firm mass in the midline of the hard palate, most often seen in young adults. Microscopically, the median palatine cyst is lined with stratified squamous epithelium that is surrounded by dense fibrous connective tissue. The median palatine cyst is treated by surgical enucleation. The prognosis is good, and recurrence is rare.

Globulomaxillary Cyst

Radiographically, a **globulomaxillary cyst** is a well-defined, pear-shaped radiolucency found between the roots of the maxillary lateral incisor and cuspid (Fig. 5.14). Although it was once thought to be a developmental fissural cyst, it is now believed to be of odontogenic epithelial origin. The size of the lesion can vary; however, when it is large enough, a divergence of the roots can result. The adjacent teeth are usually vital. Pulp testing can rule out a periapical cyst or periapical granuloma. Surgical enucleation of the globulomaxillary cyst is recommended. The diagnosis is determined by the microscopic evaluation of the lesion. The prognosis and recurrence depend on the final diagnosis.

Median Mandibular Cyst

A **median mandibular cyst** is a rare lesion. As its name indicates, it is located in the midline of the mandible. The origin of the median mandibular cyst is also unclear. Some believe it to be of odontogenic origin, ranging from odontogenic cysts to tumors. Because no mandibular midline fusion occurs, there is no evidence of epithelial entrapment. The surrounding teeth are vital. Radiographically, a well-defined radiolucency is seen below the apices of the mandibular incisors. A median mandibular cyst is treated by surgical removal; the prognosis is good, and recurrence is rare. Because there is no fissure in this region, this term should no longer be used.

Nasolabial Cyst

A **nasolabial cyst** is a soft tissue cyst with no alveolar bone involvement. The origin of this cyst is uncertain. At present it is thought to originate from the lower anterior portion of the nasolacrimal duct. The cyst is observed in adults 40 to 50 years of age; a strong predilection (4:1) exists for females.

Clinically, there may be an expansion or swelling in the mucolabial fold in the area of the maxillary canine and the floor of the nose. Usually no radiographic change is associated with this cyst. However, when the lesion is large enough, expansive pressure can cause the resorption of bone (Fig. 5.15). Microscopically, the cyst is lined with pseudostratified, ciliated columnar epithelium and multiple goblet cells. Treatment of a nasolabial cyst is surgical excision; the prognosis is good, and recurrence is rare.

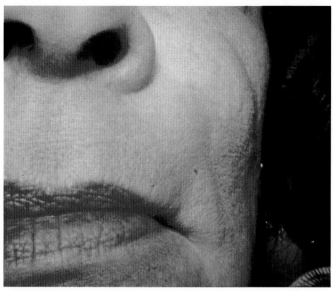

• **Figure 5.15** Nasolabial cyst causing a swelling in the nasolabial fold area.

Lymphoepithelial Cyst

A **cervical lymphoepithelial cyst** (*branchial cleft cyst*) is located on the lateral neck at the anterior border of the sternocleidomastoid muscle. They are common in children and young adults. It is composed of a stratified squamous epithelial lining surrounded by a well-circumscribed component of lymphoid tissue and connective tissue (Fig. 5.16). It appears to arise from epithelium entrapped in a lymph node during development rather than associated with a branchial cleft.

The intraoral lymphoepithelial cyst is most commonly seen in young adults on the floor of the mouth, ventral tongue, and the lateral borders of the posterior tongue (Fig. 5.16A). This lymphoepithelial cyst appears as a pinkish-yellow, raised **nodule** (a small, solid mass that can be detected through palpation) when seen intraorally. The lumen may contain a creamy material.

Treatment of a cervical lymphoepithelial cyst (branchial cleft cyst) and an intraoral lymphoepithelial cyst consists of surgical excision, and the prognosis is good.

Epidermal Cyst

An **epidermal cyst** presents as a raised nodule in the skin of the face or neck. Microscopically, the cyst is lined by keratinizing epithelium that resembles the epithelium of skin (epidermis). The cyst lumen is usually filled with keratin scales. Most epidermal cysts are thought to originate from the epithelium of the hair follicle. On occasion, when located in the skin of the cheek, the nodule may be noted intraorally from the buccal mucosal aspect and the skin. An epidermoid cyst is treated by surgical excision, and the prognosis is good.

Dermoid Cyst and Benign Cystic Teratoma

A **dermoid cyst** is a developmental cyst that is often present at birth or noted in young children. It is more common in other parts of the body than in the head and neck. When the dermoid cyst occurs in the oral cavity, it is usually found in the anterior floor of the mouth. The cyst may cause displacement of the tongue and may have a doughlike consistency when palpated.

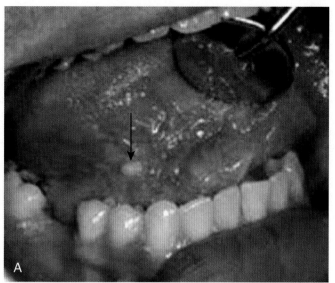

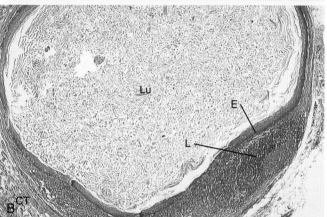

• **Figure 5.16 A,** Clinical lymphoepithelial cyst. **B,** Microscopic appearance of a lymphoepithelial cyst, showing the lumen (Lu), epithelial lining (E), surrounding lymphocytes (L), and connective tissue (CT) (low power). (**A** courtesy Dr. A. Ross Kerr.)

Microscopically, the dermoid cyst is lined by orthokeratinized, stratified squamous epithelium surrounded by a connective tissue wall. The lumen is usually filled with keratin. Hair follicles, sebaceous glands, and sweat glands may be seen in the cyst wall. A **benign cystic teratoma** has a cystic component that resembles the dermoid cyst. In addition, teeth, bone, muscles, and nerve tissue may be found in the wall of this lesion. Teeth are usually not found in the malignant form of the teratoma. Treatment of the dermoid cyst is surgical excision; the prognosis is good, and malignant transformation has been reported but is extremely rare.

Thyroglossal Tract Cyst

A **thyroglossal tract (duct) cyst** forms along the same tract that the thyroid gland follows in development, from the area of the foramen cecum to its permanent location in the neck (Fig. 5.17). Most of these cysts occur below the hyoid bone. The epithelial lining varies with location. Cysts above the hyoid bone are usually lined with stratified squamous epithelium, and those below the hyoid bone with ciliated columnar epithelium. Thyroid tissue may also be found within the connective tissue wall.

The thyroglossal tract cyst is most often initially diagnosed in young individuals under 20 years of age. There is no sex predilection. Clinically, if this cyst is located below the hyoid bone, it presents as a smooth bulge or swelling in the area of the midline of the neck. If located on the posterior aspect of the tongue, a smooth, rather firm mass of tissue is present, which can vary in size from a few millimeters to several centimeters. The patient may complain of dysphagia (difficulty in swallowing) or difficulty when extending the tongue. When large, this cyst may be fluctuant and moves up and down when the patient swallows.

Treatment of a thyroglossal tract cyst consists of complete excision of the cyst and the tract, usually including a portion of the hyoid bone and muscle tissue along the thyroglossal tract.

This is referred to as a *Sistrunk procedure.* In general, the prognosis is good, but a few cases of malignant transformation have been reported.

Pseudocysts

Pseudocysts are intraosseous lesions that appear as radiolucencies. They are called "cysts," but they are not true cysts because they are not lined by epithelium.

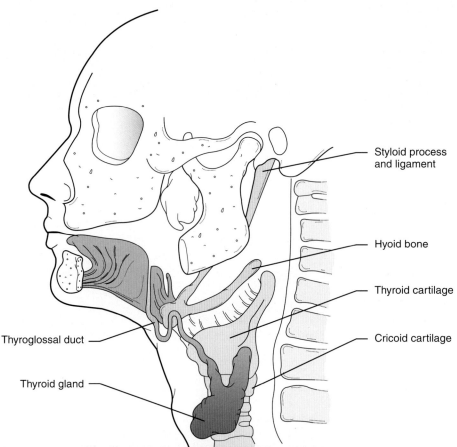

Styloid process and ligament

Hyoid bone

Thyroid cartilage

Cricoid cartilage

Thyroglossal duct

Thyroid gland

A

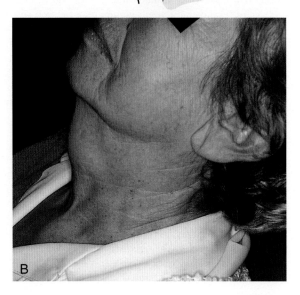

B

• **Figure 5.17** A, The thyroglossal tract extends from the area of the foramen cecum on the tongue to the lower part of the neck. **B,** A thyroglossal tract cyst is the cause of this enlargement at the midline of the neck.

Stafne Defect

A **Stafne defect** (**lingual mandibular bone concavity** or **static bone cyst**) is not a true cyst because it is not a pathologic cavity and is not lined with epithelium. Therefore it is often referred to as a *pseudocyst.* Clinically, an anatomic depression may be felt on the posterior lingual area of the mandible. There is a significant predilection for men. Although developmental, they are most often seen in adults and rare in children. Radiographically, a well-defined radiolucency is observed in the posterior region of the mandible, inferior to the mandibular canal. The radiolucency is caused by the lingual depression in the mandible, which is filled with normal salivary gland tissue (Fig. 5.18A). The salivary gland tissue may be an extension of the sublingual gland. The lesion is usually asymptomatic and remains static over time.

This developmental defect requires no treatment. A sialogram can be used to identify salivary gland tissue. However, a computed tomography (CT) scan will demonstrate the mandibular invagination that results in the well-defined radiolucency (Fig. 5.18B).

If any question exists about the diagnosis, the patient is monitored until it is determined that no enlargement of the radiolucency has occurred. If the radiolucency occurs above the mandibular canal, a biopsy may be indicated to establish the diagnosis and differentiate this pseudocyst from cysts and tumors having a predilection for that location.

Simple Bone Cyst

A **simple bone cyst** (**traumatic bone cyst, hemorrhagic bone cyst**) is a pathologic cavity in bone that is not lined with epithelium. The cause is uncertain; when it occurs in the jaws, an association with trauma has been suggested. The lesion is found most often in young individuals, and there is no sex predilection. The mandible is the most common location. The lesion is observed radiographically as a well-defined unilocular or multilocular radiolucent lesion that characteristically shows scalloping around the roots of teeth (Fig. 5.19).The scalloping is unique, but not a diagnostic feature of the simple bone cyst. It is usually asymptomatic and is discovered on routine radiographs. Surgical intervention reveals a void within the bone. A curettage is performed on the wall lining the void to establish bleeding. The void or space fills up with bone 6 months to 1 year after the surgical procedure. The prognosis is excellent, and recurrence is unusual.

Aneurysmal Bone Cyst

An **aneurysmal bone cyst** is a pseudocyst that consists of blood-filled spaces surrounded by multinucleated giant cells and fibrous connective tissue (similar to a giant cell granuloma). There is no epithelial lining. The radiolucent lesion has a multilocular appearance that is often described as a "honeycomb" or "soap bubble." It is usually seen in individuals less than 30 years of age, and a slight predilection is reported for females. When in the jaws, the mandible is more commonly affected than the maxilla. The clinical presentation may include expansion of the involved bone with a sudden enlargement of the involved bone. When the maxilla is involved, the lesion can involve the sinus and cause nasal obstruction. Microscopically, the aneurysmal bone cyst is related

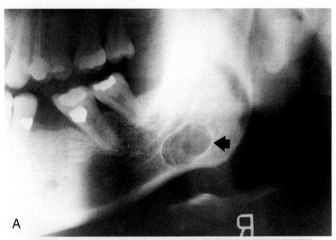

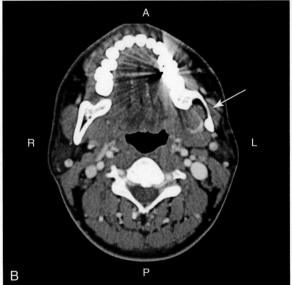

• **Figure 5.18 A,** Panoramic radiograph of a lingual mandibular bone concavity (Stafne bone cyst). Arrow points to a well-circumscribed radiolucency inferior to the mandibular canal. **B,** Axial computerized tomography (CT) image showing a depression in the bone of the left mandible (*arrow*). This results in a well-circumscribed radiolucency on a panoramic radiograph that is called a Stafne (static) bone cyst. (Courtesy Dr. K.C. Chan.)

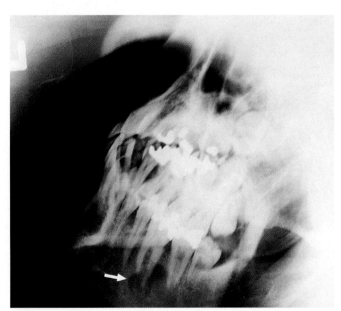

• **Figure 5.19** Extraoral radiograph showing a simple (traumatic) bone cyst in the mandible with its unique radiolucent characteristic, scalloping around the roots. (Courtesy Dr. Edward V. Zegarelli.)

to the central giant cell granuloma and is discussed in detail in Chapter 8.

Developmental Abnormalities of Teeth

Abnormalities in the Number of Teeth

Anodontia

Anodontia is the congenital lack of teeth. Total anodontia (lack of all teeth) is a rare condition that may affect either the deciduous (uncommon) or the permanent dentition. Because development of both deciduous and permanent teeth begins before birth, their failure to develop is congenital. However, teeth may not be identified as missing until the time of normal eruption or initial radiographic examination. Total anodontia is often associated with the hereditary disturbance hereditary hypohydrotic ectodermal dysplasia, which is described in Chapter 6. Missing teeth require prosthetic replacement.

Hypodontia

Hypodontia is the lack of one or more teeth. This developmental anomaly is rather common and may affect either deciduous or permanent teeth (Fig. 5.20). Any tooth in either dentition may be missing. The permanent dentition is most commonly affected. Hypodontia rarely occurs in the deciduous dentition. The teeth most often missing are the maxillary and mandibular third molars, the maxillary lateral incisors, and the mandibular second premolars. Teeth are often missing bilaterally. The mandibular incisor is the tooth most commonly missing in the deciduous dentition. Teeth are identified as congenitally lacking by careful clinical and radiographic examination along with a thorough patient history.

Oligodontia is a subcategory of hypodontia in which six or more teeth (excluding third molars) are congenitally missing.

Missing teeth tend to be **familial** (i.e., affecting more members of a family than would be expected by chance). In addition, factors such as jaw lesions in infancy and radiation therapy during tooth formation may result in the destruction of tooth germs and the subsequent lack of affected teeth. Microdontia may be associated with hypodontia.

Missing teeth may require prosthetic replacement. Their absence can also result in problems in occlusion caused by drifting or tipping of teeth. Orthodontic evaluation and treatment may be necessary. In addition, congenitally missing teeth may be a component of a syndrome; a syndrome is a group of findings that

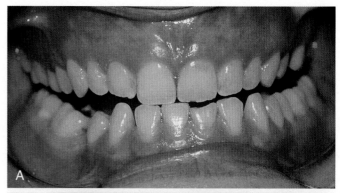

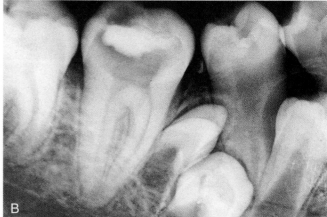

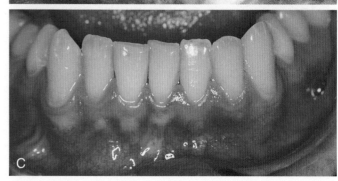

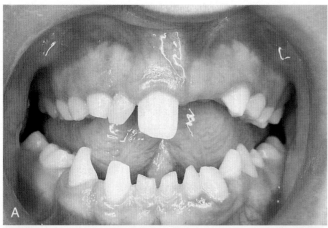

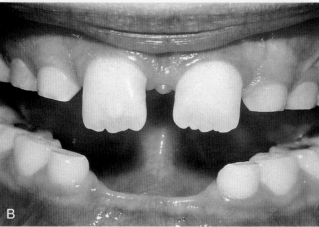

• **Figure 5.20** A and B, Hypodontia. Teeth that are missing were not extracted; they never developed. (**A** courtesy Dr. George Blozis; **B** courtesy Dr. Margot Van Dis.)

• **Figure 5.21** A, Supernumerary teeth. This patient has four maxillary lateral incisors. **B**, Radiograph showing unerupted supernumerary teeth. **C**, Supernumerary mandibular incisor. (**A** courtesy Dr. Margot Van Dis; **B** courtesy Dr. George Blozis.)

occur together. Some of these syndromes are Down syndrome, ectodermal dysplasia, Ellis–van Creveld syndrome, and Gorlin syndrome. These syndromes are discussed in Chapter 6 of this text. Patients with congenitally missing teeth should be evaluated for other abnormalities.

Supernumerary Teeth

Supernumerary teeth are extra teeth found in the dental arches (Fig. 5.21). *Supernumerary* means more than the normal or regular number. *Hyperdontia* refers to an increased number of teeth. Supernumerary teeth result from either the formation of extra tooth buds in the dental lamina or the cleavage of already existing tooth buds and may occur in either the deciduous or the permanent dentition. Extra teeth are most often seen in the maxilla and may occur singly or in multiples and unilaterally or bilaterally. Some studies have shown a higher prevalence in American blacks.

Typically the supernumerary tooth is smaller than a normal-size tooth and often does not erupt. Most are discovered on radiographs as incidental findings. A supernumerary tooth may or may not resemble a normal tooth in shape and position.

The most common supernumerary tooth is called the **mesiodens,** which is located between the maxillary central incisors at or near the midline. It is usually a small tooth with a conical crown and short roots (Fig. 5.22). It may occur singly or in pairs

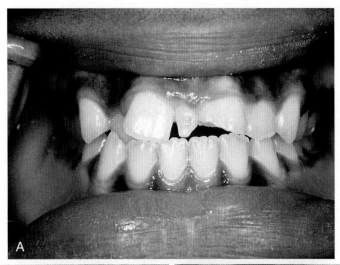

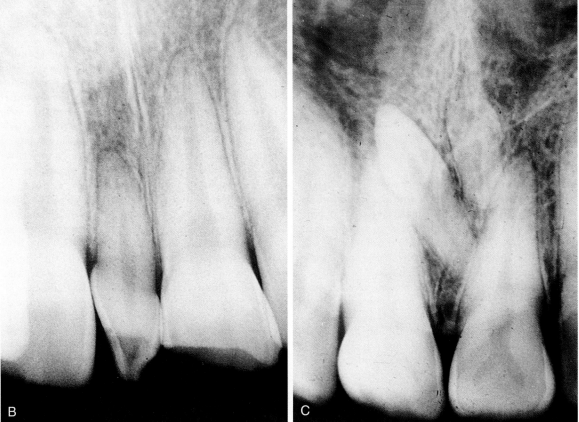

• **Figure 5.22 A,** Mesiodens seen between the maxillary central incisors. **B,** Radiograph of an erupted mesiodens. **C,** Radiograph showing a pair of inverted impacted mesiodens. (**A** and **B** courtesy Dr. George Blozis.)

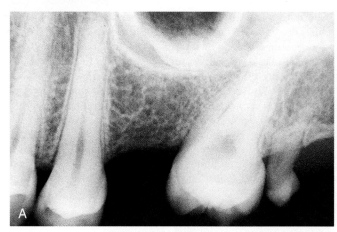
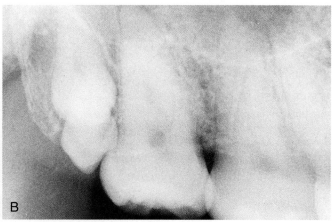

• **Figure 5.23 A,** Small erupted microdont distal to the maxillary second molar. **B,** Radiograph of a third molar microdont and distomolar. (**A** courtesy Dr. Margot Van Dis; **B** courtesy Dr. George Blozis.)

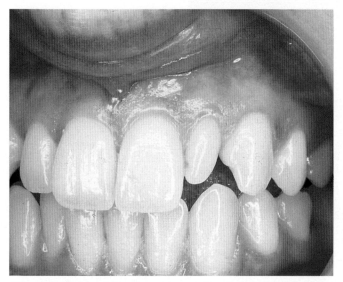

• **Figure 5.24** Peg-shaped lateral incisor. (Courtesy Dr. George Blozis.)

and may be inverted when seen on a radiograph. The mesiodens can erupt or remain embedded or impacted.

The second most common supernumerary tooth is the maxillary fourth molar, which is also called a **distomolar** or **distodens** because it is located distal to the third molar (Fig. 5.23). The distomolar can look like a miniature third molar or be of normal third-molar size and shape. It rarely erupts into the oral cavity and is usually discovered on a radiograph. The distomolar is the most common supernumerary tooth in American blacks.

Natal teeth are accessory teeth that are present at birth, and most of these are mandibular incisors. Neonatal teeth erupt during the first month of life.

Other supernumerary teeth include mandibular and maxillary premolars; maxillary lateral incisors; and the maxillary paramolar, a small rudimentary tooth that occurs buccal to the third molar. Erupted supernumerary teeth can cause crowding, malpositioning of adjacent teeth, or noneruption of normal teeth; therefore removal is often necessary. Nonerupted supernumerary teeth should be extracted because a risk exists for cyst development around the crown. Multiple supernumerary teeth may be a component of a syndrome such as cleidocranial

dysplasia or Gardner syndrome. These syndromes are described in Chapter 6.

Abnormalities in the Size of Teeth

Microdontia

Microdontia is a developmental anomaly in which one or more teeth in the dentition are smaller than normal. The term is derived from the Greek words *mikros,* meaning small, and *odontos,* meaning tooth. Microdontia is classified as true generalized microdontia, generalized relative microdontia, or microdontia involving a single tooth.

True microdontia is seen in Down syndrome and the pituitary dwarf and is extremely rare. Resulting generally from a lack of growth hormone produced by the pituitary gland, all the teeth are smaller than normal. In relative microdontia normal-size teeth appear small in large jaws. Heredity plays a role in generalized relative microdontia. For example, a child may inherit large jaws from one parent and normal-size teeth from the other, resulting in the illusion of small teeth. This is really **macrognathia** (enlarged jaw) and not microdontia. Microdontia involving a single tooth is far more common than true microdontia or relative microdontia. The maxillary lateral incisor and the maxillary third molar are the teeth most often affected (Fig. 5.24). These teeth are the ones that are most often congenitally missing. The maxillary lateral incisors often appear peg shaped, with the mesial and distal tooth surfaces converging toward the incisal edge. This "peg lateral" is smaller than normal, tends to occur bilaterally, has short roots, and is thought to be familial. The maxillary third-molar microdont typically appears small but normally shaped. Microdonts are identified clinically if erupted or radiographically if unerupted. For cosmetic reasons "peg lateral" or other erupted microdonts may be restored to resemble teeth of normal size and shape. Composites, laminates, or crowns provide excellent esthetic results. Impacted microdonts should be surgically removed to prevent cyst formation.

Macrodontia

Macrodontia is an uncommon developmental anomaly in which one or more teeth in a dentition are larger than normal. The term is derived from the Greek words *macros,* meaning large, and *odontos,* meaning tooth. Macrodontia is classified in the same

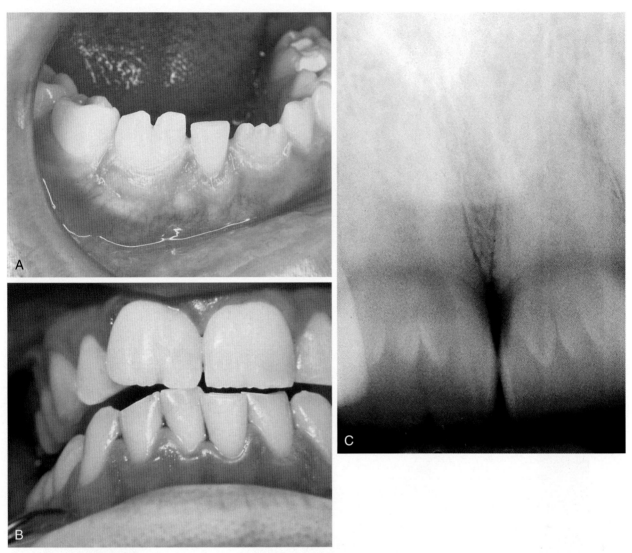

• **Figure 5.25** **A,** Clinical picture of gemination in a mandibular cuspid. **B,** Gemination seen in a maxillary central incisor. **C,** Radiograph of the same maxillary central incisor. (**A** courtesy Dr. George Blozis.)

manner as microdontia: true macrodontia, relative macrodontia, and macrodontia involving a single tooth.

True generalized macrodontia is rare and is seen occasionally in cases of pituitary gigantism. Relative generalized macrodontia is seen in individuals with normal or slightly larger-than-normal teeth in small jaws and is generally caused by the patient's inheriting tooth size from one parent and jaw size from the other. Macrodontia affecting a single tooth is uncommon.

Abnormalities in the Shape of Teeth

Gemination

Gemination is an uncommon developmental anomaly that occurs when a single tooth germ attempts to divide and results in the incomplete formation of two teeth. *Geminate* means paired or occurring in twos. The cause of this aborted twinning of a single tooth germ is unknown. Gemination is seen more frequently in the deciduous dentition, but does occur in the permanent dentition. Gemination most often affects anterior teeth and is most often seen in the deciduous mandibular incisors and the permanent maxillary incisors. In general, it is more commonly seen in the maxilla.

Clinically, gemination appears as two crowns joined together by a notched incisal area (Fig. 5.25). Radiographically, usually one single root and one common pulp canal exist, but this is not always true. The patient has a full complement of teeth.

A geminated tooth poses an esthetic problem, particularly when it occurs in the maxillary anterior region. It also poses a prosthetic challenge. Therefore treatment usually involves alteration of the tooth so that it resembles a normal tooth in size and shape.

Fusion

Fusion results from the union of two normally separated adjacent tooth germs. The cause of fusion is uncertain; heredity, external pressure, and crowding all have been suggested. Fusion of adjacent teeth can be complete or incomplete, depending on the stage of tooth development at the time of contact. Early contact of developing tooth germs can result in a single large tooth; later contact can result in the union of crowns only or the union of roots only. True fusion always involves confluence of dentin. Fusion is most often seen in the maxilla and tends to occur in the anterior region; the incisors are the teeth most often affected. Fusion of deciduous teeth occurs more often than fusion of permanent teeth.

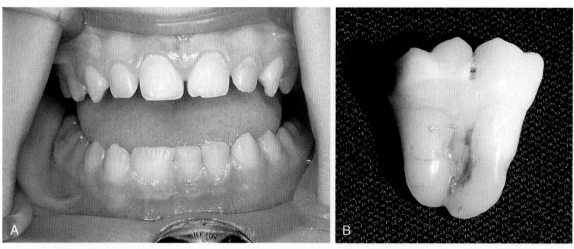

• **Figure 5.26** **A,** Clinical picture of fusion involving a permanent mandibular lateral incisor. **B,** Fusion of mandibular molars. (**A** courtesy Dr. George Blozis; **B** courtesy Dr. Rudy Melfi.)

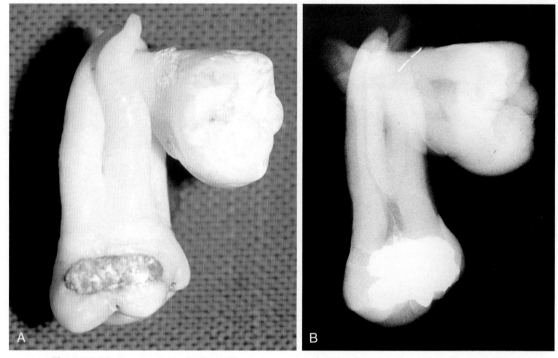

• **Figure 5.27** Concrescence illustrated in a photograph **(A)** of extracted teeth and in a corresponding radiograph **(B)**. (Courtesy Dr. George Blozis.)

Clinically, fused teeth appear as a single large crown that occurs in place of two normal teeth and may exhibit an observable separation (Fig. 5.26). Radiographically, either separate or fused roots and root canals are seen. To differentiate fusion from gemination, the teeth must be counted. If the neighboring teeth of the tooth in question are present, the tooth is geminated; if a neighboring tooth is lacking, the tooth in question is fused. Fusion can occur between two adjacent normal teeth or between a normal tooth and a supernumerary tooth. It may be difficult to distinguish between a geminated tooth and the fusion of a normal tooth to a supernumerary tooth.

As with geminated teeth, fused teeth may present esthetic and occlusal problems; they also pose a restorative challenge. Treatment involves alteration of the size and shape of the tooth and may involve replacement of one of the fused teeth.

Hypercementosis

Hypercementosis is defined as excessive cementum on the roots of teeth. It is also referred to as *cemental hyperplasia.* It occurs in adults, and the incidence and amount increase with age. It is a feature associated with several local and systemic factors. It is frequently seen in Paget disease of bone. No treatment is necessary for hypercementosis.

Concrescence

In dentistry, **concrescence** is a condition in which two adjacent teeth are united by cementum only. It is actually a form of fusion that takes place after tooth formation is complete and is usually discovered as an incidental radiographic finding (Fig. 5.27). The cause of concrescence is thought to be crowding or trauma that results in the close approximation of adjacent tooth roots.

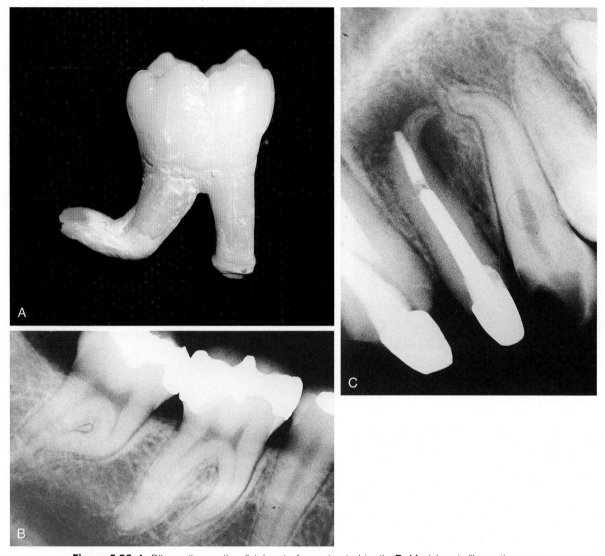

• **Figure 5.28 A,** Dilaceration on the distal root of an extracted tooth. **B,** Mesial root dilaceration on a mandibular second molar. **C,** Radiograph of root dilaceration in maxillary lateral incisor and cuspid. (**A** courtesy Dr. Rudy Melfi.)

Subsequent cementum deposition acts to fuse the two adjacent roots. Concrescence is most often seen in adjacent maxillary molars and adjacent supernumerary teeth and may involve erupted, unerupted, or impacted teeth. Concrescence generally does not require treatment. If one of the teeth joined by cementum requires extraction, extraction of the fused neighbor is inevitable. However, if the extraction of involved teeth is difficult, fracture of the associated alveolar bone may result.

Dilaceration

In dentistry, **dilaceration** refers to an abnormal curve or angle in the root or, less frequently, the crown of a tooth (Fig. 5.28). Most are idiopathic. It has been suggested that this dental anomaly may be caused by trauma to the tooth germ during root development. The position of the calcified portion of the tooth is changed, and the remainder of the tooth forms at an angle. A dilaceration can appear anywhere along the root portion of a tooth and can occur in any tooth in either the deciduous or the permanent dentition. A root dilaceration is usually discovered as an incidental radiographic finding.

Dilacerations do not require treatment. However, they may cause problems if extraction or endodontic therapy becomes necessary. The importance of a preoperative radiograph is obvious.

Enamel Pearl

Ectopic enamel refers to enamel that is found on unusual areas, most commonly the tooth root. The **enamel pearl,** or **enameloma,** is a small, spherical enamel projection located on a root surface (Fig. 5.29). This developmental anomaly is thought to occur as a result of the abnormal displacement of ameloblasts during tooth formation. The enamel pearl is usually found on permanent maxillary molars, with fewer on mandibular molars. It is attached to cementum near the root bifurcation or trifurcation area. On occasion, it is located near the cemento-enamel junction. Most have been reported in the Asian population. The enamel pearl may consist of enamel only or enamel, dentin, and pulp.

The enamel pearl is an uncommon finding. It appears radiographically as a small, spherical radiopacity. Sometimes the enamel pearl may be mistaken for calculus. In general, no treatment is necessary for this anomaly. Removal may be necessary if

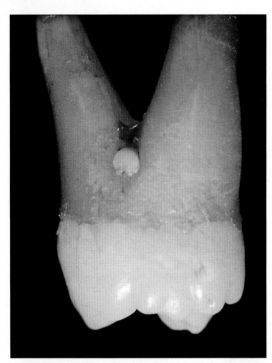

• **Figure 5.29** Enamel pearl in the furcation area. (Courtesy Dr. Rudy Melfi.)

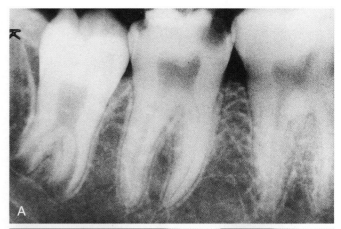

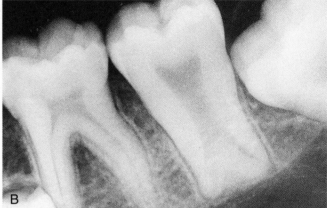

• **Figure 5.31 A,** Taurodont in the mandibular third molar. **B,** Taurodont in the mandibular second molar. (**A** courtesy Dr. Margot Van Dis; **B** courtesy Dr. George Blozis.)

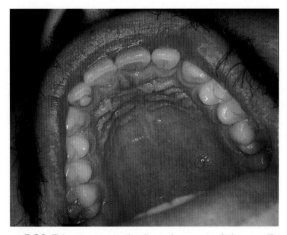

• **Figure 5.30** Talon cusp on the lingual aspect of the maxillary right lateral permanent incisor.

periodontal problems occur in the furcation area when an enamel pearl is present.

Talon Cusp

A **talon cusp** is an accessory cusp located in the area of the cingulum of a maxillary or mandibular permanent incisor (Fig. 5.30). It is most common on the maxillary lateral incisor. The talon cusp is said to resemble an eagle's talon. It often projects lingually from the cemento-enamel junction halfway to the incisal edge of the involved tooth. It is composed of normal enamel and dentin and contains some pulp tissue. Frequently a caries-susceptible fissure is present between the cusps. Removal of the talon cusp is often indicated because it interferes with

occlusion. If pulp tissue is present, endodontic therapy would be necessary.

Taurodontism

Taurodontism is a term used to describe a developmental dental anomaly in which the teeth exhibit elongated, large pulp chambers and short roots (Fig. 5.31). A tooth that exhibits taurodontism is called a **taurodont.** Taurodontism means "bull-like" teeth. The term was first used to describe teeth that resembled those of cud-chewing animals. Although the cause of taurodontism is uncertain, a variety of causes have been suggested, ranging from a primitive pattern of tooth development to the developmental failure of the Hertwig epithelial root sheath to invaginate at the proper level. It may be an isolated entity or a component of a syndrome.

Taurodontism is uncommon and seen in both the deciduous and most often permanent dentitions; it usually affects a single molar tooth or several molars in the same quadrant. Taurodontism can occur unilaterally or bilaterally. The crown of the tooth appears clinically normal. A taurodont is identified by its characteristic radiographic appearance. The tooth tends to have a radiolucent stretched appearance, and the pulp chamber is greatly enlarged and elongated without a constriction at the cemento-enamel junction. The roots appear short, with the furcation located near the apices. No treatment is indicated for

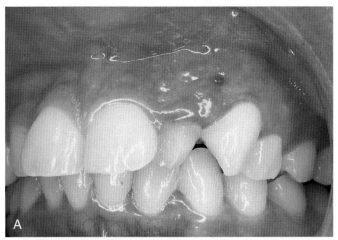

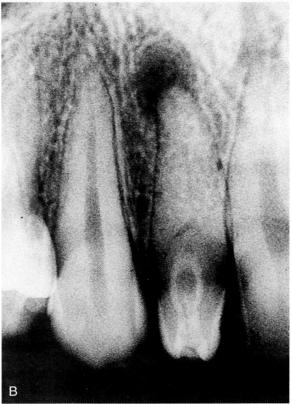

• **Figure 5.32 A,** Clinical illustration of dens in dente in maxillary lateral incisor. **B,** Radiograph of dens in dente in maxillary lateral incisor. (**A** courtesy Dr. George Blozis.)

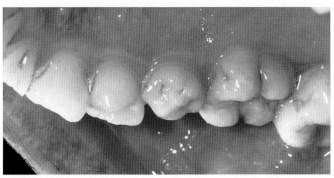

• **Figure 5.33** Dens evaginatus of maxillary premolar. (Courtesy Dr. Margot Van Dis.)

taurodontism. Taurodontism is classified as mild, moderate, or severe depending on how far apically the base of the pulp chamber extends. This is helpful in epidemiologic research. Taurodontism has been observed in syndromes such as Down syndrome, ectodermal dysplasia, Ellis–van Creveld syndrome, Klinefelter syndrome, hypophosphatasia, and several other conditions.

Dens Invaginatus

Dens invaginatus, also called **dens in dente,** is a developmental anomaly that results when the enamel organ invaginates into the crown of a tooth before mineralization (Fig. 5.32). **Invaginate** means that one portion infolds into another portion of a structure. Two forms of dens invaginatus have been described: coronal and radicular. Coronal dens invaginatus is seen most often in permanent maxillary lateral incisors. The invagination can be type I, which is within the crown; type II, which extends below the cemento-enamel junction; and type III that goes through the root and perforates the root laterally in the apical third. Sometimes in dens invaginatus, the invagination is very large, and radiographically, it will appear as "a tooth within a tooth," thus the name *dens in dente.* An elongated bulb or pear-shaped mass of enamel is seen in dentin surrounded by a radiolucent area. This defect typically is confined to the coronal third of the tooth, but in some cases it extends to include the entire root length (types II and III). Clinically, a dens in dente may appear as either a normally shaped or malformed crown that exhibits a deep pit or crevice in the area of the cingulum. The invaginated toothlike structure retains communication with the outside of the tooth via the pit or crevice visible on the crown surface. Radicular dens invaginatus is rare.

Dens invaginatus customarily affects a single tooth. The maxillary lateral incisor is the most frequently affected tooth, and when affected it is often peg shaped. Anterior teeth, particularly the maxillary and mandibular incisors, are more commonly affected than the posterior teeth. The dens invaginatus is vulnerable to caries, pulpal infection, and necrosis as a result of the communication between the oral cavity and the invaginated area of the tooth. Consequently the dens invaginatus is often nonvital and is seen in association with a periapical lesion (periapical cyst, periapical granuloma, periapical abscess). If the dens invaginatus is detected shortly after eruption, a prophylactic restoration can be placed in the deep pit or crevice to prevent caries and subsequent pulpal necrosis. A nonvital dens in dente may be treated endodontically. A malformed crown can be restored with composite materials or a full-coverage crown.

Dens Evaginatus

Dens evaginatus (central tubercle, occlusal pearl, accessory tubercle) is an accessory enamel cusp found on the occlusal surface of the tooth (Fig. 5.33). This rare developmental anomaly occurs most often on the mandibular premolars and is usually bilateral. When affected, they are called *tuberculated premolars.* Molars, cuspids, and incisors can also be affected. Dens evaginatus is thought to result from the proliferation and outpouching of enamel epithelium during tooth development. It occurs rarely in whites and most often in Asians, the Inuit, and Native Americans.

Clinically, the dens evaginatus appears as a small, rounded lobe of enamel on the occlusal surface of a mandibular premolar between the buccal and lingual cusps. A pulp horn may extend into this extra cusp. Sometimes, with occlusal wear, these teeth may experience periapical necrosis. The dens evaginatus may not require treatment. However, it can cause occlusal problems, and endodontic treatment may be necessary.

Supernumerary Roots

Supernumerary roots (extra roots) can involve any tooth (Fig. 5.34). No cause for this developmental anomaly has been identified. External pressure, trauma, and metabolic dysfunction during root development have been suggested. Supernumerary roots are not uncommon and tend to occur in teeth that exhibit root formation after birth. The multirooted teeth most often affected are the maxillary and mandibular third molars. The single-rooted teeth most often affected are the mandibular bicuspids and cuspids. Supernumerary roots may exhibit dilaceration and are diagnosed radiographically.

In general, no treatment is indicated for supernumerary roots. However, they become clinically significant if extraction of the involved tooth or endodontic therapy becomes necessary.

Abnormalities of Tooth Structure

Enamel Hypoplasia

Enamel hypoplasia is the incomplete or defective formation of enamel, resulting in the alteration of tooth form or color. **Hypoplasia** is defined as the incomplete development of an organ or tissue. Enamel hypoplasia results from a disturbance of or damage to ameloblasts during enamel matrix formation (Box 5.1). Enamel hypoplasia can affect either the deciduous or permanent dentition.

Enamel hypoplasia that is inherited is called **amelogenesis imperfecta.** Amelogenesis imperfecta is described in detail in Chapter 6. The factors that cause enamel hypoplasia by injuring the sensitive ameloblasts during enamel formation are discussed in this chapter.

Enamel Hypoplasia Caused by Febrile Illness or Vitamin Deficiency

Ameloblasts are one of the most sensitive cell groups in the body. It is believed that any serious systemic disease or severe nutritional deficiency is capable of producing enamel hypoplasia. Febrile illnesses (measles, chickenpox, and scarlet fever) and vitamin deficiencies (vitamins A, C, and D) that occur during the time of

tooth formation can result in a type of enamel hypoplasia characterized by pitting of the enamel. Only the crowns of teeth that are developing at the time of the febrile illness or vitamin deficiency are affected.

This type of hypoplasia usually involves the permanent central incisors, laterals, cuspids, and first molars, which are the teeth that form during the first year of life. One or more horizontal rows of tiny, deep pits are seen traversing the affected tooth surface. The number and rows of pits may vary, depending on the extent and severity of injury to the ameloblasts. These enamel pits tend to stain and appear unsightly (Fig. 5.35).

Teeth affected with enamel hypoplasia of the pitting type may be restored with composites during childhood and later with porcelain veneers or full-crown coverage.

Enamel Hypoplasia Resulting From Local Infection or Trauma

Enamel hypoplasia of a permanent tooth may result from infection of a deciduous tooth. A single tooth is usually affected and is referred to as a **Turner tooth.** A carious deciduous tooth with periapical involvement can disturb the ameloblasts of the underlying permanent tooth. The severity of the defect depends on the

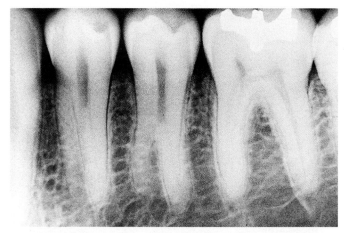

• **Figure 5.34** Supernumerary roots in mandibular premolars.

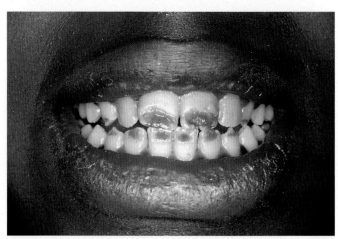

• **Figure 5.35** Enamel hypoplasia. In this patient the enamel hypoplasia follows a pattern that is suggestive of a systemic problem such as a high fever.

> • **BOX 5.1** **Factors That Can Cause Enamel Hypoplasia**

- Amelogenesis imperfecta
- Febrile illness (measles, chickenpox, and scarlet fever)
- Vitamin deficiency (vitamins A, C, and D)
- Local infection of a deciduous tooth
- Ingestion of fluoride
- Congenital syphilis
- Birth injury, premature birth
- Idiopathic factors

severity of the deciduous tooth infection, the degree of periapical tissue involvement, and the stage of development of the underlying permanent tooth.

The teeth most often affected are the permanent premolars. Anterior teeth are not usually affected. However, traumatic injury to a deciduous anterior tooth may cause a Turner tooth in the permanent dentition. In this case maxillary central incisors are more frequently involved. The clinical appearance of the affected tooth depends on the extent of the injury. The color of the enamel of these teeth may range from yellow to brown, or severe pitting and deformity may be involved. These enamel defects can frequently be identified radiographically before the eruption of the involved tooth. An anterior Turner tooth may be restored to provide an improved esthetic appearance; a posterior Turner tooth may require a restoration to provide improved function.

Enamel Hypoplasia Resulting From Fluoride Ingestion

Enamel hypoplasia resulting from fluoride ingestion, or **dental fluorosis,** occurs as a result of the patient ingesting high concentrations of fluoride during tooth formation, usually in drinking water. Affected teeth exhibit a mottled discoloration of enamel (Fig. 5.36). *Mottling* refers to irregular areas of discoloration. The more fluoride ingested, the more severe the mottling. The optimal amount of fluoride in drinking water is 0.7 ppm. This is the national standard according to the U.S. Department of Health and Human Services. Ingestion of water with a fluoride concentration two to three times the recommended amount results in mild fluorosis that appears as white flecks and chalky opaque areas of enamel. Ingestion of water containing four times the recommended amount of fluoride causes brown or black staining and a pitted or overall corroded enamel appearance. Fluoride supplements are only recommended for children in nonfluoridated areas.

All permanent teeth are involved in this type of enamel hypoplasia. The teeth affected by fluorosis are generally decay resistant. To improve the esthetic appearance of these teeth, bleaching, bonding, composites, porcelain veneers, or full-coverage crowns can be used.

Enamel Hypoplasia Resulting From Congenital Syphilis

Syphilis is a contagious sexually transmitted disease caused by the spirochete *Treponema pallidum.* It is described in detail in Chapter

4. **Congenital syphilis** is transmitted from an infected mother to her fetus via the placenta. Children with congenital syphilis have numerous developmental anomalies and may be blind, deaf, or paralyzed. In utero infection with *T. pallidum* results in enamel hypoplasia of the permanent incisors and first molars. This is so rare that a lengthy discussion is not necessary.

The affected incisors are shaped like screwdrivers: broadest at the middle third and narrow incisally, with a notched incisal edge (Fig. 5.37A). They are called **Hutchinson incisors.** First molars appear as irregularly shaped crowns with a narrow occlusal surface made up of multiple tiny globules of enamel instead of cusps (Fig. 5.37B). Because of their berrylike appearance, these molars are called **mulberry molars.** Not every case of congenital syphilis exhibits these dental findings, and similarly shaped teeth may be seen in individuals without congenital syphilis.

Treatment to improve the esthetic appearance of these teeth includes full-coverage crowns.

Enamel Hypoplasia Resulting From Birth Injury, Premature Birth, or Idiopathic Factors

Enamel hypoplasia can occur as a result of trauma or change of environment at the time of birth or in premature infants. In addition, many cases of enamel hypoplasia do not have an identifiable cause despite careful and thorough history taking. The ameloblast is a sensitive cell that is easily damaged. For this reason even a mild illness or systemic problem can result in enamel hypoplasia. Such illnesses may be so insignificant that they are not known to the patient or remembered by the patient's parents. To improve the esthetic appearance of these teeth, composites, porcelain veneers, or full-coverage crowns can be used.

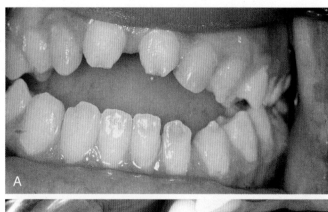
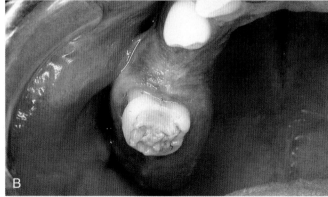

• **Figure 5.37** A, Hutchinson incisors. B, Mulberry molars. (Courtesy Dr. George Blozis.)

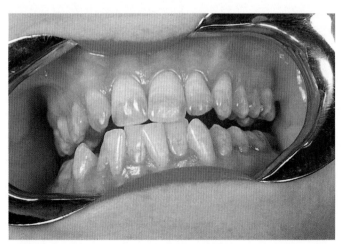

• **Figure 5.36** Mottled enamel. The discoloration of the enamel in this patient occurred as a result of high fluoride intake.

Enamel Hypocalcification

Enamel hypocalcification is a developmental anomaly that results in a disturbance of the maturation of the enamel matrix. It usually appears as a localized, chalky white spot on the middle third of smooth crowns. The underlying enamel may be soft and susceptible to caries. The cause of enamel hypocalcification is uncertain; however, trauma during the maturation of enamel matrix has been suggested. Bleaching, composites, porcelain veneers, or full-coverage crowns can be used to improve the esthetic appearance of these teeth.

Endogenous Staining of Teeth

Endogenous or **intrinsic staining of teeth** occurs as a result of the deposition of substances circulating systemically during tooth development. For example, ingestion of tetracycline during tooth development causes a yellowish-green discoloration of dentin that is visible through the enamel. At the time of eruption the teeth fluoresce under ultraviolet light. Later the tetracycline is oxidized, the color changes from yellowish to brown, and the teeth no longer fluoresce. Other conditions such as rhesus (Rh) incompatibility (erythroblastosis fetalis), neonatal liver disease, and congenital porphyria (an inherited metabolic disease) also cause endogenous staining of teeth.

Regional Odontodysplasia

Regional odontodysplasia, or **ghost teeth,** is an unusual developmental anomaly in which one or several teeth in the same quadrant are malformed, are usually unerupted, and radiographically exhibit a marked reduction in radiodensity and a characteristic ghostlike appearance (Fig. 5.38). Very thin enamel and dentin are present with an enlarged pulp. On occasion, the enamel is not even visible on the radiograph. The pulp chambers of these teeth are extremely large. Either the teeth do not erupt or eruption is incomplete. If these malformed "teeth" erupt into the oral cavity, they are typically nonfunctional.

Regional odontodysplasia can affect either the deciduous or the permanent dentition. The maxilla, especially the anterior maxilla, is more often involved than the mandible. The cause of regional odontodysplasia is idiopathic; changes in the vascular supply during tooth development is the most accepted theory. There is a slight predilection for females. Extraction usually is the treatment of choice for ghost teeth. In adults, implants have been placed to restore function if several adjacent teeth in one quadrant are affected.

Abnormalities of Tooth Eruption

Impacted and Embedded Teeth

Impacted teeth are teeth that cannot erupt because of a physical obstruction. **Embedded teeth** are those that do not erupt because of a lack of eruptive force. An impacted tooth is one of the most common developmental defects occurring in humans. Any tooth can be impacted. The most commonly impacted teeth are the maxillary and mandibular third molars, the maxillary cuspids, the maxillary and mandibular premolars, and supernumerary teeth. Impacted teeth are identified radiographically (Fig. 5.39).

Third-molar impactions are classified according to the position of the tooth: mesioangular, distoangular, vertical, and horizontal. The most common position of an impacted third molar is mesioangular. The crown of the third molar points in a mesial direction and is in contact with the second molar, which is preventing its eruption. In a distoangular impaction the crown of the third molar points in a distal direction toward the ramus, and the roots of the impacted tooth are adjacent to the distal root of the second molar. In a vertical impaction the crown of the third molar is in a normal position for eruption, but eruption is prevented by the distal aspect of the second molar or by the anterior border of the ramus. In a horizontal impaction the crown of the third molar is seen in a horizontal position relative to the inferior border of the mandible.

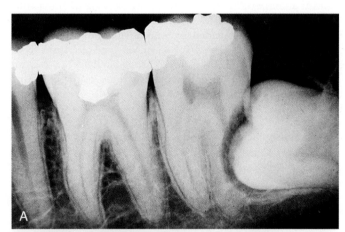
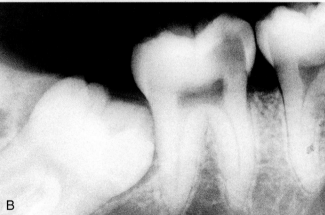

• **Figure 5.39** **A,** Horizontal impaction of the third molar. **B,** Mesioangular impaction of the third molar.

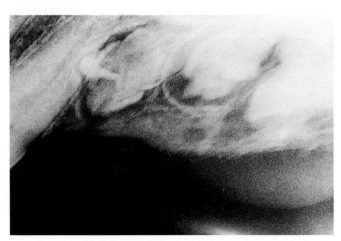

• **Figure 5.38** Regional odontodysplasia.

Teeth can be completely impacted in bone with no communication with the oral cavity, or they can be partially impacted. In a partial impaction the tooth lies partly in soft tissue and partly in bone. Partially impacted teeth often have communication with the oral cavity and are susceptible to infections, that is, pericoronitis. For unknown reasons some completely impacted teeth undergo resorption. This resorption usually begins in the crown portion of the tooth, and the tooth is slowly replaced by bone. Radiographically this resorption should not be confused with caries. Caries of an impacted tooth is impossible unless communication with the oral cavity occurs.

Impacted teeth are surgically removed to prevent odontogenic cyst and tumor formation or damage (resorption) to adjacent teeth or because the bone (in some cases) may be more susceptible to fracture. Partially impacted third molars are removed to prevent infections. Studies have shown that the optimal time to extract impacted third molars is between the ages of 12 and 24 years. With increased age a greater incidence of nerve paresthesia exists.

Ankylosed Teeth

Ankylosed teeth (or *submerged teeth*) are deciduous teeth in which bone has fused to cementum and dentin, preventing exfoliation of the deciduous tooth and eruption of the underlying permanent tooth (Fig. 5.40). However, the permanent premolar may be congenitally missing. Deciduous molars are most often affected by ankylosis. The cause is unknown; trauma and infection of the periodontal ligament have been suggested.

Initially the tooth erupts into the oral cavity into normal occlusion. The ankylosed tooth is not exfoliated. When the permanent teeth erupt, those adjacent to the ankylosed tooth have taller occlusocervical heights. Compared with the adjacent teeth, the ankylosed tooth appears submerged and has a different, more solid sound when percussed.

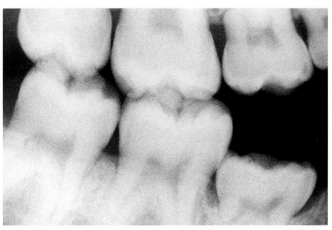

• **Figure 5.40** Ankylosis of deciduous molar. (Courtesy Dr. Margot Van Dis.)

The presence of an ankylosed tooth is usually suspected on the basis of the clinical appearance and is confirmed radiographically. The periodontal ligament space is lacking or indistinct because of the union of bone and cementum, and the tooth usually exhibits root resorption. Ankylosis may be seen in permanent teeth that have been avulsed and reimplanted.

Extraction of ankylosed deciduous teeth may be necessary at some point to allow eruption of the underlying permanent tooth if it is present. If not, sometimes these ankylosed deciduous teeth maintain the space until a permanent restoration, like a fixed bridge or implant, can be considered. Extraction of ankylosed permanent teeth is often necessary to prevent malocclusion, caries, and periodontal disease.

Selected References

Books

Alley KE, Melfi RC: *Permar's oral embryology and microscopic anatomy,* ed 10, Baltimore, 2000, Lippincott Williams & Wilkins.

Darby M: *Darby's comprehensive review of dental hygiene,* ed 8, St. Louis, 2016, Elsevier.

Langlais RP, Miller CS: *Color atlas of common oral diseases,* ed 3, Baltimore, 2003, Lippincott Williams & Wilkins.

Miller BF: *Miller-Keane encyclopedia and dictionary of medicine, nursing, and allied health, revised reprint,* ed 7, Philadelphia, 2005, Saunders.

Neville BW, Damm DD, Allen CM, et al: *Oral and maxillofacial pathology,* ed 4, St. Louis, 2016, Elsevier.

Regezi JA, Sciubba JJ, Jordan RCK: *Oral pathology: clinical-pathologic correlations,* ed 7, St. Louis, 2017, Elsevier.

Regezi JA, Sciubba JJ, Pogrel MA: *Atlas of oral and maxillofacial pathology,* Philadelphia, 2000, Saunders.

Scheid RC: *Woelfel's dental anatomy: its relevance to dentistry,* ed 7, Baltimore, 2007, Lippincott Williams & Wilkins.

Journal Articles

Alexander WN, Lilly GE, Irby WB: Odontodysplasia, *Oral Surg Oral Med Oral Pathol* 22:814, 1966.

Alfors E, Larson A, Sjögren S: The odontogenic keratocyst: a benign cystic tumor?, *J Oral Maxillofac Surg* 42:10, 1984.

Al-Talabani NG, Smith CJ: Experimental dentigerous cysts and enamel hypoplasia: their possible significance in explaining the pathogenesis of dentigerous cysts, *J Oral Pathol* 9:82, 1980.

Antonogiou GN, Sándor GK, Koidou VP, et al: Nonsyndromic and syndromic keratocystic odontogenic tumors: systematic review and meta-analysis of recurrences, *J Craniomaxillofac Surg* 42(7):e364, 2014.

Baker BR: Pits of the lip commissures in Caucasoid males, *Oral Surg Oral Med Oral Pathol* 21:56, 1966.

Barker GR: A radiolucency of the ascending ramus of the mandible associated with invested parotid salivary gland material and analogous with a Stafne bone cavity, *Br J Oral Maxillofac Surg* 26:81, 1988.

Baum BJ, Cohen MM: Patterns of size reduction in hypodontia, *J Dent Res* 50:779, 1971.

Bhargava D, Deshpande A: Keratocystic odontogenic tumor (KCOD)—a cyst to a tumor, *Oral Maxillofac Surg* 16:163, 2012.

Bodin I, Julin P, Thomsson M: Hyperdontia III: supernumerary anterior teeth, *Dentomaxillofac Radiol* 10:35, 1981a.

Bodin I, Julin P, Thomsson M: Hyperdontia IV: supernumerary premolars, *Dentomaxillofac Radiol* 19:99, 1981b.

Brannon RB: The odontogenic keratocyst—a clinicopathologic study of 312 cases. I. Clinical features, *Oral Surg Oral Med Oral Pathol* 42:54, 1976.

Brannon RB: The odontogenic keratocyst—a clinicopathologic study of 312 cases. II. Histologic features, *Oral Surg Oral Med Oral Pathol* 43:233, 1977.

Buchner A, Hansen LS: Lymphoepithelial cysts of the oral cavity: a clinicopathologic study of 38 cases, *Oral Surg Oral Med Oral Pathol* 50:441, 1980.

Burton DJ, Saffos RO, Scheffer RB: Multiple bilateral dens in dente as a factor in the etiology of multiple periapical lesions, *Oral Surg Oral Med Oral Pathol* 49:496, 1980.

Carter L, Carney Y, Perez-Pudlewski D: Lateral periodontal cyst: multifactorial analysis of a previously unreported series, *Oral Surg Oral Med Oral Pathol Oral Radiol Endod* 81:210, 1996.

Cavanha AO: Enamel pearls, *Oral Surg Oral Med Oral Pathol* 19:373, 1965.

Chi AC, Neville BW, Klinger BJ: A multilocular radiolucency, *J Am Dent Assoc* 138:1102, 2007.

Chi AC, Owings JR, Muller S: Peripherial odontogenic keratocyst: report of two cases and a review of the literature, *Oral Surg Oral Med Oral Pathol Oral Radiol Endod* 99:71–78, 2005.

Christ TF: The globulomaxillary cyst—an embryologic misconception, *Oral Surg Oral Med Oral Pathol* 30:515, 1970.

Conklin WW: Bilateral dens invaginatus in the mandibular incisor region, *Oral Surg Oral Med Oral Pathol* 45:905, 1978.

Dachi SF, Howell FV: A survey of 3874 routine full-mouth radiographs. II. A study of impacted teeth, *Oral Surg Oral Med Oral Pathol* 14:1165, 1961.

Darling AI, Levers BGH: Submerged human deciduous molars and ankylosis, *Arch Oral Biol* 18:1021, 1973.

Dean HT, Arnold FA: Endemic dental fluorosis or mottled teeth, *J Am Dent Assoc* 30:1278, 1943.

Dehlers FAC, Lee KW, Lee EC: Dens evaginatus (evaginated odontoma), *Dent Pract* 17:239, 1967.

Delany GM, Goldblatt LI: Fused teeth: a multidisciplinary approach to treatment, *J Am Dent Assoc* 103:732, 1981.

DiFiore PM, Hartwell GR: Median mandibular lateral periodontal cysts, *Oral Surg Oral Med Oral Pathol* 63:545, 1987.

Duncan WK, Helpin ML: Bilateral fusion and gemination: a literature analysis and case report, *Oral Surg Oral Med Oral Pathol* 64:82–87, 1987.

Eisenbud LE, Attie J, Garlick J, et al: Aneurysmal bone cyst of the mandible, *Oral Surg Oral Med Oral Pathol* 64:202, 1987.

el-Mofty SK, Shannon MT, Mustoe TA: Lymph node metastasis in spindle cell carcinoma arising in an odontogenic cyst, *Oral Surg Oral Med Oral Pathol* 71:209, 1991.

Everett FG, Wescott WB: Commissural lip pits, *Oral Surg Oral Med Oral Pathol* 14:202, 1961.

Fantasia JE: Lateral periodontal cyst: an analysis of 46 cases, *Oral Surg Oral Med Oral Pathol* 48:237, 1979.

Fowler CB, Kessler HP, Kahn M: Glandular odontogenic cyst: analysis of 46 cases with special emphasis on microscopic criteria for diagnosis, *Head Neck Pathol* 5:364, 2011.

Freedman PD, Lumerman H, Gee JK: Calcifying odontogenic cyst, *Oral Surg Oral Med Oral Pathol* 40:93, 1975.

Gardner DG: The dentinal changes in regional odontodysplasia, *Oral Surg Oral Med Oral Pathol* 38:887, 1974.

Gardner DG: An evaluation of reported cases of median mandibular cysts, *Oral Surg Oral Med Oral Pathol* 65:208, 1988.

Gardner DG, Girgis SS: Taurodontism, shovel-shaped incisors and the Klinefelter syndrome, *J Can Dent Assoc* 8:372, 1978.

Gardner DG, Sapp JP: Regional odontodysplasia, *Oral Surg Oral Med Oral Pathol* 35:351, 1973.

Grahnen H, Granath LE: Numerical variations in primary dentition, *Odontol Revy* 12:342, 1961.

Grahnen H, Larsson PG: Enamel defects in deciduous dentition of prematurely born children, *Odontol Revy* 9:143, 1958.

Hamner JE III, Witko CJ, Metro PS: Taurodontism: report of a case, *Oral Surg Oral Med Oral Pathol* 18:409, 1964.

Henderson HZ: Ankylosis of primary molars: a clinical, radiographic, and histologic study, *J Dent Child* 46:117, 1979.

Hernandez GA, Castro A, Castro G, et al: Aneurysmal bone cyst versus hemangioma of the mandible, *Oral Surg Oral Med Oral Pathol* 76:790, 1993.

Holt RD, Brook AH: Taurodontism: a criterion for diagnosis and its prevalence in mandibular first molars in a sample of 1115 British school children, *J Int Assoc Dent Child* 10:41, 1979.

Howell RE, Handlers JP, Aberle AM, et al: CEA immunoreactivity in odontogenic tumors and keratocysts, *Oral Surg Oral Med Oral Pathol* 66:576, 1988.

Jasmin J, Ionesco-Benaiche N, Muller M: Latent fluorides: report of a case, *J Dent Child* 62:220, 1995.

Keith A: Problems relating to the teeth of the earlier forms of prehistoric man, *Proc R Soc Med* 6(Pt 3):103, 1913.

Kelly JR: Gemination, fusion, or both?, *Oral Surg Oral Med Oral Pathol* 45:326, 1978.

King RC, Smith BR, Burk JL: Dermoid cyst in the floor of the mouth, *Oral Surg Oral Med Oral Pathol* 78:567, 1994.

Kitchin PC: Dens in dente, *J Dent Res* 15:1176, 1935.

Krolls SO: Donalhue AH: Double-rooted maxillary primary canines, *Oral Surg Oral Med Oral Pathol* 49:379, 1980.

Leamas R, Jimenez-Planas A: Taurodontism in premolars, *Oral Surg Oral Med Oral Pathol* 75:501, 1993.

MacDonald-Jankowski DS: Glandular odontogenic cyst: systematic review, *Dentomaxillofac Radiol* 39:127, 2010.

Mathewson RJ, Siegel MJ, McCanna DL: Ankyloglossia: a review of the literature and a case report, *J Dent Child* 33:238, 1966.

Maurette PE, Jorge J, deMoraes M: Conservative treatment protocol of the odontogenic keratocyst, *J Oral Maxillofac Surg* 64:379, 2006.

Mellor JK, Ripa LW: Talon cusp: a clinically significant anomaly, *Oral Surg Oral Med Oral Pathol* 29:224, 1970.

Milazzo A, Alexander SA: Fusion, gemination, oligodontia and taurodontism, *J Pedod* 6:194, 1982.

Mlynarczyk G: Enamel pitting: a common symptom of tuberous sclerosis, *Oral Surg Oral Med Oral Pathol* 71:63, 1991.

Morningstar CH: Effect of infection of deciduous molar on the permanent tooth germ, *J Am Dent Assoc* 24:786, 1937.

Partridge M, Towers JF: The primordial cyst (odontogenic keratocyst): its tumor-like characteristics and behavior, *Br J Oral Maxillofac Surg* 25:271, 1987.

Pendrys DG: Dental fluorosis in perspective, *J Am Dent Assoc* 122:63, 1991.

Ray GE: Congenital absence of permanent teeth, *Br Dent J* 90:213, 1951.

Reaume CE, Sofie VL: Lingual thyroid: review of the literature and a report of a case, *Oral Surg Oral Med Oral Pathol* 45:841, 1978.

Redman RS: Respiratory epithelium in an apical periodontal cyst of the mandible, *Oral Surg Oral Med Oral Pathol* 67:77, 1989.

Rushton MA: Invaginated teeth (dens in dente): contents of the invagination, *Oral Surg Oral Med Oral Pathol* 11:1378, 1958.

Rushton MA: Odontodysplasia: "ghost teeth", *Br Dent J* 119:109, 1965.

Sapp PJ, Stark M: Self-healing traumatic bone cysts, *Oral Surg Oral Med Oral Pathol* 69:597, 1990.

Shafer WG: Dens in dente, *NY Dent J* 19:220, 1953.

Siponen M, Neville BW, Damm DD, et al: Multifocal lateral periodontal cysts: a report of 4 cases and review of the literature, *Oral Surg Oral Med Oral Pathol Oral Radiol Endod* 111:225, 2011.

Suchina JA, Ludington JR Jr, Madden RM: Dens invaginatus of a maxillary lateral incisor: endodontic treatment, *Oral Surg Oral Med Oral Pathol* 68:467, 1989.

Tolson G, Czuszak CA, Billman MA, et al: Report of a lateral periodontal cyst and gingival cyst in the same patient, *J Periodontol* 67:541, 1996.

Trope M: Root resorption of dental and traumatic origin: classification based on etiology, *Pract Periodontics Aesthet Dent* 10:515, 1998.

van Gool AV: Injury to the permanent tooth germ after trauma to the deciduous predecessor, *Oral Surg Oral Med Oral Pathol* 35:2, 1973.

Vorheis JM, Gregory GT, McDonald RE: Ankylosed deciduous molars, *J Am Dent Assoc* 44:68, 1952.

Weinmann JP, Svoboda JF, Woods RW: Hereditary disturbances of enamel formation and calcification, *J Am Dent Assoc* 32:397, 1945.

Yip WK: The prevalence of dens evaginatus, *Oral Surg Oral Med Oral Pathol* 38:80, 1974.

Yoshikazu S, Tanimoto K, Wada T: Simple bone cyst: evaluation of contents with conventional radiography and computed tomography, *Oral Surg Oral Med Oral Pathol* 77:296, 1994.

Review Questions

1. Which term refers to a defect present at birth?
   a. Anomaly
   b. Inherited defect
   c. Congenital defect
   d. Developmental defect

2. Which term refers to the origin and tissue formation of teeth?
   a. Odontogenesis
   b. Dentinogenesis
   c. Amelogenesis
   d. Cementogenesis

3. Which term refers to the joining of teeth by cementum *only*?
   a. Fusion
   b. Gemination
   c. Twinning
   d. Concrescence

4. Which teeth are most often missing?
   a. Canines
   b. Deciduous second molars
   c. Third molars
   d. Premolars

5. Which tooth is the most common supernumerary tooth?
   a. Mesiodens
   b. Distomolar
   c. Paramolar
   d. Hutchinson incisor

6. Which teeth most often appear smaller than normal?
   a. Mandibular premolars
   b. Maxillary lateral incisors
   c. Mandibular lateral incisors
   d. Mandibular third molars

7. Which term refers to the developmental anomaly that arises when a single tooth germ attempts to divide and results in the incomplete formation of two teeth?
   a. Fusion
   b. Gemination
   c. Concrescence
   d. Dilaceration

8. Which term refers to the developmental anomaly that arises from the union of two normally separated adjacent tooth germs?
   a. Twinning
   b. Gemination
   c. Fusion
   d. Dilaceration

9. Which term refers to an abnormal angulation or curve in the root or crown of a tooth?
   a. Fusion
   b. Gemination
   c. Concrescence
   d. Dilaceration

10. Which term refers to a developmental anomaly in which teeth exhibit elongated, large pulp chambers and short roots?
    a. Dens invaginatus
    b. Dens evaginatus
    c. Taurodontism
    d. Dilaceration

11. Which developmental anomaly is often associated with a nonvital tooth and periapical lesions?
    a. Dens invaginatus
    b. Dens evaginatus
    c. Taurodontism
    d. Talon cusp

12. Which of the following teeth most often exhibit supernumerary roots?
    a. Maxillary first premolars
    b. Maxillary third molars
    c. Mandibular first molars
    d. Maxillary first molars

13. Which one of the following describes the appearance of enamel hypoplasia resulting from a febrile illness or vitamin deficiency?
    a. Pitting defects
    b. Yellowish-brown discoloration
    c. Blackish-brown staining
    d. Chalky white spots

14. Which one of the following is associated with enamel hypoplasia resulting from congenital syphilis?
    a. Turner tooth
    b. Hutchinson incisors
    c. Taurodont
    d. Dens evaginatus

15. Which one of the following describes the appearance of enamel hypocalcification?
    a. Pitting defects
    b. Yellowish-brown discoloration
    c. Blackish-brown stains
    d. Chalky white spots

16. Which term describes a tooth that has not erupted because of a lack of eruptive force?
    a. Ankylosed
    b. Impacted
    c. Embedded
    d. Fused

17. Which teeth are most often impacted?
    a. Distomolars
    b. Maxillary and mandibular first molars
    c. Mandibular cuspids
    d. Mandibular third molars

18. Which term describes a tooth in which bone has fused to cementum and dentin and prevents the eruption of an underlying permanent tooth?
    a. Concrescence
    b. Embedded
    c. Ankylosed
    d. Fused

19. Which cyst is *not* an odontogenic cyst?
    a. Dentigerous cyst
    b. Primordial cyst
    c. Median palatal cyst
    d. Lateral periodontal cyst

20. The most common cause of the radicular cyst is:
    a. Caries
    b. Trauma
    c. Malignant infiltration
    d. Food impaction

21. Which cyst is an odontogenic intraosseous cyst that forms around the crown of a developing tooth?
    a. Coronal cyst
    b. Dentigerous cyst
    c. Lateral periodontal cyst
    d. Eruption cyst

22. Which cyst develops in place of a tooth?
    a. Dentigerous cyst
    b. Primordial cyst
    c. Follicular cyst
    d. Odontogenic keratocyst

23. Which cyst is characterized by its unique microscopic appearance and frequent recurrence?
    a. Residual cyst
    b. Stafne bone cyst
    c. Odontogenic keratocyst
    d. Eruption cyst

24. The lateral periodontal cyst is defined by its location. In which area is the lateral periodontal cyst most commonly found?
    a. Mandibular third molar area
    b. Maxillary tuberosity area
    c. Between the maxillary premolars
    d. Between the mandibular cuspid and first premolar

25. The teeth are vital with all of the following cysts *except:*
    a. Nasopalatine canal cyst
    b. Cyst of the palatine papilla
    c. Dentigerous cyst
    d. Periapical cyst

26. Which cyst is characteristically pear shaped?
    a. Globulomaxillary cyst
    b. Median palatal cyst
    c. Incisal canal cyst
    d. Median mandibular cyst

27. Which of the following describes a radicular cyst left behind after extraction of the offending tooth?
    a. Periodontal cyst
    b. Gingival cyst
    c. Odontogenic cyst
    d. Residual cyst

28. With which cyst may the patient complain of dysphagia?
    a. Thyroglossal tract cyst
    b. Median palatal cyst
    c. Static bone cyst
    d. Traumatic bone cyst

29. Which cyst is considered a pseudocyst?
    a. Odontogenic keratocyst
    b. Traumatic bone cyst
    c. Lymphoepithelial cyst
    d. Primordial cyst

30. In addition to the odontogenic keratocyst, which lesion would the hygienist suspect if a radiograph revealed a multilocular radiolucency?
    a. Globulomaxillary cyst
    b. Aneurysmal bone cyst
    c. Stafne bone cyst
    d. Periapical cyst

31. Which term refers to the adhesion of the tongue to the floor of the mouth?
    a. Ankylosis
    b. Ankyloglossia
    c. Anodontia
    d. Amelogenesis

32. Which location is the most common for lip pits?
    a. Commissure
    b. Philtrum
    c. Nasolabial groove
    d. Labiomental groove

33. Which term refers to an ectopic mass of thyroid tissue located on the posterior dorsal tongue between the foramen cecum and the epiglottis?
    a. Thyroid cyst
    b. Thyroid tumor
    c. Lingual tonsil
    d. Lingual thyroid

34. Which term refers to the total absence of all teeth?
    a. Anodontia
    b. Hypodontia
    c. Hyperdontia
    d. Microdontia

35. Which term refers to the lack of one or more teeth?
    a. Anodontia
    b. Hypodontia
    c. Hyperdontia
    d. Microdontia

36. Which tooth is the second most common supernumerary tooth?
a. Taurodont
b. Mesiodens
c. Paramolar
d. Distomolar

37. Which term refers to abnormally small teeth?
a. Taurodontia
b. Macrodontia
c. Microdontia
d. Hypodontia

38. Which term refers to abnormally large teeth?
a. Taurodontia
b. Acromegaly
c. Macrodontia
d. Hypodontia

39. Which location is the most likely for an enamel pearl?
a. Maxillary molars
b. Maxillary second premolar
c. Mandibular premolars
d. Mandibular molars

40. Which location is the most likely for a talon cusp?
a. Canines
b. Incisors
c. Molars
d. Premolars

41. Which term refers to an accessory cusp located on the occlusal surface of a tooth?
a. Mulberry cusp
b. Talon cusp
c. Dens invaginatus
d. Dens evaginatus

42. Which term refers to the enamel hypoplasia of a permanent tooth that results from infection of a deciduous tooth?
a. Hutchinson tooth
b. Talon tooth
c. Turner tooth
d. Gorlin tooth

43. Which term refers to the irregular areas of discoloration that result from fluoride ingestion?
a. Pitting defects
b. Developmental defects
c. Mottling defects
d. Extrinsic staining

44. Which term refers to teeth that appear ghostlike on a dental radiograph?
a. Taurodontism
b. Enamel hypocalcification
c. Regional odontodysplasia
d. Enamel hypoplasia

45. Which term refers to teeth that cannot erupt because of physical obstruction?
a. Fused
b. Ankylosed
c. Embedded
d. Impacted

46. All of the following cause endogenous staining of teeth except one. Which one is the exception?
a. Tetracycline
b. Rhesus incompatibility
c. Penicillin
d. Neonatal liver disease

47. Enamel hypoplasia results from damage to the:
a. Odontoblasts
b. Ameloblasts
c. Fibroblasts
d. Cementoblasts

48. Hutchinson incisors and mulberry molars are associated with:
a. Odontodysplasia
b. Congenital syphilis
c. Neonatal liver disease
d. Febrile illnesses

49. Natal teeth are teeth that present:
a. 2 months in utero
b. At birth
c. After 1 month
d. At 6 months

50. When a patient is missing six teeth without including third molars, the condition is specifically termed:
a. Hyperdontia
b. Oligodontia
c. Hypodontia
d. Microdontia

51. A taurodont has which one of the following characteristics?
a. Talon cusp
b. Elongated pulp chambers
c. Long roots
d. Supernumerary roots

52. Fluoride ingestion causing enamel hypoplasia can affect which of the following?
a. Maxillary posterior teeth
b. All teeth
c. One tooth
d. Mandibular incisors

53. Accelerated growth hormone produced by the pituitary before closure of the epiphyseal plates is called:
a. Cretinism
b. Acromegaly
c. Graves disease
d. Gigantism

54. Teeth that do not erupt due to physical obstruction are:
a. Ankylosed
b. Impacted
c. Embedded
d. Fused

55. All of the following cysts within bone are pseudocysts except one. Which one is the exception?
a. Aneurysmal
b. Simple
c. Dentigerous
d. Traumatic

56. The diagnosis of radicular cyst is made by:
a. Radiographic imaging
b. Microscopic examination
c. Pulp testing
d. Clinical report of just pain

57. Dentigerous cysts are most commonly found on which unerupted or impacted tooth?
a. Maxillary canine
b. Distomolar
c. Mandibular third molar
d. Maxillary third molar

Chapter 5 Synopsis

Condition/Disease	Cause	Age/Race/Sex	Location
Ankyloglossia	Developmental	*	Tongue/floor of mouth
Commissural lip pits *Paramedian lip pits*	Developmental	*	Commissures of the lips (corners of the mouth)
Lingual thyroid *Thyroid neoplasm*	Developmental	*	Posterior, dorsal tongue Between foramen caecum and epiglottis
Dentigerous cyst *Ameloblastoma* *Odontogenic keratocyst* *Adenomatoid odontogenic tumor*	Developmental	Young adults	Around the crown of an unerupted, impacted, or developing tooth
Eruption cyst *Dentigerous cyst* *Fistula*	Developmental	Children	Soft tissue around the crown of an erupting tooth
Primordial cyst *Odontogenic keratocyst*	Developmental	Young adults	Develops in place of a tooth Mandibular third-molar area most common site
Odontogenic keratocyst (keratocystic odontogenic tumor) *Ameloblastoma* *Aneursymal bone cyst*	Developmental (dental lamina)	Most common ages, 20–30 yr	Posterior mandible most common site
Lateral periodontal cyst (LPC) and botryoid cyst (BC) *Radicular cyst*	Developmental (dental lamina)	Affects men more than women Median age, 50–60 yr	Lateral aspect of tooth root Mandibular cuspid-premolar area
Gingival cyst *Fistula (parulis)* *Fordyce granules* *Mucocele*	Developmental (dental lamina)	Median age, 50–60 yr	Soft tissue of mandibular cuspid–premolar area

NOTE: Items listed in *italics* under a specific condition/disease should be considered in a differential diagnosis.
N/A, Not applicable.
*Specific information not included in text.

58. The paramedian lip pit occurs:
   a. In the commissure
   b. In the midline area of the lower lip
   c. In the center of the upper lip
   d. On the mucosa of the upper lip

59. Which one of the following cysts in bone is a variant of the lateral periodontal cyst?
   a. Gingival
   b. Botryoid
   c. Odontogenic keratocyst
   d. Primordial

60. Which one of the following is clearly essential for the diagnosis of an odontogenic keratocyst?
   a. Radiographic features
   b. History of the lesion
   c. Degree of clinical expansion
   d. Histopathologic features

Clinical Features	Radiographic Features	Microscopic Features	Treatment	Diagnostic Process
Complete or partial fusion of the lingual frenum of the tongue to the floor of the mouth or lingual gingiva of mandibular incisors	N/A	N/A	Surgical removal of a portion of the lingual frenum	Clinical
Tiny blind tracts are present at the corner of the lips	N/A	N/A	None	Clinical
A mass of tissue at the midline posterior to the circumvallate papillae	N/A	Normal thyroid tissue	Usually none, may be the individual's only functioning thyroid tissue Removal may be indicated if the mass is large	Clinical Laboratory (to identify thyroid tissue)
When larger, can displace teeth	Well-defined unilocular radiolucency	Cyst lined by cuboidal to squamous epithelium	Removal of cyst and associated tooth	Radiographic Microscopic
Swelling at the site of erupting tooth	N/A	Cyst lined by cuboidal to squamous epithelium	Usually none Tooth erupts through cyst	Radiographic Microscopic (erupting tooth)
Asymptomatic	Well-defined radiolucency	Cyst lined by cuboidal to squamous epithelium	Surgical removal of the cyst	Radiographic
When large, may cause buccal expansion	Well-defined, usually multilocular radiolucency	Cyst lined by thin corrugated parakeratotic squamous epithelium 8-10 cell-layers thick Prominent, palisaded basal cell layer with flat interface between the epithelium and connective tissue	Surgical removal of the cyst with peripheral osseous curettage (recurrence high)	Microscopic
Asymptomatic	LPC has unilocular radiolucency BC has multilocular radiolucency	Cyst lined by thin nonkeratinized squamous epithelium with focal thickenings	Surgical removal	Microscopic Radiographic
Bulge or swelling of attached gingiva or interdental papillae	N/A	Cyst lined by thin nonkeratinized squamous epithelium that may have focal thickenings	Surgical removal	Clinical Microscopic

Continued

Chapter 5 Synopsis—cont'd

Condition/Disease	Cause	Age/Race/Sex	Location
Glandular odontogenic cyst	Developmental	Median age, 40–50 yr	Most common in anterior maxilla and posterior mandible
Nasopalatine canal cyst (incisal canal cyst) *Periapical pathosis* *Radicular cyst*	Developmental	Affects men more than women Ages, 40–60 yr	Anterior maxilla Nasopalatine canal Incisive papillae
Median palatine cyst *Pleomorphic adenoma*	Developmental	*	Midline of hard palate posterior to the palatine papilla
Globulomaxillary cyst *Giant cell granuloma* *Radicullar cyst*	Unclear	*	Between maxillary lateral incisor and cuspid
Median mandibular cyst *Traumatic bone cyst*	Unknown	*	Midline of mandible
Nasolabial cyst	Developmental	Ratio of women to men: 4:1 Adult ages, 40–50 yr	Soft tissue of face Nasolabial fold area (maxillary canine, floor of the nose area)
Cervical lymphoepithelial cyst (branchial cleft cyst) and intraoral lymphoepithelial cyst *Lymphangioma* *Oropharyngeal squamous cell carcinoma*	Developmental epithelium (entrapped in lymph node or lymphoid tissue)	*	Lateral neck at the anterior border of the sternocleidomastoid muscle Intraoral: lateral border of the posterior tongue and floor of mouth
Epidermal cyst	Epithelium of hair follicle	*	Skin of the face and neck
Dermoid cyst *Ranula*	Developmental	Present at birth or in young children	Anterior floor of mouth
Thyroglossal tract cyst *Dermoid cyst* *Branchial cyst* *Thyroid neoplasm*	Developmental	Usually diagnosed at 20 yr of age	Along the thyroglossal tract from the foramen cecum to the normal location of the thyroid gland below the hyoid bone
Static bone cyst (Stafne bone defect) *Primordial cyst*	Developmental depression on the lingual aspect of the posterior mandible Can be unilateral or bilateral	Predilection for men	Anterior to angle of ramus Inferior to the mandibular canal

NOTE: Items listed in *italics* under a specific condition/disease should be considered in a differential diagnosis.
N/A, Not applicable.
*Specific information not included in text.

Clinical Features	Radiographic Features	Microscopic Features	Treatment	Diagnostic Process
May cause enlargement of bone	Unilocular or multilocular radiolucency	Microscopic cyst lined by cuboidal-columnar epithelium with microcysts and focal thickenings	Surgical removal	Radiographic Microscopic
Asymptomatic Pink bulge at the incisive papillae area	Well-circumscribed radiolucency between the maxillary central incisors Open heart shaped	Cyst lined by squamous or respiratory epithelium Blood vessels and small nerves in cyst wall	Surgical removal	Radiographic Microscopic
If large, swelling at midline of hard palate	Unilocular radiolucency	Cyst lined by stratified squamous epithelium surrounded by dense fibrous connective tissue	Surgical removal	Radiographic Microscopic
Asymptomatic	Pear-shaped radiolucency	Cyst lining varies from squamous to cuboidal to respiratory epithelium	Surgical removal	Radiographic Microscopic
Asymptomatic If very large, may cause expansion of lingual aspect of mandible	Well-circumscribed radiolucency below the apices of the mandibular incisors	Cyst lined by squamous epithelium	Surgical removal	Radiographic Microscopic
Expansion or swelling in nasolabial fold area or in mucolabial fold area	N/A	Cyst lined by respiratory epithelium (pseudostratified ciliated columnar epithelium with goblet cells)	Surgical removal	Clinical Microscopic
Branchial cyst appears as a bulbous area on the lateral neck Intraoral: pink-yellow well-delineated raised nodule	N/A	Cyst lined by stratified squamous epithelium surrounded by lymphoid tissue	Surgical removal	Microscopic
Localized, firm movable swelling	N/A	Cyst lined by keratinized stratified squamous epithelium Lumen filled with keratin scales	Surgical removal	Microscopic
If large, can displace tongue Doughlike consistency	N/A	Cyst lined by stratified squamous epithelium surrounded by a connective tissue wall Hair follicles and glands seen in cyst wall	Surgical removal	Microscopic
If below the hyoid bone, bulge or swelling in the midline of the neck	N/A	Cyst lined by epithelium Thyroid tissue in connective tissue wall of cyst	Surgical removal Complete excision of cyst and tract	Microscopic
Asymptomatic	Well-circumscribed radiolucency in the mandible below the inferior alveolar canal	Not a true cyst (pseudocyst) Normal salivary gland tissue found within depression	No treatment	Radiographic

Continued

Chapter 5 Synopsis—cont'd

Condition/Disease	Cause	Age/Race/Sex	Location
Simple bone cyst (traumatic bone cyst) *Aneurysmal bone cyst*	Unclear Trauma suggested as possible cause	Age: teenage and young adults	Mandible
Aneurysmal bone cyst *Odontogenic keratocyst* *Ameloblastoma*	Unclear Often associated with other bone lesions	Age: <30 yr Affects women more than men	Posterior maxilla or mandible
Anodontia	Developmental	*	Throughout arches
Hypodontia	Developmental	*	Maxillary third molars Mandibular third molars Maxillary lateral incisors Mandibular second premolars
Supernumerary teeth	Developmental	*	Maxilla > mandible
Mesiodens	Developmental	*	Near/at midline between maxillary central incisors
Distomolar	Developmental	*	Distal to third molars
Microdontia	Developmental	*	Maxillary lateral incisors Peg lateral is the most common Maxillary third molars
Macrodontia	Developmental	*	Any tooth
Gemination	Developmental	*	Primary > permanent Anterior > posterior
Fusion	Developmental	*	Primary > permanent Anterior > posterior Incisors
Concrescence *Hypercementosis*	Developmental	*	Maxillary molars
Dilaceration	Developmental	*	Any tooth
Enamel pearl *Dens evaginatus*	Developmental	*	Maxillary molars (furcation area)

NOTE: Items listed in *italics* under a specific condition/disease should be considered in a differential diagnosis.
N/A, Not applicable.
*Specific information not included in text.

Clinical Features	Radiographic Features	Microscopic Features	Treatment	Diagnostic Process
Usually asymptomatic Occasionally enlargement of bone	Radiolucency Characteristic scalloping around the roots of teeth	Not a true cyst (pseudocyst) Space in bone not lined by epithelium	Surgical intervention	Surgical
Expansion of involved bone	Multilocular radiolucency "Honeycomb" or "soap bubble" appearance	Not a true cyst Blood-filled spaces surrounded by multinucleated giant cells and cellular connective tissue	Surgical removal and supplemental cryotherapy	Microscopic
Absence of all primary or permanent teeth	All teeth absent	N/A	Prosthetic replacement of missing teeth	Clinical Radiographic
Absence of one or more teeth	Absence of one or more teeth	N/A	Prosthetic replacement of missing teeth	Clinical Radiographic
Presence of one or more extra teeth; usually smaller than normal; may be erupted or unerupted	One or more extra teeth	N/A	Extraction may be necessary	Clinical Radiographic
Most common extra tooth; may be erupted or unerupted/impacted Usually appear conical and small	Extra tooth seen at the midline of the anterior maxilla	N/A	Extraction No treatment	Clinical Radiographic
Second most common supernumerary tooth May be erupted (appears small) or impacted	Extra tooth distal to third molar	N/A	No treatment Extraction	Clinical Radiographic
Affected tooth appears smaller than normal One or more teeth may be affected	Tooth smaller than normal	N/A	If erupted, restore to resemble a normal-size tooth	Clinical Radiographic
Affected tooth appears larger than normal One or more teeth may be affected	Tooth larger than normal	N/A	No treatment	Clinical Radiographic
Tooth appears larger than normal Large crown (appears bifid) Normal number of teeth present	Appears as a single tooth with a bifid crown and one common root canal	N/A	If esthetic problems, alteration of tooth to resemble normal-size tooth	Clinical Radiographic
Adjacent teeth are fused together Large crown is seen	Appears as a single large crown with separate or fused roots and root canals	N/A	If esthetic problem, alteration of tooth to resemble normal-size tooth	Clinical Radiographic
Cannot observe clinically	Appears as though the roots of adjacent teeth are connected	N/A	No treatment	Radiographic
Cannot observe clinically	Appears as a sharp bend in a tooth root	N/A	No treatment	Radiographic
Cannot observe clinically	Appears as a small sphere of enamel on a tooth root	N/A	No treatment	Radiographic

Continued

Chapter 5 Synopsis—cont'd

Condition/Disease	Cause	Age/Race/Sex	Location
Talon cusp *Normal cingulum*	Developmental	*	Incisors
Taurodontism	Developmental	*	Molars
Dens in dente (dens invaginatus) *Dens evaginatus* *Periapical pathosis*	Developmental	*	Anterior > posterior Maxillary and mandibular incisors Maxillary lateral incisors
Dens evaginatus *Enamel pearl* *Enameloma*	Developmental	*	Mandibular premolars, molars, cuspids, incisors
Supernumerary roots	Developmental	*	Maxillary and mandibular third molars, mandibular premolars, and cuspids
Enamel hypoplasia *Amelogenesis imperfecta*	Febrile illness or vitamin deficiency during tooth development Local infection or trauma during tooth development Fluoride ingestion during tooth development Congenital syphilis Birth injury, premature birth, idiopathic factors	*	Permanent central and lateral incisors, cuspids, first molars Permanent maxillary incisors and mandibular premolars All permanent teeth Permanent incisors and molars Any teeth
Enamel hypocalcification *Amelogenesis imperfecta*	Trauma to enamel during maturational phase	*	Any teeth
Endogenous staining of teeth *Fever* *Fluorosis* *Syphilis*	Ingestion of tetracycline or systemic disturbance during tooth development	*	Any teeth
Regional odontodysplasia *Complex odontoma*	Developmental	*	Several teeth in the same quadrant Primary or permanent teeth Maxilla > mandible
Impacted teeth *Embedded teeth*	Developmental	*	Maxillary and mandibular third molars Maxillary cuspids
Ankylosed teeth *Embedded teeth*	Developmental	*	Most common: deciduous molars

NOTE: Items listed in *italics* under a specific condition/disease should be considered in a differential diagnosis.

N/A, Not applicable.

*Specific information not included in text.

Clinical Features	Radiographic Features	Microscopic Features	Treatment	Diagnostic Process
Crown appears normal facially An accessory cusp is located in the area of the cingulum	Appears as a tooth with abnormally short roots and low furcation area Pulp chamber is abnormally large	N/A	Removal of cusp and restoration of tooth if cusp interferes with occlusion	Clinical
Cannot observe clinically Crown appears normal	Pulp chamber is enlarged and elongated Roots are short with the furcation near the apices	N/A	No treatment	Radiographic
Tooth may appear normal or peg shaped	Enamel invagination noted with crown of involved tooth	N/A	If tooth is vital, placement of a prophylactic restoration If nonvital, root canal therapy	Clinical Radiographic
Accessory enamel cusp seen on occlusal surface	May see pulp horn extending in accessory cusp	N/A	No treatment	Clinical
Cannot observe clinically	Visible extra root(s)	N/A	No treatment	Radiographic
Crowns have one or more rows of tiny deep pits and stains	N/A	N/A	If necessary, restoration can be placed to improve appearance	Clinical
Crowns have a yellowish-brown color; pitting and enamel deformity may be present	N/A	N/A	If necessary, restoration can be placed to improve appearance	Clinical
Crowns have a mottled discoloration ranging from chalky white spots to brown-black staining	N/A	N/A	Restoration or bleaching can be used to produce a more esthetic appearance	Clinical
Hutchinson incisors are screwdriver shaped	N/A	N/A	Full-coverage crowns	Clinical
Mulberry molars resemble berries	N/A	N/A		Clinical
Crowns may have pitting, grooves, or staining Crowns have chalk-white spots on the middle third	N/A	N/A	If necessary, restoration can be placed to improve appearance	Clinical
With tetracycline staining, crowns appear yellowish-green or brownish-gray	N/A	N/A	If necessary, restoration can be used to improve appearance	Clinical
Affected teeth do not erupt or eruption is incomplete	Reduced radiodensity of involved teeth Teeth appear "ghostlike" with large pulp chambers and thin enamel	*	Extraction	Clinical Radiographic
Teeth do not erupt	Impacted teeth are surrounded by bone	N/A	Surgical removal	Clinical Radiographic
A primary ankylosed tooth prevents the eruption of the permanent tooth	Ankylosed teeth do not exhibit a periodontal ligament space	N/A	Extraction	Clinical Radiographic

6

Genetics

HEDDIE O. SEDANO

OBJECTIVES

After studying this chapter, the student will be able to:

1. Define each of the words in the vocabulary list for this chapter.
2. Define and discuss chromosomes.
3. Do the following related to normal cell division:
   - State the purpose of mitosis.
   - Explain the four stages of mitosis.
   - State the purpose of meiosis.
   - Explain the two steps of meiosis.
4. Explain what is meant by the Lyon hypothesis and give an example of its clinical significance.
5. Discuss the molecular composition of chromosomes, including deoxyribonucleic acid and ribonucleic acid.
6. Explain the two types of chromosomal abnormalities, as well as what is meant by a gross chromosomal abnormality, and give three examples of syndromes that result from gross chromosomal abnormalities.
7. Do the following related to patterns of inheritance:
   - List the four inheritance patterns described in this chapter.
   - Explain what is meant by X-linked inheritance.
8. State the inheritance pattern and describe the oral manifestations and, if appropriate, the characteristic facies for each of the following inherited disorders that affect the gingiva and periodontium: cyclic neutropenia, chronic neutropenia, Papillon-Lefèvre syndrome, focal palmoplantar and gingival hyperkeratosis, gingival fibromatosis, and Laband syndrome.
9. State the inheritance pattern and describe the oral manifestations and, if appropriate, the characteristic facies for each of the following inherited disorders affecting the jawbones and facies: cherubism, Ellis–van Creveld syndrome (chondroectodermal dysplasia), cleidocranial dysplasia, Gardner syndrome, mandibulofacial dysostosis (Treacher Collins syndrome), nevoid basal cell carcinoma syndrome, osteogenesis imperfecta, torus mandibularis, torus palatinus, and maxillary exostosis.
10. State the inheritance pattern and describe the oral manifestations and, if appropriate, the characteristic facies for each of the following inherited disorders affecting the oral mucosa: cleft lip and palate, hereditary hemorrhagic telangiectasia (Osler-Rendu–Parkes Weber syndrome), multiple mucosal neuroma syndrome, pheochromocytoma, neurofibromatosis of von Recklinghausen, Peutz-Jeghers syndrome, and white sponge nevus (Cannon disease).
11. State the inheritance pattern and describe the oral manifestations and, if appropriate, the characteristic facies for each of the following inherited disorders affecting the teeth: amelogenesis imperfecta, dentinogenesis imperfecta, dentin dysplasia, hypohidrotic ectodermal dysplasia, hypophosphatasia, hypophosphatemic vitamin D–resistant rickets, pegged or absent maxillary lateral incisors, and taurodontism.

❖ Vocabulary

Alleles (ə-lēlz′) Genes that are located at the same level or locus in the two chromosomes of a pair and that determine the same functions or characteristics.

Amino acid (ə-me′no as′id) An organic compound containing an amino group NH2; amino acids are the main component of proteins.

Autosomes (aw′to-sōmz) (adjective, autosomal) Nonsex chromosomes, which are identical for men and women.

Barr body (bahr bod′e) Condensed chromatin of the inactivated X chromosome, which is found at the periphery of the nucleus of cells in women.

Carrier (kar′e-ər) In genetics, a heterozygous individual who is clinically normal but who can transmit a recessive trait or characteristic; also, a person who is homozygous for an autosomal-dominant condition with low penetrance.

Centromere (sen′tro-mēr) The constricted portion of the chromosome that divides the short arms from the long arms.

Chromatid (kro′mə-tid) Either of the two vertical halves of a chromosome that are joined at the centromere.

Chromatin (kro′mə-tin) A general term used to refer to the material (deoxyribonucleic acid [DNA]) that forms the chromosomes.

Chromosome (kro′mo-sōm) Structures located in the nucleus of cells and on which genes are found.

Codon (ko′don) The sequence of three bases in DNA that encodes an amino acid.

Coloboma (kälə'bōmə) A congenital defect of the eye; notch on the outer area of the lower lid.

Consanguinity (kon″san-gwin′ĭ-te) Blood relationship; in genetics the term is generally used to describe a mating or marriage between close relatives.

Deoxyribonucleic acid (de-ok″se-ri″bo-noo-kle′ik as′id) DNA; a substance composed of a double chain of polynucleotides, with both chains coiled around a central axis to form a double helix; it is the basic genetic code or template for amino acid formation.

Diploid (dip′loid) Having two sets of chromosomes; the normal constitution of somatic cells.

Dominant (dom′ĭ-nənt) In genetics, a trait or characteristic that is manifested when it is carried by only one of a pair of homologous chromosomes.

Expressivity (ek″sprĕ-siv′ĭ-te) The degree of clinical manifestation of a trait or characteristic.

Facies (fa′she-ēz) The appearance of the face.

Gamete (gam′ēt) Spermatozoon or ovum.

Gene (jēn) Hereditary units, transmitted from one generation to another, that are made up of a sequence of nucleotides and located on a chromosome.

Genetic heterogeneity (jə-net′ik het″ər-o-jə-ne′ĭ-te) Having more than one inheritance pattern.

Haploid (hap′loid) Having a single set of chromosomes; a gamete is haploid.

Heterozygote (het″ər-o-zi′gōt) (adjective, heterozygous) An individual with two different genes at the allele loci.

Homozygote (ho″mo-zi′gōt) (adjective, homozygous) An individual with identical genes at the allele loci.

Hypertelorism (hi″pər-te′lor-iz-əm) A condition in which there is greater-than-normal distance between two paired organs; ocular hypertelorism, a condition marked by a greater-than-normal distance between the eyes.

Hypodontia (hi″po-don′shə) A developmental condition marked by fewer than normal teeth; also called *partial anodontia.*

Hypohidrosis (hi′po-hi-dro′sis) Abnormally diminished secretion of sweat.

Hypotrichosis (hi′po-trĭ-ko′sis) The presence of less than the normal amount of hair.

Hypoplastic (hi″po-plas′tik) Underdeveloped.

Karyotype (kar′e-o-tīp) A photomicrographic representation of a person's chromosomal constitution arranged according to the Denver classification.

Locus (lo′kəs) (plural, loci) The position occupied by a gene on a chromosome.

Meiosis (mi-o′sis) Two-step cellular division of the original germ cells, which reduces the chromosomes from 4n DNA to 1n DNA.

Metaphase (met′ə-faz) Phase of cellular division in which the chromosomes are lined up evenly along the equatorial plane of the cell and in which they are most visible.

Mitochondria (mi″to-kon′dre-ə) Cytoplasmic organelles that have their own DNA in a circular chromosome.

Mitochondrial DNA (mi″to-kon′dre-əl DNA) Unique DNA that is maternally inherited.

Mitosis (mi-to′sis) Way in which somatic cells divide so that the two daughter cells receive the same number of identical chromosomes.

Multifactorial inheritance (mul″tĭ-fak-tor′e-əl in-her′ĭ-təns) The type of hereditary pattern seen when there is more than one genetic factor involved and, sometimes, when there are also environmental factors participating in the causation of a condition.

Mutation (mu-ta′shən) A permanent change in the arrangement of genetic material.

Nondisjunction (non-disjungk′chən) In genetics, when chromosomes that are crossing over do not separate; therefore both migrate to the same cell.

Oligodontia (ol″ĭ-go-don′she-ə) A condition in which more than six teeth are developmentally absent.

Oogenesis (o″o-jen′ə-sis) The process of formation of female germ cells (ova).

Ovum (o′vəm) (plural, ova) Egg; mature feminine germ cell.

Penetrance (pen′ə-trəns) The frequency with which a heritable trait is exhibited by individuals carrying the gene or genes that determine that trait.

Phenotype (fe′noh-tīp) The entire physical, biochemical, and physiologic makeup of an individual; genotype is the genetic composition, and phenotype is its observable appearance.

Pseudoanodontia (soo″do-an ədon′she-ə) A condition in which the teeth develop but do not erupt.

Recessive (re-ses′iv) A trait or characteristic that shows clinically when a double-gene dose (homozygosity) exists in autosomal chromosomes or a single-gene dose exists in males if the trait is X-linked.

Ribonucleic acid (ri″bo-noo-kle′ik as′id) RNA; single strands of polynucleotides found in all cells; different types of RNA have different functions in the production of proteins by the cell.

Ribosome (ri′bo-sōm) Cytoplasmic organelles in which proteins are formed on the basis of the genetic code provided by RNA.

Spermatogenesis (sper″mə-to-jen′ə-sis) The process of formation of spermatozoa (sperm).

Spermatozoon (sper″mə-to-zo′on) (plural, spermatozoa) A mature male germ cell.

Syndrome (sin′drōm) A set of signs or symptoms (or both) occurring together.

Taurodontism (taw″ro-don′tizm) A genetic, heterogeneous condition of molar teeth with dominant and recessive inheritance patterns characterized by an enlarged pulp chamber, apical displacement of the pulpal floor, and no constriction at the level of the cemento-enamel junction.

Translocation (trans″lo-ka′shən) The portion of a chromosome attached to another chromosome.

Trisomy (tri′so-me) A pair of chromosomes with an identical extra chromosome.

G enetics is the science that studies inheritance and the expression of inherited traits. The main objectives of this chapter are to introduce some of the basic concepts of genetics and present the clinical manifestations of some inherited oral disorders of interest to the dental hygienist. The descriptions of many syndromes are included. As explained in previous chapters, a **syndrome** is a distinctive association of signs and symptoms occurring together in the same patient. The syndromes included in this chapter are inherited. However, other syndromes such as acquired immunodeficiency syndrome (AIDS) are acquired, not inherited. In addition, the fact that an alteration is found as part of a syndrome does not mean that it cannot also occur independently. For example, cleft lip and palate occur as components of several syndromes and can also occur independently. The classification of syndromes is difficult because they are composed of several associated anomalies and the anomalies that compose the syndrome may not be present consistently in all patients with the same syndrome.

The term **phenotype** is used often in this chapter. It refers to the physical, biochemical, and physiologic traits of an individual. A phenotype can occur as a result of genetic factors or from a combination of genetic factors and environmental influences.

In this chapter, as in previous chapters, basic concepts are discussed first. These concepts are followed by descriptions of specific inherited disorders.

Chromosomes

The hereditary units that are transmitted from one generation to another are called **genes.** They are found on **chromosomes,** which are located in the nucleus of the cell. Using a microscope, one can see chromosomes clearly only when the nucleus and cell are dividing (Fig. 6.1). At other times the genetic material is dispersed in the nucleus (see Fig. 6.1). Each cell of the human body, with the exception of mature germ cells (ova and spermatozoa), has 46 chromosomes. Half of these chromosomes are derived from the father, and the other half from the mother.

Chromosomes contain deoxyribonucleic acid (DNA), which directs the production of **amino acids,** polypeptides, and proteins by the cell. In addition, DNA has the ability to duplicate itself (self-replication). It creates exact copies of itself, and through the process of cell division cells identical to the original cell are formed.

Normal Cell Division

Mitosis

All cells in the body, with the exception of ova and spermatozoa, are called **somatic cells.** Cellular division is achieved by **mitosis** during a part of the life span of the somatic cell, called the **mitotic cycle.** The function of mitosis is to create an exact copy of each chromosome and, through division of the original cell, distribute an identical set of chromosomes to each daughter cell. After each cell division is completed and before the next division can occur, the cell enters the **gap 1 (G₁) phase,** which is followed by the **S phase,** in which replication of the DNA takes place. The **gap 2 (G₂) phase** follows the S phase and ends when mitotic division begins. The cell cycle is illustrated in Fig. 6.2.

Stages of Mitosis

Mitosis is composed of four stages: (1) prophase, (2) metaphase, (3) anaphase, and (4) telophase. In each of these four stages, the chromosomes are distributed in a specific arrangement. In **metaphase** the chromosomes stain intensely and are arranged almost symmetrically at both sides of the center, or equatorial plane, of the cell. The appearance of a metaphase chromosome resembles the letter *X* (Fig. 6.3), having a pair of "long arms" also known as *q arms* (see Fig. 6.3, *3*) and a pair of "short arms" also known as *p arms* (see Fig. 6.3, *1*). The size of the chromosome at metaphase and the length of the long and short arms vary from chromosome to chromosome. The constriction present in all chromosomes, which joins the short and long arms, is called the **centromere** (see Fig. 6.3, *2*). During metaphase chromosomes are actually formed by two identical vertical halves, each composed of either left or right short and long arms and half of the centromere. Each of

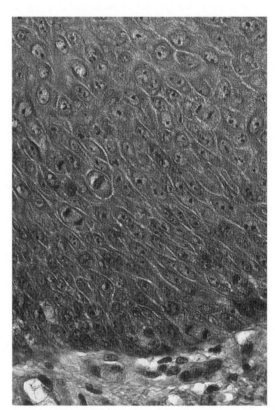

• **Figure 6.1** High-power photomicrograph shows several dividing cells with visible chromosomes and also nuclei of cells with scattered chromatin.

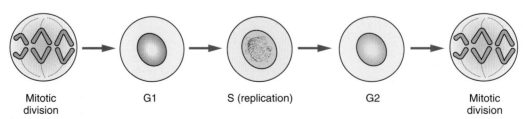

Mitotic division   G1   S (replication)   G2   Mitotic division

• **Figure 6.2** Schematic representation of the mitotic cycle shows the end of mitosis, followed by the G1, S, and G2 phases and the next mitosis.

these identical halves is called a **chromatid** (see Fig. 6.3, *4*). At metaphase each chromatid contains one molecule of DNA; therefore the DNA content of each chromosome is doubled (Fig. 6.4). When cell division takes place, each chromosome splits vertically at the centromere; 46 chromatids (which now become chromosomes) form one daughter cell, and the other 46 chromatids form a second daughter cell. During prophase the chromosomes are lining up toward metaphase; in anaphase and telophase the chromatids are in the process of splitting.

Meiosis

Primitive germ cells (oogonia, spermatogonia) have 46 chromosomes. Mature germ cells (ova, spermatozoa) have 23 chromosomes. **Meiosis** is a two-step special type of cell division in which the primitive germ cells reduce their chromosome number by half and become mature germ cells. The primitive germ cells have two chromosomes for each pair and are called **diploid.** The suffix *-ploid* refers to the number of sets of chromosomes, and its prefix

refers to the degree of ploidy. In diploid *di-* indicates two. The mature germ cells (or **gametes**) have half the number of chromosomes and are called **haploid.** During the period in which the cell is not in division, the DNA content of diploid cells is designated 2n DNA; in metaphase it is double, or 4n DNA. After the two stages of meiosis have been completed, the 4n DNA is reduced to 1n DNA. The two steps are called **first meiosis** and **second meiosis.** This reduction is necessary to maintain the normal number of human chromosomes. A new embryo must have 46 chromosomes per cell, as did its parents. Therefore the union of germ cells needs to result in 46 chromosomes. If two cells with 46 chromosomes were combined, the resulting cell would have 92 chromosomes.

First Meiosis

Before the first meiosis in the primitive germ cells, a replication of DNA occurs that is similar to that observed in the S phase of somatic cells. After replication the members of each pair of chromosomes line up next to each other in an intimate point-by-point relationship (Fig. 6.5A). This pairing does not occur in mitosis. After pairing, the two chromosomes establish actual contact at different locations. These contacts are known as **chiasmata** (meaning X shaped) and determine points of crossing over (Fig. 6.5B). This crossing over achieves the exchange of

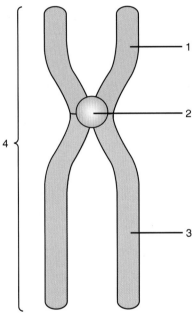

• **Figure 6.3** Autosomal chromosome at metaphase shows *(1)* short arm, *(2)* centromere, *(3)* long arm, and *(4)* chromatid.

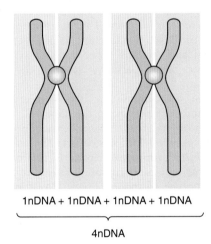

1nDNA + 1nDNA + 1nDNA + 1nDNA

4nDNA

• **Figure 6.4** Pair of autosomal chromosomes at metaphase. Each chromatid represents 1n DNA.

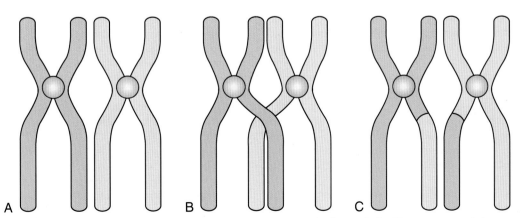

• **Figure 6.5** Homologous autosomal chromosomes line up in first meiosis **(A)**, cross over during metaphase of first meiosis **(B)**, and exchange segments after crossing over **(C)**.

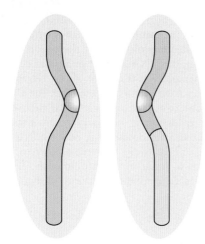

• **Figure 6.6** Two haploid cells after second meiosis, each having 1n DNA.

chromosome segments between a chromatid of one chromosome and a chromatid of the other chromosome of a pair (between homologous chromosomes) (Fig. 6.5C). This special aspect of the first meiosis takes place at metaphase. After metaphase of the first meiotic division, the chromosomes separate from each other, but no splitting of the centromere occurs. The chromosomes remain intact, and each member of the pair migrates to one of the new cells, each of which contains 23 chromosomes but twice the final amount of DNA. During this migration chromosomes of the paternal and maternal lines segregate at random, thus ensuring diversity of the species by creating a new combination of chromosomes.

On occasion, the chromosomes that were crossing over do not separate, and both migrate to the same cell. This is known as **nondisjunction** and results in the formation of a germ cell with an extra chromosome. If this occurs and that cell (either an **ovum** or a **spermatozoon**) participates in the formation of an embryo, three chromosomes (**trisomy**) instead of two result. An example of this type of abnormality is **Down syndrome,** also called **trisomy 21,** in which three of chromosome 21 are found instead of two. Trisomy has been reported for several different chromosomes.

In a female embryo **oogenesis** (ovum development) starts around the third month of prenatal life, and the future ova remain suspended, crossing over from about the time of birth until the time ovulation starts. At the beginning of ovulation the first meiosis is completed. Nondisjunction is more prevalent in female oogenesis than in male **spermatogenesis.** This is probably because of the period of prolonged crossing over; therefore the older the woman, the greater the chance of shedding a trisomic ovum and of bearing a child with Down syndrome or other trisomy.

Second Meiosis

The second stage of meiosis is essentially a mitotic division in which each chromosome splits longitudinally. No replication of DNA occurs before the second meiosis. After the splitting, two cells are formed, each containing the right amount of DNA (1n DNA) (Fig. 6.6).

Nondisjunction can occur during the first and second meiosis. If it occurs in second meiosis, a chromosome does not split, and one daughter cell has a full chromosome, and the other has none.

Immediately after fertilization, the chromosomes of the ovum and spermatozoon, each having 1n DNA, condense independently and form round structures, each known as a *pronucleus.* The DNA in these pronuclei replicates, forming a set of 23 full chromosomes for each, the maternal and paternal pronuclei. When the membranes of these pronuclei break, the 46 chromosomes mix at random, initiating the first cellular division (mitosis) that starts the development of the new embryo.

Lyon Hypothesis

The sex chromosomes are designated XX in women and XY in men. During the early period of embryonic development (possibly by the end of the second week), the genetic activity of one of the X chromosomes in each cell of a female embryo is inactivated. The inactivation is a random process affecting either the X chromosome derived from the mother or the X chromosome derived from the father. Activated chromosomes are dispersed in the nucleus. The inactivated chromosome remains contracted when the cell is not dividing and forms a structure known as the **Barr body.**

Barr bodies are only seen in female cells. The Barr body can be seen easily under the light microscope, especially in cytologic smears, including those obtained from the oral mucosa. The Barr body appears as a dark dot at the periphery of the nucleus (Fig. 6.7).

This inactivation of one of the X chromosomes in a female embryo was postulated by Mary Lyon and is known as the **Lyon hypothesis.** This hypothesis has interesting clinical implications for female **carriers** of conditions caused by genes located on the X chromosome, which are explained later in this chapter.

Molecular Composition of Chromosomes

Deoxyribonucleic Acid

Chromosomes contain **deoxyribonucleic acid (DNA).** DNA contains the basic code or template that carries all genetic information. The basic unit of DNA is called a **nucleotide,** which is formed by a nitrogen-containing base, a five-carbon sugar (deoxyribose), and a phosphate. Four bases are found in DNA: adenine (A), guanine (G), thymine (T), and cytosine (C). These chains of polynucleotides are coiled to form a structure called a **double helix** (Fig. 6.8). In DNA the base adenine is always bound to the base thymine, and guanine is always bound to cytosine. This is a consistent arrangement and is identical in all species from bacteria to humans, with just a few exceptions. Therefore the ratio of adenine to thymine (A/T) is always equal, and the same is true for the ratio of guanine to cytosine (G/C). In humans G/C pairs are about four times more frequent than A/T pairs. In Fig. 6.8, the polynucleotide chains run vertically in opposite directions. Therefore a sequence of adenine, guanine, and cytosine (AGC) is always matched by the opposing sequence of thymine, cytosine, and guanine (TCG).

In Fig. 6.8, the horizontal steps of the polynucleotide chains are nucleotides. Each pair of nucleotides is joined by a hydrogen bond, indicated by the dotted lines This arrangement is repeated horizontally to form the polynucleotide double spiral staircase (or helix) appearance of DNA (see Fig. 6.8).

Each sequence of three bases is called a **codon.** It encodes an amino acid. Several amino acids form a polypeptide, and one or

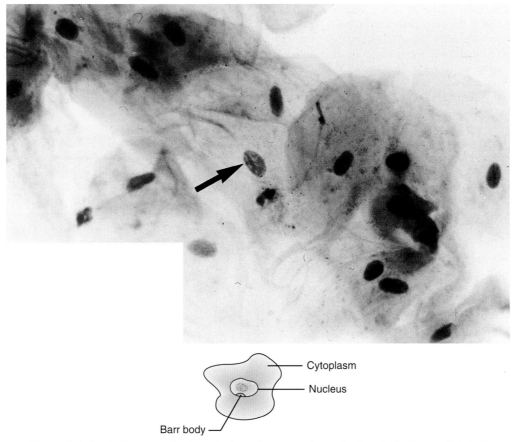

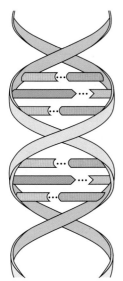

• **Figure 6.7** Cytologic preparation from the buccal mucosa shows the Barr body (the small dark dot on the nuclear membrane [*arrow*]) at the periphery of the nucleus of a desquamated epithelial cell from a woman's buccal mucosa. (Courtesy Dr. Carl J. Witkop.)

• **Figure 6.8** Schematic representation of the DNA double helix.

more polypeptides form a protein. A gene is often equated with the unit that forms a polypeptide.

DNA has the unique capability of self-replication, which is achieved by unwinding its double chain like the plaits of a braid. Each separated chain serves as a blueprint for another chain.

Mitochondrial DNA is found in the circular chromosome of the **mitochondria,** and it is maternally inherited. This is the DNA present in the cytoplasmic mitochondrial organelles of the ovum. Mitochondrial DNA is passed from the mother to all her offspring, regardless of sex.

Ribonucleic Acid

To produce amino acids, polypeptides, and proteins, the genetic code contained in the DNA is transcribed into **ribonucleic acid (RNA),** which differs from DNA in that it is a single strand (in its simplest form), its sugar is a ribose (the sugar in DNA is deoxyribose), and the base uracil (U) replaces the thymine (T) in DNA.

Types of Ribonucleic Acid

The four types of RNA are (1) messenger RNA (mRNA), (2) transfer RNA (tRNA), (3) ribosomal RNA (rRNA), and (4) heterogeneous nuclear RNA (hnRNA). RNA can be found in both the nucleus and the cytoplasm of a cell.

The first type of RNA, **mRNA,** is a blueprint of the genetic DNA for the coding of proteins. It carries the message for the DNA to **ribosomes** in the cytoplasm, in which proteins are produced. The second type of RNA, **tRNA,** transfers amino acids from the cytoplasm to the mRNA, positioning amino acids in the proper sequence to form polypeptides and hence proteins. The third type of RNA, **rRNA,** combines with several polypeptides to form ribosomes. The fourth type of RNA, **hnRNA,** is found within the nucleus and is the precursor of mRNA.

In the production of a protein (Fig. 6.9) the mRNA carries the genetic code for the formation of that protein to the ribosomes. The tRNA brings amino acids to the ribosomes from the cellular cytoplasm. The amino acid sequence forms proteins according to the genetic code, and these proteins exit the ribosomes as they are formed.

Genes and Chromosomes

Genes in a chromosome are located in a linear manner. The genes in both members of a pair of chromosomes (homologous chromosomes) govern the same functions or dictate the same characteristics. The genes that are located at the same level (or **locus**) in homologous chromosomes and that dictate the same functions or characteristics are called **alleles.**

The manifestations (phenotype) of a gene action are not necessarily the same from one individual to another. This is best explained with the ABO blood group system. The locus can be occupied by either the factor that determines the blood group A

or the factor that determines the blood group B. If it is empty, it results in the blood group O. The locus is always the same, and the three genes govern the same function; however, the clinical result is different. In this situation the trait or condition is said to have multiple alleles. For example, if both loci are AA or if they are AO, the person is said to have blood group A. If both loci are BB or BO, the person is said to have blood group B. If the loci are AB or BA, the person is said to have blood group AB. Only if both the loci are empty does the person have blood group O. The locus always controls the blood group, but the group depends on the alleles that are either present or lacking in each person.

When the allelic genes are identical, the person is said to be homozygous for that gene, or a **homozygote.** Using the ABO blood group system again as an example, a person with AA, BB, or OO would be homozygous. When the genes are different (e.g., AB, AO, or BO), the person is said to be heterozygous for that gene, or a **heterozygote.** If a gene can express its effect clinically with a single dose (heterozygous), as in the combination AO = blood group A, the characteristic is said to be **dominant.** If the gene needs a double dose to exhibit its action (homozygous), the resulting characteristic or function is said to be **recessive.** For example, only the combination OO results in the blood group O.

Chromosomal Abnormalities

Abnormalities of chromosomes can be divided into two categories: (1) molecular abnormalities and (2) gross abnormalities. Molecular alterations occur at the DNA level and are not detectable microscopically. Most inherited disorders represent examples of molecular changes (**mutations**) at the level of one or both allelic genes. Examples of these conditions are presented later in this chapter.

Gross chromosomal alterations can be observed in a karyotype. A **karyotype** (Figs. 6.10 and 6.11) is a photographic

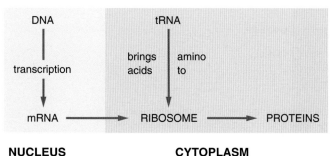

• **Figure 6.9** Production (synthesis) of protein from DNA.

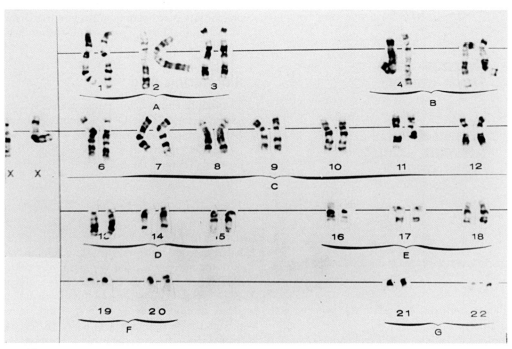

• **Figure 6.10** Karyotype from a female shows the 22 pairs of autosomal chromosomes and the pair of X chromosomes. (Courtesy Dr. Jaroslav Cervenka.)

representation of a person's chromosomal constitution. Clinicians can create a karyotype by culturing cells from blood, skin, or other tissues. One method uses peripheral blood by placing it in a test tube with heparin to avoid coagulation and centrifuging it. After centrifugation the white blood cells (leukocytes) are deposited at the bottom of the tube. The leukocytes are removed and placed in a culture medium containing phytohemagglutinin, which is a substance that enhances mitosis. Because chromosomes are best observed when cell division is arrested at metaphase, colchicine is added to the culture after 72 hours of culture at 37°C to stop mitosis at metaphase. This also prevents the centromere from dividing. A hypotonic solution is then added to the culture to make the cells swell. The cells are then fixed (preserved) and stained and observed under the microscope. Examples of well-defined mitoses are chosen and photographed. The photograph is enlarged, and each chromosome is cut out of the photographic print. When stained, the chromosomes have a bandlike appearance that allows an accurate identification of each. These cutouts are then pasted on a special chart to construct the karyotype.

Gross Chromosomal Abnormalities

Alterations in Number and Structure of Chromosomes

Gross chromosomal abnormalities are caused by either alterations in chromosome number, which are almost always a result of nondisjunction (explained earlier), or alterations in structure, which develop because of chromosomal breaks or abnormal rearrangements. The following illustrate alterations in number:

- **Euploid:** A complete second set of chromosomes, the total number being 92. This is incompatible with life.
- **Polyploid:** Three (triploid) or four (tetraploid) complete sets of chromosomes. This has been described occasionally in humans and is incompatible with life.

- **Aneuploid:** Any extra number of chromosomes that do not represent an exact multiple of the total chromosome complement (e.g., trisomy [a pair with an identical extra chromosome] and monosomy [a missing chromosome from a pair]).

Examples of structural abnormalities include the following:

- **Deletion:** The loss of part of a chromosome.
- **Translocation:** A portion of a chromosome is attached to another chromosome.
- **Inversion:** A portion of a chromosome is upside-down.
- **Duplication:** A chromosome is larger than normal; the extra segment is identical to a segment of the normal chromosome.

Clinical Syndromes Resulting From Gross Chromosomal Abnormalities

Trisomy 21

Trisomy 21, also known as **Down syndrome,** is the most frequent of the trisomies. Ninety-five percent of cases of Down syndrome are the result of nondisjunction, mostly associated with late maternal age at the time of conception.

Slanted eyes characterize the **facies** (the appearance of the face). Patients are generally shorter than normal, and heart abnormalities are present in more than 30% of individuals with trisomy 21. The intelligence level varies from near normal to markedly low.

Fissured tongue (see Fig. 1.19) is frequently present in patients with trisomy 21, and macroglossia may also be seen (Fig. 6.12). Premature loss of teeth, especially the mandibular central incisors, caused by alveolar bone loss is seen frequently. Gingival and periodontal disease has been reported in 90% of affected individuals. **Hypodontia** (fewer teeth than normal), abnormally shaped teeth, and anomalies in eruption with malposition and crowding of teeth are common findings. Dental hygienists play an important role in the maintenance of oral health in these patients.

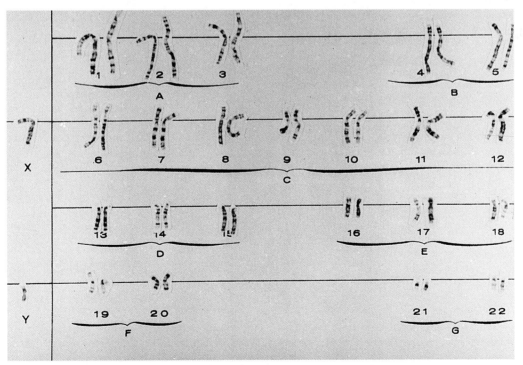

• **Figure 6.11** Karyotype from a male shows the 22 pairs of autosomal chromosomes and the X and Y chromosomes. (Courtesy Dr. Jaroslav Cervenka.)

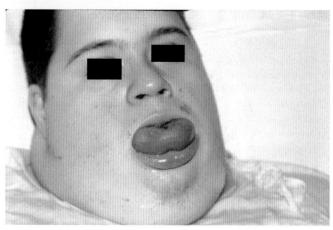

• **Figure 6.12** Macroglossia in a patient with Down Syndrome. (Courtesy Dr. Sanford Fenton).

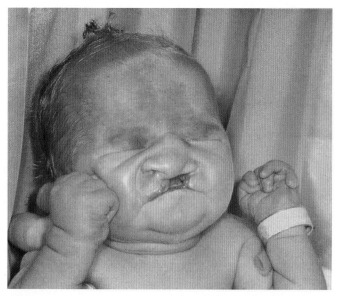

• **Figure 6.13** Newborn with Trisomy 13. Cleft lip, frontal hemangioma, and abnormal position of fingers should be noted.

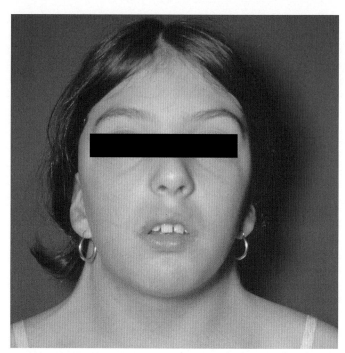

• **Figure 6.14** Patient with Turner Syndrome. Note the webbing of the neck.

Trisomy 13

Trisomy 13 is characterized by multiple abnormalities in various organs. Seventy percent of live-born infants die within the first 7 months of life. Characteristic clinical findings include bilateral cleft lip and palate, microphthalmia (small eyes) or anophthalmia (no eyes), superficial hemangioma of the forehead or nape of the neck, growth retardation, severe mental handicap, polydactyly of hands and feet (supernumerary digits), clenching of the fist with the thumb under the fingers, rocker-bottom feet, heart malformations, and several anomalies of the external genitals. The facial appearance is quite striking because of the cleft lip, cleft palate, and ocular abnormalities (Fig. 6.13).

Turner Syndrome

Patients with Turner syndrome have a female phenotype, and in the majority of cases the karyotype has the normal 44 autosomal chromosomes and only one X chromosome. A normal female would have two X chromosomes: one from the mother and one from the father. Most cases of Turner syndrome are the result of

nondisjunction of the X chromosome in the paternal gamete. Clinically, these women are of short stature and have webbing of the neck and edema of the hands and feet (Fig. 6.14). They frequently exhibit a low hairline on the nape of the neck. The chest is broad with wide-spaced nipples. The aorta frequently is abnormal, and body hair is sparse. The external genitals appear infantile, and generally the ovaries are not developed; therefore these individuals have primary amenorrhea (abnormal temporary or permanent cessation of the menstrual cycle). Smears taken from the oral mucosa demonstrate the lack of Barr bodies.

Klinefelter Syndrome

Klinefelter syndrome occurs when an ovum carrying two X chromosomes is fertilized by a spermatozoon with a Y chromosome; therefore the fertilized ovum will have two X chromosomes plus a Y chromosome. The majority of cases result from nondisjunction of the X chromosome, generally in the ova of older women. Affected individuals have a male phenotype, and the condition cannot be detected clinically until after puberty. These patients are taller than normal and have wide hips and female pubic hair distribution. About 50% have gynecomastia (development of female breasts), and intelligence levels are lower than normal in 10% of affected individuals. The penis appears normal, but the testes are smaller and harder than normal and lack seminiferous tubules.

The maxilla is slightly **hypoplastic** (underdeveloped). Buccal smears reveal the presence of one Barr body.

Variations of Klinefelter syndrome also occur; they are represented by karyotypes containing XXXY or XXXXY. The greater the number of X chromosomes, the more pronounced the clinical manifestations and the lower the level of intelligence. The maxilla becomes increasingly hypoplastic with increasing number of X chromosomes. Buccal smears show one Barr body for each extra X chromosome.

Cri du Chat (Cat Cry) Syndrome and Wolf-Hirschhorn Syndrome

Cri du chat (cat cry) syndrome and Wolf-Hirschhorn syndrome are examples of abnormalities caused by deletions. The cri du chat syndrome results from a deletion on the short arm of chromosome 5, and the Wolf-Hirschhorn syndrome results from a deletion on the short arm of chromosome 4. Newborns with a chromosome 5 deletion exhibit a catlike cry at birth and are mentally retarded. No oral abnormalities occur. Most newborns with the deletion in the short arm of chromosome 4 have a cleft palate and intelligence quotients of less than 30.

Patterns of Inheritance

Because loci are present in both **autosomal** and X chromosomes and because of a double- and single-dose effect, four possible inheritance patterns exist. Dominant genes need only a single dose, and recessive genes need a double dose. The inheritance patterns are autosomal dominant, autosomal recessive, X-linked dominant, and X-linked recessive. Autosomal chromosomes include all chromosomes except those that determine sex (X and Y). The Y chromosome participates only in the differentiation of the masculine gonads.

Autosomal-Dominant Inheritance

A condition with autosomal-dominant inheritance is transmitted vertically from one generation to the next. Males and females are equally affected. When a person has a gene for the condition, the risk of having an affected offspring is 50% for each pregnancy. Genetic risk is always a mathematical estimate of probability governed by chance. Therefore none, less than half, half, more than half, or all of the offspring could be affected by a condition that is transmitted by autosomal-dominant inheritance.

An individual can carry a gene with a dominant effect without presenting any clinical manifestations. This is referred to as **lack of penetrance.** This situation can be explained partially by the presence of modifying genes in the same or other chromosomes. The clinical manifestations in autosomal-dominant disorders frequently vary among affected individuals. This is known as *variable expressivity*. **Penetrance** refers to the number of individuals affected, and **expressivity** pertains to the degree to which an individual is affected.

Autosomal-Recessive Inheritance

As stated previously, individuals exhibiting an autosomal-recessive trait must be homozygous for the gene. Clinically normal parents of affected children are heterozygous, and both are carriers of the trait. They are not generally recognized as carriers until after the birth of an affected child. If the enzymatic defect is known, carriers can be recognized before the birth of a child by assessing levels of the responsible enzyme in clinically normal members of a family with the trait. For parents who are carriers of the same recessive trait, the risk of having an affected child is 25%, the risk of having a homozygous normal child is 25%, and the chance of having a heterozygous carrier is 50% for each pregnancy. As in other inheritance patterns, risk is a mathematical estimate of the probability of an event occurring. If both parents are homozygous (have two of the genes of the trait) for a recessive trait, they would be expected to be affected, and all their children would be affected equally because they would also be homozygous (have two of the same genes) for the trait. In humans this type of situation is quite rare because individuals affected by the same recessive trait usually do not mate.

In genetics **consanguinity** means a familial relationship and is generally used to describe matings or marriages between close relatives, usually including first cousins. In the United States marriage or mating between very close relatives (parent-offspring, brother-sister, uncle-niece, aunt-nephew) is illegal, and in most states marriage of first cousins is also illegal. However, consanguineous matings occur sporadically. The chance of having deleterious genes in common increases between close relatives. When consanguinity exists between the members of a family, the chance of the offspring being homozygous for a deleterious gene increases. The closer the degree of consanguinity, the greater the risk.

X-Linked Inheritance

Women have two X chromosomes and therefore can be either heterozygous or homozygous for a gene that is located on the X chromosome. Thus in women X-linked traits can be dominant or recessive. Men have only one X and one Y chromosome. If a deleterious gene occurs on the X chromosome in a male, the condition or trait will be seen clinically, regardless of the dominant or recessive behavior of the same gene in women. The man's X chromosome is transmitted to all of his daughters and to none of his sons. The X chromosome in his sons comes from the mother. Consequently no male-to-male (from father to son) transmission of X-linked traits occurs. Some X-linked dominant traits are lethal in males. Females probably survive because of the action of the allelic normal gene on the second X chromosome. All offspring, male and female, of a woman homozygous for a dominant X-linked condition will be affected with the condition. This is because all of her X chromosomes contain that gene (and all offspring receive an X chromosome). Because the gene is dominant, only one of the genes is necessary for that condition to occur. A mother who is a carrier of an X-linked recessive trait has a 50% risk of having an affected son and a 50% risk of having a carrier daughter. This is because both daughters and sons have a 50% risk of getting the X chromosome with the gene for that condition. Again, the reader should remember that risk is a mathematical prediction. A male affected with an X-linked trait will have no affected sons because he does not give the X chromosome to his sons. All of his daughters will be either carriers or affected, depending on the recessive or dominant nature of the trait, because all daughters will receive his X chromosome.

Lyon Hypothesis and X-Linked Recessive Traits

As discussed previously, according to the Lyon hypothesis, one of the X chromosomes in the female is genetically cancelled at an early stage of embryonic development. This cancellation affects X chromosomes from both maternal and paternal lines. If a female embryo is a carrier of an X-linked recessive trait, half of the X chromosomes have the normal gene, and the other half have the abnormal gene (allele) for the given trait before cancellation occurs. Classic hemophilia (hemophilia A) is a good example. Hemophilia A is inherited as an X-linked recessive condition. In this disorder blood does not coagulate because of the low or almost nonexistent levels of factor VIII (antihemophilic globulin) in circulating blood. Males with the abnormal gene have a severe coagulation defect. In the female carrier some of the cancelled X chromosomes have the abnormal gene, and others have the normal one. The female carrier is a mosaic (i.e., she has both normal and abnormal X chromosomes). Because cancellation is random, the number of X chromosomes that remain genetically active and contain the normal or abnormal gene will vary. The female carrier's levels of factor VIII are often reduced; however, this reduction and the length of coagulation time vary, depending on the number of X chromosomes that contain the abnormal gene and remain genetically active. Although female carriers of the gene for hemophilia do not have as severe a problem as males, they tend to bleed more than usual after extraction of teeth or scaling and curettage. The variation in the bleeding problem in female carriers of the gene for hemophilia reflects the Lyon hypothesis. Other inherited disorders that reflect this hypothesis are described in detail later in this chapter. They include the X-linked type of amelogenesis imperfecta and hypohidrotic ectodermal dysplasia.

Genetic Heterogeneity

The term **genetic heterogeneity** is used when a condition has more than one inheritance pattern and differences in the degree of clinical manifestations for each of the inherited varieties. Amelogenesis imperfecta (described later in the chapter) is a condition that illustrates genetic heterogeneity.

In general, alterations in structural proteins (complex substances formed by one or more polypeptides) are inherited as a dominant trait, whereas alterations in enzymatic proteins (a protein inducing changes in other body substances) are inherited in a recessive manner; however, exceptions to this rule are seen.

Physical characteristics can be inherited as either dominant or recessive traits. The term **recessive** does not mean deleterious or abnormal. Instead it means that the individual must be homozygous for the trait to be seen. For example, in the ABO blood group system, blood group O is recessive, whereas groups A and B are dominant. However, no blood group is abnormal.

Genes can be codominant. Again, a good example is the ABO blood group. A and B are dominant over O, but when A and B are allelic, the result is blood group AB, in which both genes are exhibited. This is called **codominance.**

The four inheritance patterns refer to the characteristics that are governed by the action of one gene. This is called **single-gene inheritance. Oligogenic inheritance** refers to characteristics or traits that are inherited by the participation of several genes. These conditions show greater clinical variation than do those inherited through single-gene action. Characteristics such as tooth shape and form and eye color are determined by oligogenic inheritance. Most physical characteristics are oligogenic. The various genes that participate in determining a trait or condition can be located in the same chromosome or in different chromosomes.

Multifactorial Inheritance

The term **multifactorial inheritance** is used to describe a type of hereditary pattern seen when more than one genetic factor is involved and when environmental factors participate in the cause of a condition.

Examples of Inherited Disorders

All of the inherited disorders described in this section include oral and dental alterations and are discussed by location—gingiva and periodontium, jawbones and facies, oral mucosa, and teeth. Patients affected with these genetic abnormalities should receive routine dental hygiene care to maintain oral health. Specific dental hygiene management considerations are included only if they are unique to the disorder described.

Inherited Disorders Affecting the Gingiva and Periodontium

Most of the disorders included here are rare. However, they exhibit severe gingival or periodontal alterations (or both); therefore the dental hygienist should be aware of the disorders and their clinical manifestations.

Cyclic Neutropenia. The inheritance pattern of **cyclic neutropenia** is autosomal dominant; the responsible gene has been identified and is called *ELA-2* (neutrophil elastase gene). This gene is located on the short arm of chromosome 19. In the chromosome mapping system its location is designated as 19p13.3. The disorder is characterized by a cyclic decrease in the number of circulating neutrophilic leukocytes (neutrophils); a decrease in the number of circulating neutrophils is called **neutropenia.** The cycles usually occur in intervals of 21 to 27 days, but in some patients the interval may be extended to several months. These episodes of neutropenia generally persist for 2 to 3 days.

The clinical manifestations are related to the decrease in neutrophils. Systemic manifestations of cyclic neutropenia include fever, malaise, sore throat, and occasional cutaneous infections. Oral manifestations consist of severe ulcerative gingivitis or gingivostomatitis (Fig. 6.15). In addition to the gingiva, areas of ulceration can occur on the tongue and surfaces of the oral mucosa. The ulcers are of variable size and have a craterlike appearance. They are very painful and have a bleeding base. In general, the oral lesions are infected secondarily. When neutrophils return to normal, the oral lesions tend to improve.

Patients with cyclic neutropenia are usually managed by first determining the frequency of the cycles through periodic neutrophil counts and then instituting preventive antibiotic therapy to protect against secondary opportunistic infections. Over time, episodes of neutropenia and associated ulcerative gingivitis lead to severe periodontal disease, with loss of alveolar bone, tooth mobility, and exfoliation of teeth. Treatment should be initiated when the circulating neutrophil count is normal to reduce the risk of complications such as gingival hemorrhage and secondary infection. Dental hygiene care, including frequent appointments for removal of local irritants and maintenance of optimal oral hygiene, reduces the risk of opportunistic infections in patients with cyclic neutropenia.

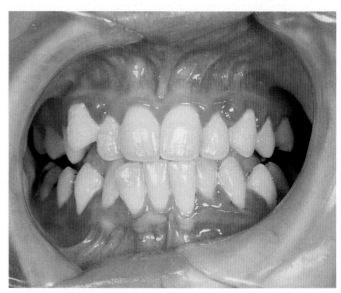

• **Figure 6.15** Hypertrophic gingivitis with areas of gingival recession is exhibited in a patient with Cyclic Neutropenia.

Patients with cyclic neutropenia are treated periodically with granulocyte colony-stimulating factor (G-CSF), which reduces the symptoms and results in substantial clinical improvement.

Chronic neutropenia, also known as *Kostmann syndrome,* is another variety of neutropenia that is inherited as an autosomal-recessive condition. In this syndrome the neutropenia is constant and not cyclic. The intraoral manifestations of Kostmann syndrome may be similar to those of the cyclic variety but are constantly present and require systemic treatment The responsible gene is still unknown, and it is also treated with periodic G-CSF.

Papillon-Lefèvre Syndrome. **Papillon-Lefèvre syndrome** has an autosomal-recessive inheritance pattern and is characterized by marked destruction of the periodontal tissues (periodontoclasia) of both dentitions with premature loss of teeth and hyperkeratosis of the palms of the hands and soles of the feet (palmar and plantar hyperkeratosis). Parents are generally heterozygous for the trait and unaffected. However, a homozygous parent would be affected.

The gene for this syndrome has been mapped to the long arm of chromosome 11 regions 14 to 21 (11q14-21). These patients are normal at birth except for a reddening of the palms of the hands and soles of the feet. Teeth erupt in normal sequence, position, and time. At about 1.5 to 2 years of age, a marked gingivoperiodontal inflammatory process develops, characterized by edema, bleeding, alveolar bone resorption, and mobility of teeth with consequent exfoliation. A red, scaly keratosis develops on the palms and soles concurrent with these oral lesions and occasionally extends to the dorsal surfaces of the hands and feet. The oral lesions are complicated by superimposed inflammation, and radiographs reveal marked alveolar bone resorption with vertical pockets. The extensive bone loss results in teeth that appear to be floating in soft tissue when viewed radiographically. Teeth are lost in the same sequence in which they erupted. When the last tooth is lost, the gingiva regains a normal appearance.

The lesions on the hands and feet remain as reddish-white, scaly, thick areas of hyperkeratinization (Fig. 6.16). The permanent dentition begins to erupt at the proper time. At about 8 or 9 years of age the gingivoperiodontal destruction is repeated in the same manner as occurred in the primary dentition (Fig. 6.17). All permanent teeth are lost before 14 years of age. The gingiva again resumes a normal appearance.

The peripheral blood neutrophil count is depressed in all patients with Papillon-Lefèvre syndrome. This suggests that the neutrophils may be an important factor in the pathogenesis of severe periodontal disease in these patients. Retinoid therapy markedly improves the skin condition but has no effect on the periodontal disease in patients with this syndrome. To date all therapeutic attempts at preventing the gingival and periodontal destruction and subsequent loss of teeth have been unsuccessful. The basic defect that causes the condition is unknown. Peripheral

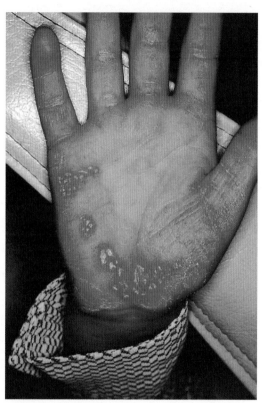

• **Figure 6.16** Areas of hyperkeratinization of the palms are exhibited in a patient with Papillon-Lefèvre Syndrome. (From Sedano HO, Sauk JJ, Gorlin RJ: *Oral manifestations of inherited disorders,* Boston, Butterworths, 1977. Used with permission.)

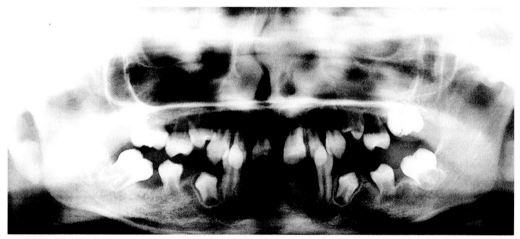

• **Figure 6.17** Papillon-Lefèvre Syndrome. Panoramic radiograph shows marked periodontal destruction with alveolar bone resorption in the patient in Fig. 6.16. (From Sedano HO, Sauk JJ, Gorlin RJ: *Oral manifestations of inherited disorders,* Boston, Butterworths, 1977. Used with permission.)

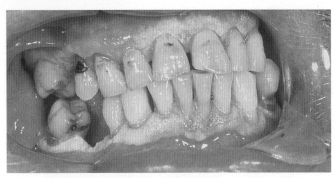

• **Figure 6.18** Marked hyperkeratosis follows the normal contour of the gingiva in Focal Palmoplantar and Gingival Hyperkeratosis. (From Sedano HO, Sauk JJ, Gorlin RJ: *Oral manifestations of inherited disorders,* Boston, Butterworths, 1977. Used with permission.)

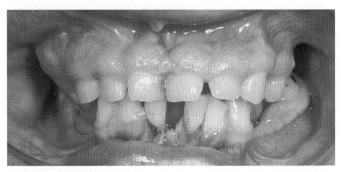

• **Figure 6.19** Gingival hypertrophy is shown in a patient with isolated Gingival Fibromatosis.

blood neutrophil chemotaxis has been reported to be depressed in patients with Papillon-Lefèvre syndrome. This decreased chemotaxis suggests that neutrophils may play a role in periodontal destruction in patients with this syndrome. Current research suggests bacterial and viral involvement as the initiating factors for the periodontal destruction. It has been suggested that the genetic component of Papillon-Lefèvre syndrome is a predisposition rather than the main determinant of periodontal disease.

The skin manifestations remain for life, but treatment with retinoid (oral etretinate) has proven somewhat effective in controlling the hyperkeratinization. These patients do not have any other abnormalities.

Focal Palmoplantar and Gingival Hyperkeratosis. Areas of hyperkeratinization of the palms and soles and marked hyperkeratinization of the labial and lingual gingiva characterize **focal palmoplantar** and **gingival hyperkeratosis**. This syndrome has an autosomal-dominant inheritance pattern. The palmar and plantar hyperkeratosis starts at the tips of the fingers and toes and extends to the surface of the palms and soles. This process increases with age and becomes localized, with calluses forming on the weight-bearing areas.

The oral hyperkeratinization is bandlike and a few millimeters in width (Fig. 6.18). It follows the normal festooned contour of the gingiva. The free gingiva is not affected. Palatal and lingual mucosa occasionally can be affected with areas of hyperkeratinization. These changes start in childhood and increase with age. The rest of the oral cavity is normal.

Gingival Fibromatosis. Gingival fibromatosis is a component of several inherited syndromes. The gingival enlargement generally develops early in life, and within a few years the teeth are completely covered. The fibromatosis is composed of very firm tissue with a granular corrugated surface. In general, the color is paler than that of the normal gingiva and results from the marked collagenization of the fibrous connective tissue. The extensive gingival enlargement leads to protrusion of the lips.

In addition to isolated gingival fibromatosis (Fig. 6.19), which has an autosomal-dominant inheritance pattern and no other associated abnormalities, gingival fibromatosis is a component of a number of syndromes. Because of the gingival involvement, several of these syndromes, although rare, are described here. However, only those that are well known and occur most frequently are included.

Dental hygiene care can reduce the risk of secondary inflammation and infection in patients with gingival fibromatosis.

Laband Syndrome. The inheritance pattern of **Laband syndrome** is autosomal dominant. In addition to gingival fibromatosis, patients have dysplastic or absent nails and malformed nose and ears because of soft and pliable cartilage formation, hepatosplenomegaly (enlarged liver and spleen), and hypoplasia of terminal phalanges of the fingers and toes with a resultant froglike appearance.

Gingival Fibromatosis With Hypertrichosis, Epilepsy, and Mental Retardation Syndrome. Gingival fibromatosis with hypertrichosis, epilepsy, and mental retardation syndrome has an autosomal-dominant inheritance pattern. Hypertrichosis (excessive growth of hair), especially of the eyebrows, extremities, genitals, and sacral region, characterize gingival fibromatosis with hypertrichosis, epilepsy, and mental retardation syndrome. Epilepsy and mental retardation can also occur in this syndrome but are inconsistent features.

Gingival Fibromatosis With Multiple Hyaline Fibromas. Gingival fibromatosis with multiple hyaline fibromas has an autosomal-dominant inheritance pattern and is also known as the *Murray-Puretic-Drescher syndrome.* In addition to gingival fibromatosis, it is characterized by hypertrophy of the nail beds and multiple hyaline fibrous tumors developing on the nose, chin, head, back, fingers, thighs, and legs. These tumors on the extremities can produce contractures of various joints, including hips, knees, shoulders, and elbows.

Inherited Disorders Affecting the Jawbones and Facies

Cherubism. The inheritance pattern of **cherubism** is autosomal dominant with marked penetrance (when the gene is present, the clinical manifestations are usually seen) in males and variable expressivity and incomplete penetrance in females (females are generally less severely affected). The gene for cherubism has been mapped to the short arm of chromosome 4 region 16 (4p16). The first clinical manifestation is a progressive bilateral facial swelling that appears when the patient is between 1.5 and 4 years of age. This change can affect either the mandible or the maxilla, but involvement of the mandible is most common. Displacement of the eyes is evident when the maxilla is affected. This, added to the bilateral deformity, produces the characteristic cherubic facial appearance that is responsible for the name of the syndrome. Increased distance between the eyes (**ocular hypertelorism**) is always present in affected patients. The eyes tilt upward showing more sclera than normal below the iris. Radiographs of the jaws show a typical "soap-bubble" or multilocular appearance (Fig. 6.20), which usually occupies the ascending ramus and coronoid process of the mandible and extends into the molar and premolar

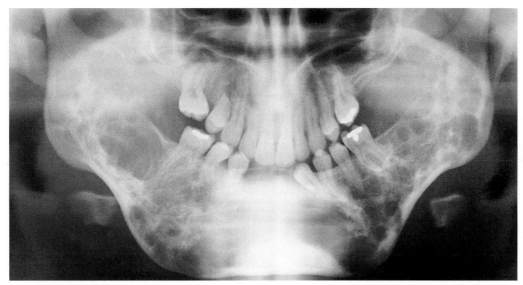

• **Figure 6.20** Panoramic radiograph of the jaws shows typical bilateral soap-bubble image in a patient with Cherubism. (From Young WG, Sedano HO: *Atlas of oral pathology,* Minneapolis, University of Minnesota Press, 1981. Used with permission.)

areas, but does not involve the condyle. Severe cases can involve the full mandible, but the condyle is always spared. When the maxilla is affected, the changes are observed at the level of the tuberosity and involve the antrum.

These areas of bone radiolucency are occupied by fibrous connective tissue containing multinucleated giant cells. The microscopic appearance resembles a central giant cell granuloma. The central giant cell granuloma is described in Chapter 8. The bone lesions interfere with tooth development and eruption. Most of these patients have **pseudoanodontia** (teeth falsely appear to be lacking), especially of molars and premolars, because of delayed eruption.

The size of the jaws tends to increase rapidly until about puberty and then generally remains stable. After the individual reaches 20 or 30 years of age, radiographs show an almost-normal bone appearance, with a few areas of increased bone density. The facial deformity remains for life, and in some patients it can be quite striking.

Ellis–van Creveld Syndrome. Ellis–van Creveld syndrome has an autosomal-recessive inheritance pattern. The gene for this has been mapped to the short arm of chromosome 4 region 16 (4p16). Affected individuals are dwarfs because of distal shortening of the extremities. One third of these patients are mildly mentally handicapped. The hands show polydactyly (supernumerary digits) on the ulnar side, and fingernails and toenails are hypoplastic and deformed. Other skeletal anomalies include curvature of the legs and feet. Fifty percent of affected individuals have congenital heart defects. Anomalies of the external genitals, especially in males, are also observed.

The oral manifestations are consistent and characteristic, and include fusion of the anterior portion of the maxillary gingiva to the upper lip from canine to canine. Thus the anterior maxillary vestibular sulcus is lacking (Fig. 6.21). This anomaly induces a V-notch appearance in the midline of the upper lip. The anterior lower alveolar ridge presents a serrated appearance caused by thick frenula, which start at the vestibular sulcus and traverse the alveolar ridge. The central incisors of both maxilla and mandible are

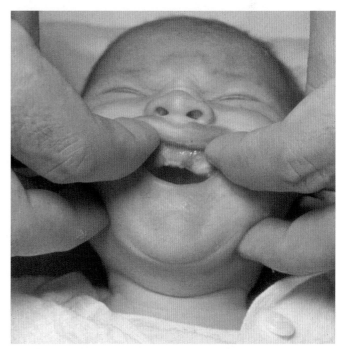

• **Figure 6.21** Infant with Ellis–van Creveld Syndrome (Chondroectodermal Dysplasia). The anterior maxillary vestibular sulcus is absent.

generally lacking and are replaced by a centrally located abnormal tooth. Most of the teeth have a conical shape and exhibit enamel hypoplasia. More than 50% of newborns with this syndrome have natal teeth.

Cleidocranial Dysplasia. The inheritance pattern of **cleidocranial dysplasia** is autosomal dominant; however, about half of the cases are isolated examples caused by either spontaneous mutation or a gene with poor penetrance. The gene for this syndrome has been mapped to the short arm of chromosome 6 region 21 (6p21). The cranium develops a mushroom shape because the fontanelles remain open. This makes the face appear small. Frontal, parietal, and occipital enlargement is quite noticeable. Skull radiographs reveal the open fontanelles, which are often open for life. The paranasal sinuses are lacking or hypoplastic. The neck is long and narrow because of unilateral or bilateral aplasia (lack of development) or hypoplasia of the clavicles. Affected individuals are able to approximate their shoulders to the midline because of this clavicular alteration. Various other bone anomalies can also be present.

The premaxilla is generally underdeveloped, resulting in pseudoprognathism. Radiographic features include many supernumerary teeth, sometimes even simulating a third dentition (Fig. 6.22), and the teeth are crowded in the jaws and do not erupt. The supernumerary teeth also interfere with the eruption of normal teeth, resulting in pseudoanodontia. A lack of cellular cementum has been reported in patients with this syndrome. Multiple cysts can develop in association with the impacted teeth. About 1% of affected patients have cleft lip, cleft palate, or both.

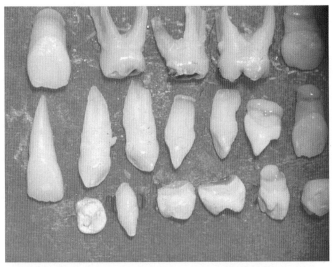

• **Figure 6.22** Multiple extracted supernumerary teeth from a patient with Cleidocranial Dysplasia.

Gardner Syndrome. Gardner syndrome, also known as *familial colorectal polyposis,* has an autosomal-dominant inheritance pattern with variable expressivity and marked penetrance. The adenomatous polyposis coli gene is responsible for Gardner syndrome and is located on the long arm of chromosome 5 regions 21 to 22 (5q21-22). One of the basic components is the presence of osteomas in various bones, especially the frontal bones, mandible, and maxilla. When they expand, osteomas of the facial skeleton obliterate the sinuses and induce facial asymmetry. Osteomas can also occur in the long bones of the skeleton but with less frequency than in the bones of the face.

In addition to osteomas, multiple odontomas can occur in the jawbones, especially the mandible (Fig. 6.23). Teeth can exhibit hypercementosis and fail to erupt.

The most serious component of this syndrome is the presence of multiple colorectal polyps, which become malignant at age 30 years and after. Polyposis primarily affects the colon and rectum and generally develops before puberty. Some authors advocate intestinal resection when the polyps appear because their malignant transformation into adenocarcinoma is invariable, especially with increasing age.

Mandibulofacial Dysostosis. The inheritance pattern of **mandibulofacial dysostosis,** also known as *Treacher Collins syndrome,* is autosomal dominant with incomplete penetrance and variable expressivity. The gene for this syndrome has been mapped to the long arm of chromosome 5 regions 32 to 33.1 (5q32-33.1). The facies shows downward sloping of the palpebral fissures, a hypoplastic nose, hypoplastic malar bones with hypoplasia or absence of the zygomatic process, abnormal and misplaced ears, and a receding chin. The mouth appears fishlike, with downward sloping of the lip commissures. The lower eyelids show a cleft (**coloboma**) of the outer third, with a lack of lashes medial to it. The ears may exhibit tags, which on occasion can also be seen near the angle of the mouth.

Deafness is a consistent feature resulting from a lack of otic ossicles. Mental development is within normal limits; difficulty in learning arises from deafness. Oral manifestations include a markedly hypoplastic mandible with flattened condyles and coronoid processes and an obtuse mandibular angle. Teeth are malposed, and malocclusion with open bite is quite evident. The palate

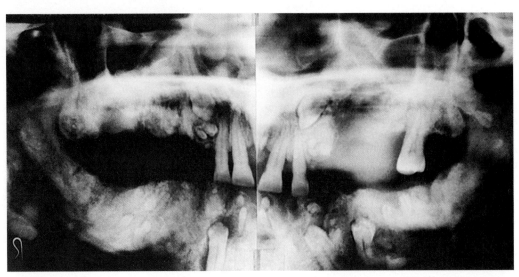

• **Figure 6.23** Panoramic radiograph of a patient with Gardner Syndrome shows multiple osteomas and odontomas. (Courtesy Dr. Carl J. Witkop.)

is high, or a cleft is present in about 30% of affected patients (Fig. 6.24). Gingival disease is common and is related to the dental abnormalities.

Nevoid Basal Cell Carcinoma Syndrome. The **nevoid basal cell carcinoma syndrome**, also known as *Gorlin syndrome*, has an autosomal-dominant inheritance pattern with high penetrance and variable expressivity. The gene for this syndrome maps to the long arm of chromosome 9 region 22.3 (9q22.3). The facies are characterized by mild **ocular hypertelorism** (increased distance between the eyes) and mild prognathism, with frontal and parietal bossing (enlargement) and a broad nasal root.

The cutaneous manifestations, which are called **nevi**, typically are basal cell carcinomas. The term *nevus* (plural, *nevi*), as defined here, is a congenital lesion characterized by skin pigmentation. These basal cell carcinomas are a major component of this syndrome. They appear early in life and continue to develop over the

nose, eyelids, cheeks, neck, arms, and trunk. They can be flesh-colored or pale-brown papules that develop singly or in clusters. Histologically, they are basal cell carcinomas. The palms and soles show small pits that become filled with dirt and appear as dark spots on those surfaces.

The oral manifestations of this syndrome consist of multiple cysts of the jaws (Fig. 6.25) that microscopically are odontogenic keratocysts (keratocystic odontogenic tumor) (see Chapter 5). These cysts vary in size; they can be very large and have a marked tendency to recur after surgical removal. On occasion, an ameloblastoma arises in these cysts as part of this syndrome. The cysts develop as early as 5 to 6 years of age in some affected patients and interfere with normal development of the jawbones and teeth.

A great variety of skeletal anomalies have been reported in association with the nevoid basal cell carcinoma syndrome, the most constant being bifurcation or splaying of one or more ribs. Other frequent abnormalities of bone include shortening of the metacarpals, spina bifida occulta (defective closure of the bone encasement of the spinal cord), and kyphoscoliosis (a combination of scoliosis, which is a lateral curving of the spine, and kyphosis, which is an abnormal vertical curvature of the spine or "hunchback").

Many different neoplasms have been reported in association with this syndrome. Medulloblastoma (brain tumor) has been seen in many cases. Children surviving the medulloblastoma eventually present other manifestations of the syndrome. Other, less frequent findings include calcified ovarian fibromas and mesenteric cysts.

Osteogenesis Imperfecta. **Osteogenesis imperfecta** is known to have an autosomal-dominant inheritance pattern with variable expressivity. However, only 30% of patients have a family history of this condition. The remaining 70% represent sporadic cases and cases suggesting autosomal-recessive inheritance. The basic defect is produced by different mutations affecting the genes that encode for type I collagen, resulting in abnormally formed bones that fracture easily. The genes responsible for the inherited varieties of osteogenesis imperfecta are mapped as follows: collagen type I α_2 is in the long arm of chromosome 7 region 22.1 (7q22.1);

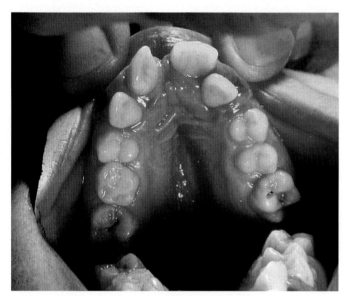

• **Figure 6.24** Markedly high-arched palate and malpositioned teeth in a patient with Mandibulofacial Dysostosis.

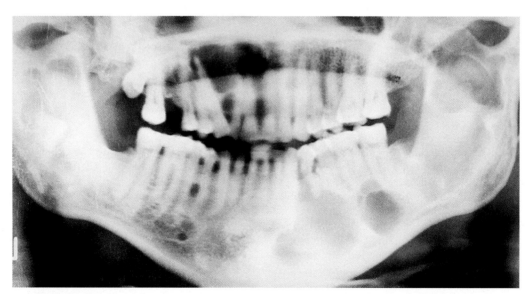

• **Figure 6.25** Multiple mandibular radiolucencies in a patient with Nevoid Basal Cell Carcinoma Syndrome. These lesions are odontogenic keratocysts (keratocystic odontogenic tumors).

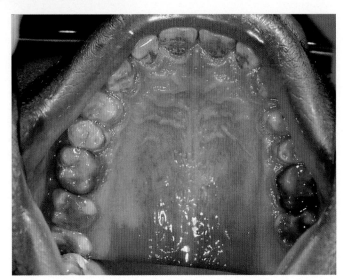

• **Figure 6.26** Patient with Osteogenesis Imperfecta. Teeth are yellowish with chipped enamel.

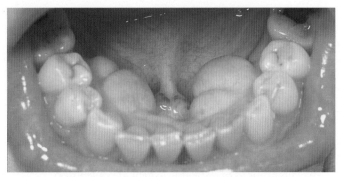

• **Figure 6.27** Bilateral lobulated Mandibular Tori.

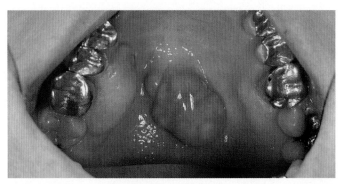

• **Figure 6.28** Torus Palatinus.

collagen type I α_1 is in the long arm of chromosome 17 region 21.31-22.05 (17q21.31-22.05). Osteogenesis imperfecta occurs in about 1 in 20,000 births, and major syndromes have been classified into four types: I, II, III, and IV.

The clinical manifestations vary markedly from patient to patient. The sporadic cases tend to be more severe than those with an autosomal-dominant inheritance pattern. The basic defect involves collagen and results in abnormally formed bones that fracture easily. Multiple spontaneous bone fractures are the main clinical complication of this syndrome. In the congenital form newborns can have several fractured bones at birth. Infants with this condition have experienced fractures just by being moved. In the most severe cases all bones can be affected, presenting a plethora of abnormalities, including bowing of the legs, curvature of the spine (kyphosis and scoliosis), deformity of the skull, shortening of arms and legs, deafness in a few cases, and other abnormalities. In the mildest cases individuals show only blue sclerae (a blue appearance of the white of the eye).

The oral manifestation of this syndrome is a dentinogenesis imperfecta–like condition (a description of dentinogenesis imperfecta follows later in this chapter). This clinical feature does not occur in all cases of osteogenesis imperfecta. Primary teeth are affected in 80% of patients, whereas permanent teeth are affected in only 35% of these individuals (Fig. 6.26). The crowns, roots, and pulp chambers generally are smaller than normal. Teeth appear opalescent or translucent at the time of eruption, but they darken with age. The enamel is lost because the abnormal dentin cannot provide adequate support.

Torus Mandibularis. Mandibular tori (singular, torus) have an autosomal-dominant inheritance pattern with variable expressivity and marked penetrance. This anomaly can be unilateral or bilateral. These tori occur on the lingual aspect of the mandible in the area of the premolar teeth (Fig. 6.27). Occurrence before age 15 years is extremely rare. The size of the torus is variable, and occasionally it can be multilobulated. Mandibular tori are symptomless and generally require no treatment. Surgical removal may be necessary if the patient needs a denture. Intraoral radiographs usually show a radiopacity in the area of the mandibular premolars if mandibular tori are present. Positioning of the film or sensor may be difficult when attempting to radiograph these areas.

Torus Palatinus. Autosomal dominance with variable expressivity and almost 100% penetrance characterize torus palatinus. A bony overgrowth occurs at the midline of the hard palate (Fig. 6.28). A marked predilection exists for women (2 : 1), and a higher prevalence exists among Native Americans, including the Inuit. Torus palatinus becomes evident around the time of puberty and is only rarely seen in children younger than 14 years of age. The size of this anomaly varies from nearly undetectable to large masses that occupy almost the entire surface of the hard palate. Some palatal tori are multilobular. Torus palatinus is symptomless. However, the surface mucosa is thin and easily traumatized. The torus may need to be removed if the patient needs a full denture.

Maxillary Exostosis. Exostoses have an autosomal-dominant inheritance pattern. **Maxillary exostoses** represent tori that generally develop on the buccal aspect of the maxillary alveolar ridge, usually in the molar and premolar area (Fig. 6.29). They are generally symptomless unless traumatized. They may be single, multiple, unilateral, or bilateral and occur less frequently than either palatal or mandibular tori.

Inherited Disorders Affecting the Oral Mucosa

Isolated Cleft Palate and Cleft Lip With or Without Cleft Palate. The majority of cases of facial clefting are multifactorial in origin; they occur in about 1 in 800 births. A large number of inherited syndromes can include cleft lip and palate or isolated cleft palate as a component. When clefting is part of an inherited syndrome, its occurrence within affected families will be in accordance with the inheritance pattern of the syndrome. Most of these syndromes are very rare. **Cleft lip-palate** and **congenital lip pits** (Van der Woude syndrome) is the syndrome that is considered to occur most frequently; therefore it is the only one described here. It has an autosomal-dominant inheritance pattern

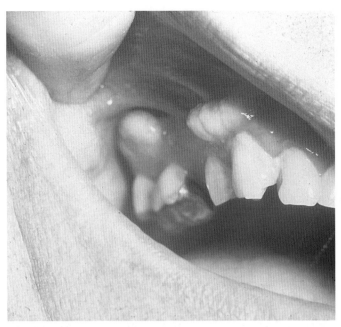

• **Figure 6.29** Maxillary Exostoses are inherited as autosomal dominant.

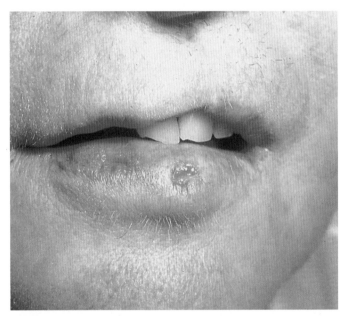

• **Figure 6.30** Paramedial Pits in the lower lip. Note the scar of the repaired cleft of the left upper lip.

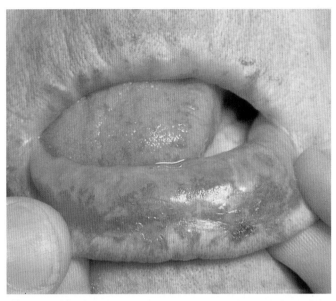

• **Figure 6.31** Multiple telangiectases of lips and tongue in a patient with Hereditary Hemorrhagic Telangiectasia. Gingival bleeding can be profuse in cases like this. (From Sedano HO, Sauk JJ, Gorlin RJ: *Oral manifestations of inherited disorders,* Boston, Butterworths, 1977. Used with permission.)

with 80% penetrance for any of its components. In the majority of cases the gene has been mapped to the long arm of chromosome 1 regions 32 to 41 (1q32-41). The labial pits (Fig. 6.30) are bilateral and are located near the midline of the vermilion border of the lower lip. They may be 3 mm or more in diameter and generally finish in a blind end. On occasion, they exude saliva because of their association with a labial minor salivary gland. These pits are rarely unilateral, and the clefting is bilateral in about 80% of patients. Some patients without clefting have agenesis (lack of development) of the maxillary lateral incisors or peg lateral incisors. Other oral findings that have been seen include fibrous adhesions between the maxilla and mandible, a cleft uvula, and ankyloglossia.

Hereditary Hemorrhagic Telangiectasia. The inheritance pattern of **hereditary hemorrhagic telangiectasia,** also known as *Osler-Rendu–Parkes Weber syndrome,* is autosomal dominant. Studies indicate that this syndrome may have two different responsible loci: one at the long arm of chromosome 9 (9q3) and the other in chromosome 12. It is characterized by multiple capillary dilations of the skin and mucous membranes (Fig. 6.31). The skin of the face shows numerous pinpoint and spiderlike telangiectases, especially on the lips, eyelids, and around the nose. The scalp and ears are also affected. Similar lesions are present in the nasal mucosa and are responsible for frequent and sometimes serious nosebleeds (**epistaxis**; plural, **epistaxes**) that can last for several days. Any organ or mucous membrane can be the site of telangiectasia.

Telangiectases of the oral mucosa are especially prominent on the tip and anterior dorsum of the tongue. The palate, gingiva, and buccal mucosa are often affected but to a lesser degree. Hemorrhage from sites in the oral cavity, mainly the lips and tongue, is second in frequency to epistaxis. Gingival bleeding has been reported and is a possible complication of dental hygiene treatment. The risk of gingival hemorrhage should be a concern of the dental hygienist when treating a patient with this syndrome.

Multiple Mucosal Neuroma Syndrome. The combination of multiple mucosal neuromas, medullary carcinoma of the thyroid gland, and pheochromocytoma is identified as multiple endocrine neoplasia, type 2B (MEN 2B). The inheritance pattern is autosomal dominant with decreased penetrance. This syndrome is the result of mutations in the receptor tyrosine kinase that maps to chromosome 10q11.2. Patients are tall with characteristic thick, large lips and often everted upper eyelids. The mucosal neuromas are prominent on the lips and anterior dorsal surface of the tongue (Fig. 6.32). They generally appear in the first few years of life. In addition, neuromas can occur on the buccal mucosa and the eyelids. The mucosal neuromas are seen as multiple, mobile, firm

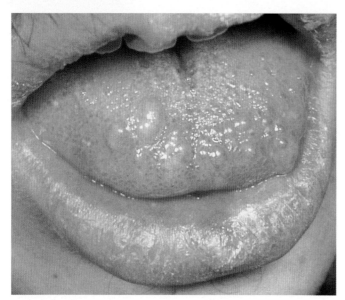

• **Figure 6.32** Patient with Multiple Endocrine Neoplasia, type 2B (MEN 2B) syndrome with multiple mucosal neuromas on the tip of the tongue and upper lip. (From Sedano HO, Sauk JJ, Gorlin RJ: *Oral manifestations of inherited disorders,* Boston, Butterworths, 1977. Used with permission.)

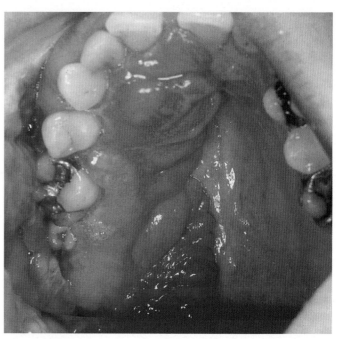

• **Figure 6.33** Multiple neurofibromas of the maxillary gingiva and palate in a patient with Neurofibromatosis of von Recklinghausen.

lumps covered by normal mucosa. Histologically, they are aggregates of nerve tissue.

Medullary carcinoma of the thyroid has been diagnosed in more than 75% of patients with this syndrome; it generally develops in the second decade of life. Metastatic lesions develop frequently, and about 20% of patients die as a consequence of metastasis. The thyroid carcinoma produces calcitonin (a hormone normally produced by the C cells of the thyroid gland). The carcinoma can be detected by evaluating plasma levels of this hormone.

Pheochromocytoma is a benign neoplasm that generally develops in ganglia around the adrenal glands. The tumor is often bilateral and is responsible for night sweats, high blood pressure, and episodes of severe diarrhea. It generally develops in the second or third decade of life. A pheochromocytoma induces increased urinary levels of epinephrine and other substances. Other findings in this syndrome have included cutaneous pigmentation and a host of skeletal abnormalities.

Early diagnosis of this syndrome is imperative because of the high malignant potential of the thyroid carcinoma. Some authors recommend preventive thyroidectomy when this syndrome is diagnosed so that the development of carcinoma is avoided. The neuromas of the oral mucosa may be the earliest visible manifestation of this syndrome.

Neurofibromatosis of von Recklinghausen. Neurofibromatosis of von Recklinghausen, also called *von Recklinghausen disease,* has an autosomal-dominant inheritance pattern and is probably a disorder of neural crest origin. The gene for this syndrome maps to the long arm of chromosome 17 region 11.2 (17q11.2). Several varieties exist; however, only the classic form is described here.

Multiple neurofibromas, which appear as papules and growths of various sizes, are seen on the facial skin, especially the eyelids. The tumors can arise anywhere, including the oral cavity, and can be present at birth or develop early in life, increasing in number and size at puberty. Malignant transformation of the neurofibromas occurs in an estimated 3% to 15% of patients with

neurofibromatosis. Neurofibromas also develop in the central nervous system, eyes, ears, viscera, and intraosseous locations. Mental disability is observed occasionally, and multiple skeletal anomalies are common.

Oral involvement is seen in about 10% of patients and is characterized by single or multiple tumors at any location in the oral mucosa, the most frequent being the lateral borders of the tongue. Gingival neurofibromas can also occur in these patients (Fig. 6.33), and intramandibular neurofibromas have been reported and present as radiolucencies in the mandible. When these involve the mandibular canal, there may be an enlargement of the mandibular foramen or a funnel-shaped widening of the mandibular canal.

Café au lait (the color of coffee with milk) pigmentation of the skin is present from the first decade of life in 90% of patients with neurofibromatosis. This pigmentation is quite marked in the axilla and can also affect other areas of the skin. Café au lait skin pigmentation generally precedes the development of the neurofibromas.

Peutz-Jeghers Syndrome. Autosomal-dominant inheritance characterizes **Peutz-Jeghers syndrome,** also called *hereditary intestinal polyposis syndrome.* The gene for this syndrome maps to the short arm of chromosome 19 region 13.3 (19p13.3). It consists of multiple melanotic macular pigmentations of the skin and mucosa, which are associated with gastrointestinal polyposis. The pigmentations occur around the eyes, nose, and mouth (Fig. 6.34). These macules are a few millimeters in diameter and vary in number and degree of pigmentation. They tend to diminish with age. Intraorally, larger areas of pigmentation are observed on the lips and buccal mucosa of about 98% of affected patients.

Pigmentation of the hands, nasal mucosa, and eyes can also occur. The intestinal polyps are hamartomas (an abnormal growth of normal tissue in its normal location). They develop mostly in the small intestine; only rarely do they undergo malignant transformation.

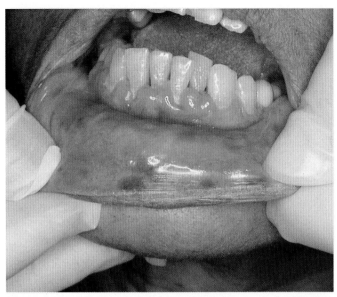

• **Figure 6.34** Multiple small- to medium-size pigmented macules on the labial mucosa of a patient with Peutz-Jeghers Syndrome.

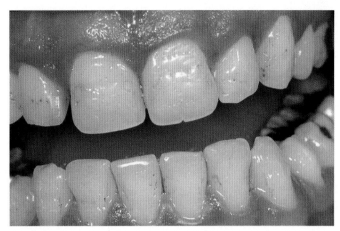

• **Figure 6.35** Pitted Autosomal-Dominant Amelogenesis Imperfecta. Multiple pits on the labial surface of the teeth should be noted. Some of the pits have been filled with composite. (From Young WG, Sedano HO: *Atlas of oral pathology*, Minneapolis, University of Minnesota Press, 1981. Used with permission.)

White Sponge Nevus. Autosomal-dominant inheritance with complete penetrance characterizes **white sponge nevus** (also called *Cannon disease* or *familial white folded mucosal dysplasia*). The cause of white sponge nevus is a mutation in the mucosal keratin pair K4 or K13. The disorder can be present at birth or develop around puberty. Clinically, it is characterized by a white, corrugated, soft, folding oral mucosa. The buccal mucosa is always affected, and in most patients the lesions are bilateral. A thick layer of keratin, which at times desquamates and leaves a raw mucosal surface, produces the whitening. Other areas of the oral mucosa can also be affected, but the free gingiva is spared.

Inherited Disorders Affecting the Teeth

Amelogenesis Imperfecta. A group of inherited conditions affecting the enamel of teeth and having no associated systemic defects characterizes **amelogenesis imperfecta.** Witkop and Sauk classified amelogenesis imperfecta into four types:

- *Type I:* Hypoplastic amelogenesis imperfecta
- *Type II:* Hypocalcified amelogenesis imperfecta
- *Type III:* Hypomaturation amelogenesis imperfecta
- *Type IV:* Hypoplastic-hypomaturation amelogenesis imperfecta

The *hypoplastic type* of amelogenesis imperfecta is characterized by tooth enamel that does not develop to a normal thickness because of failure of the ameloblasts to lay down enamel matrix properly. On radiographs the abnormal enamel contrasts with dentin. Several varieties of this type of amelogenesis imperfecta are further classified according to their clinical presentation: pitted, local, smooth, rough, and enamel agenesis. Combined with the clinical appearance, the classification also includes the inheritance pattern. Thus an autosomal-dominant variety and an autosomal-recessive variety exist for the local hypoplastic type. Among this group of enamel defects, the most frequent one is the pitted autosomal-dominant variety (Fig. 6.35), which is characterized by teeth that have random pits on the enamel. The size of these pits varies from pinpoint to pinhead, and the pits are observed mostly on the labial and buccal surfaces of the permanent teeth. The pits are frequently arranged in rows or columns or both. On occasion, more than one tooth has a normal clinical appearance.

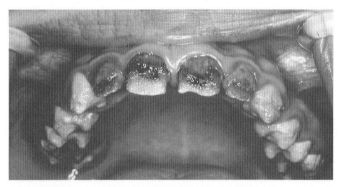

• **Figure 6.36** Loss of enamel is exhibited in the teeth of a patient with Hypocalcified Amelogenesis Imperfecta.

The gene for the local hypoplastic autosomal-dominant type of amelogenesis imperfecta maps to the long arm of chromosome 4 (4q11-13).

An autosomal-recessive type of hypoplastic amelogenesis imperfecta is also known as *enamel agenesis.* This variety is characterized by complete absence of enamel in all the teeth and lack of eruption of multiple teeth.

An enamel of normal thickness that is poorly calcified characterizes the *hypocalcified type* of amelogenesis imperfecta (Fig. 6.36). Two varieties of hypocalcified amelogenesis imperfecta exist: (1) an autosomal-dominant variety and (2) an autosomal-recessive variety. The autosomal-recessive pattern is more severe in its clinical manifestations. At eruption teeth present yellow-to-orange enamel that is very soft and rapidly lost, leaving exposed dentin. On radiographs the enamel has a moth-eaten appearance and is less radiopaque than dentin. Cervical enamel is better calcified and generally remains on the crown. Radiographically, enamel is primarily seen interproximally because the hypocalcified enamel on the occlusal surface has worn away. This type of amelogenesis imperfecta is frequently associated with an anterior open bite.

An enamel of mottled appearance but normal thickness characterizes the *hypomaturation type* of amelogenesis imperfecta. This type of amelogenesis imperfecta has been reported as due to a mutation in the *KLK4* (kallikrein) gene, which maps to 19q13.2,

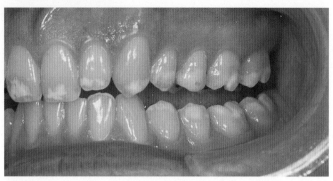

• **Figure 6.37** Uniform whitening of incisal edges and occlusal cusps is exhibited in a case of Snow-Capped Amelogenesis Imperfecta.

and also to a mutation in the *MMP20* (enamelysin) gene, which maps to 11q22.3-q23.

The hypomaturation type of amelogenesis imperfecta is characterized by large amounts of enamel matrix; therefore the enamel is softer than normal. With pressure the tip of a dental explorer will penetrate the enamel. The basic defect seems to be in the enamel rod sheath. The enamel chips easily from the crown. On radiographs it has almost the same radiodensity as dentin. Four varieties of the hypomaturation type of amelogenesis imperfecta exist; however, only the snow-capped type is discussed here.

A type of hypomaturation amelogenesis imperfecta, called *snow-capped amelogenesis imperfecta,* apparently has an X-linked recessive inheritance pattern in some families and an autosomal-dominant pattern in others. Clinically, both varieties are identical and are characterized by a hypomaturation of the surface enamel of the occlusal third of all the teeth of both dentitions. The maxillary teeth are more severely affected with this whitish discoloration (Fig. 6.37). The enamel in these areas is of regular hardness and smooth. It does not fracture or chip from the crown.

Its association with taurodontic teeth characterizes the *hypoplastic-hypomaturation type* of amelogenesis imperfecta. The thin enamel is yellow to brown and pitted. On radiographs the enamel has a radiodensity similar to dentin, and single-rooted teeth have large pulp chambers, and molar teeth appear as taurodonts.

It is generally not easy to diagnose the exact type of amelogenesis imperfecta clinically because of the frequent similarity among the different varieties. The mode of inheritance must be kept in mind, and an accurate family history should always be taken. Different mutations in several genes have been identified as responsible for some types of amelogenesis imperfecta; the genes are as follows: AMELX, AMELY, ENAM, AMELOBLASTIN, TUFTELIN, ENAMELYSIN, KALLIKREIN, and DLX3.

The prevalence of all forms of amelogenesis imperfecta in the United States has been estimated at 1 : 15,000.

Dentinogenesis Imperfecta. **Dentinogenesis imperfecta** is usually subdivided into three types. *Type I dentinogenesis imperfecta* is associated with osteogenesis imperfecta (previously described in this chapter). The other two types are not associated with osteogenesis imperfecta. The teeth in all three types have a similar clinical appearance. Type III dentinogenesis imperfecta is very rare. It is occurs in a small group of people in the Brandywine area of Maryland and is not described in this text.

Dentinogenesis imperfecta type II is also known as *hereditary opalescent dentin.* The inheritance pattern is autosomal dominant, and the gene maps to the long arm of chromosome 4 (4q13-21).

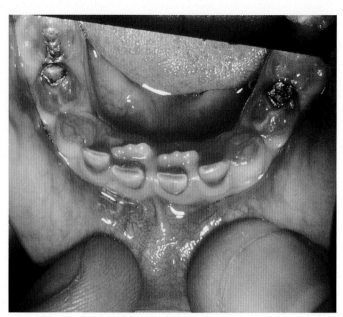

• **Figure 6.38** Opalescent bluish hue in the anterior teeth typical of Dentinogenesis Imperfecta. The yellow color seen in the molars is from exposed abnormal dentin due to loss of enamel.

Teeth have bulbous crowns with a color that varies from opalescent brown to brownish-blue (Fig. 6.38). The primary teeth are usually affected more severely than the permanent teeth. Twenty percent of patients have enamel hypoplasia as well. The dentin is very soft, which produces chipping of enamel that results in tooth attrition. On occasion, this attrition can cause the teeth to be worn down to the alveolar process. Radiographically, no pulp chambers or root canals are seen (Fig. 6.39). Roots are short and thin with periapical radiolucencies. Patients may lose teeth prematurely because of complications produced by the attrition and the short roots. The basic defect lies with the odontoblasts, which lay down an abnormal matrix and then degenerate. Cells derived from the dental pulp, which lay down abnormal dentin, later replace these odontoblasts.

Dentin Dysplasia. **Dentin dysplasia** is subdivided into type I (radicular dentin dysplasia) and type II (coronal dentin dysplasia).

Radicular Dentin Dysplasia. Teeth with normal crowns, abnormal roots, and an autosomal-dominant inheritance pattern characterize this condition. The basic defect seems to lie in a disturbance in the Hertwig epithelial root sheath, which guides the formation of the root. Radiographs show a total or partial lack of pulp chambers and root canals (Fig. 6.40). Primary and secondary dentitions are affected equally. The color of the teeth is normal. Because of the short roots, the teeth generally are exfoliated prematurely, especially in the event of even minor trauma. The pulp chambers of the permanent teeth generally are not obliterated fully and have a half-moon appearance on radiographs. Multiple periapical radiolucencies are associated with this condition.

Coronal Dentin Dysplasia. Dentin dysplasia type II has an autosomal-dominant inheritance pattern. The basic defect in this condition is a mutation in the gene termed *dentin sialophosphoprotein* (DSPP) that maps to the long arm of chromosome 4 (4q13-21). It has been shown that dentinogenesis imperfecta type II and dentin dysplasia type II share the DSPP gene loci and the proteins encoded by that gene. Translucent teeth with an amber color characterize the primary dentition. Radiographs show a lack

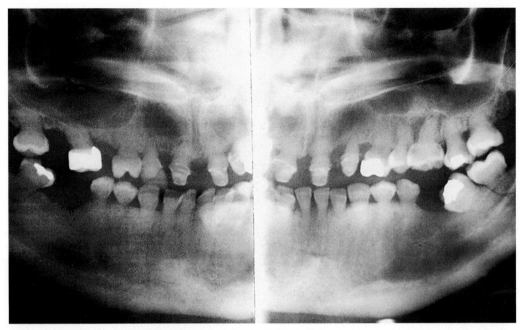

• **Figure 6.39** Panoramic radiograph of a patient with Dentinogenesis Imperfecta shows markedly short roots and almost complete lack of pulp chambers. (From Young WG, Sedano HO: *Atlas of oral pathology,* Minneapolis, University of Minnesota Press, 1981. Used with permission.)

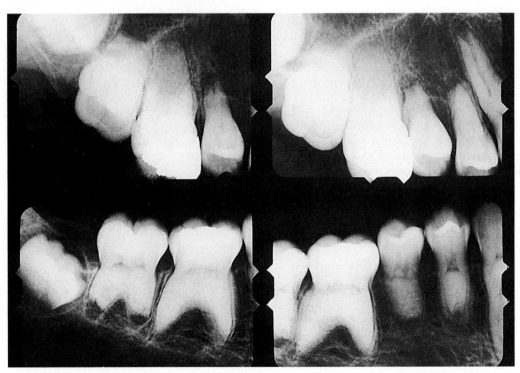

• **Figure 6.40** Radiographs of a patient with Radicular Dentin Dysplasia shows blunted and short tooth roots. The few remaining pulp chambers have a half-moon appearance. (Courtesy Dr. Carl J. Witkop.)

of pulp chambers and small root canals. Primary teeth are quite similar to those observed in dentinogenesis imperfecta. Permanent teeth present normal crown formation with normal color. Radiographs show thistle-shaped pulp chambers in single-rooted teeth and a bow-tie appearance of the pulp chambers of permanent molars (Fig. 6.41). Permanent teeth may or may not have pulp stones.

Hypohidrotic Ectodermal Dysplasia. Hypohidrotic ectodermal dysplasia represents a genetic heterogeneity. Although in the majority of families it is inherited as an X-linked recessive trait, in some families it is inherited as an autosomal-recessive trait. The clinical manifestations for both the X-linked and autosomal-recessive forms are identical. The gene for the X-linked variety of this syndrome maps to the long arm of the X chromosome region

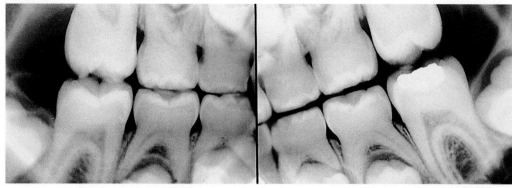

• **Figure 6.41** Obliteration and partial lack of coronal pulp chambers and small root canals can be seen in teeth of a patient affected with Coronal Dentin Dysplasia. (Courtesy Dr. Carl J. Witkop.)

12 to 13.1 (Xq12-13.1). The autosomal-recessive variety maps to the long arm of chromosome 2 (2q11-13). Some other types of ectodermal dysplasia are due to mutations in various other genes.

This entity represents the most severe form of ectodermal dysplasia. Its major components are hypodontia (partial anodontia), **hypotrichosis** (less than the normal amount of hair), and **hypohidrosis** (abnormally diminished secretion of sweat) due to a decrease in the number of sweat glands. Affected children are born without lanugo (body hair present at birth), and many have episodes of fever of unknown cause because of the almost complete lack of sweat glands. Individuals with this condition are very uncomfortable with changes in environmental temperature. Some patients die of hyperthermia (greatly increased body temperature) after prolonged exposure to the sun or heavy exercise. The clinical characteristics of this condition may not be apparent until the second year of life.

The facies are quite typical, with marked frontal bossing, depressed nasal bridge (saddle nose), protuberant lips, and almost complete lack of scalp hair. The hair that is present is usually blond, short, fine, and stiff. The skin is soft, thin, and very dry. Sebaceous glands are also lacking. Linear wrinkles and increased pigmentation are seen around the eyes and mouth. The eyelashes and eyebrows are often missing entirely. After puberty the beard generally is normal, but axillary and pubic hair are scanty.

The oral manifestations of hypohidrotic ectodermal dysplasia consist of hypodontia or, rarely, anodontia. When present, incisors and canines have small, conical crowns (Fig. 6.42). The alveolar bone is formed only when teeth are present; therefore patients lacking alveolar processes have loss of vertical dimension with markedly protruding lips. There may also be partial lack and aplasia of minor salivary glands in the buccal, labial, and lower respiratory tract mucosa.

Female carriers of the X-linked form of hypohidrotic ectodermal dysplasia have minor clinical manifestations such as thin and slightly sparse hair, cone-shaped teeth, hypodontia, and variable degrees of reduced sweating. This is in accordance with the Lyon hypothesis of variability of expression.

Hypophosphatasia. The inheritance pattern of **hypophosphatasia** is autosomal recessive. The gene for this syndrome maps to the short arm of chromosome 1 regions 36.1-34 (1p36.1-34). The basic defect in this condition is a decrease in serum alkaline phosphatase levels with increased urinary and plasma levels of phosphoethanolamine. Alkaline phosphatase participates in the process of calcification of bone and cementum; therefore these two tissues will be altered in patients with hypophosphatasia.

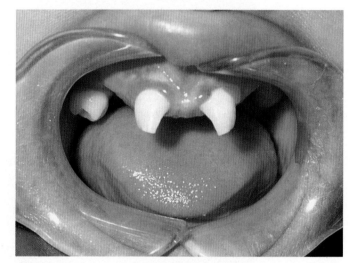

• **Figure 6.42** Patient with Hypohidrotic Ectodermal Dysplasia has only three, abnormally shaped teeth.

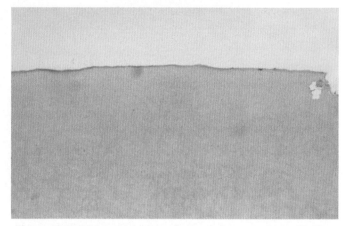

• **Figure 6.43** Histologic section of a tooth from a patient with Hypophosphatasia shows only dentin. Cementum is entirely lacking.

Agenesis, or abnormal formation of cementum, in these patients leads to spontaneous premature shedding of primary teeth, especially mandibular incisors (Fig. 6.43). Teeth are exfoliated without evidence of periodontal or gingival disease. The primary molars and permanent teeth are rarely, if ever, affected, which is probably associated with the greater mechanical fixation resulting from the larger size of their roots. The total lack of cementum observed in exfoliated teeth implies a lack of periodontal fiber attachment, with consequent exfoliation of single-rooted teeth. The most important alteration in this syndrome is the improper formation of mature bone. Therefore individuals who survive the neonatal period experience rachitic-like changes such as bowing of legs and multiple fractures.

Hypophosphatemic Vitamin D–Resistant Rickets. Hypophosphatemic vitamin D–resistant rickets, which is quite common, has an X-linked–dominant inheritance pattern and is the result of a mutation in the *PHEX* gene. It is characterized by low serum levels of phosphorus, which is caused by low absorption of inorganic phosphate in the renal tubules; rickets or osteomalacia; resistance to treatment with usual doses of vitamin D; and a lack of other abnormalities. Affected individuals generally are of short stature and have bowlegs, especially if the condition is present from childhood. Adult-onset forms also exist, and the clinical manifestations in these patients are minor or even lacking, with the exception of low serum levels of inorganic phosphate.

The characteristic radiographic oral findings are large pulp chambers with very long pulp horns. In addition, the dentin exhibits pronounced cracks that extend to the dentinoenamel junction. These cracks induce fracture of the enamel with microexposure of the pulp and subsequent pulpal infection. Eventually, infectious inflammatory pulpal disease progresses to periapical abscess formation. Gingival abscesses are also frequent. Regional lymphadenitis accompanies these processes.

Pegged or Absent Maxillary Lateral Incisors. The inheritance pattern of **pegged** or **absent maxillary lateral incisors** is generally autosomal dominant with variable expressivity. The lateral incisor can be small, peg shaped, or congenitally lacking, either unilaterally or bilaterally (Fig. 6.44). Both primary and secondary dentitions can be affected, but mostly the latter. This condition has a prevalence of 1% to 3% in the white population and about 7% in Asians. In addition, the premolar teeth are congenitally lacking in 10% to 20% of affected individuals.

Taurodontism. Taurodontism is a genetic heterogeneous condition with dominant and recessive inheritance. It is characterized by very large, pyramid-shaped molars with large pulp

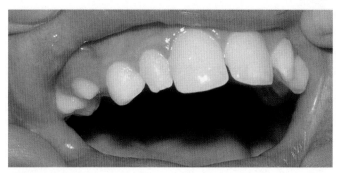

• **Figure 6.44** Pegged Maxillary Lateral Incisors. The conical shape should be noted.

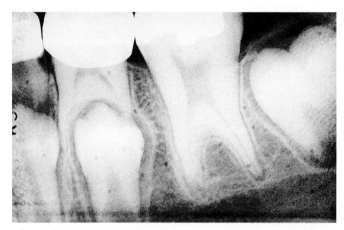

• **Figure 6.45** Intraoral radiograph of Taurodontic Teeth shows large pulp chambers and low bifurcation of the roots in this pyramid-shaped molar.

chambers (Fig. 6.45). Taurodontism is most frequent among Native Americans, including the Inuit. The furcation of the roots is displaced apically, and these teeth are classified according to the degree of furcation displacement. Taurodontism is frequently found in Klinefelter syndrome and is associated with many other syndromes as well.

Selected References

Books

Cummings MR: *Human heredity: principles and issues*, ed 7, Stamford, 2006, Brooks/Cole-Cengage Learning.

Fitzgerald MJT, Fitzgerald M: *Human embryology*, London, 1994, Saunders.

Hennekam RCM, Krantz ID, Allanson JE: *Gorlin's syndromes of the head and neck*, ed 5, New York, 2010, Oxford University Press.

Neussbaum RL, McInnes RR, Willard HF: *Thompson and Thompson genetics in medicine*, ed 11, Philadelphia, 2016, Saunders.

Neville BW, Damm DD, Allen CM, et al: *Oral and maxillofacial pathology*, ed 4, St. Louis, 2016, Elsevier.

Sadler TW: *Langman's medical embryology*, ed 11, Philadelphia, 2010, Lippincott Williams & Wilkins.

Sapp JP, Eversole LR, Wisocki GP: *Contemporary oral and maxillofacial pathology*, ed 2, St. Louis, 2004, Mosby.

Witkop CJ, Sauk JJ, Stewart R, et al: Heritable defects of enamel. In *Oral facial genetics*, St Louis, 1976, Mosby, pp 151–226.

Young WG, Sedano HO: *An atlas of oral pathology*, Minneapolis, 1981, University of Minnesota Press.

Journal Articles

Bala Subramanyam S, Naga Sujata D, Sridhar K, et al: Nevoid basal cell carcinoma syndrome: a case report and review, *J Maxillofac Oral Surg* 14:11–15, 2015.

Bianchi ML: Hypophosphatasia: an overview of the disease and its treatment, *Osteoporos Int* 26(12):2743–2757, 2015.

Chen Y, Fang L, Yang X: Cyclic neutropenia presenting as recurrent oral ulcers and periodontitis, *J Clin Pediatr Dent* 37:307–308, 2013.

Dale DC, Welte K: Cyclic and chronic neutropenia, *Cancer Treat Res* 157:97–108, 2011.

de La Dure-Molla M, Philippe Fournier B, Berdal A: Isolated dentinogenesis imperfecta and dentin dysplasia: revision of the classification, *Eur J Hum Genet* 2:445–451, 2015.

Dyasanoor S, Naik S: Clinicoradiologic features of cherubism: a case report and literature review, *Gen Dent* 62:12–15, 2014.

Foster BL, Ramnitz MS, Gafni RI, et al: Rare bone diseases and their dental, oral, and craniofacial manifestations, *J Dent Res* 93:7S–19S, 2014.

Hopp RN, de Siqueira DC, Sena-Filho M, et al: Oral vascular malformation in a patient with hereditary hemorrhagic telangiectasia: a case report, *Spec Care Dentist* 33:150–153, 2013.

Koruyucu M, Bayram M, Tuna EB, et al: Clinical findings and long-term managements of patients with amelogenesis imperfecta, *Eur J Dent* 4:546–552, 2014.

Lu RF, Men HX: Severe periodontitis in a patient with cyclic neutropenia: a case report of long-term follow-up, *Chin J Dent Res* 15:159–163, 2012.

Sreeramulu B, Shyam ND, Ajay P, et al: Papillon-Lefèvre syndrome: clinical presentation and management options, *Clin Cosmet Investig Dent* 15(7):75–81, 2012.

Tripathi AK, Dete G, Saimbi CS, et al: Management of hereditary gingival fibromatosis: a 2 years follow-up case report, *J Indian Soc Periodontol* 19:342–344, 2015.

Review Questions

1. Which one of the following is associated with cyclic neutropenia?
   a. Exfoliating teeth because of short roots
   b. Chipping away of enamel
   c. Diminished number of circulating neutrophils
   d. Premature loss of primary teeth

2. The so-called "enamel agenesis" is one of which type of amelogenesis imperfecta?
   a. Hypocalcified
   b. Hypomaturation
   c. Hypoplastic-hypomaturation
   d. Hypoplastic

3. Two characteristic clinical components of mandibulofacial dysostosis are:
   a. Lack of clavicles and delayed teeth eruption
   b. Hypodontia and dysplastic nails
   c. Hypoplastic mandible and deafness
   d. Cleft lip and fistulas of lower lip

4. Which of the following is *true* for von Recklinghausen disease?
   a. Patients may have gingival neurofibromas.
   b. It is inherited as an autosomal-recessive trait.
   c. Patients experience a generalized whitening of the oral mucosa.
   d. Patients have multiple fibromatoses.

5. Which one of the following is characteristically associated with teeth with large pulp chambers?
   a. Coronal dentin dysplasia
   b. Dentinogenesis imperfecta
   c. Hypophosphatasia
   d. Pitted autosomal-dominant amelogenesis imperfecta

6. Which one of the following statements is *true* when comparing cyclic neutropenia and Kostmann syndrome?
   a. The oral lesions in cyclic neutropenia are more severe.
   b. Both conditions are inherited as autosomal dominant.
   c. Both conditions are associated with capillary fragility.
   d. The oral lesions in Kostmann syndrome are always present unless systemic treatment is instituted.

7. A 9-year-old boy exhibits markedly swollen red and bleeding gingiva. In addition, he has tooth mobility, and the intraoral radiographs show marked alveolar bone atrophy with vertical periodontal pockets. Which of the following will be found in this child if he were to have Papillon-Lefèvre syndrome?
   a. Lack of anterior vestibular sulcus
   b. Diminished sweating
   c. Palmar and plantar hyperkeratosis
   d. Blue sclerae

8. The karyotype of a patient with Turner syndrome shows:
   a. 43 autosomes and XYY
   b. 44 autosomes and XO
   c. 44 autosomes and XYY
   d. 44 autosomes and XXY

9. The major concern for a dental hygienist when treating a patient with Osler-Rendu–Parkes Weber syndrome should be:
   a. Severe infections
   b. Epithelial desquamation
   c. Spontaneous ulcerations
   d. Gingival hemorrhage

10. The characteristic finding in permanent teeth affected with coronal dentin dysplasia is:
    a. Large, square pulp chambers in molars
    b. Thistle-shaped pulp chambers in incisors
    c. Crowns with amber color
    d. Markedly short roots

11. Radiographs of a patient with radicular dentin dysplasia show:
    a. Taurodontic teeth
    b. Large pulp chambers with long pulp horns
    c. Pulp chambers with a half-moon appearance
    d. Internal resorption of teeth

12. Hypotrichosis means:
    a. Increased number of sweat glands
    b. Diminished number of sweat glands
    c. Increased amount of hair
    d. Decreased amount of hair

13. Snow-capped amelogenesis imperfecta have teeth with:
    a. Short, blunted roots
    b. White hypocalcified enamel at the incisal and occlusal thirds
    c. A thin, brown enamel
    d. Obliterated pulp chambers

14. The most frequently exfoliated teeth in patients with hypophosphatasia are the:
    a. Mandibular permanent incisors
    b. Mandibular primary incisors
    c. Maxillary primary molars
    d. Maxillary primary incisors

15. A gamete is the result of the process of:
    a. The S phase
    b. Meiosis
    c. Mitosis
    d. Prophase

16. Which of the following is the most serious component of Gardner syndrome?
    a. Teeth hypercementosis
    b. Mandibular odontomas
    c. Colorectal polyposis
    d. Multiple osteomas

17. Patients with hypophosphatasia characteristically have:
    a. Increase in serum alkaline phosphatase levels
    b. Obliterated pulp chambers
    c. Marked gingival keratinization
    d. Absence of root cementum

18. A 14-year-old boy is seen in consultation because of bilateral mandibular swelling. Radiographs show a bilateral multilocular lesion in the ascending mandibular rami. The mother of this patient has similar findings. The most likely diagnosis is:
    a. Cleidocranial dysplasia
    b. Nevoid basal cell carcinoma syndrome
    c. Ellis–van Creveld syndrome
    d. Cherubism

19. The order of the four stages of mitosis is:
    a. Prophase, metaphase, anaphase, telophase
    b. Metaphase, prophase, telophase, anaphase
    c. Anaphase, metaphase, telophase, prophase
    d. Prophase, telophase, metaphase, anaphase

20. The constriction that joins the short and long arms of each chromosome is called the:
    a. Chromatid
    b. Equatorial plate
    c. Centromere
    d. Chiasmata

21. In dentinogenesis imperfecta type II, teeth have:
    a. Roots that are short and thin
    b. Dilacerated roots
    c. Hard, dense dentin
    d. Markedly brittle enamel

22. Torus mandibularis and torus palatinus are:
    a. Sporadic traits
    b. Inherited as an autosomal-dominant trait
    c. Inherited as an autosomal-recessive trait
    d. More prevalent in males

23. The Papillon-Lefèvre syndrome is inherited according to a (an):
    a. X-linked recessive pattern
    b. Autosomal-dominant pattern
    c. Autosomal-recessive pattern
    d. X-linked dominant pattern

24. Hypothetically, an autosomal-dominant trait would be clinically present in:
    a. 25% of the offspring of an affected parent
    b. 50% of the offspring of an affected parent
    c. 75% of the offspring of an affected parent
    d. Only in males, never in female offspring

25. Which one of the following is characteristically associated with oral ulcerations?
    a. Gardner syndrome
    b. Gorlin syndrome
    c. Kostmann syndrome
    d. Peutz-Jeghers syndrome

26. The most frequent site of hemorrhage in patients with hereditary hemorrhagic telangiectasia is the:
    a. Lip mucosa
    b. Gingiva
    c. Nasal mucosa
    d. Eyelids

27. Barr bodies are seen at the:
    a. Nuclear periphery of all cells in women
    b. Periphery of the cytoplasm in all human cells
    c. Nuclear periphery of all human cells
    d. Periphery of the cytoplasm in all cells from women

28. Which one of the following is typically found in the MEN 2B syndrome?
    a. Carcinoma of the pancreas
    b. Pheochromocytoma
    c. Basal cell carcinomas
    d. Carcinoma of the colon

29. A 19-year-old woman is diagnosed with cleidocranial dysplasia. She has absent clavicles and a mushroom-shaped skull. Which of the following conditions is she also most likely to have?
    a. Large pulp chambers
    b. Taurodontism
    c. Supernumerary teeth
    d. Pegged lateral incisors

30. Trisomy refers to:
    a. One extra chromosome in each pair
    b. Three extra chromosomes
    c. The presence of two extra X chromosomes in a male
    d. A pair of chromosomes with an identical extra chromosome

31. Patients with hypohidrotic ectodermal dysplasia characteristically have:
   a. Blue sclerae
   b. Excessive amounts of hair
   c. Hypodontia
   d. Multiple tongue nodules

32. Which of the following is a component of the Peutz-Jeghers syndrome?
   a. Multiple jaw cysts
   b. Multiple pigmented macules on the lower lip and mucosa
   c. Multiple nodules on the tip of the tongue
   d. Multiple supernumerary teeth

33. In all inherited varieties of gingival fibromatosis, the gingival enlargement is characterized by a marked:
   a. Alveolar bone hypertrophy
   b. Collagenization of the connective tissue
   c. Hyperplasia of the covering epithelium
   d. Chronic inflammatory cellular infiltrate

34. Karyotype refers to:
   a. A portion of a chromosome attached to an another chromosome
   b. A pair of chromosomes with an identical extra chromosome
   c. A microphotograph showing a person's chromosomes from a single cell
   d. The position occupied by a gene in a chromosome

35. Taurodontic teeth:
   a. Have long roots
   b. Have thistle-shaped pulp chambers
   c. Are pyramidal in shape
   d. Are supernumerary

36. Cannon disease is also known as:
   a. White sponge nevus
   b. Gingival fibromatosis
   c. Chronic neutropenia
   d. Cherubism

Chapter 6 Synopsis

Condition/Disease	Cause	Age/Race/Sex	Location
Trisomy 21	One extra chromosome no. 21	From birth	Systemic
Trisomy 13	One extra chromosome no. 13	From birth	Systemic
Turner syndrome	One X chromosome missing	From birth Women	Systemic
Klinefelter syndrome	One or more extra X chromosomes	From birth Men	Systemic
Cat cry syndrome	Deletion 5p	From birth M = F	Systemic
Cyclic neutropenia	AD, gene ELA-2, 19p13.3	From birth M = F	Oral mucosa and periodontium
Papillon-Lefèvre syndrome	AR, 11q14-21	From birth M = F	Gingiva, periodontal ligament, palms and soles
Focal palmoplantar and gingival hyperkeratosis	AD	From birth M = F	Gingiva, palms and soles
Laband syndrome	AD	From birth M = F	Gingiva
Gingival fibromatosis, hypertrichosis, epilepsy, and mental retardation syndrome	AD	From birth M = F	Gingiva, hair, central nervous system
Gingival fibromatosis with multiple hyaline fibromas	AD	From birth M = F	Gingiva, nails, mucosa, and skin

AD, Autosomal dominant; *AR,* autosomal recessive; *CL/P,* cleft lip with or without cleft palate; M = F, occurs in men and women equally; G-CSF, granulocyte-colony stimulating factor.
*No significant information.

37. The cause of all forms of labial and palatal clefting is considered to be:
a. Multifactorial
b. Environmental
c. Autosomal recessive
d. Autosomal dominant

38. Odontogenic keratocysts are a clinical component of:
a. Cherubism
b. Pegged lateral incisors
c. Nevoid basal cell carcinoma syndrome
d. Neurofibromatosis of von Recklinghausen

39. Patients with an X-linked hereditary condition:
a. Are generally affected more severely if they are men
b. Are always XYY
c. Have cells with an extra Barr body
d. Are always women

40. The Lyon hypothesis is demonstrated by:
a. X-linked dominant traits
b. X-linked recessive traits
c. Autosomal-dominant traits
d. Autosomal-recessive traits

41. All of the following are characteristics of cherubism except one. Which one is the exception?
a. Pseudoanodontia
b. Autosomal dominant
c. Ocular hypertelorism
d. Autosomal recessive

42. All of the following are involved in cherubism except one. Which one is the exception?
a. Coronoid process
b. Condyle
c. Posterior mandible
d. Ascending ramus

43. In which one of the following conditions can the shoulders be brought forward to the midline due to hypoplastic clavicles?
a. Cherubism
b. Ellis--von Creveld syndrome
c. Turner syndrome
d. Cleidocranial dysplasia

Clinical Features	Radiographic Features	Microscopic Features	Treatment	Diagnostic Process
Slanted eyes, gingivoperiodontitis, fissured tongue, hypodontia	None	None	Root planing, scaling	Karyotype shows trisomy 21
Bilateral CL/P, polydactyly, microphthalmia	Extra fingers in hand	None	None	Karyotype shows trisomy 13
Short stature, webbing of neck, edema of hands	None	No Barr bodies in buccal smear	None	Karyotype shows absent X chromosome
Tall stature, gynecomastia	Hypoplastic maxilla	One Barr body, in buccal smear	None	Karyotype shows two X chromosomes
Catlike cry, severe mental retardation	None	None	Dental care for mentally handicapped	Karyotype shows deletion of short arm of chromosome 5
Gingivitis, periodontitis, ulcers, hemorrhage	Alveolar bone loss, pocket formation	Diminished neutrophils in peripheral blood	Root planing, scaling, antibiotics, G-CSF	Clinical and blood studies
Teeth mobility, pockets, palmoplantar hyperkeratosis	Alveolar bone loss, severe periodontal disease	Profuse inflammatory infiltrate of soft dental tissues	Root planing, scaling, tooth fixation, retinoid for skin lesions	Clinical, genetic evaluation
Keratosis of gingiva, palms and soles	None	Hyperorthokeratosis of affected areas	Maintenance of oral hygiene	Clinical and family history
Marked gingival hyperplasia, abnormal nails, short fingers and toes	Hypoplasia of terminal phalanges of fingers and toes	Profuse fibrosis and increase collagen of affected gingiva	Maintenance of oral hygiene, surgical remodeling of gingiva (recurrence)	Clinical and family history
Gingival hyperplasia, abundant body hair, epilepsy	None	Profuse fibrosis and increased collagen affect gingiva	Maintenance of oral hygiene, surgical remodeling of gingiva (recurrence)	Clinical and family history
Gingival hyperplasia, hypertrophy of nails, multiple tumors	None	Fibrosis of gingiva, hyaline fibromas	Maintenance of oral hygiene, removal of fibromas	Clinical and family history

Continued

Chapter 6 Synopsis—cont'd

Condition/Disease	Cause	Age/Race/Sex	Location
Cherubism	AD, 4p16	From birth M = F	Mandible bilaterally
Ellis–van Creveld syndrome (chondroectodermal dysplasia)	AR, 4p16	From birth M = F	Gingiva, teeth, alveolar ridge, hands
Cleidocranial dysplasia	AD, 6p21	From birth M = F	Teeth, clavicles, skull
Gardner syndrome	AD, 5q21-22	From birth M = F	Maxilla and mandible
Mandibulofacial dysostosis	AD, 5q32-33.1	From birth M = F	Mandible, teeth, ears
Nevoid basal cell carcinoma syndrome	AD, 9q22.3	From birth M = F	Mandible, maxilla, skin
Osteogenesis imperfecta	AD, multiple genes involved	From birth M = F	Skeleton teeth
Hereditary hemorrhagic telangiectasia	AD, 9q3 and 12	Starts after teens M = F	Mucous membranes and skin
Multiple mucosal neuroma syndrome	AD, 10q11.2	From birth M = F	Oral mucosa, especially tongue
Neurofibromatosis of von Recklinghausen	AD, 17q11.2	From birth M = F	Skin, oral mucosa, especially tongue
Peutz-Jeghers syndrome	AD, 19p13.3	From birth M = F	Skin, oral mucosa, small intestine
White sponge nevus (also called Cannon disease)	AD, mutation in mucosal keratin K4 or K13	From birth or develops at puberty M = F	Buccal mucosa
Amelogenesis imperfecta: pitted hypoplastic	AD	Visible when teeth erupt M = F	All primary and permanent teeth
Amelogenesis imperfecta: hypocalcified type	AD and AR	When teeth erupt M = F	All primary and permanent teeth

AD, Autosomal dominant; *AR,* autosomal recessive; CL/P, cleft lip with or without cleft palate; M = F, occurs in men and women equally; G-CSF, granulocyte-colony stimulating factor.
*No significant information.

Clinical Features	Radiographic Features	Microscopic Features	Treatment	Diagnostic Process
Bilateral enlargement of face	Multiple bilateral radiolucencies of mandibular ramus	Multinucleated giant cells in a loose connective tissue	Lesions fill in after puberty	Clinical and family history Radiographic
Absent upper vestibule, serrated lower alveolar ridge, polydactyly	Thinning of enamel	None	Reconstruction of upper vestibule, amputation of extra fingers	Clinical and family history
Supernumerary teeth, absent clavicles, open fontanelles	Multiple impacted teeth	Absent cellular cementum	Extractions, orthodontia	Clinical and family history Radiographic
Multiple osteomas, colon polyps, adenocarcinoma	Odontomas and osteomas in jaws	Osteoma Colorectal cancer	Surgery for polyps and/or carcinoma, odontomas, osteomas	Clinical and family history Radiographic
Hypoplastic mandible, malposed teeth, deafness	Obtuse mandibular angle, small condyle	None	Plastic surgery, orthodontia; maintenance of oral hygiene	Clinical and family history Radiographic
Multiple: odontogenic keratocysts and basal cell carcinoma	Multiple radiolucencies of the jaws; bifid rib	Review odontogenic keratocyst and basal carcinoma	Surgical removal of cysts and basal cell carcinomas	Clinical and family history Radiographic Microscopic
Blue sclera, multiple spontaneous bone fractures, multiple skeletal deformities, dentinogenesis imperfecta–like teeth	Small teeth: crowns and roots, small pulp chambers, skeletal changes	*	*	Clinical and family history Radiographic
Telangiectases, gingival bleeding	None	Capillary dilations	Care must be taken during scaling because of marked bleeding tendency	Clinical and family history
Multiple nodes on tongue tip, lips, and cheek mucosa	None	Neuromas Thyroid carcinoma Pheochromocytoma	Preventive thyroidectomy and excision of oral neurofibromas	Clinical and family history Microscopic
Multiple nodes on tongue and other mucosa	Spine anomalies Radiolucencies in the mandible	Neurofibroma	Surgical removal of neurofibromas	Clinical and family history Microscopic
Pigmented macules in perioral skin and oral mucosa	Intestinal polyps	Melanin apposition in skin and oral mucosa	Removal of intestinal polyps if needed	Clinical and family history
Bilateral whitening of buccal mucosa	None	Thick layer of orthokeratin and clear cells	Maintenance of oral hygiene	Clinical and family history Microscopic
Random pinpoint pits on labial and lingual surfaces	Enamel thinner than normal	Abnormal enamel matrix, thinner than normal	Esthetic dentistry, operative procedures	Clinical and family history
Cheesy soft enamel, rapidly lost, anterior open bite	Enamel has "moth-eaten" appearance	Enamel of normal thickness, poorly calcified	Jacket crowns, metal crowns, esthetic dentistry	Clinical and family history

Continued

Chapter 6 Synopsis—cont'd

Condition/Disease	Cause	Age/Race/Sex	Location
Amelogenesis imperfecta: hypomaturation type	AD, AR, and X-linked recessive	When teeth erupt, AD and AR, M = F X-linked, more often men	All primary and permanent teeth
Amelogenesis imperfecta: snow-capped (hypomaturation)	AD and X-linked recessive	When teeth erupt, AD, M = F X-linked, more often men	All primary and permanent teeth
Dentinogenesis imperfecta	AD, 4q13-21	When teeth erupt	All primary and permanent teeth
Radicular dentin dysplasia	AD	When teeth erupt	All primary and permanent teeth
Coronal dentin dysplasia	AD, 4q13-21	When teeth erupt	All primary teeth
Hypohidrotic ectodermal dysplasia	X-linked recessive, Xq12-13.1 AR, 2q11-13	From birth X-linked, all males AR, M = F	Skin, sweat glands, hair, both dentitions
Hypophosphatasia	AR, 1p36.1-34	From birth M = F	Bones, teeth
Hypophosphatemic vitamin D–resistant rickets	X-linked dominant	From birth More often men	Bones, teeth

AD, Autosomal dominant; AR, autosomal recessive; CL/P, cleft lip with or without cleft palate; M = F, occurs in men and women equally; G-CSF, granulocyte-colony stimulating factor.
*No significant information.

Clinical Features	Radiographic Features	Microscopic Features	Treatment	Diagnostic Process
Enamel softer than normal and chips easily	Enamel has same radiolucency as dentin	Large amounts of enamel matrix	Jacket crowns, metal crowns, esthetic dentistry	Clinical and family history
White discoloration of surface enamel of occlusal one third of all teeth	None	Not available	Esthetic dentistry if the patient wants it	Clinical and family history
Bulbous crowns, opalescent brown-bluish crowns	Short pointed roots, absent pulp chambers	Abnormal globular dentin, trapped odontoblasts	Esthetic dentistry, crowns, operative procedures	Clinical and family history
Normal crowns in size and color	Short pointed roots, absent pulp chambers	Abnormal tubular dentin and osteodentin	Prosthesis if teeth are lost	Family history Radiographic
Primary teeth amber in color, permanent teeth normal in color	Primary: absent pulp chambers Permanent molars: "bow tie" pulp Uniradicular teeth: "thistle-shaped" pulp	Abnormal dentin in primary teeth, permanent teeth with pulp stones	Regular dental and dental hygiene care	Clinical and family history Radiographic
Few teeth formed Hypotrichosis Hypohydrosis Frontal bossing Depressed nasal bridge Protuberant lips	Almost no teeth present	Reduced and abnormal sweat pores	Dental implants and/or dental prosthesis	Clinical and family history Radiographic
Premature loss of primary anterior teeth	Large pulp chambers	Absence of root cementum	Space retainers or dental prosthesis	Clinical and family history Radiographic
Multiple periapical radiolucencies (cyst, granuloma)	Large pulp chambers, large pulp horns	Abnormal globular dentin, large cracks in dentin	Endodontics and regular dental hygiene care	Clinical and family history Radiographic

7

Neoplasia

ANNE CALE JONES, JOAN ANDERSEN PHELAN, AND OLGA A.C. IBSEN

OBJECTIVES

After studying this chapter, the student will be able to:

1. Define each of the words in the vocabulary list for this chapter.
2. Describe neoplasia, including its causes.
3. Explain the classification of tumors, including the difference between a benign tumor and a malignant tumor.
4. Do the following related to the names and treatment of tumors:
   - Discuss how prefixes and suffixes are combined to form names of tumors, as well as give examples.
   - List tumors according to their tissue or cell of origin.
   - Discuss the different ways in which tumors are treated.
5. Do the following related to epithelial tumors:
   - List and describe the three different types of epithelial tumors in the oral cavity.
   - Define each of the following tumors of squamous epithelium, describe the clinical features of each, and explain how they are treated: papilloma, squamous cell carcinoma, verrucous carcinoma, and basal cell carcinoma.
   - Define and discuss leukoplakia and erythroplakia.
   - Explain the concept of epithelial dysplasia and the microscopic significance of this premalignant condition.
6. Define each of the following salivary gland tumors, describe the clinical features of each, and explain how they are treated: pleomorphic adenoma, monomorphic adenoma, mucoepidermoid carcinoma, and adenoid cystic carcinoma.
7. Define each of the following odontogenic tumors, describe the clinical features of each, and explain how they are treated: ameloblastoma, calcifying epithelial odontogenic tumor, adenomatoid odontogenic tumor, calcifying cystic odontogenic tumor, odontogenic myxoma, central cementifying and ossifying fibromas, benign cementoblastoma, ameloblastic fibroma, ameloblastic fibro-odontoma, and odontoma.
8. Define each of the following peripheral odontogenic tumors, describe the clinical features of each, and explain how they are treated: lipoma, neurofibroma, schwannoma, granular cell tumor, congenital epulis, rhabdomyosarcoma, hemangioma (benign vascular malformation), lymphangioma, and Kaposi sarcoma.
9. Define each of the following tumors of melanin-producing cells, describe the clinical features of each, and explain how they are treated: melanocytic nevi and melanoma.
10. Define each of the following tumors of bone and cartilage, describe the clinical features of each, and are treated: osteoma, osteosarcoma, chondrosarcoma, leukemia, lymphoma, and multiple myeloma.
11. Describe metastatic tumors.

◆ Vocabulary

Aberrant (ab-ar′ənt) Deviating from the usual or natural type; atypical.

Anaplastic (an″ə-plas′tik) Characterized by a loss of differentiation of cells and their orientation to one another; a characteristic of malignant tumors.

Bence Jones proteins (bens-jōnz pro′tēnz) Fragments of abnormal immunoglobulins excreted in the urine of patients with multiple myeloma.

Benign (be-nīn′) A condition that is not life threatening, not cancerous, not malignant.

Benign tumor (be-nīn′ too′mor) A tumor that is not malignant and favorable for treatment and recovery.

Carcinoma (kahr″sĭ-no′mə) Malignant tumor of the epithelium.

Central (sen′trəl) In oral pathology, describing a tumor or lesion occurring within bone.

Dysplasia (dis-pla′zhə) Disordered growth; alteration in size, shape, and organization of adult cells.

Encapsulated (en-kap′su-lāt-əd) Surrounded by a dense band of fibrous connective tissue.

Enucleation (ē-noo′klē-ā′shən) Complete surgical removal without cutting into the lesion.

Erythroplakia (ĕ-rith″ro-pla′ke-ah) A clinical term used to describe an oral mucosal lesion that appears as a smooth red patch or a granular red and velvety patch.

Excision (ek-sizh′ən) Surgical removal.

Hyperchromatic (hi″pər-kro-mat′ik) Microscopic staining that is more intense than normal.

Hyperplasia (hi″pər-pla′zhə) Abnormal increase in the number of cells in an organ or tissue.

Immunoglobulin (im″u-no-glob′u-lin) A protein, also called an *antibody*, synthesized by plasma cells in response to a specific antigen.

Idiopathic (id″e-o-path′ik) Occurring without known cause.

In situ (in si′tu) Confined to the site of origin without invasion of neighboring tissues.

Invasion (in-va′shən) Infiltration and active destruction of surrounding tissues.

Leukoplakia (loo″ko-pla′ke-ə) Clinical term used to identify a white, plaquelike lesion of the oral mucosa that cannot be wiped off or diagnosed as any other disease.

Malignant (mə-lig′nənt) Tending to produce death, able to metastasize; describing cancer.

Malignant tumor (mə-lig′nənt too′mor) Cancer; a tumor that is resistant to treatment and may cause death; a tumor that has the potential for uncontrolled growth and dissemination or recurrence, or both.

Metastasis (mə-tas′tə-sis) (plural, metastases [mə-tas′tə-sez]) Transport of neoplastic cells to parts of the body remote from the primary tumor and the establishment of new tumors at those sites.

Metastatic tumor (met″ə-stat′ik too′mor) Tumor formed by cells that have been transported from the primary tumor to sites not connected with the original tumor.

Mitotic figure (mi-tot′ik fig′ər) A term used in microscopy to describe dividing cells caught in the process of mitosis (mi-to′sis).

Monoclonal spike (mon″o-klōn′əl spīk) An elevation of a single type of immunoglobulin; detected by a process called *immunoelectrophoresis.*

Neoplasia (ne″o-pla′zhə) New growth; the formation of tumors by the uncontrolled proliferation of cells.

Neoplasm (ne′o-plaz-əm) Tumor; a new growth of tissue in which growth is uncontrolled and progressive.

Neoplastic (ne″o-plas′tik) Pertaining to the formation of tumors by the uncontrolled proliferation of cells.

Neurilemmoma (noor″ĭ-lĕ-mo′mah) A peripheral nerve sheath tumor; also called a *schwannoma.*

Nevus (ne′vəs) (plural, nevi [ne′vi]) A benign tumor consisting of melanocytes (nevus cells); also a circumscribed, usually pigmented, congenital malformation of the skin or oral mucosa.

Odontogenic (o-don″to-jen′ik) Tooth forming.

Oncology (ong-kol′ə-je) The study of tumors or neoplasms.

Pedunculated (pə-dung′ku-lāt-əd) Attached by a stalk.

Peripheral (pə-rif′ər-əl) In oral pathology, describing a lesion that occurs on the gingiva or alveolar mucosa.

Pleomorphic (ple″o-mor′fik) Occurring in various forms.

Primary tumor (pri′mar-e too′mor) Original tumor; the source of metastasis.

Sarcoma (sahr-ko′mə) Malignant tumor of the connective tissue.

Sessile (ses′il) Attached by a broad base.

Tumor (too′mor) Neoplasm; also, a swelling or enlargement.

Undifferentiated (ən-dif″ər-en′she-āt-əd) Absence of normal differentiation; anaplasia; a characteristic of some malignant tumors.

Waldeyer ring (vahl′di-er ring) A ring of lymphatic tissue formed by the two palatine tonsils, the pharyngeal tonsil, the lingual tonsil, and intervening lymphoid tissue.

Description of Neoplasia

Neoplasia means new growth. It is a process in which cells exhibit abnormal and uncontrolled proliferation. A **neoplasm** is a mass of such cells. Although the word **tumor** means swelling, it is commonly used as a synonym for a neoplasm. The study of tumors is called **oncology.** *Onco* in Greek means swelling or mass.

For neoplasia to occur, an irreversible change must take place in the cells, and this change must be passed on to new cells, resulting in uncontrolled cell multiplication. In most cases the initial stimulus that triggers the process of cell change is not known. Regulatory processes maintain the size of normal tissues. The regulatory processes that maintain the size of normal tissues do not function correctly in a neoplasm; therefore it exhibits unlimited and unregulated growth.

Unlike **hyperplasia,** neoplasia is an uncontrolled abnormal process. With hyperplasia, normal cells proliferate in a normal arrangement in response to tissue damage, and the proliferation stops when the stimulus is removed. Although the size of the tissue may be greater than normal, the growth of the tissue is still under control. Reactive lesions such as the irritation fibroma, denture-related hyperplasia (epulis fissuratum), and pyogenic granuloma are examples of hyperplasia (see Chapter 2). In contrast, neoplasia is a completely abnormal process; the cells are abnormal, and the proliferation of these cells is uncontrolled and unlimited.

Causes of Neoplasia

Many agents—principally chemicals, viruses, and radiation—have been shown to cause **neoplastic** transformation of cells in the laboratory. Hundreds of chemicals have been shown to cause cancer in animals. In addition, certain chemicals, viruses such as Epstein-Barr virus (EBV) and human papillomavirus (HPV), and radiation have been shown to cause specific types of cancer in humans. Neoplastic transformation may also occur spontaneously secondary to a genetic mutation. Viruses that cause tumors are called **oncogenic** viruses. Radiation from sunlight (ultraviolet rays), x-rays, nuclear fission, or other sources is well established as a cancer-producing agent in humans.

Classification of Tumors

Tumors are divided into two categories: **benign** and **malignant.** A **benign tumor** or neoplasm remains localized. It may be **encapsulated,** which means that it is walled off by surrounding fibrous connective tissue. Sometimes a benign tumor can invade adjacent structures, but it does not have the ability to spread to distant sites. In contrast, a **malignant tumor** invades and destroys surrounding tissue and has the ability to spread throughout the body (**metastasis**). **Cancer** is synonymous with malignancy.

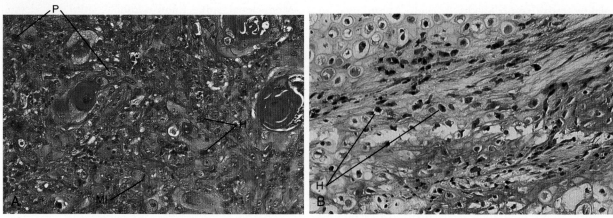

• Figure 7.1 Photomicrographs of malignant tumors show pleomorphic (P) and hyperchromatic (H) nuclei and mitotic figures (MI). **A,** Squamous cell carcinoma. **B,** Osteosarcoma.

TABLE 7.1	Comparison of Benign and Malignant Tumors	
Benign	**Malignant**
Usually well differentiated	Well differentiated to anaplastic
Usually slow growth	Slow to rapid growth
Mitotic figures are rare	Mitotic figures may be numerous
Usually encapsulated	Invasive and unencapsulated
No metastasis	Metastasis likely

TABLE 7.2	Names of Tumors	
Tissue of Origin	**Benign Tumor**	**Malignant Tumor**
Epithelium		
Squamous cells	Papilloma	Squamous cell or epidermoid carcinoma
Basal cells	Basal cell carcinoma	
Glands or ducts	Adenoma	Adenocarcinoma
Neuroectoderm		
Melanocytes	Nevus	Melanoma
Connective Tissue		
Fibrous	Fibroma	Fibrosarcoma
Cartilage	Chondroma	Chondrosarcoma
Bone	Osteoma	Osteosarcoma
Fat	Lipoma	Liposarcoma
Endothelium		
Blood vessels	Hemangioma	Angiosarcoma
Lymphatic vessels	Lymphangioma	Lymphangiosarcoma
Muscle		
Smooth muscle	Leiomyoma	Leiomyosarcoma
Striated muscle	Rhabdomyoma	Rhabdomyosarcoma

Benign tumors most often resemble normal cells, whereas malignant tumors vary in their microscopic appearance. Malignant tumors composed of neoplastic cells that resemble normal cells are called *well-differentiated tumors.* Malignant tumors may also be *poorly differentiated.* The cells of these tumors have only some of the characteristics of the tissue from which they were derived. Still others may be **undifferentiated** or **anaplastic** and do not resemble at all the tissue from which they were derived. Fig. 7.1 illustrates two examples of malignant tumors: a malignant tumor of squamous epithelium (Fig. 7.1A) and a malignant tumor of bone (Fig. 7.1B). Malignant tumors are often composed of cells that vary in size and shape **(pleomorphic)**. The nuclei of these cells are darker than those of normal cells **(hyperchromatic)** and exhibit an increased nuclear-to-cytoplasmic ratio (see Fig. 7.1). Normal and abnormal **mitotic figures** are seen in the nucleus of the neoplastic cells (see Fig. 7.1). Abnormal mitotic figures are those that are not dividing normally; therefore the shape of the dividing nucleus does not follow the shape of a normal mitotic figure. Table 7.1 compares benign and malignant tumors.

Names of Tumors

The prefix of the name of a tumor is determined by the cell or tissue of origin. The suffix *-oma* is used to indicate a tumor. The prefix of the name of a benign or malignant tumor is also determined by the cell or tissue of origin. For example, a benign tumor of fat is called a **lipoma,** and a benign tumor of bone is called an **osteoma.** Malignant tumors are named in a similar fashion. Malignant tumors of epithelial origin are called **carcinomas,** and malignant tumors of connective tissue origin are called **sarcomas.** Therefore a malignant tumor of squamous epithelium is called a **squamous cell carcinoma** or an **epidermoid carcinoma,** and a malignant tumor of bone is called an **osteosarcoma** (osteogenic sarcoma). Carcinomas are about 10 times more common than sarcomas. Table 7.2 lists tumors according to their tissue or cell of origin. The names of some malignant tumors sound like benign tumors. Lymphoma, melanoma, and myeloma sound benign, but are always malignant.

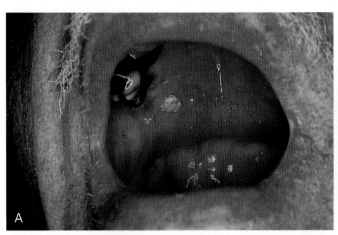
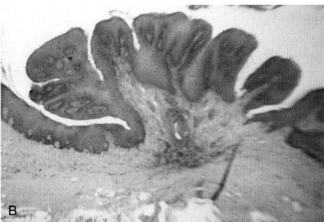

• **Figure 7.2 A,** Clinical appearance of a papilloma of the oral mucosa shows a cauliflower-like appearance and rough surface resulting from fingerlike projections. **B,** Microscopic appearance of a papilloma shows fingerlike projections surfaced by squamous epithelium and supported by thin cores of fibrous connective tissue.

Treatment of Tumors

Benign tumors generally are treated by surgical **excision,** which can be accomplished through **enucleation** or by wide local excision. Malignant tumors are treated by surgery, chemotherapy, or radiation therapy. Often a combination of two or three of these modalities is used.

Because there are many different types of tissue in the oral cavity, numerous tumors can arise in this location. These neoplasms can be either benign or malignant. In this chapter the neoplasms are classified according to their tissue of origin. Benign tumors are described first, followed by their malignant counterparts.

Epithelial Tumors

Three different types of **epithelial** tumors occur in the oral cavity: (1) tumors derived from squamous epithelium, (2) tumors derived from salivary gland epithelium, and (3) tumors derived from **odontogenic** epithelium.

Tumors of Squamous Epithelium

Papilloma

The **papilloma** is a benign tumor of squamous epithelium that arises as a small, exophytic, **pedunculated,** or **sessile** growth. These tumors are composed of numerous papillary projections that may be either white or the color of normal mucosa (Fig. 7.2A). The color of the lesion depends on the amount of surface keratin; the more keratin produced by the squamous epithelial cells, the whiter the lesion appears clinically.

They are often described as cauliflower-like in appearance. Most cases arise on the soft palate or tongue. A papilloma may occur at any age, and an equal sex predilection is noted. Microscopic examination demonstrates numerous fingerlike or papillary projections composed of normal stratified squamous epithelium surfaced by a thickened layer of keratin. A central core of fibrous connective tissue supports each papillary projection (Fig. 7.2B).

Other oral lesions that may resemble a papilloma clinically are a verruca vulgaris (common wart) and condyloma acuminatum (venereal wart). These two lesions are caused by HPV and are described in Chapter 4. They are differentiated from the papilloma by microscopic examination. Special procedures can be used to identify specific viral particles within these lesions. Evidence suggests that low-risk HPV (types 6 and 11) are involved in the etiology of oral squamous papillomas, but microscopic evidence of HPV infection is generally not present in these lesions.

A papilloma is treated by surgical excision, which must include the base of the growth. With adequate excision, the papilloma usually does not recur.

Premalignant Lesions

Leukoplakia

In any discussion of premalignant lesions of the oral mucosa, it is important to define the term **leukoplakia.** Leukoplakia is a clinical term and does not refer to a specific microscopic appearance. It is defined as a white plaquelike lesion of the oral mucosa that cannot be rubbed off and cannot be diagnosed clinically as a specific disease (Fig. 7.3A-B).

Leukoplakia is sometimes called **idiopathic** *leukoplakia* to indicate that the specific cause of the lesion is not known. The white lesion illustrated in Fig. 7.4 is more accurately called **smokeless tobacco-associated keratosis** rather than a leukoplakia because the direct cause of the lesion is known.

The microscopic appearance of leukoplakia varies; therefore a biopsy is essential to establish a definitive diagnosis. Most leukoplakias are the result of hyperkeratosis (thickening of the keratin layer) or a combination of epithelial hyperplasia (thickening of the prickle cell or spinous layer) and hyperkeratosis and are not considered premalignant. When examined microscopically, a leukoplakia may also show epithelial **dysplasia,** a premalignant condition, or even squamous cell carcinoma, a malignant tumor of squamous epithelium. Depending on the study, approximately 5% to 25% of leukoplakias examined microscopically demonstrate epithelial dysplasia. Studies have also revealed that a leukoplakia found on the floor of the mouth, ventrolateral tongue, soft

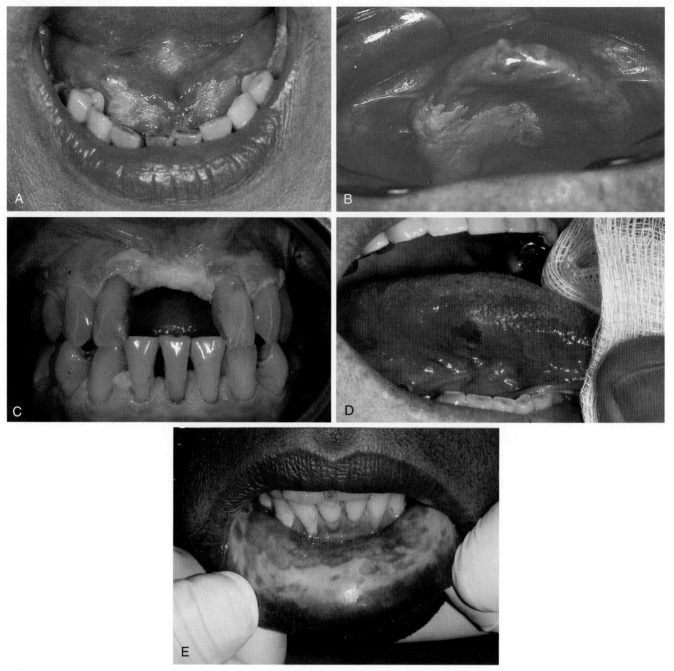

• **Figure 7.3** Clinical appearance of leukoplakia. **A,** Floor of the mouth. **B,** Maxillary alveolar mucosa and palate. The cause of these lesions could not be identified. **C,** Proliferative verrucous leukoplakia. The patient died as a result of malignant transformation to squamous cell carcinoma. **D,** Clinical appearance of eythroplakia. This case was diagnosed microscopically as squamous cell carcinoma. **E,** Oral submucous fibrosis. Fibrosis has led to limited range of motion and blanching of the oral mucosa. (**C** and **E** courtesy of Dr. A. Ross Kerr, NYU College of Dentistry. **D** reprinted with permission from SAVVY SUCCESS: Volume II: Patient Care, Flanders, NJ.)

palate, and lip is more likely to represent epithelial dysplasia or squamous cell carcinoma than leukoplakia occurring in other oral mucosal sites.

When a white lesion is identified in the oral cavity, the first goal is to identify the cause. Any associated irritation should be removed. If the lesion does not resolve, a biopsy and microscopic examination of the tissue must be performed. Any white lesion that is diagnosed as epithelial dysplasia should be completely removed. When leukoplakia is found on the floor of the mouth, ventrolateral tongue, soft palate, or lip, the lesion should be completely removed, regardless of the microscopic appearance, because there is an increased risk of squamous cell carcinoma developing in these locations.

A specific form of leukoplakia called **proliferative verrucous leukoplakia** is characterized by the development of persistent, slowly spreading, rough-surfaced, keratotic plaques (Fig. 7.3C). This type of leukoplakia persists even after surgical removal and has a high risk of the development of squamous cell carcinoma. The histopathologic characteristics of this type of leukoplakia include a verrucous surface with varying degrees of epithelial

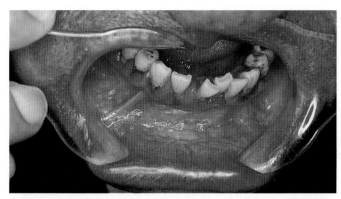

• **Figure 7.4** Clinical appearance of a white lesion that was associated with smokeless tobacco (smokeless tobacco–associated keratosis). This lesion developed on the lower labial mucosa at the site where the tobacco was held.

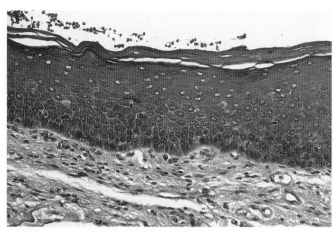

• **Figure 7.5** Microscopic appearance of epithelial dysplasia. Loss of the normal stratification of the epithelium, hyperplasia of the basal cells, and enlarged, hyperchromatic nuclei are seen.

dysplasia. Proliferative verrucous leukoplakia frequently involves the gingiva.

The treatment of leukoplakia depends on the microscopic diagnosis. The treatment of epithelial dysplasia and squamous cell carcinoma is discussed in the sections that follow.

Erythroplakia

Erythroplakia is a clinical term used to describe an oral mucosal lesion that appears as a smooth red patch or a granular red and velvety patch (see Fig. 7.3D). A lesion that shows a mixture of red and white areas is generally called **speckled leukoplakia** rather than erythroplakia. Most cases of erythroplakia occur in the floor of the mouth, tongue, and soft palate. Erythroplakia is much less common than leukoplakia. In one study 60 cases of leukoplakia were seen for every 1 case of erythroplakia. When examined microscopically, more than 90% of cases of erythroplakia demonstrate epithelial dysplasia or squamous cell carcinoma. Because of these microscopic findings, erythroplakia is considered a more serious clinical finding than leukoplakia (a biopsy must be performed to establish a definitive diagnosis). Treatment of erythroplakia depends on the microscopic diagnosis.

Oral Submucous Fibrosis

Oral submucous fibrosis is a chronic oral mucosal disease that is associated with betel-quid and areca-nut chewing. Malignant transformation of oral submucous fibrosis to squamous cell carcinoma has been reported to be between 2% and 8%. Areca-nut and betel-quid chewing is prevalent in the Indian subcontinent and Southeast Asia and among immigrants in the United States from these areas. Epithelial changes range from atrophy to hyperplasia and hyperkeratosis resulting in clinical features that vary from erythema to leukoplakia. Increased deposition of collagen in the oral mucosa results in severe restriction of movement of the oral mucosal tissues (Fig. 7.3E).

Epithelial Dysplasia

Epithelial dysplasia is a microscopic diagnosis that indicates disordered growth. It is considered a premalignant condition. Lesions that microscopically exhibit epithelial dysplasia frequently precede squamous cell carcinoma. Unlike squamous cell carcinoma, the cellular changes in epithelial dysplasia may revert to normal if the stimulus, such as tobacco smoking, is removed. Epithelial dysplasia may present clinically as an erythematous

(red) lesion (erythroplakia), a white lesion (leukoplakia), or a mixed erythematous and white lesion (speckled leukoplakia). These lesions often arise in the floor of the mouth or tongue. The term **dysplasia** may also be used to describe lesions that occur in tissues other than epithelium. These lesions are developmental and characterized by disordered growth. They are not considered premalignant lesions.

Microscopic examination of epithelial dysplasia demonstrates abnormal maturation of epithelial cells with disorganization of the epithelial layers, including hyperplasia of the basal cells, and epithelial cells with enlarged and hyperchromatic nuclei, increased nuclear-to-cytoplasmic ratios, abnormal keratinization, and increased numbers of normal and abnormal mitotic figures (Fig. 7.5). Microscopically, epithelial dysplasia differs from squamous cell carcinoma in that there is no **invasion** of the abnormal epithelial cells through the basement membrane into the underlying connective tissue. Severe dysplasia involving the full thickness of the epithelium is called carcinoma **in situ.**

All dysplastic lesions should be excised surgically. Close long-term follow-up examinations are indicated because of the potential for recurrence.

Squamous Cell Carcinoma

Squamous cell carcinoma, or epidermoid carcinoma, is a malignant tumor of squamous epithelium. It is the most common primary malignancy of the oral cavity and, like other malignant tumors, can infiltrate adjacent tissues and metastasize to distant sites. Squamous cell carcinoma usually metastasizes to lymph nodes of the neck and then to more distant sites such as the lungs and liver. Clinically, squamous cell carcinoma usually presents as an exophytic ulcerative mass (Fig. 7.6A-C), but early tumors may be white and plaquelike (leukoplakia), red and plaquelike (erythroplakia), or a mixture of red and white areas (speckled leukoplakia). Squamous cell carcinoma can infiltrate and destroy bone (Fig. 7.6D).

The essential microscopic feature of a squamous cell carcinoma is the invasion of tumor cells through the epithelial basement membrane into the underlying connective tissue (Fig. 7.7A). Invasive sheets and nests of neoplastic squamous cells characterize this tumor. Although squamous cell carcinoma is a malignant

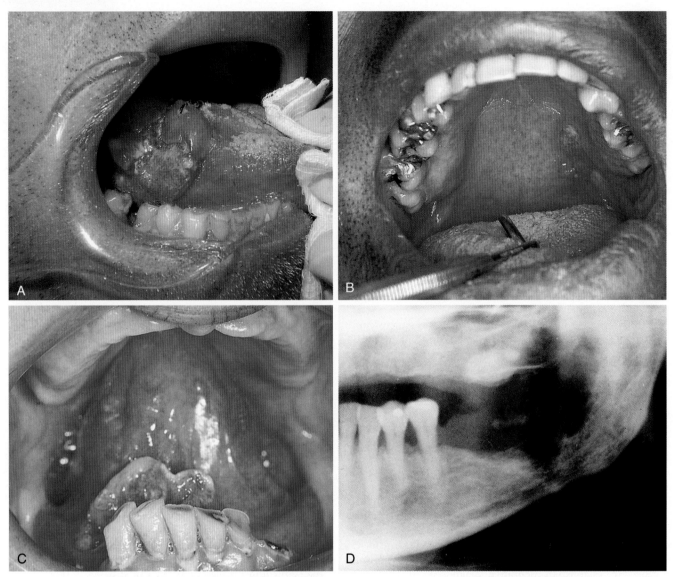

• **Figure 7.6 A,** Clinical appearance of a squamous cell carcinoma of the posterolateral tongue shows an exophytic, ulcerated mass. **B,** Clinical appearance of a squamous cell carcinoma on the left side of the soft palate and facies. **C,** Clinical appearance of a squamous cell carcinoma on the floor of the mouth. **D,** Left side of a panoramic radiograph shows destruction of the mandible by a squamous cell carcinoma. (**C** courtesy Dr. Edward V. Zegarelli.)

tumor, it often exhibits features that allow the cells to be recognized as squamous epithelial cells. In well-differentiated tumors these features are easily recognized; however, they may not be easily recognized in a poorly differentiated squamous cell carcinoma. Because keratin is a product of squamous epithelium, well-differentiated tumors show keratin formation. In addition to normal surface keratin, the keratin may be seen in individual cells within the tumor and as structures called **keratin pearls** (Fig. 7.7B). The neoplastic cells are not normal cells. They contain large hyperchromatic nuclei and numerous mitotic figures. Some of the mitotic figures appear normal, whereas others are bizarre.

Squamous cell carcinomas may occur anywhere in the oral cavity, but the most sites of involvement are the floor of the mouth, ventrolateral tongue, soft palate, and tonsillar pillar. The clinical appearance of squamous cell carcinoma occurring in several different locations is seen in Fig. 7.6.

Squamous cell carcinomas may occur on the vermilion border of the lips and skin of the face (Fig. 7.8). In this location they are associated with sun exposure (actinic cheilitis and actinic keratosis) and tend to be more common in individuals with fair skin. The prognosis for squamous cell carcinoma of the lips and skin is much better than that for squamous cell carcinoma of the oral mucosa. Sun exposure causes recognizable changes of the vermilion border of the lips. The color changes from dark and uniform to mottled grayish-pink. The interface of the vermilion border and the skin becomes blurred, and linear fissures are seen at right angles to the line of the interface. Microscopically, damage from ultraviolet rays as a result of sun exposure is seen as changes that range from degeneration of the collagen under the epithelium to a condition called **solar** or **actinic cheilitis,** in which mild-to-severe epithelial dysplasia occurs. Solar or actinic cheilitis is also described in Chapter 2. Avoidance of sun exposure and the use

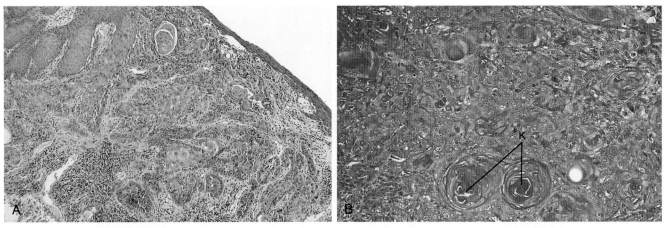

• **Figure 7.7 A,** Microscopic appearance (low power) of a squamous cell carcinoma shows infiltration of the tumor into the connective tissue. **B,** High-power photomicrograph shows abnormal keratinization and keratin pearls (K).

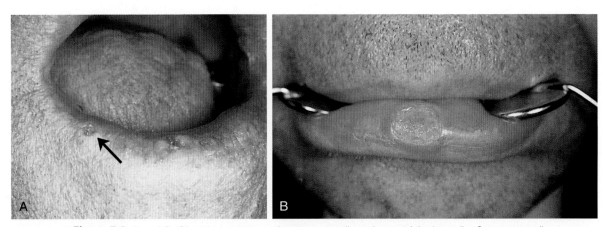

• **Figure 7.8 A and B,** Clinical appearance of squamous cell carcinoma of the lower lip. Squamous cell carcinoma (*arrow*) is seen with actinic (solar) cheilitis in **(A).** (Courtesy Dr. Edward V. Zegarelli.)

of a sun-blocking agent are important in preventing the damaging effects of sunlight.

The majority of squamous cell carcinomas occur in patients over 40 years of age. In the past, more men than women have developed squamous cell carcinoma; however, in the last 30 years there has been an increased incidence of squamous cell carcinoma in women. This is most likely a result of the increased number of women who smoke and the fact that women outnumber men in older age groups.

Risk Factors

Several risk factors have been associated with the development of squamous cell carcinoma. The cause of oral squamous cell carcinoma is multifactorial; more than a single factor is needed to produce malignancy. The most significant is tobacco—including cigar, pipe, and cigarette smoking; snuff dipping; and tobacco chewing. The proportion of smokers is much higher among patients with oral squamous cell carcinoma than among the general population. Alcohol consumption appears to add to the risk of oral squamous cell carcinoma, especially in individuals who also use tobacco products. High-risk types of HPV have been identified in squamous cell carcinomas of the oropharynx and have been suggested to be important factors in the pathogenesis of these cancers. HPV 16 has been identified in more than 90%

of HPV-positive oropharyngeal carcinomas. There is evidence that HPV contributes to the transformation of normal epithelial cells into malignant epithelial cells (HPV infection is discussed in Chapter 4). There is no evidence that chronic irritation (e.g., an ill-fitting denture) is an initiating factor in the development of oral cancer. As described earlier, chronic exposure to ultraviolet light (sunlight) results in actinic cheilitis and increases the risk of squamous cell carcinoma of the lips (particularly the lower lip).

Treatment and Prognosis

Squamous cell carcinoma generally is treated by surgical excision. Radiation therapy or chemotherapy may be used in combination with surgery. On occasion, radiation therapy is used alone. The prognosis of squamous cell carcinoma is related to the size and location of the tumor and the presence or absence of metastases. The smaller the tumor is at the time of treatment, the better the prognosis. For oral squamous cell carcinoma, determining the size of the tumor and the presence or absence of cervical lymph node involvement and distant **metastasis** is important in predicting the patient's prognosis. These are assessed using a system called the **TNM staging system;** the higher the stage, the worse the prognosis (Box 7.1 and Table 7.3). Metastasis to cervical lymph nodes is associated with a much poorer prognosis, as is the presence of distant metastasis. Therefore it is important to clinically

T: Tumor

T_1: Tumor less than 2 cm in diameter
T_2: Tumor 2 to 4 cm in diameter
T_3: Tumor larger than 4 cm in diameter
T_4: Tumor invading adjacent structures

N: Node

N_0: No palpable nodes
N_1: Ipsilateral (same side as primary tumor) palpable nodes (same side as tumor)
N_2: Contralateral (opposite side from primary tumor) or bilateral nodes
N_3: Fixed palpable nodes

M: Metastasis

M_0: No distant metastasis
M_1: Clinical or radiographic evidence of metastasis

Adapted from International Union against Cancer: TNM classification of malignant tumours (Sobin LH, Wittekind C, eds.), ed 6, New York, Wiley-Liss, 2002.

TABLE 7.3 **TNM Staging System**

Stage	Tumor	Node	Metastasis
I	T_1	N_0	M_0
II	T_2	N_0	M_0
III	T_3	N_0	M_0
	T_1	N_1	M_0
	T_2	N_1	M_0
	T_3	N_1	M_0
IV	T_1	N_2	M_0
	T_2	N_2	M_0
	T_3	N_2	M_0
	T_1	N_3	M_0
	T_2	N_3	M_0
	T_3	N_3	M_0
	T_4	N_0	M_0

Stage IV includes any patients with M_1.

Adapted from International Union against Cancer: TNM classification of malignant tumours (Sobin LH, Wittekind C, eds.), ed 6, New York, Wiley-Liss, 2002.

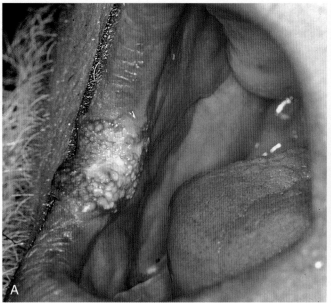
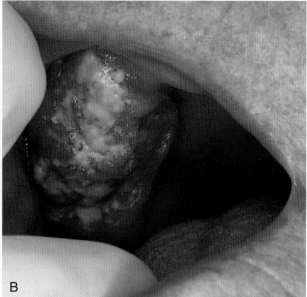

• **Figure 7.9** **A,** Clinical appearance of a verrucous carcinoma occurring on the commissure and anterior buccal mucosa. **B,** Maxillary alveolar ridge.

identify asymptomatic areas of leukoplakia and erythroplakia while they are small and to remove all potentially premalignant lesions. Compared with patients with HPV-negative squamous cell carcinoma, patients with HPV-positive tumors have been reported to have a better response to radiation therapy and chemotherapy.

Patients who have undergone radiation therapy for malignant tumors of the head and neck often experience severe xerostomia (dry mouth) as a result of radiation damage to salivary gland tissue. These patients require preventive dental care consisting of nutritional counseling, topical fluoride application, and meticulous home care. Oral manifestations of therapy for oral cancer are discussed in Chapter 9.

Verrucous Carcinoma

Verrucous carcinoma is a specific type of squamous cell carcinoma that is separated from other squamous cell carcinomas because it has a much better prognosis. Verrucous means "wart-like." Clinically, it appears as a slow-growing exophytic tumor with a pebbly white and red surface (Fig. 7.9). Most cases occur in men over 55 years of age and involve the vestibule and buccal mucosa. The use of smokeless tobacco products has been associated with the development of verrucous carcinoma. Microscopic examination demonstrates a tumor composed of numerous papillary epithelial proliferations. The spaces between these papillary projections are filled with keratin (keratin plugging). The

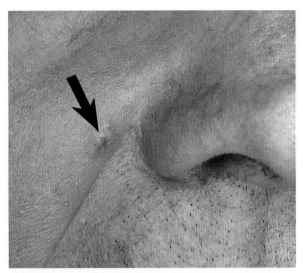

• **Figure 7.10** Clinical appearance of a basal cell carcinoma (*arrow*), illustrating the characteristic "rolled" borders.

epithelium is well differentiated, does not contain atypical cells, and exhibits broad-based rete pegs that penetrate deeply into the connective tissue. The epithelial basement membrane is intact, and the tumor does not show invasion of tumor cells through the basement membrane, as is seen in squamous cell carcinoma. This is the reason that verrucous carcinoma has a better prognosis compared with squamous cell carcinoma.

Verrucous carcinoma is treated by surgical excision. Although it is a carcinoma, it usually does not metastasize; therefore the prognosis is better for verrucous carcinoma than for squamous cell carcinoma. However, if it is not treated, it can cause extensive local damage; there is also a risk of the development of infiltrating squamous cell carcinoma. Close long-term follow-up examinations are necessary for patients with this condition.

Basal Cell Carcinoma

Basal cell carcinoma is a malignant skin tumor associated with sun exposure. This particular neoplasm does not occur in the oral cavity. Basal cell carcinoma frequently arises on the skin of the face and appears as a nonhealing ulcer with characteristic rolled borders (Fig. 7.10). The ulcer develops a crusted surface that suggests healing, but the ulcer persists. A basal cell carcinoma begins as a small 0.5-cm ulcer but will continue to enlarge slowly with destruction of underlying structures; metastasis is extremely rare. Most cases occur in white adults, especially those with fair complexions, blond or red hair, and blue or green eyes. There is no sex predilection.

A basal cell carcinoma is composed of a proliferation of basal cells derived from the surface stratified squamous epithelium. Microscopic examination demonstrates nests and islands of basal epithelial cells in the underlying connective tissue. In most cases the tumor cells are well differentiated.

Basal cell carcinoma is a locally invasive tumor that can become quite large and disfiguring if it is not removed. Surgical excision is the treatment of choice, and radiation therapy may be used to treat large lesions. Only rarely does a basal cell carcinoma metastasize. As a general rule, a patient should be referred to an oral and maxillofacial surgeon or dermatologist to have a biopsy performed on any nonhealing ulcer of the skin or lips that has been present for more than 2 weeks.

Salivary Gland Tumors

Benign and malignant tumors may arise in either the major or minor salivary glands. Tumors may occur within the parotid, submandibular, or sublingual glands; or they may involve any of the minor salivary glands located throughout the oral cavity. Intraorally, minor salivary gland tumors are located most commonly at the junction of the hard and soft palates. They may also occur on the labial and buccal mucosa, the retromolar area, the floor of the mouth, and rarely on the tongue (Fig. 7.11). Tumors of minor salivary gland origin are much more common in the upper lip than in the lower lip.

Because the origin of these tumors is glandular epithelium, benign tumors of salivary gland origin are called **adenomas.** Although some malignant salivary gland tumors are called **adenocarcinomas,** most have more specific names such as adenoid cystic carcinoma and mucoepidermoid carcinoma. All salivary gland tumors are diagnosed on the basis of their microscopic appearance. A biopsy and microscopic examination of the tissue are required to establish a specific diagnosis.

Pleomorphic Adenoma (Benign Mixed Tumor)

The **pleomorphic adenoma** is a benign salivary gland tumor. It is the most common salivary gland neoplasm and accounts for about 90% of all benign salivary gland tumors. Microscopic examination reveals an encapsulated tumor composed of tissue that appears to be a mixture of both epithelium and connective tissue (Fig. 7.12). For this reason this tumor is often called a **benign mixed tumor.** The connective tissue–like part can vary from loose and dense fibrous connective tissue with a myxoid appearance to tissue that resembles cartilage. The tissue that looks like connective tissue is derived from a salivary gland cell called a **myoepithelial cell.**

The most common extraoral location for the pleomorphic adenoma is the parotid gland. The most common intraoral site is the palate. However, these tumors may occur wherever salivary gland tissue is present. Clinically, the pleomorphic adenoma appears as a slowly enlarging, nonulcerated, painless, dome-shaped mass (see Fig. 7.11A and C). The surface can be ulcerated if traumatized. Its size can range from a few to several centimeters. Most pleomorphic adenomas occur in individuals over 40 years of age, and a female predilection has been noted. Pleomorphic adenomas have also been reported in children.

A pleomorphic adenoma is treated by surgical excision. The extent of the surgery depends on the location of the tumor. Clinicians treat parotid gland tumors by removing the part of the parotid gland (partial parotidectomy) containing the tumor, whereas minor salivary gland tumors are treated by more conservative surgical excision. A pleomorphic adenoma grows by extension of projections of tumor into the surrounding tissue. Therefore some tumors are difficult to remove completely. Recurrence rates vary and are related to the adequacy of the initial surgical removal. A small percentage (2% to 4%) of long-standing pleomorphic adenomas have been reported to undergo malignant transformation; this occurrence is known as a **carcinoma ex (arising in a) pleomorphic adenoma.**

Monomorphic Adenomas

The term **monomorphic adenoma** has been used for a group of benign encapsulated salivary gland tumors that occur less

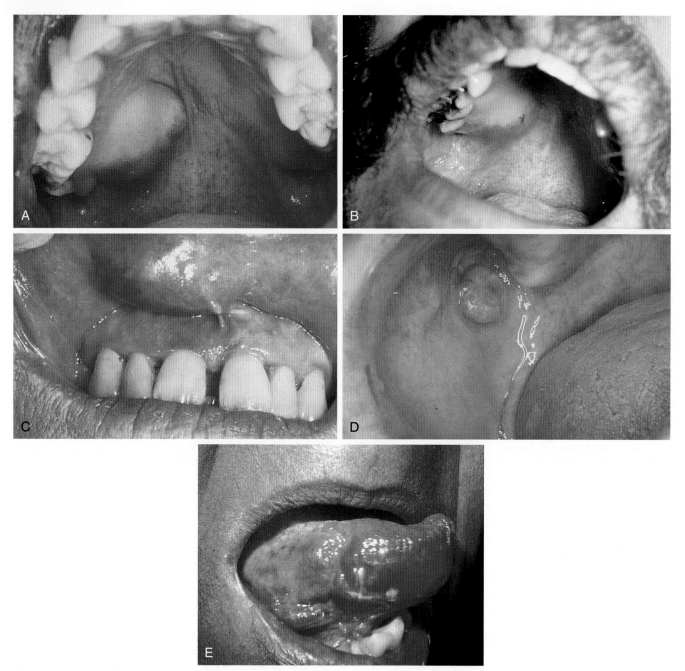

• **Figure 7.11** **A,** Benign salivary gland tumor of the palate (pleomorphic adenoma). **B,** Malignant salivary gland tumor of the palate (adenoid cystic carcinoma). Biopsy site should be noted. **C,** Benign salivary gland tumor of the upper lip (pleomorphic adenoma). **D,** Malignant salivary gland tumor of the buccal mucosa (mucoepidermoid carcinoma). **E,** Malignant salivary gland tumor of the tongue (adenoid cystic carcinoma).

frequently than pleomorphic adenoma. They are composed of a uniform pattern of epithelial cells (Fig. 7.13). These tumors do not have the connective tissue–like component seen in a pleomorphic adenoma. Recently more specific names rather than monomorphic adenoma have been used for this group of tumors. **Canalicular** and **basal cell adenoma** are monomorphic-type adenomas that are named for the microscopic pattern of the tumor. These tumors occur most commonly in adult women, with a predilection for the upper lip and buccal mucosa. A **papillary cystadenoma lymphomatosum** is another benign, encapsulated

salivary gland tumor with a distinctive uniform histopathologic pattern It is also called a **Warthin tumor.** Microscopic examination of this particular variant demonstrates an encapsulated tumor composed of two types of tissue: epithelial and lymphoid (Fig. 7.14). The epithelial component is neoplastic. It lines papillary projections that protrude into cystic structures. Sheets of lymphocytes surround the cystic structures. In some cases the lymphoid component demonstrates germinal center formation. A Warthin tumor presents as a painless, soft, and compressible or fluctuant mass, almost always located in the parotid gland. This tumor often

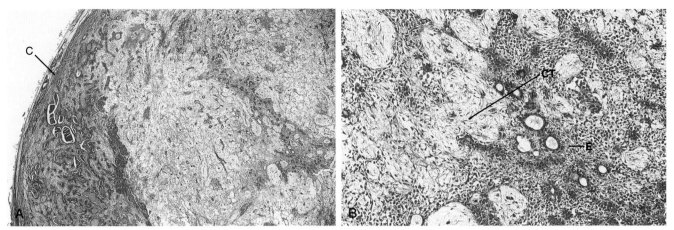

• **Figure 7.12** Microscopic appearance of a pleomorphic adenoma. **A,** Low-power photomicrograph shows a capsule (C). **B,** High-power photomicrograph shows a mixture of epithelium (E) and connective tissue (CT).

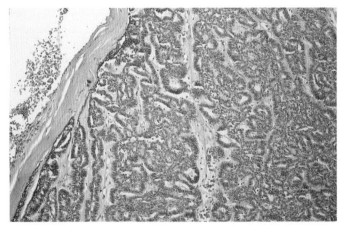

• **Figure 7.13** Microscopic appearance (low power) of a portion of a monomorphic adenoma shows a capsule and a uniform pattern of epithelial cells.

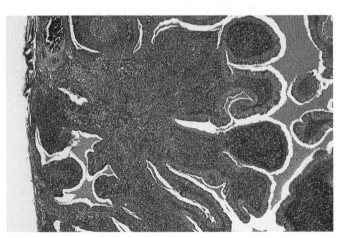

• **Figure 7.14** Microscopic appearance of a portion of a papillary cystadenoma lymphomatosum (Warthin tumor) shows spaces lined by epithelium and surrounded by sheets of lymphocytes.

develops bilaterally and occurs predominantly in adult men. A higher incidence it noted in individuals who smoke. Intraoral examples are very rare.

Canalicular adenoma, basal cell adenoma, and papillary cystadenoma lymphomatosum (Warthin tumor) are treated by surgical excision. Recurrence is rare.

Adenoid Cystic Carcinoma (Cylindroma)

The **adenoid cystic carcinoma** (see Fig. 7.11E) is a malignant tumor of salivary gland origin that can originate from either major or minor salivary gland tissue. It is unencapsulated and infiltrates surrounding tissue. This tumor is composed of small, deeply staining, uniform epithelial cells arranged in perforated round-to-oval islands. The microscopic appearance of adenoid cystic carcinoma has been likened to that of Swiss cheese (Fig. 7.15). These round and oval islands represent cylinders of tumor; therefore this tumor has also been called a **cylindroma.** Although it is malignant, pleomorphic cells and mitotic figures are rarely seen. Malignancy is recognized on the basis of the unique microscopic features. The adenoid cystic carcinoma is a slow-growing malignant tumor.

The most common extraoral site for an adenoid cystic carcinoma is the parotid gland. The most common intraoral site is the palate. Most tumors appear as slowly growing masses that can exhibit surface ulceration (see Fig. 7.11B and E). Pain is often present, even before the swelling, because of the tendency of these tumors to surround nerves. Adenoid cystic carcinoma is more common in women than in men and is a tumor of adults; the majority of cases are diagnosed in the fifth and sixth decades of life.

The treatment of choice for adenoid cystic carcinoma is complete surgical excision. Radiation treatment has been attempted and has been shown to be of benefit in some cases. However, recurrence and persistent local invasion are common. Metastasis occurs late in the course of the disease. About 30% of patients experience cervical lymph node involvement. Distant metastases, most often involving the lungs, may occur after many years. In these cases the prognosis is poor.

Mucoepidermoid Carcinoma

Mucoepidermoid carcinoma is a malignant salivary gland tumor. It is an unencapsulated, infiltrating tumor composed of a combination of mucous cells interspersed with squamouslike epithelial cells called **epidermoid cells** (Fig. 7.16). Most studies show that the mucoepidermoid carcinoma represents the most common malignant salivary gland neoplasm.

Mucoepidermoid carcinomas involving the major glands occur most often in the parotid gland, whereas minor gland tumors are most common on the palate. Mucoepidermoid carcinomas may also occur in other intraoral locations, but much less commonly than the palate. They appear clinically as slowly enlarging masses (see Fig. 7.11D). On occasion, a mucoepidermoid carcinoma may arise centrally within bone (Fig. 7.16B), usually in the mandibular premolar and molar region. In this location it appears as either a unilocular or multilocular radiolucency (Fig. 7.16B). A central mucoepidermoid carcinoma is derived from either salivary gland tissue trapped within bone or the transformed epithelial lining of a dentigerous cyst (a developmental odontogenic cyst that forms around the crown of an unerupted or impacted tooth; see Chapter 5).

A mucoepidermoid carcinoma may occur over a wide age range. Although it usually occurs in adults after middle age, this tumor is the most common malignant salivary gland neoplasm in children. A female predilection is noted.

Treatment of a mucoepidermoid carcinoma depends on the location, size, and histopathologic features and consists of complete surgical excision, with close, long-term follow-up for signs of recurrence and metastasis. Neck dissection is indicated if patients have clinical evidence of metastasis to cervical lymph nodes. Radiation therapy may be used for high-grade (more anaplastic) tumors. The behavior of any one tumor is difficult to predict and is related to the microscopic appearance of the tumor. Low-grade tumors have a 92% 5-year survival rate after initial treatment. For high-grade tumors, only 49% of patients survive 5 years after the initial treatment.

Other Malignant Salivary Gland Tumors

In addition to the adenoid cystic and mucoepidermoid carcinomas, several other malignant salivary gland tumors exist, including polymorphous low-grade adenocarcinoma (lobular carcinoma), acinic cell adenocarcinoma, and other adenocarcinomas not otherwise specified.

Odontogenic Tumors

Odontogenic tumors are derived from tooth-forming tissues. Tooth formation results from an interaction between odontogenic epithelium and odontogenic mesenchyme. Some odontogenic tumors are composed of epithelium only, some are composed of mesenchymal tissue only, and others are composed of a mixture of both elements. Most odontogenic tumors are benign. Malignant odontogenic tumors occur but are rare. Table 7.4 presents a

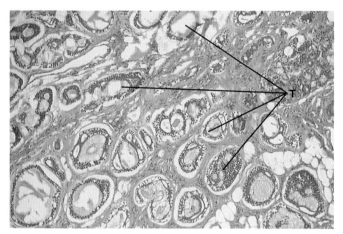

• **Figure 7.15** Microscopic appearance of an adenoid cystic carcinoma shows perforated islands of uniform cells. Tumor (T) is seen infiltrating the adjacent adipose tissue.

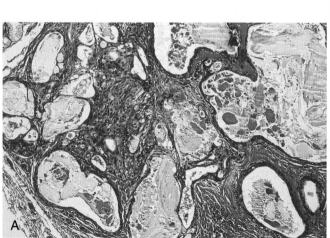

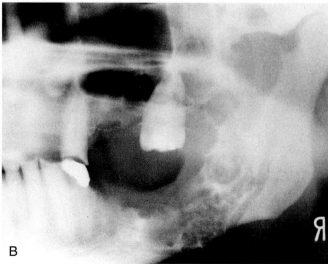

• **Figure 7.16 A,** Microscopic appearance (low power) of a mucoepidermoid carcinoma shows cystic structures, mucous cells, and epidermoid cells. **B,** Radiograph of a central mucoepidermoid carcinoma shows a multilocular radiolucency.

TABLE 7.4 Classification of Central Odontogenic Tumors		
Epithelial Odontogenic Tumors	**Mesenchymal Odontogenic Tumors**	**Mixed Odontogenic Tumors**
Ameloblastoma	Odontogenic myxoma	Ameloblastic fibroma
Calcifying epithelial odontogenic tumor (CEOT)	Cementifying fibroma	Ameloblastic fibro-odontoma
Adenomatoid odontogenic tumor (AOT)	Ossifying fibroma	Odontoma
Calcifying cystic odontogenic tumor	Cementoblastoma	

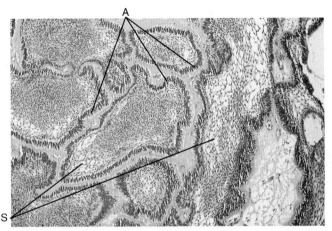

• **Figure 7.17** Microscopic appearance (low power) of a follicular ameloblastoma shows dental follicle–like islands composed of epithelial cells consisting of peripheral ameloblast-like cells (A) and stellate reticulum–like areas (S).

classification scheme for odontogenic tumors based on the derivation of the odontogenic tissue.

Epithelial Odontogenic Tumors

Ameloblastoma

The **ameloblastoma** is a benign, slow-growing but locally aggressive epithelial odontogenic tumor that may arise in either the maxilla or the mandible. It is an unencapsulated tumor that infiltrates into surrounding tissue and can cause extensive destruction. When it occurs in the maxilla, death can result from direct extension into the brain and adjacent vital structures. An ameloblastoma is composed of ameloblast-like epithelial cells that surround areas resembling stellate reticulum. These cells are arranged in either dental follicle–like islands or interconnecting strands (Fig. 7.17).

The classic radiographic appearance of an ameloblastoma is a multilocular soap bubble–like or honeycombed radiolucency (Fig. 7.18). In smaller tumors the radiolucency may be unilocular. An ameloblastoma may arise anywhere in the jaws and can occur in association with a dentigerous cyst (Fig. 7.19). However, 80% of ameloblastomas arise in the mandible, most often in the molar and ramus area. The molar area is also the most common location when they occur in the maxilla. The tumor may cause expansion of bone. The initial presentation is usually that of a slowly developing, asymptomatic swelling of the affected bone. The age range

of individuals affected is broad, but most ameloblastomas occur in adults. No sex predilection is noted.

Ameloblastomas are treated by complete surgical removal. Recurrence is common. On occasion, these tumors occur in the gingiva and do not involve bone, in which case they are called **peripheral ameloblastomas.** These are also treated by surgical excision and differ from the central ameloblastomas in that they generally do not recur.

Calcifying Epithelial Odontogenic Tumor

The **calcifying epithelial odontogenic tumor,** also known as a **Pindborg tumor,** is a benign epithelial odontogenic tumor that occurs much less frequently than the ameloblastoma. It is a unique odontogenic tumor because the proliferating cells do not resemble odontogenic epithelium. The tumor is composed of islands and sheets of polyhedral (multisided) epithelial cells. Deposits similar to amyloid are seen in the tumor, and calcifications are seen within these deposits. The amyloid-like material is thought to represent a form of abnormal enamel protein (Fig. 7.20A). Radiographically, a calcifying epithelial odontogenic tumor appears as a unilocular or multilocular radiolucency (Fig. 7.20B). Calcifications that form within the tumor appear as radiopacities within the radiolucency.

The majority of patients affected with this tumor are adults. However, the calcifying epithelial odontogenic tumor affects a broad age range that extends from young adults to elderly individuals. No sex predilection is noted. Reports of this tumor occurring in the mandible are twice as common as reports of it occurring in the maxilla. Although it can occur anywhere in the maxilla or mandible, the bicuspid and molar areas are the most common locations.

Treatment of a calcifying epithelial odontogenic tumor depends on the size and location of the tumor and involves complete surgical excision. Recurrence has been reported, but the recurrence rate is lower than that for an ameloblastoma.

Adenomatoid Odontogenic Tumor

The **adenomatoid odontogenic tumor** (AOT) is an encapsulated, benign epithelial odontogenic tumor that has a distinctive age, sex, and site distribution. It also differs from the other epithelial odontogenic tumors in that it does not recur. Approximately 70% of AOTs occur in females under the age of 20, and 70% involve the anterior maxilla and mandible. The maxilla is more commonly involved than the mandible. Many AOTs are associated with the crown of an unerupted tooth, commonly impacted canines. Although a localized swelling may be present, most are asymptomatic and are discovered on a routine radiographic examination.

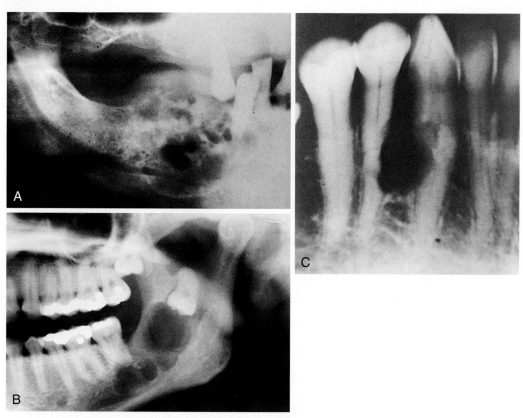

• **Figure 7.18** **A and B,** Radiographs of ameloblastomas showing multilocular radiolucencies in the molar area of the mandible. **C,** Radiograph of an ameloblastoma shows a small but multilocular radiolucency in the mandibular cuspid and bicuspid region.

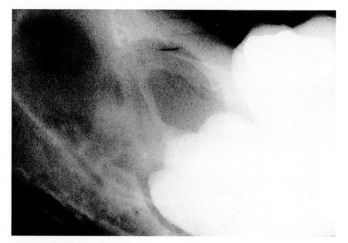

• **Figure 7.19** Radiograph of an ameloblastoma that formed in association with an impacted tooth and dentigerous cyst.

Radiographically, an AOT appears as a well-circumscribed radiolucency (Fig. 7.21B). Because of the frequent association with an impacted tooth, an AOT often simulates a dentigerous cyst. However, unlike the dentigerous cyst, the AOT extends beyond the cemento-enamel junction and can involve 50% to 60% of the root. As calcifications form within the tumor, radiopaque areas of varying size are visible on radiographs.

Microscopic examination reveals a dense, fibrous connective tissue capsule surrounding ductlike structures, whorls, and large masses of cuboidal and spindle-shaped epithelial cells (Fig. 7.21A). The ductlike structures are one of the distinctive features of this tumor and are the reason for the name **adenomatoid,** or glandlike. These structures are not ducts but actually ameloblast-like cells that resemble ducts because of their circular arrangement. Eosinophilic material is seen in the centers of these structures, and calcifications also form in this tumor.

The clinician should treat an AOT conservatively by enucleation. The tumor is removed in its entirety because it is easily separated from the surrounding bone. Recurrence is rare.

Calcifying Odontogenic Cyst (Calcifying Cystic Odontogenic Tumor)

The calcifying odontogenic cyst is part of a group of lesions that are characterized by odontogenic epithelium–containing "ghost" cells. The World Health Organization classification includes this group of lesions as odontogenic tumors. The cystic variant of these ghost cell lesions accounts for the majority of these and is commonly called the *calcifying odontogenic cyst.* The solid variants are called *ghost cell tumors.* The calcifying odontogenic cyst affects a broad age range, but is most commonly seen in individuals younger than 40 years of age. No significant sex predilection is noted, and lesions occur equally in the maxilla and mandible.

Microscopic examination usually reveals a cystic structure lined by odontogenic epithelium with an associated and

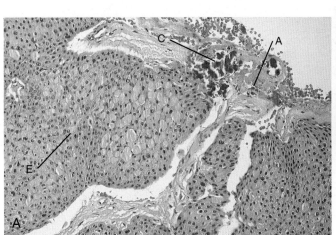

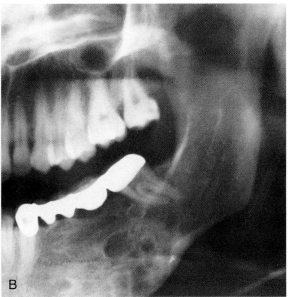

• **Figure 7.20** Calcifying epithelial odontogenic tumor. **A,** Microscopic appearance (low power) of a calcifying epithelial odontogenic tumor shows sheets of epithelial cells (E), amorphous material (A), and calcifications (C). **B,** Radiograph of a calcifying epithelial odontogenic tumor shows a multilocular radiolucency.

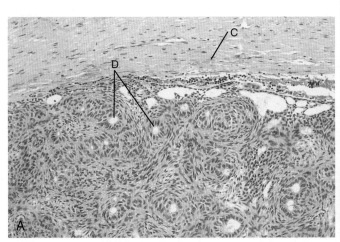

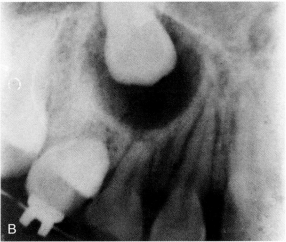

• **Figure 7.21** Adenomatoid odontogenic tumor. **A,** Microscopic appearance of a portion of an adenomatoid odontogenic tumor shows the capsule (C), epithelial cells, and ductlike structures (D). **B,** Radiograph of an adenomatoid odontogenic tumor shows a unilocular radiolucency surrounding the crown of an unerupted maxillary cuspid. (Note that the radiolucency extends beyond the cemento-enamel junction.)

characteristic ghost cell keratinization (Fig. 7.22A). The epithelium resembles that seen in an ameloblastoma, consisting of ameloblast-like cells and stellate reticulum–like areas. The ghost cells that are characteristic of this lesion exhibit a clear central area. They are thought to represent degenerating epithelial cells or an **aberrant** (atypical) form of keratinization. The solid variant is similar to the cystic variant with the absence of a defined cystic structure.

The calcifying odontogenic cyst presents radiographically as a well-defined, unilocular or multilocular radiolucency (Fig. 7.22B). Calcifications can occur and are seen as radiopaque areas within the radiolucency.

A calcifying odontogenic cyst is treated by surgical enucleation. Although a few recurrences have been reported, they usually do not recur. The solid variant may exhibit more aggressive behavior and should be treated by a more extensive surgical procedure.

Mesenchymal Odontogenic Tumors

Odontogenic Myxoma

The **odontogenic myxoma** is a benign mesenchymal odontogenic tumor that occurs most often in individuals between 10 and 29 years of age. No sex predilection is noted.

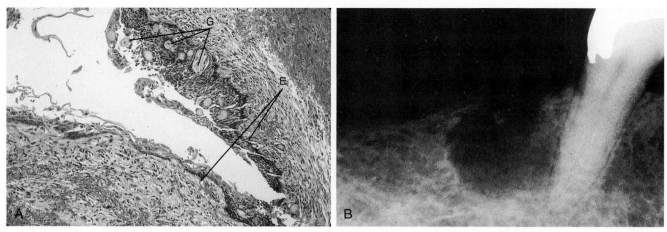

• **Figure 7.22** Calcifying odontogenic cyst. **A,** Microscopic appearance of a calcifying odontogenic cyst shows a cystic structure lined by odontogenic epithelium (E) with associated ghost cells (G). **B,** Radiograph of a calcifying odontogenic cyst shows a unilocular radiolucency of the mandible.

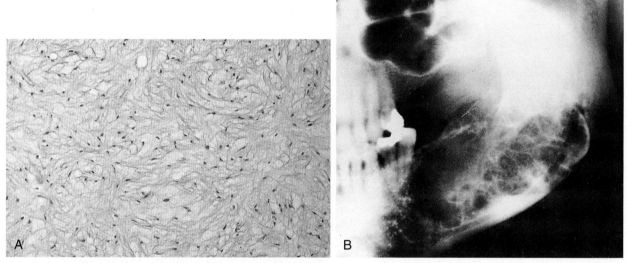

• **Figure 7.23** **A,** Photomicrograph of an odontogenic myxoma shows background substance containing widely dispersed cells with long cytoplasmic processes. **B,** Radiograph of an odontogenic myxoma shows a multilocular, honeycombed radiolucency.

Radiographically, the odontogenic myxoma may appear unilocular or multilocular, but most often presents as a multilocular, honeycombed radiolucency. The radiographic margins may be scalloped or may be poorly defined (Fig. 7.23B). The tumor may become quite large and cause tooth displacement. Although most cases occur in the posterior mandible, the odontogenic myxoma may arise anywhere in the maxilla or mandible. Microscopic examination reveals a nonencapsulated infiltrating tumor composed of a pale-staining mucopolysaccharide ground substance that contains dispersed cells with long cytoplasmic processes (Fig. 7.23A). This tissue closely resembles tissue seen in the dental papilla, the mesenchymal component of tooth-forming tissue.

The odontogenic myxoma is treated by complete surgical excision. The extent of the surgery depends on the size of the tumor. The recurrence rate is approximately 25%, and most recurrences take place within 2 years of treatment.

Central Cementifying Fibroma and Central Ossifying Fibroma

The **central cementifying fibroma** and **central ossifying fibroma** are benign, well-circumscribed tumors classified as fibro-osseous lesions. They are considered variants of the same neoplasm because they are both composed of fibrous connective tissue and calcifications. In the central cementifying fibroma the calcifications are rounded and globular and are considered to be cementoid material (Fig. 7.24A), whereas in the central ossifying fibroma the calcifications more closely resemble bone trabeculae. Some tumors have a mixture of globular calcifications resembling cementum and bone trabeculae. These tumors are called **central cemento-ossifying fibromas.** This particular variant results from the potential of periodontal ligament cells to produce either cementum or bone.

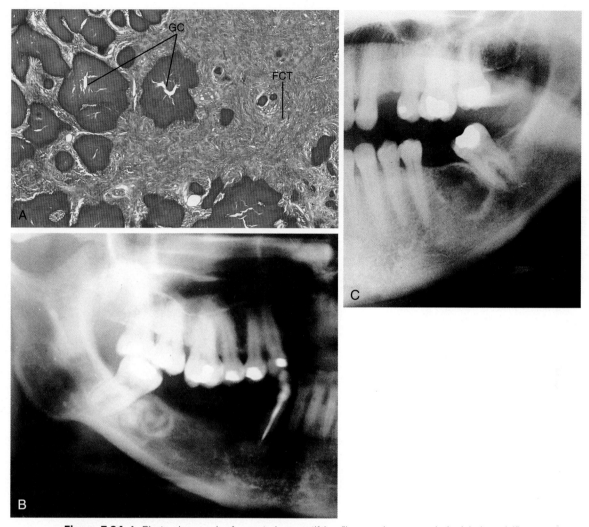

• **Figure 7.24** **A,** Photomicrograph of a central cementifying fibroma shows rounded, globular calcifications (GC) and cellular fibrous connective tissue (FCT). **B,** Radiograph of a central cementifying fibroma shows a radiolucent and radiopaque lesion. **C,** Radiograph of a central cementifying fibroma shows a well-circumscribed radiolucent lesion.

The tumor usually occurs in adults in the third and fourth decades of life. Women are affected more often than men. Affected patients may be asymptomatic or demonstrate bone expansion or facial asymmetry. Radiographically, central cementifying fibroma and central ossifying fibroma are well defined and demonstrate a radiolucent-to-radiopaque appearance, depending on the amount of calcified tissue that is present (Fig. 7.24B-C). The neoplasms tend to have a circular appearance and grow circumferentially as they increase in size. The majority of cases occur in the mandible.

Other benign fibro-osseous lesions, such as periapical cemento-osseous dysplasia and fibrous dysplasia, may be histologically identical to central cementifying fibroma and central ossifying fibroma. The radiographic appearance of each of these lesions is important in distinguishing them from one another. Benign fibro-osseous lesions are described in Chapter 8.

Central cementifying fibroma and central ossifying fibroma are treated by surgical excision. Because these lesions are well delineated, they separate easily from the surrounding bone. Recurrence is rare.

Cementoblastoma

The **cementoblastoma** is a benign cementum-producing neoplasm that is fused to the root or roots of a vital tooth. It has been called a "true cementoma." The tumor typically occurs in young adults; most cementoblastomas occur in patients under 30 years of age. Unlike other odontogenic tumors, pain is a frequent symptom. The radiographic appearance is distinctive and consists of a well-defined radiopaque mass fused to the tooth root surrounded by a radiolucent halo (Fig. 7.25). The radiolucent halo represents the periodontal ligament. Early in its development this lesion may be radiolucent and mimic inflammatory periapical disease. The neoplasm is usually seen in continuity with the root or roots of a mandibular molar or premolar tooth. Obliteration of the apex of the affected tooth is common. Occasional cases may cause localized bone expansion. Microscopic examination reveals a proliferation of cellular cementum fused to the root or roots of the affected tooth.

Treatment of the cementoblastoma consists of enucleation of the tumor and removal of the involved tooth. It does not recur.

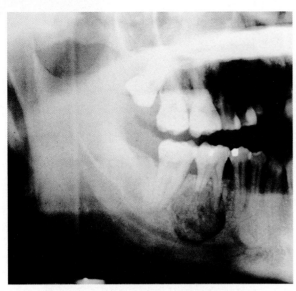

• **Figure 7.25** Radiograph of a benign cementoblastoma shows a well-circumscribed radiopaque mass surrounded by a radiolucent halo and attached to the roots of a mandibular first molar.

Mixed Odontogenic Tumors

Ameloblastic Fibroma

The **ameloblastic fibroma** is a benign, mixed odontogenic tumor that consists of both epithelium and mesenchymal tissue. It occurs in young children and adults. Most cases occur in individuals younger than 20 years of age. A male sex predilection is noted. The most common location is the mandibular bicuspid and molar region. Most patients are asymptomatic, but bone expansion or swelling may be noted. Radiographically, the ameloblastic fibroma appears as either a well-defined or poorly defined unilocular or multilocular radiolucency (Fig. 7.26B).

Histologic examination demonstrates a nonencapsulated odontogenic tumor composed of strands and small islands of ameloblast-like epithelial cells set in myxoid tissue that resembles the dental papilla (Fig. 7.26A).

An ameloblastic fibroma is treated by surgical excision, and the recurrence rate is low.

Ameloblastic Fibro-Odontoma

The **ameloblastic fibro-odontoma** is a benign odontogenic tumor that has features of both an ameloblastic fibroma and an odontoma. Most cases occur in young adults, with an average age of 10 years. No sex predilection is noted. The ameloblastic fibro-odontoma typically arises in the posterior jaws and is often asymptomatic. However, some patients may experience swelling of the affected area.

Radiographic examination reveals a well-delineated radiolucent lesion that may be unilocular or multilocular. Calcifications of various sizes and shapes are noted within the radiolucency. These calcifications represent tooth formation.

Microscopic examination demonstrates features similar to those described for the ameloblastic fibroma combined with structures that resemble teeth. Therefore various amounts of enamel, dentin, cementum, and pulp tissue are produced.

The ameloblastic fibro-odontoma is a well-circumscribed lesion that usually separates easily from the surrounding bone. It is treated by conservative surgical excision, and recurrence is unusual.

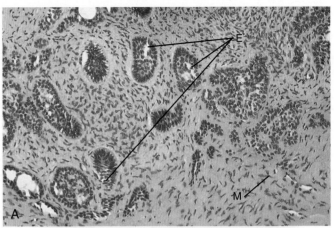

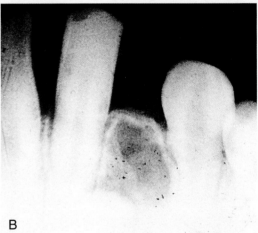

B

• **Figure 7.26** A, Microscopic appearance of an ameloblastic fibroma shows a combination of odontogenic epithelium (E) and mesenchymal tissue (M). B, Radiograph of an ameloblastic fibroma shows a poorly defined unilocular radiolucency.

Odontoma

The **odontoma** is an odontogenic tumor composed of mature enamel, dentin, cementum, and pulp tissue. The odontoma is the most common odontogenic tumor. Two types of odontomas are recognized: compound and complex. A **compound odontoma** consists of a collection of numerous small teeth. Although compound odontomas may consist of many small teeth, they do not exhibit unlimited growth potential. They are more accurately described as developmental lesions (hamartomas) rather than true tumors. A **complex odontoma** consists of a mass of enamel, dentin, cementum, and pulp that does not resemble a normal tooth.

Most odontomas are detected in adolescents and young adults. No sex predilection is noted. The compound odontoma is usually located in the anterior maxilla, and the complex odontoma most commonly occurs in the posterior mandible. The most common clinical manifestation of an odontoma is the failure of a permanent tooth to erupt. Most odontomas are small, but large lesions can cause swelling, displace teeth, and prevent the eruption of a permanent tooth. Odontomas may be associated with impacted or unerupted teeth, and with odontogenic cysts and tumors.

Radiographically, compound odontomas appear as a cluster of numerous miniature teeth surrounded by a radiolucent halo (Fig. 7.27). A complex odontoma appears as a radiopaque mass surrounded by a thin radiolucent halo (Fig. 7.28).

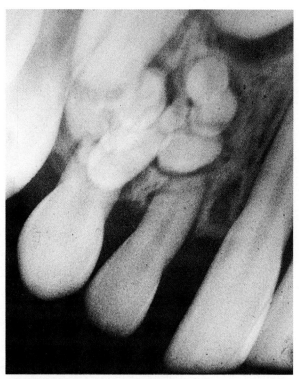

• **Figure 7.27** Radiograph of a compound odontoma shows a collection of numerous, small, toothlike radiopacities surrounded by a radiolucent halo.

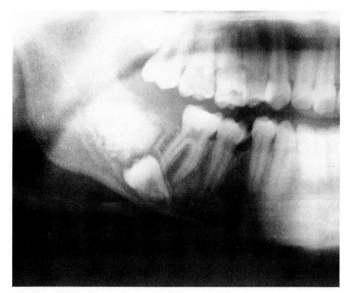

• **Figure 7.28** Radiograph of a complex odontoma shows a radiopaque mass surrounded by a radiolucent halo.

Treatment of an odontoma consists of surgical excision. They generally do not recur.

Peripheral Odontogenic Tumors

Several of the odontogenic tumors have been reported to occur on the gingiva without underlying bone involvement. The peripheral ameloblastoma and the peripheral calcifying epithelial odontogenic tumor have been reported to occur on the gingiva

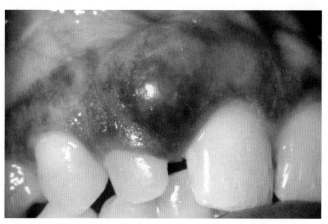

• **Figure 7.29** Clinical appearance of a peripheral ameloblastomas. (Courtesy Dr. Kean K. White.)

(Fig. 7.29). The peripheral odontogenic fibroma is composed of a combination of fibrous tissue and islands or stands of odontogenic epithelium. Calcifications may occasionally be present. Although rare, these peripheral odontogenic tumors are important to the dental hygienist because of their gingival location. Treatment is surgical excision. Recurrence is rare.

Tumors of Soft Tissue

Tumors of soft tissue include benign and malignant tumors of adipose (fat) tissue, nerve, muscle, blood vessels, and lymphatic vessels.

Lipoma

The lipoma is a benign tumor of mature fat cells (adipose tissue). Clinically, it appears as a yellowish mass that is surfaced by a thin layer of epithelium (Fig. 7.30A). Because of this thin epithelium, a delicate pattern of blood vessels is usually seen on its surface. The majority of lipomas occur in individuals over 40 years of age, and no sex predilection is noted. The most common intraoral locations are the buccal mucosa and the vestibule. Microscopic examination reveals a well-delineated tumor composed of lobules of mature fat cells that are uniform in size and shape (Fig. 7.30B). The lipoma is treated by surgical excision and generally does not recur.

Tumors of Nerve Tissue

Neurofibroma and Schwannoma

The **neurofibroma** (Fig. 7.31A) and the **schwannoma** are benign tumors derived from nerve tissue. The schwannoma is also called a **neurilemmoma.** A schwannoma is derived from Schwann cells, and a neurofibroma is derived from Schwann cells and perineural fibroblasts. Both of these cells are components of the connective tissue surrounding a nerve. Although the neurofibroma and schwannoma are distinct tumors microscopically, they are quite similar in their clinical presentation and behavior and therefore are discussed together. The tongue is the most common intraoral location. On occasion, macroglossia (tongue enlargement) may occur as a result of growth of these tumors in this location. Schwannomas have been reported to occasionally cause a complaint of pain. Neurofibromas and schwannomas may occur at

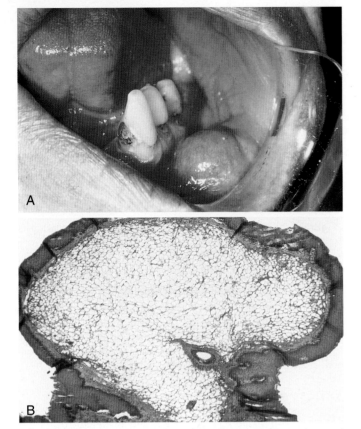

• **Figure 7.30** **A,** Clinical appearance of a lipoma. **B,** Photomicrograph of a lipoma shows mature fat cells. (**A** courtesy Dr. Edward V. Zegarelli.)

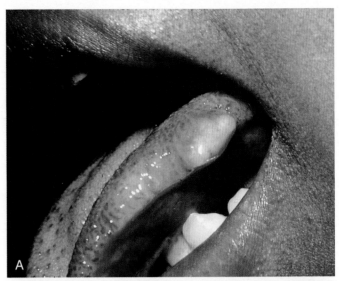

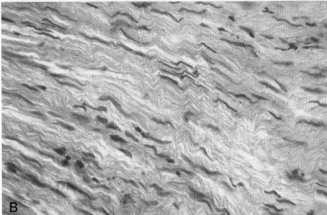

• **Figure 7.31** **A,** Clinical appearance of a neurofibroma shows a nonulcerated mass on the lateral border of the tongue. **B,** Photomicrograph of a neurofibroma.

any age, and no sex predilection is noted. Microscopic examination of a neurofibroma reveals a fairly well-delineated but unencapsulated proliferation of spindle-shaped Schwann cells and perineural fibroblasts (Fig. 7.31B). A schwannoma is composed of spindle-shaped Schwann cells arranged in palisaded whorls around a central pink zone. A connective tissue capsule surrounds the schwannoma.

A neurofibroma and a schwannoma are both treated by surgical excision. They generally do not recur. Malignant tumors of nerve tissue occur but are extremely rare; most cases arise from a preexisting neurofibroma.

Multiple neurofibromas occur in a genetically inherited disorder known as **neurofibromatosis of von Recklinghausen** or von Recklinghausen disease. Patients with this syndrome have numerous neurofibromas on the skin, in internal organs, and within bone, including the mandible. Malignant nerve sheath tumors have been reported to arise in about 5% of individuals with this syndrome. Other abnormalities are also seen in neurofibromatosis of von Recklinghausen. This syndrome is genetically inherited and is described in detail in Chapter 6.

Granular Cell Tumor

The **granular cell tumor** is a benign tumor composed of large cells with a granular cytoplasm. This tumor most likely arises from a neural or primitive mesenchymal cell. The granular cell tumor most often occurs on the tongue, followed by the buccal mucosa. It appears as a painless, nonulcerated nodule (Fig. 7.32A). Most cases occur in adults, and a female sex predilection is noted.

Microscopic examination reveals large oval-shaped cells with a granular cytoplasm. The granular cells are found in the connective tissue and between striated muscle fibers (Fig. 7.32B). The overlying surface epithelium may exhibit pseudoepitheliomatous hyperplasia (PEH), which is a benign proliferation of epithelium into the connective tissue (Fig. 7.32C) that may be mistaken for squamous cell carcinoma. This tumor is treated by surgical excision and does not recur.

Congenital Epulis

The **congenital epulis,** or congenital epulis of the newborn, is a benign neoplasm composed of cells that closely resemble those seen in the granular cell tumor. The neoplasm most likely arises from a primitive mesenchymal cell. This tumor is present at birth and appears as a sessile or pedunculated mass on the gingiva, usually on the anterior maxillary gingiva. Most cases occur in girls, suggesting a hormonal component in the development of this lesion.

The congenital epulis is treated by surgical excision and does not recur. Occasional examples have regressed without treatment.

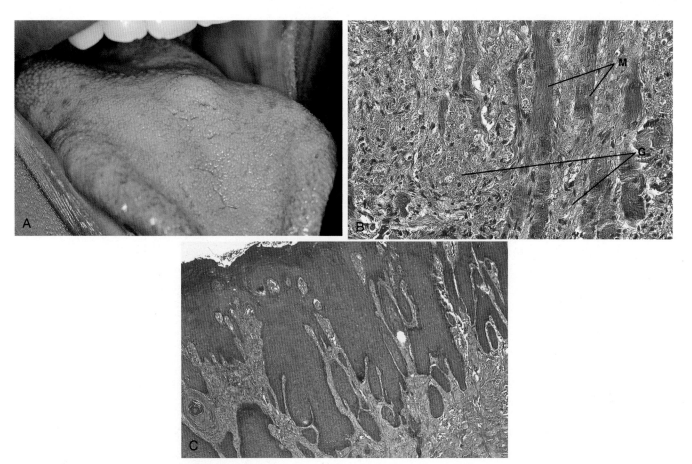

• **Figure 7.32** **A,** Clinical appearance of a granular cell tumor of the tongue shows a nonulcerated mass. **B,** Photomicrograph of a granular cell tumor showing granular cell(s) (G) between striated muscle fiber(s) (M). **C,** Photomicrograph of a granular cell tumor, showing overlying pseudoepitheliomatous hyperplasia. (**A** courtesy Dr. Sidney Eisig.)

Tumors of Muscle

Tumors of muscle are extremely uncommon in the oral cavity. The **rhabdomyoma,** a benign tumor of striated muscle, has been reported to occur on the tongue. The **leiomyoma,** a benign tumor of smooth muscle, may occur in association with blood vessels. These tumors are called **vascular leiomyomas** and occasionally occur in the oral cavity.

The **rhabdomyosarcoma,** a malignant tumor of striated muscle, is the most common malignant soft tissue tumor of the head and neck in children. It typically occurs in individuals under 10 years of age and has a male sex predilection. It is a rapidly growing, destructive tumor. The rhabdomyosarcoma is an aggressive malignant tumor that is best treated by a combination of multidrug chemotherapy, radiation therapy, and surgery. Despite treatment, the prognosis is poor.

Vascular Tumors

The **hemangioma,** or vascular malformation, is a benign proliferation of capillaries. It is a common vascular lesion considered by many to represent a developmental lesion rather than a tumor because a hemangioma does not exhibit unlimited growth potential. Some contain numerous small capillaries and are called **capillary hemangiomas.** Others contain larger blood vessels and are called **cavernous hemangiomas** (Fig. 7.33D).

Most hemangiomas are present at birth or arise shortly thereafter (Fig. 7.33A). More than half of the hemangiomas that occur in the body occur in the head and neck area. The tongue is the most common intraoral location. Involvement of the tongue often leads to marked enlargement. Hemangiomas are more common in girls than in boys. When they occur in adults, they should be referred to as a *vascular malformation.* In this age group they most likely arise as a response to trauma and represent an abnormal proliferation of blood vessels during the healing process (Fig. 7.33B-C). They appear as variably sized, deep-red or blue lesions that frequently blanch when pressure is applied.

Many hemangiomas undergo spontaneous remission. Others can enlarge rapidly because of hemorrhage, thrombosis, or inflammation. Treatment is variable and includes surgery or the injection of a sclerosing solution into the lesion. Injection of a sclerosing solution into the lesion will cause it to shrink in size or resolve.

Lymphangioma

The **lymphangioma** is a benign tumor of lymphatic vessels. It is less common than the hemangioma. Most lymphangiomas are congenital (present at birth), and half arise in the head and neck area. No sex predilection is noted. The most common intraoral location is the tongue, where a lymphangioma presents as an ill-defined mass with a pebbly surface. Involvement of the tongue may lead to macroglossia. A cystic lymphangioma in the neck is

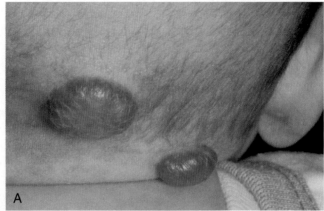

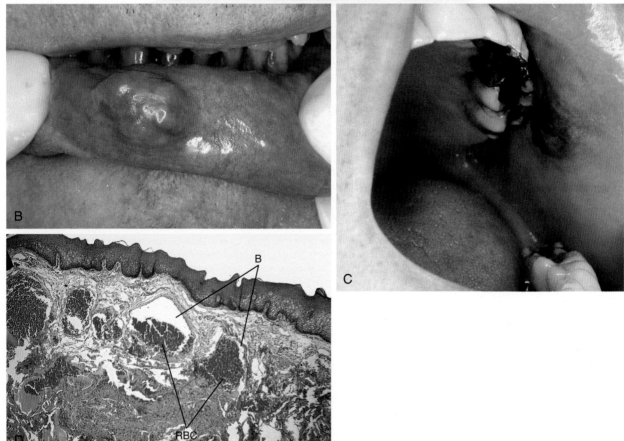

• **Figure 7.33** Hemangioma. **A,** Infant with two red, nodular masses on the posterior scalp and neck (strawberry hemangioma). Clinical appearance of a vascular malformation of the lower lip **(B)** and of the buccal mucosa **(C). D,** Microscopic appearance of a cavernous hemangioma showing large dilated blood vessels (B) filled with red blood cells (RBC). (**A** from Neville BW, Damm DD, Allen CM: *Oral and maxillofacial pathology,* ed 4, St Louis, 2016, Elsevier.)

called a **cystic hygroma.** It is usually present at birth or develops shortly thereafter.

Lymphangiomas are generally treated by surgical excision and tend to recur. Unlike a hemangioma, a lymphangioma will not shrink in size after injection with a sclerosing solution.

Malignant Vascular Tumors

Malignant vascular tumors arising from endothelial cells include an **angiosarcoma** and **Kaposi sarcoma**. An **angiosarcoma** typically arises on the skin of the head and neck in older individuals; they may occur in the oral cavity, but are extremely rare in this location. **Kaposi sarcoma** is a malignant vascular tumor and may arise in multiple sites, including the skin and oral mucosa. Classic Kaposi sarcoma occurs as multiple purplish tumors of the lower extremities in older men. The neoplasm progresses slowly, usually resolves with low doses of radiation, and rarely causes death.

With the advent of the human immunodeficiency virus (HIV) epidemic in the 1980s, Kaposi sarcoma appeared in a much more aggressive form. In HIV-positive patients these lesions are often seen in the oral cavity, where they present as purple macules, plaques, or exophytic tumors. The hard palate and gingiva are the most common intraoral sites. Kaposi sarcoma associated with HIV infection is described in Chapter 4 (see Fig. 4.37). It may also occur in patients with other forms of immunodeficiency, specifically patients who have received immunosuppressive drug therapy as a result of organ transplantation.

Kaposi sarcoma is caused by a human herpesvirus that is called both *human herpesvirus type 8* and *Kaposi sarcoma–associated herpesvirus*. Men are affected more often than women. Microscopic examination reveals a neoplasm composed of spindle-shaped cells mixed with slitlike spaces containing red blood cells.

Kaposi sarcoma is treated by surgical excision, radiation therapy, chemotherapy, or a combination of these therapies. In HIV-positive patients recurrence is common, and the disease may progress rapidly.

Tumors of Melanin-Producing Cells

Melanocytic Nevus

The word **nevus** (plural, **nevi**) has two meanings. Here the word is used to mean a benign tumor of melanocytes (melanin-producing cells), which are called **nevus cells.** Nevus also refers to a pigmented congenital (present at birth) lesion. A hemangioma present at birth is an example of this second type of nevus.

Melanocytic nevi can arise on the skin or the oral mucosa. Intraoral tumors consist of tan-to-brown macules or papules that occur most often on the hard palate. The buccal mucosa is the second most common intraoral location (Fig. 7.34). They occur twice as often in women as in men and are usually first identified in individuals between 20 and 50 years of age. Most pigmented lesions that occur in the oral cavity are benign. Pigmented lesions that exhibit ulceration, an increase in size, or a change in shape or color may be malignant.

The ABCDE's (*A*symmetry, *B*order, *C*olor, *D*iameter, *E*volving) of melanoma should be considered when assessing pigmented lesions of the skin. Lesions that show these characteristics should be further evaluated to rule out melanoma. These include lesions that are **A**symmetric (i.e., one half is different from the other), lesions that have irregular **B**orders, lesions in which the **C**olor varies from tan to black and possibly red or blue, lesions that have **D**iameters larger than 6 mm, and lesions that are **E**volving (i.e., changing in size, shape, or color).

A biopsy, followed by microscopic examination, is indicated for pigmented lesions of unknown cause, unknown duration, or recent onset. Surgical excision is the treatment of choice for intraoral melanocytic nevi. Recurrence is rare.

Melanoma

Melanoma is a malignant tumor of melanocytes (Fig. 7.35). Although the name *melanoma* suggests that a benign counterpart exists, all melanomas are malignant. Most melanomas arise on the skin as a result of prolonged exposure to sunlight. Primary melanoma of the oral cavity is rare. However, melanomas that arise on the skin may metastasize to the oral cavity.

Melanoma usually presents as a rapidly enlarging, blue-to-black mass. The neoplasm demonstrates an aggressive and unpredictable behavior with early metastasis. The most common

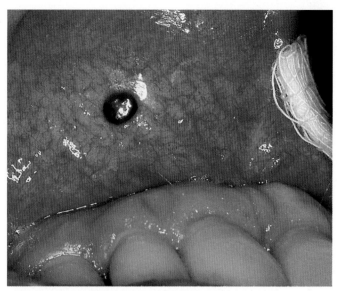

• **Figure 7.34** Clinical appearance of a melanocytic nevus shows a well-defined pigmented lesion on the labial mucosa.

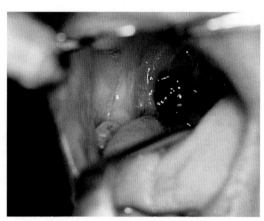

• **Figure 7.35** Clinical appearance of a malignant melanoma shows a darkly pigmented lesion in the area of the faucees. (Courtesy Dr. Edward V. Zegarelli.)

intraoral locations are the palate and maxillary gingiva. These neoplasms usually occur in adults older than 40 years of age.

Melanomas are treated by wide surgical excision. Chemotherapy may be used in conjunction with surgery. The prognosis for oral melanoma is poor.

Tumors of Bone and Cartilage

Osteoma

An osteoma is an asymptomatic benign tumor composed of normal compact bone. It is a slow-growing tumor that appears radiographically as either a sharply defined radiopaque mass within bone (endosteal) or a delineated mass attached to the outer surface of the bone (periosteal) (Fig. 7.36). A large osteoma within bone may cause expansion of the involved bone. No sex predilection is noted. The most common location within the jaws is the posterior mandible. Tumors are commonly located in the frontal

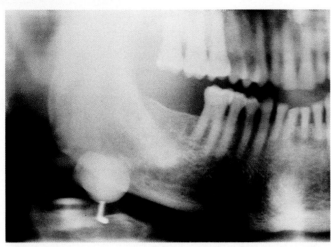

• **Figure 7.36** Radiograph of an osteoma shows a radiopacity of the posterior mandible. (Courtesy Dr. Sidney Eisig.)

sinuses. Multiple osteomas are a component of Gardner syndrome, which is transmitted genetically and described in Chapter 6. Osteomas are treated by surgical excision and generally do not recur.

Osteosarcoma

Osteosarcoma (osteogenic sarcoma) is a malignant tumor of bone-forming tissue. It is the most common primary malignant tumor of bone in patients under 40 years of age. Tumors that involve the long bones occur at an average age of 27 years, whereas the average age of occurrence for tumors that involve the jaws is about 37 years of age. These tumors occur in the mandible twice as frequently as in the maxilla and are more common in men than in women. Patients may experience a diffuse swelling or mass that is often painful (Fig. 7.37A). Some patients present initially with a toothache or tooth mobility. Paresthesia of the lip is common in tumors involving the mandible.

The radiographic appearance of an osteosarcoma varies from radiolucent to radiopaque (Fig. 7.37B). It is usually a destructive, poorly defined lesion and may or may not involve the adjacent soft tissue. In some cases, asymmetric widening of the periodontal ligament space and a sunburst pattern may be seen radiographically. Microscopic examination of this tumor shows pleomorphic and hyperchromatic cells and abnormal bone formation. Abnormal cartilage formation may also be present (Fig. 7.37C).

At present, osteosarcomas are treated with preoperative multi-agent chemotherapy followed by surgery. Jaw tumors frequently recur after treatment. Only about 20% of patients with an osteosarcoma of the jaws survive 5 years.

Tumors of Cartilage

Cartilaginous tumors of the jawbones are extremely rare and are more likely to be malignant than benign. A **chondroma** is a benign tumor of cartilage. A **chondrosarcoma** is a malignant tumor of cartilage (Fig. 7.38). A chondrosarcoma may occur in either the maxilla or the mandible and is more common in men than in women. Most patients have enlargement of the affected bone.

Chondrosarcomas are treated by wide surgical excision. Radiation therapy and chemotherapy are not effective. The prognosis is poor. Only about 30% of patients with chondrosarcoma involving the jaws survive 5 years after the diagnosis.

Tumors of Blood-Forming Tissues

Leukemia

Leukemia comprises a broad group of disorders characterized by an overproduction of atypical white blood cells. The atypical white blood cells proliferate in the bone marrow and then spill into the circulating blood and tissues. Several types of leukemia are classified according to the kind of cells that are proliferating: myelocytes, lymphocytes, or monocytes.

Leukemias are divided into two forms: acute and chronic. Acute leukemia is common in children and young adults and is characterized by a proliferation of immature white blood cells (blasts). Chronic leukemia is characterized by an excess proliferation of mature white blood cells and most frequently occurs in middle-aged adults. Because immature white blood cells proliferate faster than mature white blood cells, acute leukemias generally have a more aggressive clinical course and require immediate treatment, whereas chronic leukemias generally have a more slowly progressive clinical course. In general, leukemia occurs more often in men than in women.

Although oral involvement may occur in any type of leukemia, the monocytic variant most often demonstrates oral lesions. A common oral manifestation of monocytic leukemia is diffuse gingival enlargement with persistent bleeding (Fig. 7.39). (Leukemia is further described in Chapter 9.)

The treatment of leukemia consists of chemotherapy, radiation therapy, and corticosteroids. The prognosis depends on the type of leukemia and the extent of disease.

Lymphoma (Non-Hodgkin Lymphoma)

Lymphoma is a malignant tumor of lymphoid tissue. Numerous types of lymphoma exist, each of which is differentiated on the basis of microscopic findings with immunohistochemical and genetic testing to identify the specific types of malignant lymphocytes. The characteristic clinical presentation is gradual enlargement of the involved lymph nodes. Rarely, a lymphoma may present as a primary lesion in the oral soft tissues or bone. However, most lymphomas involve either lymph nodes or aggregates of lymphoid tissue that are located anywhere in the digestive tract from the oral cavity to the anus. In the oral cavity, lymphoid tissue is located at the base of the tongue, soft palate, and pharynx (**Waldeyer ring**). Common locations for intraoral lymphoma are the tonsillar pillar area and the posterior hard palate. When a lymphoma arises in bone, it presents as a destructive, poorly defined radiolucency. Lymphomas usually occur in adults and are more common in men than in women.

Lymphoma is treated by radiotherapy, chemotherapy, or a combination of these therapies. Surgery is not a good option to treat lymphoma because patients often have systemic involvement at the time of diagnosis. The prognosis depends on the type of lymphoma and the extent of involvement.

Multiple Myeloma

Multiple myeloma is a systemic, malignant proliferation of plasma cells that causes destructive lesions in bone. The neoplastic

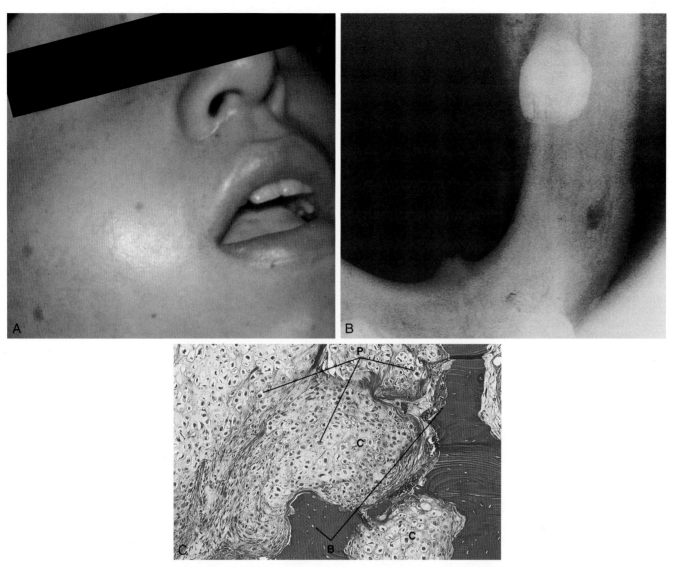

• **Figure 7.37 A,** Clinical appearance of an osteogenic sarcoma shows swelling. **B,** Radiograph of an osteogenic sarcoma in the left molar area shows a poorly defined radiopaque lesion. **C,** Microscopic appearance of an osteogenic sarcoma shows pleomorphic (P) and hyperchromatic cells, abnormal cartilage (C), and bone formation (B).

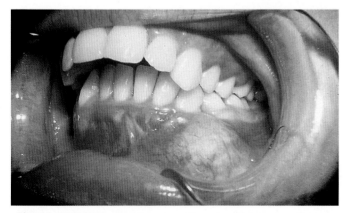

• **Figure 7.38** Clinical appearance of a chondrosarcoma shows an exophytic mass in the anterior mandible.

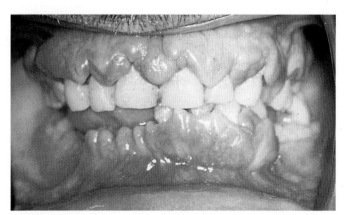

• **Figure 7.39** Clinical appearance of a patient with leukemic infiltration of the gingiva, resulting in diffuse enlargement. (Courtesy Dr. Edward V. Zegarelli.)

plasma cells produce large amounts of **immunoglobulin.** Most patients are older than 40 years of age, and the disease occurs most commonly in the seventh decade of life. Men are affected more often than women. Patients usually experience bone pain and swelling. Pathologic fracture of an involved bone is common and typically occurs in bones weakened as a result of their destruction by the proliferation of neoplastic plasma cells (Fig. 7.40A).

Radiographically, the involved bones show multiple radiolucent lesions. The disease can involve the skull, spine, ribs, pelvis, long bones, and jaws. The mandible is affected more often than the maxilla (Fig. 7.40B). Most patients have an elevation of a single type of immunoglobulin, which is detected by a process called *immunoelectrophoresis.* This elevation is called a **monoclonal spike.** Patients may have fragments of immunoglobulins in the urine. These fragments are called **Bence Jones proteins.** The tumors are composed of sheets of well-to-poorly differentiated plasma cells.

A localized tumor of plasma cells in soft tissue is called an **extramedullary plasmacytoma.** Although these are rare tumors, they are more common in the head and neck region than anywhere else in the body. Many patients with extramedullary plasmacytoma will eventually develop multiple myeloma. Therefore patients with a single tumor of plasma cells must be evaluated to determine whether the lesion is solitary or part of multiple myeloma.

Patients with multiple myeloma are treated with chemotherapy, radiation therapy, autologous stem cell transplantation, and immunotherapy. New treatment modalities have dramatically improved the prognosis for patients with multiple myeloma. Systemic bisphosphonate medication is used to prevent bone destruction. Oral complications related to this treatment are discussed in Chapter 9.

Metastatic Tumors

Metastatic tumors from primary sites elsewhere in the body are rare. Most of these tumors arise from the thyroid gland, breast, lungs, prostate gland, and kidneys. The most frequent intraoral site for metastatic tumors is the mandible. Patients display various

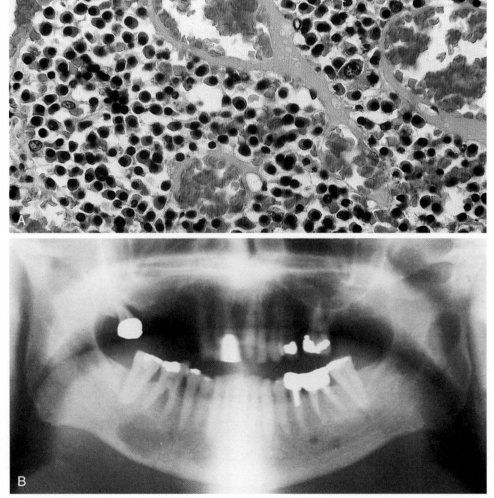

• **Figure 7.40** Multiple myeloma. **A,** Microscopic appearance of multiple myeloma shows a proliferation of plasma cells. **B,** Radiograph shows multiple radiolucent lesions of the mandible in a patient with multiple myeloma.

signs and symptoms, including pain, paresthesia or anesthesia of the lip, swelling, expansion of the affected bone, and loosening of the teeth in the involved area. Metastatic lesions usually appear several years after the primary lesion is discovered. On occasion, the oral metastatic tumor is the first manifestation of a **primary tumor** elsewhere. Most patients are adults, and men are affected more often than women.

The radiographic appearance of metastatic tumors varies (Fig. 7.41). Lesions are usually poorly defined and radiolucent. The roots of the involved teeth may show a spiked appearance. Metastatic tumors from the breast, prostate gland, and lungs may form bone and therefore may show areas of radiopacity.

Microscopically, a metastatic tumor resembles the primary malignancy. Most metastatic tumors in the jaws are epithelial in origin and are adenocarcinomas.

Chemotherapy and radiation therapy are used to alleviate the discomfort of metastatic tumors in the jaws. The prognosis for patients with tumors that have metastasized to the jaws is poor. Systemic bisphosphonate medication is used to prevent bone destruction in patients with tumors such as breast and prostate cancer that metastasize to bone. Oral complications related to this treatment are discussed in Chapter 9.

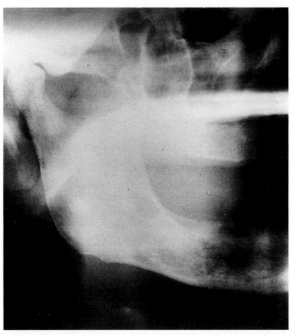

• **Figure 7.41** Radiograph shows diffuse radiolucent and radiopaque changes resulting from metastatic carcinoma of the prostate gland.

Selected References

Books

Barnes L, Eveson JW, Reichart P, et al, editors: *World Health Organization classification of tumours: pathology and genetics of head and neck tumours*, Lyon, France, 2005, IARC Press.

Kumar V, Abbas AK, Aster JC: *Robbins basic pathology*, ed 9, St Louis, 2013, Saunders.

Neville BW, Damm DD, Allen CM: *Oral and maxillofacial pathology*, ed 4, St Louis, 2016, Elsevier.

Regezi JA, Sciubba JJ, Jordan RCK: *Oral pathology: clinical-pathologic correlations*, ed 7, St Louis, 2017, Saunders.

Journal Articles
Tumors of Squamous Epithelium

Abbey LM, Page DG, Sawyer DR: The clinical and histopathologic features of a series of 464 oral squamous cell papillomas, *Oral Surg Oral Med Oral Pathol* 49:419, 1980.

Addante RR, McKenna SJ: Verrucous carcinoma, *Oral Maxillofac Surg Clin North Am* 18:513–519, 2006.

American Cancer Society: *Cancer facts & figures – 2007*, Atlanta, 2007, American Cancer Society, pp 1–56.

Bsoul SA, Huber MA, Terezhalmy GT: Squamous cell carcinoma of the oral tissues: a comprehensive review for oral healthcare providers, *J Contemp Dent Pract* 4:1–16, 2005.

Cleveland JL, Junger ML, Saraiya M, et al: The connection between human papillomavirus and oropharyngeal squamous cell carcinomas in the United States: implications for dentistry, *J Am Dent Assoc* 142:915, 2011.

Fantasia JE, Damm DD: Oral diagnosis: exophytic lesion of palatal mucosa: papilloma, *Gen Dent* 181:183, 2004.

Freitas MD, Blanco-Carrión A, Gándara-Vila P, et al: Clinicopathologic aspects of oral leukoplakia in smokers and nonsmokers, *Oral Surg Oral Med Oral Pathol Oral Radiol Endod* 102:199, 2006.

Gillison ML, Broutian T, Pickard RK, et al: Prevalence of oral HPV infection in the United States, 2009–2010, *JAMA* 307:693, 2012.

Kaugars GE, Pillion T, Svirsky JA, et al: Actinic cheilitis: a review of 152 cases, *Oral Surg Oral Med Oral Pathol Oral Radiol Endod* 88:181, 1999.

Warnakulasuriya KA, Ralhan R: Clinical, pathological, cellular and molecular lesions caused by oral smokeless tobacco—a review, *J Oral Pathol Med* 36:63, 2007.

Leukoplakia and Erythroplakia

Ha PK, Califano JA: The role of human papillomavirus in oral carcinogenesis, *Crit Rev Oral Biol Med* 15:188–196, 2004.

Ray JG, Ranganathan K, Chattopadhyay A: Malignant transformation of oral submucous fibrosis: overview of histopathological aspects, *Oral Surg Oral Med Oral Pathol Oral Radiol* 122:200, 2016.

Shafer WG, Waldron CA: Erythroplakia of the oral cavity, *Cancer* 36:1021, 1975.

Silverman S Jr, Gorsky M, Lozada F: Oral leukoplakia and malignant transformation: a follow-up study of 257 patients, *Cancer* 53:563, 1984.

Sugiyama M, Bhawal UK, Dohmen T, et al: Detection of human papillomavirus-16 and HPV-18 DNA in normal, dysplastic, and malignant oral epithelium, *Oral Surg Oral Med Oral Pathol Oral Radiol Endod* 95:594, 2003.

Waldron CA, Shafer WG: Leukoplakia revisited: a clinicopathologic study of 3256 oral leukoplakias, *Cancer* 36:1386, 1975.

Zain RB, Ikeda N, Gupta PC, et al: Oral mucosal lesions associated with betel quid, areca nut and tobacco chewing habits: consensus from a workshop held in Kuala Lumpur, Malaysia, November 25–27, 1996, *J Oral Pathol Med* 28:1, 1999.

Salivary Gland Tumors

Pires FR, Pringle GA, de Almeida OP, et al: Intra-oral minor salivary gland tumors: a clinicopathological study of 546 cases, *Oral Oncol* 43:463, 2007.

Waldron CA, El-Mofty SK, Gnepp DR: Tumors of the intraoral minor salivary glands: a demographic and histologic study of 426 cases, *Oral Surg Oral Med Oral Pathol* 66:323, 1988.

Yih W-Y, Kratochvil FJ, Stewart JCB: Intraoral minor salivary gland neoplasms: review of 213 cases, *J Oral Maxillofac Surg* 63:805–810, 2005.

Odontogenic Tumors

Ai-Ru L, Zhen L, Jian S: Calcifying epithelial odontogenic tumors: a clinicopathologic study of 9 cases, *J Oral Pathol* 11:399, 1982.

Buchner A, Merrell PW, Carpenter WM: Relative frequency of central odontogenic tumors: a study of 1,088 cases from northern California and comparison to studies from other parts of the world, *J Oral Maxillofac Surg* 64:1343–1352, 2006.

Courtney RM, Kerr DA: The odontogenic adenomatoid tumor: a comprehensive study of 20 new cases, *Oral Surg Oral Med Oral Pathol* 39:424, 1975.

Fregnani ER, Pires FR, Quezada RD, et al: Calcifying odontogenic cyst: clinicopathological features and immunohistochemical profile of 10 cases, *J Oral Pathol Med* 32:163–170, 2003.

Kaugars GE, Miller ME, Abbey LM: Odontomas, *Oral Surg Oral Med Oral Pathol* 67:172, 1989.

Ulmansky M, Hjørting-Hansen E, Praetorius F, et al: Benign cementoblastoma, *Oral Surg Oral Med Oral Pathol* 77:48, 1994.

Waldron CA, El-Mofty SK: A histopathologic study of 116 ameloblastomas with special reference to the desmoplastic variant, *Oral Surg Oral Med Oral Pathol* 63:441, 1987.

Zomosa X, Müller S: Calcifying cystic odontogenic tumor, *Head Neck Pathol* 4:292, 2010.

Lipoma

Furlong MA, Fanburg-Smith JC, Childers ELB: Lipoma of the oral and maxillofacial region: site and subclassification of 125 cases, *Oral Surg Oral Med Oral Pathol* 98:441, 2004.

Neurogenic Tumors

Cunha KS, Barboza EP, Dias EP, et al: Neurofibromatosis type I with periodontal manifestations: a case report and literature review, *Br Dent J* 196:457, 2004.

Vascular Tumors

Greene AK: Current concepts of vascular anomalies, *J Craniofac Surg* 23:220, 2012.

Hernandez GA, Castro A, Castro G, et al: Aneurysmal bone cyst versus hemangioma of the mandible, *Oral Surg Oral Med Oral Pathol* 76:790, 1993.

Tumors of Melanin-Producing Cells

Kerr EH, Hameed O, Lewis JS Jr, et al: Head and neck mucosal malignant melanoma: clinicopathologic correlation with contemporary review of prognostic indicators, *Int J Surg Pathol* 20:37, 2012.

Melanoma Research Foundation. What is melanoma? Available at http://www.melanoma.org/learn-more/melanoma-101/abcdes-melanoma.

Tumors of Bone

Canadian Society of Otolaryngology—Head and Neck Surgery Oncology Study Group: Osteogenic sarcoma of the mandible and maxilla: a Canadian review (1980–2000), *J Otolaryngol* 33:139, 2004.

Ottaviani G, Jaffe N: The epidemiology of osteosarcoma, *Cancer Treat Res* 152:3, 2009.

Tumors of Blood-Forming Tissues

Denz U, Haas PS, Wäsch R, et al: State of the art therapy in multiple myeloma and future perspectives, *Eur J Cancer* 42:1591–1600, 2006.

Lambertenghi-Deliliers G, Bruno E, Cortelezzi A, et al: Incidence of jaw lesions in 193 patients with multiple myeloma, *Oral Surg Oral Med Oral Pathol* 65:533, 1988.

Mhaskar R, Redzepovic J, Wheatley K, et al: Bisphosphonates in multiple myeloma, *Cochrane Database Syst Rev* (3):CD003188, 2010. Update in: *Cochrane Database Syst Rev* 5:CD003188, 2012.

Metastatic Tumors

Hashimoto N, Kurihara K, Yamasaki H, et al: Pathological characteristics of metastatic carcinoma in the human mandible, *J Oral Pathol* 16:362, 1987.

Khalili M, Mahboobi N, Shams J: Metastatic breast carcinoma initially diagnosed as pulpal/periapical disease: a case report, *J Endod* 36:922, 2010.

Review Questions

1. All of the following are associated with the neoplastic transformation of cells except one. Which one is the exception?
   a. Chemicals
   b. Sunlight
   c. Repeated trauma
   d. Viruses

2. Neoplasia involves all of the following except one. Which one is the exception?
   a. Normal arrangement of cells
   b. Irreversible cellular changes
   c. Abnormal process
   d. Uncontrolled cell multiplication

3. Which of the following statements concerning leukoplakia is *true*?
   a. Most cases are associated with a previous history of radiation therapy.
   b. Common sites for leukoplakia are the buccal mucosa and gingiva.
   c. A biopsy should be performed to establish a diagnosis.
   d. Leukoplakia is less common than erythroplakia.

4. Which of the following is a characteristic of a benign tumor?
   a. Invasive and unencapsulated
   b. Often grows rapidly
   c. Composed of well-differentiated cells
   d. Numerous abnormal mitotic figures

5. A small white exophytic lesion on the palate is a benign lesion composed of squamous epithelium. Papillary projections are arranged in a cauliflower-like appearance. It is most likely a:
   a. Congenital epulis
   b. Neurofibroma
   c. Granular cell tumor
   d. Papilloma

6. All of the following are microscopic characteristics of squamous cell carcinoma except one. Which one is the exception?
   a. Invasion of tumor cells into the connective tissue
   b. Cells with very small nuclei
   c. Cells with hyperchromatic nuclei
   d. Keratin pearls

7. Which of the following are the most common locations for intraoral squamous cell carcinoma?
   a. Upper labial mucosa, frenum, and lingual gingiva
   b. Lower labial mucosa, maxillary gingiva, and buccal mucosa
   c. Floor of the mouth, ventrolateral tongue, and soft palate
   d. Anterior tongue, mandibular gingiva, and retromolar area

8. A patient with squamous cell carcinoma of the lateral tongue exhibits metastatic disease in the liver. What clinical stage correlates with these findings?
   a. Stage I
   b. Stage II
   c. Stage III
   d. Stage IV

9. Which of the following represents an early clinical example of squamous cell carcinoma?
   a. Exophytic erythroleukoplakia
   b. Urticaria
   c. Brown macule
   d. Destructive radiolucency

10. The most appropriate treatment for epithelial dysplasia is:
    a. Radiation therapy
    b. Chemotherapy
    c. Surgical excision
    d. Observation

11. Verrucous carcinoma is differentiated from squamous cell carcinoma because it:
    a. Occurs primarily on the hard palate
    b. Responds to chemotherapy
    c. Often metastasizes
    d. Has a better prognosis

12. The most common intraoral location for salivary gland tumors is the:
    a. Gingival mucosa
    b. Anterior buccal mucosa
    c. Junction of the hard and soft palate
    d. Posterior lateral tongue

13. All of the following are examples of malignant salivary gland tumors except one. Which one is the exception?
    a. Pleomorphic adenoma
    b. Mucoepidermoid carcinoma
    c. Cylindroma
    d. Adenoid cystic carcinoma

14. All of the following statements concerning an ameloblastoma are true except one. Which one is the exception?
    a. Presents as a multilocular radiolucency
    b. Represents a benign and locally aggressive lesion
    c. Often occurs in the mandibular molar and ramus area
    d. Should be treated with radiation therapy

15. The odontogenic tumor that characteristically appears as a well-circumscribed radiolucency located in the anterior maxilla of an adolescent girl is a(n):
    a. Ameloblastic fibro-odontoma
    b. Adenomatoid odontogenic tumor
    c. Calcifying cystic odontogenic tumor
    d. Odontogenic myxoma

16. Which odontogenic tumor most closely resembles the mesenchyme of the dental follicle?
    a. Cementoblastoma
    b. Odontogenic myxoma
    c. Compound odontoma
    d. Ameloblastoma

17. Which of the following best describes the radiographic features of a cementoblastoma?
    a. Well-circumscribed radiopaque lesion with a radiolucent halo fused to the root of a vital tooth
    b. Multilocular radiolucency in the posterior mandible
    c. Unilocular radiolucent lesion around the crown of an impacted tooth
    d. Numerous toothlike structures in the anterior maxilla

18. Which of the following lesions characteristically occurs on the alveolar mucosa in newborn girls?
    a. Granular cell tumor
    b. Congenital epulis
    c. Lymphangioma
    d. Plasmacytoma

19. Human herpesvirus 8 is associated with:
    a. Herpangina
    b. Melanoma
    c. Kaposi sarcoma
    d. Schwannoma

20. A compound odontoma differs from a complex odontoma in that a compound odontoma:
    a. Is composed of several toothlike structures
    b. Has unlimited growth potential
    c. Presents as a radiopaque mass
    d. Is located in the posterior mandible

21. Which term describes a unique feature of the adenoid cystic carcinoma?
    a. Honeycombed radiolucency
    b. Histopathologic pattern described as resembling "Swiss cheese"
    c. Most common salivary gland tumor
    d. Radiolucency that scallops around tooth roots

22. A benign tumor of bone is called a(n):
    a. Osteoma
    b. Neurofibroma
    c. Hemangioma
    d. Chondroma

23. The most common malignant soft tissue tumor of the head and neck in children is:
    a. Granular cell tumor
    b. Lymphangioma
    c. Rhabdomyosarcoma
    d. Schwannoma

24. Melanoma of the oral cavity is rare; however, the most common intraoral locations are the:
    a. Dorsal and lateral tongue
    b. Floor of mouth and anterior buccal mucosa
    c. Palate and maxillary gingiva
    d. Retromolar pad and soft palate

25. Which of the following neoplasms often occurs in the buccal mucosa or vestibule?
    a. Lipoma
    b. Congenital epulis
    c. Hemangioma
    d. Granular cell tumor

26. A malignant tumor of bone-forming tissue is called:
    a. Chondrosarcoma
    b. Multiple myeloma
    c. Osteosarcoma
    d. Rhabdomyosarcoma

27. An overproduction of atypical lymphocytes in the bone marrow that results in an increase in lymphocytes in the circulating blood is called a:
    a. Lymphoma
    b. Leukemia
    c. Melanoma
    d. Plasmacytoma

28. Which of the following is a malignant tumor of lymphocytes?
    a. Multiple myeloma
    b. Lymphoma
    c. Melanoma
    d. Plasmacytoma

29. The cell type involved in multiple myeloma is a:
    a. Lymphocyte
    b. Macrophage
    c. Basophil
    d. Plasma cell

30. The most frequent intraoral site for metastatic tumors is the:
    a. Gingiva
    b. Mandible
    c. Hard palate
    d. Lateral tongue

31. Which of the following tumors is associated with von Recklinghausen disease?
    a. Schwannoma
    b. Granular cell tumor
    c. Chondroma
    d. Neurofibroma

32. Which of the following is the most common odontogenic tumor?
    a. Odontoma
    b. Ameloblastoma
    c. Ameloblastic fibroma
    d. Cementoblastoma

33. Which of the following salivary gland tumors often occurs in adult men?
    a. Pleomorphic adenoma
    b. Trabecular adenoma
    c. Warthin tumor
    d. Tubular adenoma

34. A benign tumor composed of a proliferation of capillaries is called a:
    a. Neurofibroma
    b. Hemangioma
    c. Schwannoma
    d. Lymphangioma

35. A white plaquelike lesion that cannot be rubbed off or diagnosed clinically as a specific disease is called:
    a. Squamous cell carcinoma
    b. Erythroplakia
    c. Leukoplakia
    d. Erythroleukoplakia

36. All of the following are benign lesions that histologically contain bonelike mineralized material except one. Which one is the exception?
    a. Osteoma
    b. Odontoma
    c. Chondroma
    d. Osteosarcoma

37. Which of the following neoplasms may present as diffuse gingival enlargement with persistent bleeding?
    a. Leukemia
    b. Multiple myeloma
    c. Lymphoma
    d. Congenital epulis

38. Which of the following malignancies is characterized by a monoclonal spike on immunoelectrophoresis?
    a. Osteosarcoma
    b. Rhabdomyosarcoma
    c. Multiple myeloma
    d. Leukemia

39. Which of the following malignant tumors has been reported to show a characteristic sunburst pattern on radiographic examination?
    a. Multiple myeloma
    b. Osteosarcoma
    c. Lymphoma
    d. Chondrosarcoma

40. All of the following neoplasms arise from squamous epithelium except one. Which one is the exception?
    a. Squamous cell carcinoma
    b. Verrucous carcinoma
    c. Adenoid cystic carcinoma
    d. Papilloma

41. All of the following are correct concerning solar cheilitis except one. Which one is the exception?
    a. There is a distinct demarcation between the vermilion border and skin.
    b. It appears as a mottled grayish-pink discoloration of lower lip.
    c. Linear fissures are seen at right angles to the vermilion border.
    d. It is caused by excessive exposure to sunlight.

42. Which of the following has the best long-term prognosis?
    a. Basal cell carcinoma
    b. Squamous cell carcinoma
    c. Multiple myeloma
    d. Melanoma

43. All of the following arise in the oral cavity except one. Which one is the exception?
    a. Squamous cell carcinoma
    b. Malignant melanoma
    c. Basal cell carcinoma
    d. Verrucous carcinoma

44. Which of the following may undergo malignant transformation?
    a. Granular cell tumor
    b. Neurofibroma
    c. Papilloma
    d. Hemangioma

45. Which of the following neoplasms occurs most often in males?
    a. Congenital epulis
    b. Mucoepidermoid carcinoma
    c. Pleomorphic adenoma
    d. Multiple myeloma

46. Pain is most often a symptom of a:
    a. Complex odontoma
    b. Cementoblastoma
    c. Neurofibroma
    d. Fibroma

47. Central involvement of the jaws may occur with a:
    a. Granular cell tumor
    b. Basal cell carcinoma
    c. Melanocytic nevus
    d. Mucoepidermoid carcinoma

48. Syndrome involvement may occur with a:
    a. Neurofibroma
    b. Verrucous carcinoma
    c. Pleomorphic adenoma
    d. Granular cell tumor

49. Which of the following neoplasms is most likely to occur in the mandible?
    a. Ameloblastoma
    b. Melanocytic nevus
    c. Pleomorphic adenoma
    d. Basal cell carcinoma

50. Which of the following neoplasms has the worst long-term prognosis?
    a. Basal cell carcinoma
    b. Verrucous carcinoma
    c. Mucoepidermoid carcinoma
    d. Metastatic tumor to the jaws

51. What is the most common benign salivary gland tumor?
    a. Trabecular adenoma
    b. Pleomorphic adenoma
    c. Canalicular adenoma
    d. Warthin tumor

52. All of the following are characteristic features of an ameloblastoma except one. Which one is the exception?
    a. Represents a benign tumor
    b. Most often occurs in the mandible
    c. May be radiographically multilocular
    d. Often encapsulated

53. A hemangioma is a:
    a. Malignant tumor of melanocytes
    b. Benign tumor of fat cells
    c. Benign tumor of blood vessels
    d. Malignant tumor of bone

54. What is the most common intraoral location for a neurofibroma and a schwannoma?
    a. Buccal mucosa
    b. Soft palate
    c. Gingiva
    d. Tongue

55. Which of the following are cells that produce melanin?
    a. Nevus cells
    b. Squamous cells
    c. Granular cells
    d. Mesenchymal cells

56. All of the following tumors may contain a radiopaque component except one. Which one is the exception?
    a. Adenomatoid odontogenic tumor
    b. Ameloblastic fibroma
    c. Benign cementoblastoma
    d. Complex odontoma

57. All of the following are characteristic of a malignant tumor except one. Which one is the exception?
    a. Usually unencapsulated
    b. Contains abnormal mitotic figures
    c. Composed of pleomorphic cells
    d. Usually grows very slowly

58. All of the following are types of monomorphic adenoma except one. Which one is the exception?
a. Trabecular adenoma
b. Canalicular adenoma
c. Pleomorphic adenoma
d. Papillary cystadenoma lymphomatosum

59. What is the predominant type of tissue found in Waldeyer rings?
a. Epithelial cells
b. Skeletal muscle
c. Lymphoid tissue
d. Adipose tissue

60. All of the following statements are correct concerning leukemia except one. Which one is the exception?
a. Diffuse hemorrhagic, gingival enlargement may be an oral manifestation.
b. It is characterized by an overproduction of atypical white blood cells.
c. Surgical excision is the treatment of choice.
d. It can occur in all age groups.

61. All of the following neoplasms occur in young individuals except one. Which one is the exception?
a. Ameloblastic fibroma
b. Basal cell carcinoma
c. Congenital epulis
d. Hemangioma

62. Which of the following neoplasms is derived from odontogenic mesenchyme?
a. Ameloblastoma
b. Complex odontoma
c. Adenomatoid odontogenic tumor
d. Odontogenic myxoma

63. Which salivary gland neoplasm may arise as a multilocular radiolucency in the posterior mandible?
a. Monomorphic adenoma
b. Adenoid cystic carcinoma
c. Mucoepidermoid carcinoma
d. Pleomorphic adenoma

Chapter 7 Synopsis

Condition/Disease	Cause	Age/Race/Sex	Location
Papilloma *Condyloma acuminatum* *Verruca vulgaris*	A low-risk human papillomavirus	M = F	Soft palate, tongue
Epithelial dysplasia *Erythroplakia* *Leukoplakia* *Erythroleukoplakia*	Premalignant Smoking considered a risk factor	Age: adults	Floor of mouth, tongue
Squamous cell carcinoma *Traumatic ulcer* *Deep fungal infections* *Verrucous carcinoma* *Necrotizing sialometaplasia*		Age: over 40 M > F	Most common sites: floor of mouth, tongue, lips
Verrucous carcinoma *Squamous cell carcinoma*	Neoplastic	Age: over 55 M > F	Most common sites: vestibule, buccal mucosa
Basal cell carcinoma *Squamous cell carcinoma* *Melanoma*	Neoplastic Associated with sun exposure	Age: over 40 M = F Whites	Skin of face

NOTE: Items listed in *italics* under a specific condition/disease should be considered in a differential diagnosis.
N/A, Not applicable.
*Not covered in text.

64. What benign salivary gland neoplasm is known to undergo malignant transformation?
a. Pleomorphic adenoma
b. Trabecular adenoma
c. Canalicular adenoma
d. Warthin tumor

65. Which of the following represents a slow-growing, exophytic malignant neoplasm composed of numerous papillary surface projections?
a. Basal cell carcinoma
b. Verrucous carcinoma
c. Squamous cell carcinoma
d. Mucoepidermoid carcinoma

66. A patient with an extramedullary plasmacytoma is at an increased risk of developing what disease?
a. Osteosarcoma
b. Chronic leukemia
c. Multiple myeloma
d. Acute leukemia

67. The term *vascular malformation* is used in association with which condition?
a. Kaposi sarcoma
b. Hemangioma
c. Leukemia
d. Lymphangioma

68. Which of the following is an example of a benign salivary gland tumor that has undergone malignant transformation?
a. Adenocystic carcinoma
b. Carcinoma ex pleomorphic adenoma
c. Transcarcinoma
d. Speckled leukoplakia

Clinical Features	Radiographic Features	Microscopic Features	Treatment	Diagnostic Process
Exophytic fingerlike projections	N/A	Papillary projections surfaced by stratified squamous epithelium covering connective tissue cores	Surgical excision	Microscopic
White, erythematous, or mixed white and erythematous mucosal lesion	N/A	Abnormal maturation of epithelial cells Hyperplasia of basal cells, disorganization of epithelial layers, increased nuclear/cytoplasmic ratios, cells with enlarged and hyperchromatic nuclei Abnormal keratinization Increased numbers of normal and abnormal mitotic figures No invasion of abnormal cells into underlying connective tissue	Surgical excision	Microscopic
Exophytic mass Ulcerated Leukoplakia or erythroplakia	N/A	Invasion of tumor cells through basement membrane into underlying connective tissue Pleomorphic epithelial cells, normal and abnormal mitotic figures	Surgical excision Radiation therapy Chemotherapy	Microscopic
Slow-growing exophytic mass Papillary projections	N/A	Papillary epithelial projections Well-differentiated epithelium with normal-appearing epithelial cells Broad-based rete pegs with intact basement membrane	Surgical excision	Microscopic
Nonhealing ulcer Rolled borders	N/A	Proliferation of basal epithelial cells into underlying connective tissue	Surgical excision Radiation therapy	Microscopic

Continued

Chapter 7 Synopsis—cont'd

Condition/Disease	Cause	Age/Race/Sex	Location
Pleomorphic adenoma *Monomorphic adenoma* *Mucoepidermoid carcinoma*	Neoplastic	Age: over 40 F > M	Parotid gland Most common intraoral site: palate
Monomorphic adenoma, trabecular adenoma, canalicular adenoma, Warthin tumor *Pleomorphic adenoma*	Neoplastic	Adults F > M	Most common oral sites: upper lip and buccal mucosa; Warthin tumor: parotid
Adenoid cystic carcinoma *Mucoepidermoid carcinoma*	Neoplastic	Adults F > M	Parotid gland Most common oral site: palate
Mucoepidermoid carcinoma *Adenoid cystic carcinoma*	Neoplastic	F > M	Parotid gland Most common oral site: palate Some are central in mandible
Ameloblastoma *Odontogenic myxoma* *Central mucoepidermoid carcinoma*	Neoplastic	Adults M = F	Intraosseous Peripheral tumors also occur Mandible > maxilla Posterior > anterior
Calcifying epithelial odontogenic tumor *Calcifying cystic odontogenic tumor* *Adenomatoid odontogenic tumor* *Ameloblastic fibro-odontoma*	Neoplastic	Adults M = F	Posterior mandible
Adenomatoid odontogenic tumor *Calcifying epithelial odontogenic tumor* *Calcifying odontogenic cyst* *Ameloblastic fibro-odontoma* *Dentigerous cyst*	Neoplastic	Age: 70% under 20 F > M	70% involve anterior maxilla and mandible Maxilla > mandible Usually associated with an impacted cuspid
Calcifying odontogenic cyst *Calcifying epithelial odontogenic tumor* *Adenomatoid odontogenic tumor* *Ameloblastic fibro-odontoma*	Cyst with neoplastic variant	Age: Under 40 M = F	Maxilla and mandible
Odontogenic myxoma *Ameloblastoma* *Central mucoepidermoid carcinoma*	Neoplastic	Age: 10–29 M = F	Mandible > maxilla
Central cementifying and ossifying fibroma *Focal cemento-osseous dysplasia* *Osteoma*	Neoplastic	Age: adults F > M	Mandible (90%)
Cementoblastoma *Hypercementosis*	Neoplastic	Age: younger than 25 M = F	Most occur in association with a mandibular molar

NOTE: Items listed in *italics* under a specific condition/disease should be considered in a differential diagnosis.

N/A, Not applicable.

*Not covered in text.

Clinical Features	Radiographic Features	Microscopic Features	Treatment	Diagnostic Process
Nonulcerated Dome-shaped	N/A	Encapsulated tumor Mixture of epithelium and tissue that resembles various forms of connective tissue	Surgical excision	Microscopic
Smooth-surfaced mass	N/A	Encapsulated epithelial tumor with a uniform pattern of epithelial cells	Surgical excision	Microscopic
Mass Often painful Surface may be ulcerated	N/A	Unencapsulated, infiltrating tumor composed of small, deeply staining, uniform epithelial cells arranged in perforated round-to-oval islands	Surgical excision Radiation therapy	Microscopic
Asymptomatic swelling or mass	When intraosseous, unilocular or multilocular radiolucency	Unencapsulated, infiltrating tumor composed of a combination of mucous cells and squamous-like epithelial cells	Surgical excision	Microscopic
Slow-growing Expansion of bone	Unilocular or multilocular radiolucency	Unencapsulated, infiltrating tumor composed of ameloblast-like epithelial cells surrounding areas resembling stellate reticulum	Surgical excision	Microscopic
Asymptomatic Slow-growing expansion of bone	Unilocular or multilocular radiolucency with scattered calcifications	Unencapsulated, infiltrating tumor composed of islands and sheets of polyhedral epithelial cells Calcifications and eosinophilic deposits in tumor	Surgical excision	Microscopic
Asymptomatic swelling	Well-defined radiolucency associated with an impacted tooth Radiopacities within the radiolucency	Encapsulated tumor composed of ductlike epithelial structures, masses of cuboidal and spindle-shaped epithelial cells with eosinophilic material and calcifications	Surgical excision	Microscopic
Asymptomatic swelling Root resorption	Unilocular or multilocular radiolucency Radiopacities within the radiolucency	Cyst lined with odontogenic epithelium with associated ghost cell keratinization Ameloblast-like cells and stellate reticulum-like areas	Enucleation	Microscopic
Asymptomatic expansion of bone	Multilocular, honeycombed radiolucency	Unencapsulated, infiltrating tumor composed of pale-staining substance containing widely dispersed cells with small nuclei	Surgical excision	Microscopic
Asymptomatic expansion Facial asymmetry	Well-defined unilocular lesion, varying degrees of opacities	Well-circumscribed tumor composed of fibrous connective tissue and rounded globular calcifications, bone trabeculae, or both	Surgical excision	Radiographic Microscopic
Localized expansion Painful Vital teeth	Well-defined radiopaque mass in continuity with root or roots of the affected tooth	*	Enucleation of the tumor Removal of the associated tooth	Radiographic Microscopic

Continued

Chapter 7 Synopsis—cont'd

Condition/Disease	Cause	Age/Race/Sex	Location
Ameloblastic fibroma *Odontogenic myxoma* *Central mucoepidermoid carcinoma,* *Odontogenic keratocyst (keratocystic odontogenic tumor)*	Neoplastic	Age: younger than 20 M > F	Posterior mandible
Ameloblastic fibro-odontoma *Calcifying epithelial odontogenic tumor* *Calcifying cystic odontogenic tumor* *Adenomatoid odontogenic tumor*	Neoplastic	Age: younger than 10	Posterior maxilla and mandible
Odontoma *Complex odontoma* *Calcifying epithelial odontogenic tumor* *Adenomatoid odontogenic tumor* *Ameloblastic fibro-odontoma*	Neoplastic	Age: children and young adults M = F	Most common locations: anterior maxilla, posterior mandible
Lipoma *Fibroma* *Neurofibroma* *Schwannoma*	Neoplastic	Age: most over 40 M = F	Most common intraoral locations: buccal mucosa, vestibule
Neurofibroma/schwannoma *Fibroma* *Granular cell tumor*	Neoplastic	Age: any M = F	Most common intraoral location: tongue
Granular cell tumor *Fibroma* *Neurofibroma* *Schwannoma*	Neoplastic	Age: 30–50 F > M	Most common locations: tongue, buccal mucosa
Congenital epulis *Fibroma* *Eruption cyst* *Pyogenic granuloma*	Neoplastic	Present at birth F > M	Anterior maxillary gingiva
Hemangioma/benign vascular malformation *Kaposi sarcoma* *Pyogenic granuloma*	Hemangioma: congenital or developmental Benign vascular malformation: adults; response to trauma	Hemangioma: infants Benign vascular malformation: adults F > M	Most common oral site: tongue
Lymphangioma *Hemangioma*	Neoplastic/developmental	Congenital M = F	Most common oral site: tongue
Kaposi sarcoma *Hemangioma* *Pyogenic granuloma*	Neoplastic human herpesvirus 8	M > F	Most common oral sites: hard palate and gingiva
Melanocytic nevus *Melanoma* *Melanotic macule* *Focal melanosis*	Developmental	Age: 20–50 F > M	Most common oral sites: hard palate and buccal mucosa

NOTE: Items listed in *italics* under a specific condition/disease should be considered in a differential diagnosis.

N/A, Not applicable.

*Not covered in text.

Clinical Features	Radiographic Features	Microscopic Features	Treatment	Diagnostic Process
Asymptomatic swelling	Well-defined unilocular or multilocular radiolucency	Nonencapsulated tumor composed of both strands and small islands of odontogenic epithelium and tissue that resemble the dental papilla	Surgical excision	Microscopic
Asymptomatic swelling	Well-defined radiolucency with associated calcifications Calcifications may resemble teeth	Strands and small islands of odontogenic epithelium and tissue that resemble the dental papilla combined with tooth structures	Surgical excision	Microscopic
Lack of eruption Swelling	Compound: cluster of miniature teeth Complex: radiopaque mass	Mature enamel, dentin, cementum, and pulp Compound form: multiple small teeth Complex form: irregular mass	Surgical excision	Radiographic Microscopic
Yellowish mass with delicate pattern of blood vessels on the surface	N/A	Well-delineated tumor composed of lobules of mature, uniform fat cells	Surgical excision	Microscopic
Asymptomatic nodule	N/A	Neurofibroma: well-delineated, diffuse proliferation of spindle-shaped cells Schwannoma: encapsulated proliferation of Schwann cells arranged in palisaded whorls around central pink zones	Surgical excision	Microscopic
Asymptomatic nodule	N/A	Unencapsulated tumor composed of large cells with a granular cytoplasm Overlying epithelium exhibits pseudoepitheliomatous hyperplasia (PEH)	Surgical excision	Microscopic
Sessile or pedunculated mass	N/A	Unencapsulated tumor composed of large cells with granular cytoplasm (similar to cells in granular cell tumor)	Surgical excision	Microscopic
Deep red-to-blue mass Blanches with pressure	N/A	Vascular lesion composed of numerous small capillaries or larger blood vessels	Injection of sclerosing solution Spontaneous remission Surgical excision	Clinical Microscopic
Ill-defined mass with a pebbly surface	N/A	Lesion composed of lymphatic vessels	Surgical excision	Clinical Microscopic
Purple macules, plaques Exophytic mass	N/A	Unencapsulated tumor composed of spindle-shaped cells mixed with slit-like spaces containing red blood cells	Surgical excision Radiation therapy Chemotherapy	Clinical Microscopic
Tan/brown macule or papule	N/A	Benign tumor composed of nevus cells	Surgical excision	Clinical Microscopic

Continued

Chapter 7 Synopsis—cont'd

Condition/Disease	Cause	Age/Race/Sex	Location
Melanoma *Melanocytic nevus* *Melanotic macule* *Focal melanosis*	Neoplastic	Age: over 40	Most common oral sites: hard palate and maxillary alveolus
Osteoma *Central cementifying and ossifying fibroma* *Focal cemento-osseous dysplasia*	Neoplastic	M = F	Intraosseous
Osteosarcoma *Chondrosarcoma* *Metastatic tumors* *Lymphoma*	Neoplastic	Most common primary malignant tumor of bone in patients younger than 40 M > F	Twice as frequent in mandible as in maxilla
Chondrosarcoma *Osteosarcoma* *Metastatic tumors* *Lymphoma*	Neoplastic	M > F	Maxilla and mandible
Leukemia *Pregnancy gingivitis* *Thrombocytopenia,* *Drug-related gingival enlargement*	Neoplastic	M > F	Gingiva
Lymphoma *Squamous cell carcinoma*	Neoplastic	Adults M > F	Most common oral sites: tonsillar area and posterior hard palate
Multiple myeloma *Metastatic tumors*	Neoplastic	Adults M > F	Mandible>maxilla
Metastatic tumors *Osteosarcoma* *Chondrosarcoma* *Lymphoma*	Neoplastic	Adults M > F	Mandible>maxilla

NOTE: Items listed in *italics* under a specific condition/disease should be considered in a differential diagnosis.
N/A, Not applicable.
*Not covered in text.

Clinical Features	Radiographic Features	Microscopic Features	Treatment	Diagnostic Process
Rapidly enlarging blue-and-black mass	N/A	Malignant tumor	Surgical excision	Microscopic
Asymptomatic	Sharply defined radiopaque mass	Benign, compact bone	None, unless necessary for fabrication of prosthetic appliance	Microscopic
Painful, diffuse swelling or mass Expansion of involved bone	Destructive, poorly defined radiolucency to radiopacity Asymmetric widening of the periodontal ligament space Sunburst pattern	Malignant tumor of bone*	Multiagent chemotherapy Surgical excision	Microscopic
Enlargement of involved bone	*	Malignant tumor of cartilage*	Wide surgical excision	Microscopic
Diffuse gingival enlargement with persistent bleeding	N/A	Atypical white blood cells circulating in blood and tissues	Chemotherapy Radiation therapy Corticosteroids	Laboratory Microscopic
Enlargement of involved tissue	Destructive, poorly defined radiolucent lesion	Malignant tumor of white blood cells in lymphoid tissue or extranodal tissue	Radiation therapy Chemotherapy	Laboratory Microscopic
Bone pain, swelling	Multiple radiolucent lesions	Malignant proliferation of plasma cells	Chemotherapy	Laboratory Microscopic
Pain Paresthesia Swelling Expansion of bone	Variable Usually poorly defined and radiolucent Tooth roots may show spiked appearance Some may show area of radiopacity	Resemble primary malignancy	Chemotherapy Radiation therapy	Microscopic

8

Nonneoplastic Diseases of Bone

ANNE CALE JONES, JOAN ANDERSEN PHELAN, AND OLGA A.C. IBSEN

OBJECTIVES

After studying this chapter, the student will be able to:

1. Define each of the words in the vocabulary list for this chapter.
2. Define dysplasia as it relates to bone diseases and differentiate the term from epithelial dysplasia.
3. Do the following related to benign fibro-osseous lesions:
   - Define benign fibro-osseous lesions and list the benign fibro-osseous lesions that occur in the jawbones and are described in this chapter.
   - Describe the clinical, radiographic, and microscopic features of periapical cemento-osseous dysplasia, florid cemento-osseous dysplasia, and focal cemento-osseous dysplasia.
   - Compare and contrast periapical cemento-osseous dysplasia, florid cemento-osseous dysplasia, and focal cemento-osseous dysplasia.
   - Compare and contrast monostotic fibrous dysplasia with polyostotic fibrous dysplasia.

- Compare and contrast the radiographic appearance, microscopic appearance, and treatment of fibrous dysplasia of the jaws with those of ossifying fibroma of the jaws.
- Compare and contrast the three types of polyostotic fibrous dysplasia.
4. Describe the microscopic appearance of Paget disease of bone and describe its clinical and radiographic appearance when the maxilla or mandible is involved.
5. Describe the clinical, radiographic, and microscopic features of both the central giant cell granuloma and an aneurysmal bone cyst.
6. Describe the cause of osteomalacia and rickets.

❖ Vocabulary

Benign fibro-osseous lesion (bə-nin′ fi″bro-os′e-əs le′zhən) Benign lesion of bone characterized microscopically by cellular fibrous connective tissue admixed with irregularly shaped bone trabeculae or cementoid material.

Café au lait (kah-fa′o-la′) Refers to a macular skin pigmentation that is the color of coffee with milk.

Dysplasia (dis-pla′zhə) Disordered growth; abnormal development.

Metabolic (me-tə-ˈbä-lik) Relating to the biochemical processes that occur in living organisms; metabolism.

Monostotic (mon′os-tot′ik) Involvement of a single bone.

Neoplasia (ne″o-pla″zhə) New growth; the formation of tumors by the uncontrolled proliferation of cells.

Neoplastic (ne″o-plas′tik) Pertaining to the formation of tumors by the uncontrolled proliferation of cells.

Nonneoplastic (non″neo-plas′tik) Not neoplastic.

Polyostotic (pol′e-os-tot′ik) Involvement of multiple bones.

Precocious (pri-ˈkō-shəs) Exceptionally early in development or occurrence; early.

Recontouring (rē-kontūr-ing) Shaped to fit the outline or contour.

Nonneoplastic diseases of bone that affect the maxilla and mandible fall into multiple categories. Inherited diseases that affect bone are discussed in Chapter 6, and benign and malignant neoplasms of bone are discussed in Chapter 7. The purpose of this chapter is to delineate several nonneoplastic diseases of bone that are important for a dental hygienist to understand but are not covered elsewhere in this text. These include three forms of cemento-osseous dysplasia: (1) periapical, (2) florid, and (3) focal. In addition, the dental hygienist should be familiar with the various types of fibrous dysplasia

and the clinical and radiographic features of Paget disease of bone, central giant cell granuloma, aneurysmal bone cyst, and osteomalacia.

The term **dysplasia**, as used in this chapter in the context of the three types of cemento-osseous dysplasia and fibrous dysplasia, refers to the abnormal and disordered production of cementum and bone. This term in this context should not be confused with dysplasia as used in the context of epithelial dysplasia. Epithelial dysplasia connotes a premalignant condition affecting squamous epithelium.

Benign Fibro-Osseous Lesions

Benign fibro-osseous lesions that affect the maxilla and mandible include central and peripheral cementifying and ossifying fibromas, periapical cemento-osseous dysplasia, florid cemento-osseous dysplasia, focal cemento-osseous dysplasia, and fibrous dysplasia (Box 8.1).

Periapical Cemento-Osseous Dysplasia

Periapical cemento-osseous dysplasia is a relatively common disease of unknown cause that affects periapical bone (Fig. 8.1A-B). The term **cementoma** was used in the past for this disease. However, because the disease does not represent a neoplasm, this term is inappropriate and should be avoided.

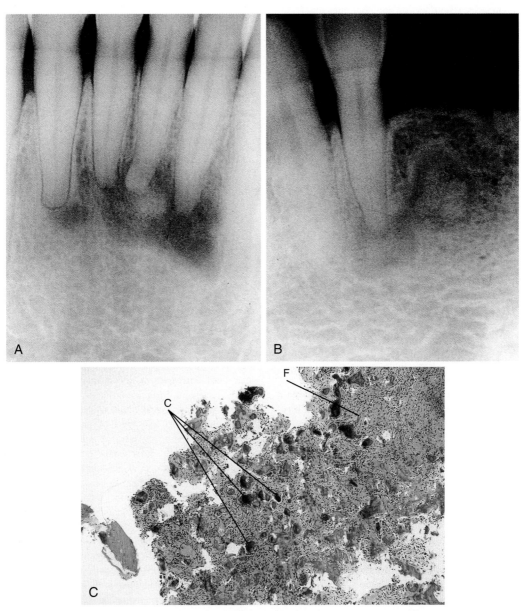

• Figure 8.1 A and **B,** Radiographs of periapical cemento-osseous dysplasia. **C,** Microscopic appearance of periapical cemento-osseous dysplasia shows a combination of cellular fibrous connective tissue (F) and calcified tissue (C).

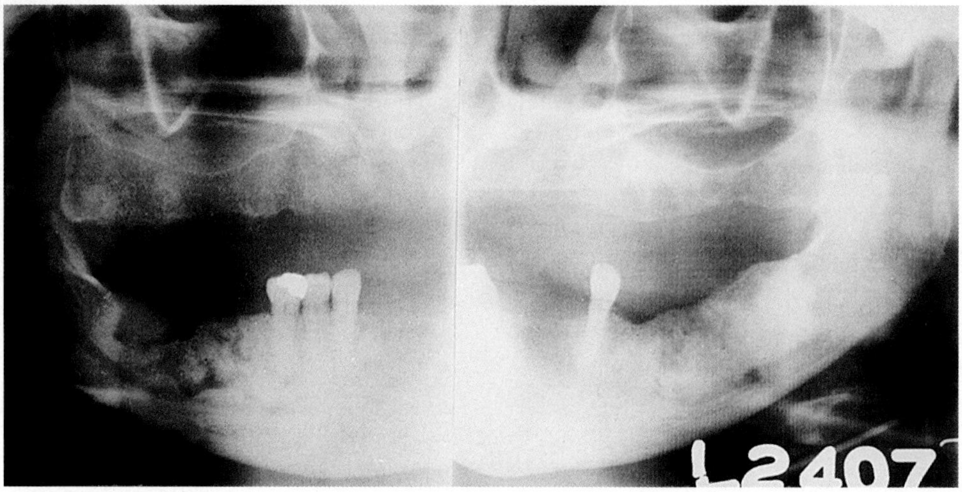

• **Figure 8.2** Florid cemento-osseous dysplasia. Panoramic radiograph shows irregular radiopaque masses in both the left and right mandible.

The lesion is asymptomatic and is discovered on routine radiographic examination. It occurs most commonly in the anterior mandible of patients older than 30 years of age. It is more common in women than men (10:1). Most studies have shown a predilection for this disease in black women. Early lesions are well circumscribed and radiolucent and may mimic periapical inflammatory disease. The bone at the apical area of multiple teeth may be involved. Teeth in the affected area are vital unless they are coincidentally carious or have been traumatized. With time the lesions become increasingly calcified; therefore older lesions are increasingly radiopaque and may appear radiolucent with central opacifications.

The diagnosis of periapical cemento-osseous dysplasia is usually established on the basis of its characteristic clinical and radiographic features. Historical and clinical information and radiographic appearance are both important in establishing the diagnosis. Pulp testing confirms that teeth are vital. A biopsy may be necessary in cases in which the characteristic radiographic features are not evident. Microscopic examination reveals a fibro-osseous lesion. Like other fibro-osseous lesions, periapical cemento-osseous dysplasia is composed of a combination of fibrous tissue and calcifications. The calcifications in this lesion may resemble bone, cementum, or both. Early lesions consist mainly of fibrous tissue, whereas long-standing lesions contain fibrous connective tissue interspersed with numerous calcifications (Fig. 8.1C). If a patient demonstrates radiographic changes characteristic of an early lesion, follow-up examinations may be necessary to ensure that a correct diagnosis was established. Once the condition is recognized, no treatment is necessary. The lesion remains asymptomatic and localized.

Florid Cemento-Osseous Dysplasia

Florid cemento-osseous dysplasia is another fibro-osseous lesion characterized by disordered cementum and bone development. This lesion characteristically involves multiple quadrants in the maxilla and mandible.

Florid cemento-osseous dysplasia occurs most often in black women older than 40 years of age. The cause of this disease is unknown. Radiographically, it differs in location from periapical cemento-osseous dysplasia in that it typically affects more than one quadrant of the maxilla and mandible, often in the posterior areas. On occasion, an early radiolucent phase similar to that seen in periapical cemento-osseous dysplasia may be identified. However, the majority of cases present as radiopaque masses of irregular opacification (Fig. 8.2). There is usually no bone expansion.

Florid cemento-osseous dysplasia is best diagnosed on the basis of its characteristic patient history, clinical presentation, and radiographic appearance (black women, radiographic changes in more than one quadrant). Asymptomatic florid cemento-osseous dysplasia does not require treatment. However, in an edentulous patient the sclerotic masses may perforate the mucosa, resulting in a communication between the oral environment and the underlying bone. This complication may lead to the development of osteomyelitis, resulting in pain and swelling. In these cases, antibiotic therapy and surgical intervention are needed.

Focal Cemento-Osseous Dysplasia

Focal cemento-osseous dysplasia is an asymptomatic fibro-osseous lesion that shares similar microscopic features with periapical cemento-osseous dysplasia and florid cemento-osseous dysplasia. However, it differs from these two lesions in that it has unique clinical and radiographic features.

Focal cemento-osseous dysplasia usually occurs in women between 30 and 50 years of age. Unlike periapical and florid cemento-osseous dysplasia, it is reported to be more common in white than black individuals. It typically arises in the posterior mandible and appears as an isolated, well-delineated, radiolucent-to-radiopaque lesion that is less than 1.5 cm in size.

Biopsy and microscopic examination usually are necessary to establish a diagnosis of focal cemento-osseous dysplasia. A characteristic surgical feature of focal cemento-osseous dysplasia is that it is composed of numerous gritty pieces of soft and hard tissue. This finding is distinctly different from the characteristic surgical features of a central cementifying or ossifying fibroma. These latter tumors present as a well-circumscribed mass of hard tissue that separates easily from the adjacent normal bone. The gritty tissue removed from focal cemento-osseous dysplasia represents fibrous connective tissue interspersed with bone trabeculae and cementum-like material. Once a definitive diagnosis has been

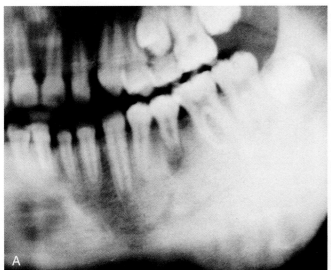
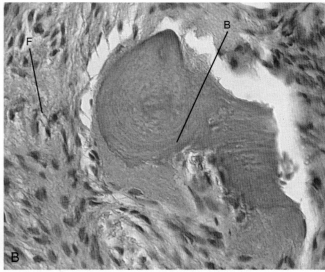

• **Figure 8.3** Fibrous dysplasia. **A,** Radiograph of fibrous dysplasia demonstrating indistinct borders that blend into the adjacent normal bone. **B,** Microscopic appearance (high power) of fibrous dysplasia shows cellular fibrous connective tissue *(F)* and irregular trabeculae of bone *(B)*. (**A** courtesy Drs. Paul Freedman and Stanley Kerpel.)

established, no further treatment is necessary. The prognosis for focal cemento-osseous dysplasia is excellent. On occasion, a focal lesion has progressed to florid cemento-osseous dysplasia.

Fibrous Dysplasia

Fibrous dysplasia is a developmental disease that is characterized by the replacement of bone with abnormal fibrous connective tissue interspersed with varying amounts of calcified material. Although the cause is unknown, several theories have been proposed. A genetic mutation (*GNAS* gene) has been identified as the underlying cause of this disorder. Several types of fibrous dysplasia exist; each type shares similar microscopic features, but the clinical presentation and associated systemic signs and symptoms differ. The extent of the disease is dependent on when in embryologic development the genetic mutation occurs. The earlier the genetic mutation occurs, the more severe the disease. Microscopically, fibrous dysplasia is classified as a benign fibro-osseous lesion. It is composed of vascularized, cellular fibrous connective tissue interspersed with irregular trabeculae of bone emerging from the connective tissue. Clinically, jaw involvement typically appears as a painless, progressive, unilateral enlargement of the maxilla or mandible. The expanding nature of the lesion may lead to malocclusion, tipping, or displacement of adjacent teeth. However, the teeth are rarely mobile. Involvement of the jaws may occur in any type of fibrous dysplasia. The classic radiographic appearance of fibrous dysplasia is a diffuse radiopacity that is described as resembling "ground glass" (Fig. 8.3A). The abnormal bone blends into the adjacent normal bone, making it difficult to determine the periphery of the lesion. A patchy radiolucency with central opacifications and a dense radiopacity have also been observed in fibrous dysplasia. The radiolucent or radiopaque appearance of fibrous dysplasia depends on the degree of calcification present in the lesion. Lesions that are primarily radiolucent contain an abundance of fibrous connective tissue with few calcifications, whereas more radiopaque lesions are composed predominantly of calcified tissue and a scant amount of fibrous connective tissue.

Types of Fibrous Dysplasia

Monostotic Fibrous Dysplasia

Monostotic fibrous dysplasia, the most common type of fibrous dysplasia, is characterized by involvement of a single bone. About 85% of cases of fibrous dysplasia are the monostotic type. The mandible and posterior maxilla are commonly affected; the maxilla is more frequently involved than the mandible. Other bones may be affected, including the ribs, femur, and tibia. Monostotic fibrous dysplasia is most commonly diagnosed in children and young adults; no sex predilection is seen. When fibrous dysplasia involves the maxilla, the disease usually extends into the maxillary sinuses and surrounding bones and is called **craniofacial fibrous dysplasia.**

Polyostotic Fibrous Dysplasia

Polyostotic fibrous dysplasia is characterized by involvement of more than one bone. It typically occurs in children under 10 years of age, and a definite female gender predilection is seen. The skull, clavicles, and long bones are often affected, and most cases are asymptomatic. When the long bones are involved, they may exhibit bowing, pathologic fractures, and pain. Patients with polyostotic fibrous dysplasia often demonstrate skin lesions. These lesions appear as light-brown macules called **café au lait spots.** Several forms of polyostotic fibrous dysplasia exist. *Craniofacial fibrous dysplasia* is the term used for polyostotic fibrous dysplasia that involves the maxilla with extension into the sinuses and adjacent zygoma, sphenoid, and occipital bones. Another form of polyostotic fibrous dysplasia is called the *Jaffe type* (or *Jaffe-Lichtenstein type*). It involves multiple bones along with associated café au lait macules on the skin. The most severe form of polyostotic fibrous dysplasia is called *Albright syndrome* (or *McCune-Albright syndrome*). This condition is characterized by endocrine abnormalities, including **precocious** (early) puberty in females and stunting or deformity of skeletal growth in both sexes as a result of early epiphyseal plate closure. Precocious puberty is exhibited by menses, pubic hair, and breast development in children as young as 2 years of age. Other complications of Albright syndrome include diabetes mellitus and hyperthyroidism. Café au lait skin macules may occur in this form of polyostotic fibrous dysplasia.

The diagnosis of fibrous dysplasia is established by correlating the microscopic findings along with the characteristic clinical features and radiographic appearance. Microscopic examination reveals a benign fibro-osseous lesion (Fig. 8.3B). The microscopic appearance is characterized by cellular fibrous connective tissue interspersed with irregularly shaped bone trabeculae. Fibrous dysplasia of the maxilla or mandible is distinguished from a central cementifying or ossifying fibroma on the basis of review of the radiographic findings. In fibrous dysplasia the radiographic changes blend into the surrounding normal bone. In a central cementifying or ossifying fibroma, a tumor that can demonstrate microscopic features similar to fibrous dysplasia, the radiographic findings consist of a well-defined lesion that is easily differentiated from the surrounding normal bone. Likewise, other fibro-osseous lesions such as periapical cemento-osseous dysplasia and florid cemento-osseous dysplasia can be distinguished from fibrous dysplasia on the basis of an examination of their distinct historical, clinical, and radiographic features. Although usually not used in diagnosis, the genetic mutation that has been identified in fibrous dysplasia is not found in the other fibro-osseous lesions. Fibrous dysplasia is treated surgically by **recontouring** the affected bone when necessary for cosmetic reasons. No treatment exists for severe and progressive polyostotic fibrous dysplasia. Radiation treatment of fibrous dysplasia is contraindicated because it has been associated with malignant transformation to osteosarcoma.

Paget Disease of Bone

Paget disease of bone, also called *osteitis deformans* and *leontiasis ossea,* is a chronic **metabolic** bone disease. It is characterized by abnormal bone metabolism, including resorption, osteoblastic repair, and remineralization of the involved bone. The cause is unknown. Several theories have been proposed, including viral, genetic, and environmental factors. The disease occurs most commonly in men over the age of 50. It typically involves the pelvis, femur, spinal column, tibia, and skull. When found in the jawbones, the maxilla is more commonly affected than the mandible.

The clinical manifestations of Paget disease of bone depend on the bone involved. Enlargement of the affected bone is common, and the patient often complains of pain. When the maxilla or mandible is involved, spacing between the teeth increases as the bone enlarges (Fig. 8.4A). Edentulous patients may complain that their dentures no longer fit. When other bones of the skull are involved, clinical manifestations include severe headache, dizziness, and deafness. These symptoms occur because the enlarging bone impinges on cranial nerves as they exit the skull. The classic radiographic appearance is a patchy radiolucency and radiopacity that has been referred to as a "cotton-wool" appearance (Fig. 8.4B). However, this occurs only in the later stages of Paget disease of bone. In earlier stages the radiographic appearance is not so specific. Hypercementosis, loss of the lamina dura, and obliteration of the periodontal ligament may also occur.

The diagnosis of Paget disease of bone involves the clinical, radiographic, and histopathologic features. Laboratory evaluation is important in establishing the diagnosis. The serum alkaline phosphatase level is significantly elevated in active disease. Serum calcium and phosphorous levels are normal. Two different measurements are used to evaluate the serum alkaline phosphatase

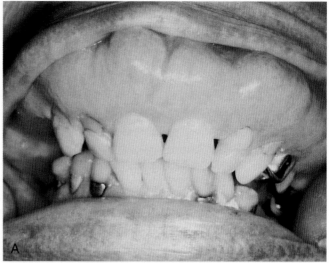

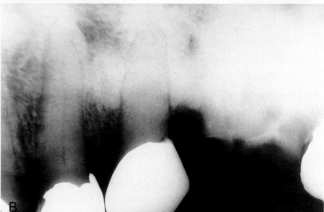

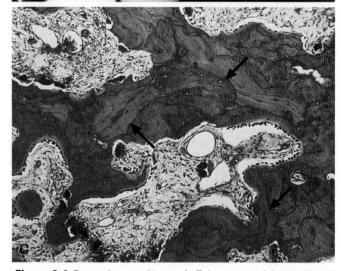

• **Figure 8.4** Paget disease of bone. **A,** Enlargement of the maxilla with spaces between the teeth. **B,** Radiograph demonstrating irregular opacification that is also referred to as a "cotton-wool" appearance. In areas, the lamina dura is obliterated. **C,** Microscopic appearance of Paget disease of bone shows bone trabeculae surfaced by numerous osteoclasts and osteoblasts. The prominent reversal lines (*arrows*) seen here characterize the mosaic pattern of bone.

level. In Bodansky units, the normal serum alkaline phosphatase value is 1.5 to 5.0. In Paget disease of bone the serum alkaline phosphatase value can be as high as 250 Bodansky units. Another measurement used to evaluate the serum alkaline phosphatase level is the King-Armstrong unit (KAU). Normal values are 5 to 10 KAU. In patients with Paget disease of bone, KAU values may be as high as 200+. Microscopic examination reveals bone trabeculae surfaced by numerous osteoclasts and osteoblasts (Fig. 8.4C). The involved bone demonstrates prominent reversal lines that result from the resorption and deposition of bone; this pattern has been described as *mosaic bone.* The connective tissue between the bone trabeculae is so well vascularized that the overlying skin may feel warm when touched. The most commonly used treatment for Paget disease of bone is a bisphosphonate. One intravenous dose of the bisphosphonate zoledronic acid has been found to be effective in keeping the disease in remission for up to 6 years. Oral complications related to bisphosphonate treatment are discussed in Chapter 9. Other treatments involve osteoclast inhibitors.

The disease is slowly progressive. Complications include fracture of the involved bone and development of malignant tumors, particularly osteosarcoma. Heart disease is a rare complication of Paget disease of bone.

Central Giant Cell Granuloma (Central Giant Cell Lesion)

The central giant cell granuloma is a nonneoplastic, intraosseous lesion of unclear pathogenesis. It has also been called a *giant cell reparative granuloma* and a *central giant cell lesion;* however, evidence that this lesion represents a reparative response is lacking. The giant cell granuloma is composed of well-vascularized fibrous connective tissue containing many multinucleated giant cells. Red blood cells, chronic inflammatory cells, and hemosiderin pigment are also seen in this lesion (Fig. 8.5A). The giant cell granuloma occurs both within gingival or alveolar soft tissue (peripheral) and within the bone of the maxilla or mandible (central). The peripheral giant cell granuloma is described in Chapter 2.

The central giant cell granuloma occurs within the maxilla or mandible, primarily in children and young adults under 30 years of age. Studies have reported its occurrence more commonly in females than in males. These lesions are most common in the anterior segments of the maxilla and mandible, more common in the mandible than the maxilla, and uncommon in the ramus of the mandible. Patients with central giant cell granulomas may complain of discomfort, but pain is not a common feature. Most central giant cell granulomas are discovered on routine radiographs. The lesion is slow growing and destructive and produces a unilocular or multilocular radiolucency in the bone. The borders of the radiolucency may be either sclerotic or ill defined (Fig. 8.5B-C). Divergence of the roots of teeth adjacent to the lesion is a common feature of a central giant cell granuloma.

Two categories of central giant cell granuloma have been described: a nonaggressive type and an aggressive type. The nonaggressive type is small, asymptomatic, and does not cause root resorption or cortical perforation. The aggressive type is large, painful, destructive, and causes root resorption and cortical perforation.

Central giant cell granulomas are generally treated by surgical removal, and they may occasionally recur. Successful treatment with intralesional corticosteroid injection has also been reported.

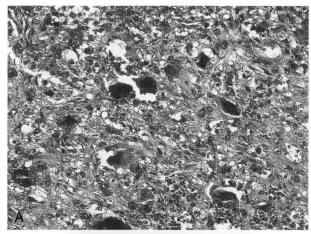

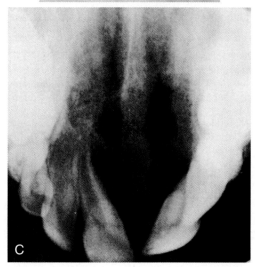

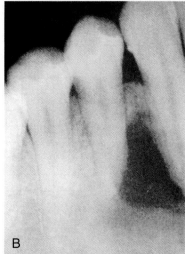

• **Figure 8.5** **A,** Microscopic appearance of a central giant cell granuloma showing the same features as a peripheral giant cell granuloma except for the absence of surface mucosa. Radiographs of two central giant cell granulomas showing multilocular radiolucencies in the mandible **(B)** and maxilla **(C).**

A lesion of bone identical to the central giant cell granuloma occurs in patients with hyperparathyroidism (discussed in Chapter 9). In patients with hyperparathyroidism, this lesion has been called a **brown tumor.** In patients with hyperparathyroidism, the lesions are not surgically removed because they resolve when the underlying disease (hyperparathyroidism) is successfully treated.

Aneurysmal Bone Cyst

An **aneurysmal bone cyst** is a pseudocyst that consists of blood-filled spaces surrounded by multinucleated giant cells and fibrous connective tissue (similar to the giant cell granuloma). Pseudocysts, including the aneurysmal bone cyst, are also discussed in Chapter 5. There is no epithelial lining. Aneurysmal bone cysts are most commonly seen in the long bones. Jaw lesions are rare. This radiolucent lesion has a unilocular or, more characteristically, a multilocular appearance that is often described as resembling a "honeycomb" or "soap bubbles." It is usually seen in individuals less than 30 years of age, and a slight female predilection has been reported. Lesions in the jaws may cause expansion of the involved bone.

A previous history of trauma to the area has been reported in some cases, but no direct correlation exists. Other reports have noted an association between the aneurysmal bone cyst and other bone lesions. It has frequently been associated with fibrous dysplasia, central giant cell granuloma, chondroblastoma, and other primary bone lesions. These other lesions may cause a change in vascularity that results in an aneurysmal bone cyst. Surgical excision and supplemental cryotherapy are the recommended treatments for an aneurysmal bone cyst. Recurrence is associated with incomplete removal of the original lesion.

Osteomalacia

Osteomalacia is a disease of bone that develops over a long period as the result of a calcium deficiency. When this disease occurs in young children, it is usually caused by a nutritional deficiency of vitamin D, and the associated disease is termed *rickets*. An inherited form of vitamin D deficiency called **hypophosphatemic vitamin D–resistant rickets** is included in Chapter 6. In adults the disease may be related to various problems such as a malabsorption syndrome, drugs, liver or kidney disease, and the chronic use of antacids. Osteomalacia may also be induced by certain tumors.

Delayed tooth eruption and periodontal disease have been associated with osteomalacia. Changes in bone trabeculation that occur in patients with osteomalacia may be subtle and difficult to detect. Due to poor bone mineralization, bones are susceptible to fracture.

Treatment is based on identification of the cause of the vitamin D deficiency and includes nutritional supplementation with vitamin D and dietary calcium.

Selected References

Books
Neville BW, Damm DD, Allen CM, et al: *Oral and maxillofacial pathology,* ed 4, St Louis, 2016, Elsevier.

Regezi JA, Sciubba JJ, Jordan RCK: *Oral pathology: clinical-pathologic correlations,* ed 7, St. Louis, 2017, Elsevier.

Journal Articles
Alsufyani NA, Lam EW: Cemento-osseous dysplasia of the jaw bones: key radiographic features, *Dentomaxillofac Radiol* 40:141, 2011.

Beylouni I, Farge P, Mazoyer JF, et al: Florid cemento-osseous dysplasia: report of a case documented with computed tomography and 3D imaging, *Oral Surg Oral Med Oral Pathol Oral Radiol Endod* 85:707, 1998.

Cohen MM Jr, Howell RE: Etiology of fibrous dysplasia and McCune-Albright syndrome, *Int J Oral Maxillofac Surg* 28:366, 1999.

Collins MT: Spectrum and natural history of fibrous dysplasia of bone, *J Bone Miner Res* 21(Suppl 2):99, 2006.

DiCaprio MR, Enneking WF: Fibrous dysplasia. Pathophysiology, evaluation, and treatment, *J Bone Joint Surg Am* 87:2005, 1848.

Dolanmaz D, Esen A, Mihmanli A, et al: Management of central giant cell granuloma of the jaws with intralesional steroid injection and review of the literature, *Oral Maxillofac Surg* 20(2):203, 2015.

Hadjipavlou AG, Gaitanis IN, Kontakis GM: Paget disease of the bone and its management, *J Bone Joint Surg* 84:160, 2002.

MacDonald-Jankowski DS: Fibro-osseous lesions of the face and jaws, *Clin Radiol* 59:11, 2004.

Ozek C, Gundogan H, Bilkay U, et al: Craniomaxillofacial fibrous dysplasia, *J Craniofac Surg* 13:382, 2002.

Polyzos SA, Anastasilakis AD, Makras P, et al: Paget's disease of bone and calcium homeostasis: focus on bisphosphonate treatment, *Exp Clin Endocrinol Diabetes* 119:519, 2011.

Regezi JA: Odontogenic cysts, odontogenic tumors, fibro-osseous, and giant cell lesions of the jaws, *Mod Pathol* 15:331, 2002.

Singer SR, Mupparapu M, Rinaggio J: Florid cemento-osseous dysplasia and chronic diffuse osteomyelitis: report of a simultaneous presentation and review of the literature, *J Am Dent Assoc* 136:927, 2005.

Siris ES, Lyles KW, Singer FR, et al: Medical management of Paget's disease of bone: indications for treatment and review of current therapies, *J Bone Miner Res* 21(Suppl 2):4, 2006.

Summerlin Don-John, Tomich CE: Focal cemento-osseous dysplasia: a clinicopathologic study of 221 cases, *Oral Surg Oral Med Oral Pathol* 78:611, 1994.

Sun ZJ, Zhao YF, Yang RL, et al: Aneurysmal bone cysts of the jaws: analysis of 17 cases, *J Oral Maxillofac Surg* 68:2122, 2010.

Triantafillidou K, Venetis G, Karakinaris G, et al: Central giant cell granuloma of the jaws: a clinical study of 17 cases and a review of the literature, *Ann Otol Rhinol Laryngol* 120:167, 2011.

Urs AB, Augustine J, Chawla H: Aneurysmal bone cyst of the jaws: clinicopathologic study, *J Maxillofac Oral Surg* 13(4):458, 2013.

Vallet M, Ralston SH: Biology and treatment of Paget's disease of bone, *J Cell Biochem* 117:289, 2015.

Whyte MP: Clinical practice: Paget disease of bone, *N Engl J Med* 355:593, 2006.

Zacharin M: The spectrum of McCune Albright syndrome, *Pediatr Endocrinol Rev* 4(Suppl):412, 2007.

Review Questions

1. A 48-year-old black woman has multiple asymptomatic, radiopaque masses in the mandible and maxilla. No expansion of bone is noted. The most likely diagnosis is:
   a. Central cementifying fibromas
   b. Florid cemento-osseous dysplasia
   c. Periapical cemento-osseous dysplasia
   d. Fibrous dysplasia

2. All of the following are examples of benign fibro-osseous lesions except one. Which one is the exception?
   a. Fibrous dysplasia
   b. Periapical cemento-osseous dysplasia
   c. Central ossifying fibroma
   d. Osteoma

3. Which of the following is characterized by precocious puberty in females?
   a. Monostotic fibrous dysplasia
   b. Jaffe-Lichtenstein–type fibrous dysplasia
   c. Albright-McCune–type fibrous dysplasia
   d. Focal cemento-osseous dysplasia

4. Periapical cemento-osseous dysplasia is located in the:
   a. Posterior mandible
   b. Posterior maxilla
   c. Anterior maxilla
   d. Anterior mandible

5. Periapical cemento-osseous dysplasia has also been known as a(n):
   a. Cementoma
   b. Odontoma
   c. Cementoblastoma
   d. Fibrous dysplasia

6. Which of the following diseases is associated with café au lait spots?
   a. Polyostotic fibrous dysplasia
   b. Paget disease of bone
   c. Monostotic fibrous dysplasia
   d. Focal cemento-osseous dysplasia

7. What is the name of the type of fibrous dysplasia that involves the maxilla and adjacent bones?
   a. Periapical
   b. Jaffe
   c. Craniofacial
   d. Monostotic

8. All of the following are features of Paget disease of bone except one. Which one is the exception?
   a. Deposition of amorphous material
   b. Resorption and osteoblastic repair
   c. Chronic metabolic bone disease
   d. Hypercementosis

9. The most characteristic radiographic appearance of fibrous dysplasia is described as a:
   a. "Cotton-wool" appearance
   b. Well-circumscribed radiopacity
   c. "Ground glass" appearance
   d. Well-circumscribed, unilocular radiolucency

10. All of the following are histologic features seen in Paget disease of bone except one. Which one is the exception?
    a. Osteoblasts and osteoclasts
    b. Bone with prominent irregular dark lines
    c. Well-vascularized fibrous connective tissue
    d. Hyperchromatic nuclei and atypical mitotic figures

11. All of the following have a characteristic radiographic appearance except one. Which one is the exception?
    a. Paget disease of bone
    b. Osteomalacia
    c. Florid cemento-osseous dysplasia
    d. Periapical cemento-osseous dysplasia

12. In patients with fibrous dysplasia, which of the following is the only recommended treatment modality?
    a. Surgery
    b. Radiation therapy
    c. Chemotherapy
    d. Sclerosing agent

13. Which of the following tests is most helpful in the diagnosis of Paget disease of bone?
    a. Immunoelectrophoresis
    b. Serum alkaline phosphatase
    c. Serum calcium
    d. Urinalysis

14. Osteomalacia is usually caused by a nutritional deficiency of:
    a. Vitamin B_{12}
    b. Vitamin D
    c. Alkaline phosphatase
    d. Potassium

15. Osteomalacia in children is called:
    a. Florid cemento-osseous dysplasia
    b. Osteogenesis imperfecta
    c. Albright syndrome
    d. Rickets

16. In which of the following diseases is there an associated increased risk of the development of osteosarcoma?
    a. Paget disease of bone
    b. Aneurysmal bone cyst
    c. Focal cemento-osseous dysplasia
    d. Giant cell granuloma

17. All the following do not describe the aneurysmal bone cyst except one. Which one is the exception?
    a. The radiographic appearance resembles a "honeycomb."
    b. It represents a true cyst.
    c. It has been associated with other primary bone lesions.
    d. It is usually treated with curettage or enucleation.

18. Leontiasis ossea and osteitis deformans are two other names for:
    a. Paget disease of bone
    b. Rickets
    c. Albright syndrome
    d. Fibrous dysplasia

19. The central giant cell granuloma:
    a. May occur on the tongue
    b. May present as a multilocular radiolucency
    c. Occurs primarily in children less than 6 years of age
    d. Is histologically the same as a periapical granuloma

20. Florid cemento-osseous dysplasia tends to affect:
    a. White women in their thirties
    b. Hispanic men over 60
    c. Black men under 30
    d. Black women over 40

21. Which one of the following is not a characteristic of Paget disease of bone?
    a. Patients may have expansion of the maxilla.
    b. It occurs primarily in young women.
    c. It may have a radiographic "cotton-wool" appearance.
    d. It has elevated serum alkaline phosphatase levels.

22. A brown tumor is associated with a(n):
    a. Aneurysmal bone cyst
    b. Fibrous dysplasia
    c. Osteomalacia
    d. Hyperparathyroidism

23. Pain is not a common feature in which one of the following conditions:
    a. Paget disease of bone
    b. Long bone involvement in polyostotic fibrous dysplasia
    c. Florid cemento-osseous dysplasia with osteomyelitis
    d. Central giant cell granuloma

24. Albright syndrome may involve all of the following characteristics except one. Which one is the exception?
    a. Precocious puberty
    b. Endocrine abnormalities
    c. Stunting or deformity of skeletal growth
    d. Characteristic loss of teeth

25. Diabetes can be associated with which one of the following:
    a. Albright syndrome
    b. Paget disease of bone
    c. Periapical cemento-osseous dysplasia
    d. Osteomalacia

26. All of the following are histologic features of benign fibro-osseous lesions except one. Which one is the exception?
    a. Calcifications that resemble bone
    b. Vascularized fibrous connective tissue
    c. Calcifications that resemble cementum
    d. Numerous multinucleated giant cells

27. All of the following are manifestations of osteomalacia except one. Which one is the exception?
    a. Delayed tooth eruption
    b. "Ground-glass" opacification
    c. Periodontal disease
    d. Altered bone trabeculation

28. Divergence of the roots of teeth is a common feature of:
    a. Paget disease of bone
    b. Osteomalacia
    c. Central giant cell granuloma
    d. Fibrous dysplasia

29. Osteomyelitis is a potential complication of:
    a. Florid cemento-osseous dysplasia
    b. Aneurysmal bone cyst
    c. Fibrous dysplasia
    d. Focal cemento-osseous dysplasia

30. All of the following occur in children or young adults except one. Which one is the exception?
    a. Rickets
    b. Paget disease of bone
    c. Fibrous dysplasia
    d. Central giant cell granuloma

31. All of the following are causes for the development of osteomalacia in adults except one. Which one is the exception?
    a. Malabsorption syndrome
    b. Liver and kidney disease
    c. Vitamin D deficiency
    d. Chronic use of antacids

32. Surgical recontouring of the affected bone is the treatment of choice for:
    a. Central giant cell granuloma
    b. Focal cemento-osseous dysplasia
    c. Paget disease of bone
    d. Fibrous dysplasia

33. Which of the following represents a generalized bone disease?
    a. Aneurysmal bone cyst
    b. Central giant cell granuloma
    c. Periapical cemento-osseous dysplasia
    d. Osteomalacia

34. Which of the following diseases is associated with the delayed eruption of teeth in children?
    a. Rickets
    b. Osteomalacia
    c. Fibrous dysplasia
    d. Central giant cell granuloma

35. Which of the following diseases often causes pain?
    a. Periapical cemento-osseous dysplasia
    b. Paget disease of bone
    c. Central giant cell granuloma
    d. Focal cemento-osseous dysplasia

36. All of the following features are characteristics of Paget disease of bone except one. Which one is the exception?
    a. Hypercementosis
    b. Mosaic bone
    c. Elevated serum alkaline phosphatase
    d. Periapical pathosis

37. The most common characteristics of race, sex, and age seen in patients with periapical cemento-osseous dysplasia are:
    a. White males over 50
    b. White females over 60
    c. Black males over 20
    d. Black females over 35

38. Which one of the following is more often diagnosed in white individuals?
    a. Florid cemento-osseous dysplasia
    b. Periapical cemento-osseous dysplasia
    c. Cementoma
    d. Focal cemento-osseous dysplasia

39. Which one of the following has characteristic features that include precocious puberty and endocrine abnormalities?
    a. Rickets
    b. Craniofacial fibrous dysplasia
    c. Paget disease of bone
    d. Albright syndrome

40. Craniofacial fibrous dysplasia, a form of polyostotic fibrous dysplasia, involves which of the following?
    a. Maxilla
    b. Mandible
    c. Femur
    d. Base of skull

41. Patients with polyostotic fibrous dysplasia exhibit skin lesions referred to as:
    a. Purple scales
    b. Bullae
    c. Café au lait pigmentation
    d. Urticaria

42. Mosaic bone describes a feature of which of the following conditions?
    a. Fibrous dysplasia
    b. Paget disease of bone
    c. Osteomalacia
    d. Florid cemento-osseous dysplasia

43. A lesion identical to the central giant cell granuloma is called a brown tumor. It is found in which of the following conditions?
    a. Hyperparathyroidism
    b. Hypothyroidism
    c. Hyperpituitarism
    d. Graves disease

Chapter 8 Synopsis

Condition/Disease	Cause	Age/Race/Sex	Location
Periapical cemento-osseous dysplasia *Periapical granuloma* *Periapical cyst*	Cause unknown	Age: >30 F > M Race: more common in blacks	Anterior mandible
Florid cemento-osseous dysplasia *Paget disease of bone*	Cause unknown	Age >40 F > M Race: more common in blacks	Multiple areas of maxilla and mandible
Focal cemento-osseous dysplasia *Periapical granuloma* *Periapical cyst* *Ossifying fibroma*	Cause unknown	Age: 30–50 F > M Race: more common in whites	Posterior mandible
Fibrous dysplasia *Ossifying fibroma*	Cause unknown	Monostotic: children and young adults; M = F Polyostotic: children; F > M	Monostotic: maxilla > mandible; ribs, femur, tibia Polyostotic: • More than one bone involved; skull, clavicles, long bones • Craniofacial type: maxilla and adjacent bones • Jaffe type: more than one bone involved • Albright syndrome: many bones involved
Paget disease of bone *Florid cemento-osseous dysplasia*	Chronic metabolic bone disease Cause unknown	Age: older than 50 M > F	Typically pelvis and spinal column When affecting the jaws: maxilla > mandible
Central giant cell granuloma *Brown tumor of hyperparathyroidism*	Unknown	Children/young adults	Within bone of maxilla and mandible Usually anterior segments
Aneurysmal bone cyst *Giant cell granuloma*	Unknown, associated with other bone diseases	Age: under 30 F > M	Within bone of the maxilla and mandible
Osteomalacia *Adults: osteoporosis*	Long-term deficiency of calcium Children: nutritional deficiency of vitamin D Adults: malabsorption syndromes, drugs, liver disease, kidney disease, chronic use of antacids	Children: rickets Adults: osteomalacia	Generalized bone disease

NOTE: Items listed in *italics* under a specific condition/disease should be considered in a differential diagnosis.
*Not covered in text

Clinical Features	Radiographic Features	Microscopic Features	Treatment	Diagnostic Process
Asymptomatic Vital teeth	Well-defined radiolucency to radiopacity at area of tooth apex	Benign fibro-osseous lesion Fibrous connective tissue with dense sclerotic masses of bone, cementum, or both	None	Historical Clinical (pulp test for tooth vitality) Radiographic
Asymptomatic	Multiple areas of radiolucency to radiopacity	Benign fibro-osseous lesion Fibrous connective tissue with dense sclerotic masses of bone, cementum, or both	None unless complicated by osteomyelitis	Historical Clinical (no expansion) Radiographic
Asymptomatic	Well-defined radiolucency to radiopacity	Fibrous connective tissue with round globular calcifications and bone trabeculae Numerous gritty pieces of soft and hard tissue	None	Radiographic Microscopic if diagnosis not certain
All types: enlargement of involved bones; maxilla/mandible involved; malocclusion, tipping, or displacement of teeth Jaffe type and Albright syndrome: • Café au lait macules on the skin • Extensive, progressive bone involvement • Endocrine abnormalities	Diffuse "ground-glass"–appearing radiolucency Abnormal bone blends into normal bone Unilocular and multilocular radiolucencies have been described	Benign fibro-osseous lesion	Surgical recontouring of affected bone for cosmetic reasons	Radiographic Clinical (unilateral expansion) Microscopic
Enlargement of the involved bone; patient may complain of pain in affected bone With involvement of maxilla or mandible, spacing between teeth increases; when edentulous, dentures no longer fit	Patchy radiolucency/radiopacity ("cotton-wool" appearance) Hypercementosis and loss of lamina are also described	Mosaic bone: reversal lines in bone with osteoblasts and osteoclasts lining the trabeculae Well-vascularized fibrous tissue	Experimental	Radiographic Clinical (bone expansion) Laboratory Elevated serum alkaline phosphatase
Usually asymptomatic	Unilocular to multilocular radiolucency Divergence of tooth roots is a common feature	Many multinucleated giant cells in well-vascularized connective tissue	Surgical excision	Microscopic
None, unless expansion of bone	Multilocular radiolucency	Blood-filled spaces surrounded by multinucleated giant cells in well-vascularized connective tissue	Surgical excision Supplemental cryotherapy	Microscopic
Children: delayed tooth eruption Pathologic fractures Periodontal disease	Subtle changes in bone trabeculation	*	Children: vitamin D and dietary calcium Adults: dependent on cause	*

9

Oral Manifestations of Systemic Diseases

OLGA A.C. IBSEN, JOAN ANDERSEN PHELAN, AND ANTHONY T. VERNILLO

OBJECTIVES

After studying this chapter, the student will be able to:

1. Define each of the words in the vocabulary list for this chapter.
2. Describe the difference between gigantism and acromegaly and list the physical characteristics of each.
3. State the oral manifestations of hyperthyroidism and hypothyroidism.
4. Describe the difference between primary and secondary hyperparathyroidism.
5. Do the following related to diabetes mellitus:
   - List the oral and systemic manifestations that occur in the uncontrolled diabetic state.
   - List the major clinical characteristics and oral manifestations of type 1 and type 2 diabetes.
   - Discuss treatment options for diabetes.
6. Define Addison disease, state some systemic features, and describe the changes that occur on the skin and oral mucosa in a patient with Addison disease.
7. Discuss Cushing syndrome.
8. Compare and contrast the cause, laboratory findings, oral manifestations, diagnosis, and treatment of each of the following blood disorders: iron deficiency anemia, pernicious anemia, thalassemia, sickle cell anemia, aplastic anemia, and polycythemia.
9. Describe the clinical features, oral manifestations, diagnosis, and treatment of both agranulocytosis and cyclic neutropenia.
10. Discuss leukemia, and compare and contrast acute and chronic leukemia.
11. Describe the clinical features, oral manifestations, diagnosis, and treatment of celiac disease.
12. Discuss bleeding disorders and state the purpose of each of the following laboratory tests: platelet count, bleeding time, prothrombin time, partial thromboplastin time, and international normalized ratio.
13. Do the following related to purpura:
    - List two causes of thrombocytopenic purpura.
    - Describe the oral manifestations of thrombocytopenia and nonthrombocytopenic purpura.
14. Define hemophilia, discuss the types of hemophilia, and describe its oral manifestations and treatment.
15. Discuss the oral manifestations of therapy for oral cancer.
16. Discuss radiation therapy, and describe the oral problems that would be expected to occur in a patient with radiation-induced xerostomia.
17. List two drugs that are associated with gingival enlargement.
18. Describe the criteria used to define bisphosphonate-associated osteonecrosis of the jaw.

❖ Vocabulary

Acromegaly (a-krō-′me-gə-lē) A disorder that is caused by chronic overproduction of growth hormone by the pituitary gland and is characterized by a gradual and permanent enlargement of bones after closure of epiphyseal plates.

Agranulocytosis (a-gran″u-lo-si-to′sis) A marked decrease in the number of granulocytes, particularly neutrophils.

Anemia (ə-ne′me-ə) A reduction in the number of red blood cells, quantity of hemoglobin, or volume of packed red blood cells to less than normal.

Apertognathia (ə -per″tog-na′the- ə) Anterior open bite.

Aplasia (ə-pla′zhə) (*adjective, aplastic*) Lack of development.

Arthralgia (ahr-thral′jə) Severe pain in a joint.

Atherosclerosis (ath″ər-o-sklə-ro′sis) The process by which lipid accumulates within the walls of large and medium-sized arteries. It leads to reduced blood flow to and death of vital organs.

Catabolism (kə-tab′o-liz-əm) Component of metabolism that involves the breakdown of tissues.

Chemotherapy (kēmō′therəpē) The treatment of disease by the use of chemical substances, especially the treatment of cancer by cytotoxic and other drugs.

Coagulation (ko-ag″u-la′shən) Formation of a clot.

Dysphagia (dis-fa′zhə) Difficulty swallowing.

Ecchymosis (ek″ĭ-mo′sis) (plural ecchymoses) A small, flat, hemorrhagic patch larger than a petechia on the skin or mucous membrane.

Epistaxis (epə′staksis) Bleeding from the nose.

Exophthalmos (ek″sof-thal′mos) An abnormal protrusion (bulging) of one or both eyes.

Fibrin (fi′brin) An insoluble protein that is essential to the clotting of blood.

Gastrectomy (ga strek″tuh′mee) Surgical removal of the stomach.

Gigantism (jī′gan‚tizəm) Excessive growth and height. Pituitary gigantism is a condition caused by increased production of growth hormone by the pituitary gland before closure of the epiphyseal plates.

Hematocrit (he-mat′ə-krit) Volume percentage of red blood cells in whole blood.

Hematoma (he″mah-to′mah) A localized swelling that is filled with blood caused by a break in the wall of a blood vessel.

Hematuria (he·ma·tu·ria) The presence of blood in the urine

Hemochromatosis (hē-mə-krō-mə-′tō-səs) A hereditary disorder of metabolism involving the deposition of iron-containing pigments in the tissues.

Hemolysis (he-mol′ə-sis) The release of hemoglobin from red blood cells by destruction of the cells.

Hemostasis (he″mo-sta′sis) Stoppage or cessation of bleeding.

Hepatomegaly (hep″ ə-to-meg′ ə-le) Enlargement of the liver.

Hormone (hor′mōn) Secreted molecules produced in the body that have a specific regulatory action on target cells that are distant from their sites of synthesis; an endocrine hormone is frequently carried by the blood from its site of release to its target.

Hypercalcemia (hi″pər-kal-se′me-ə) Excess calcium in the blood.

Hypercortisolism (hy·per·cor·ti·sol·ism) A condition caused by prolonged exposure to cortisol.

Hyperglycemia (hi″pər-gli-se′me-ə) Excess glucose in the blood.

Hypochromic (hi″po-kro′mik) Stained less intensely than normal.

Hyponatremia (hy·po·na·tre′mia) A deficiency of sodium in the blood.

Hypoglycemia (hīpōglī′sēmēə) A deficiency of glucose in the bloodstream.

Hypophosphatemia (hi″po-fos″fə-te′me-ə) A deficiency of phosphates in the blood.

Icterus (iktərəs) The technical term for jaundice.

International Normalized Ratio (INR) A system established by the World Health Organization (WHO) and the International Committee on Thrombosis and Hemostasis for reporting the results of blood coagulation (clotting) tests.

Ischemia (is′kēmēə) An inadequate blood supply to an organ or part of the body, especially the heart muscles.

Insulin (in′sə-lin) A hormone produced in the pancreas by beta cells in the islets of Langerhans; insulin regulates glucose metabolism and is the major fuel-regulating hormone.

Insulin shock (in′sə-lin shok) Profound hypoglycemia, or low blood sugar, that necessitates emergency intervention.

Ketoacidosis (ke″to-as″ĭ-do′sis) Accumulation of acid in the body resulting from the accumulation of ketone bodies.

Leukopenia (‚lü-kə-′pē-nē-ə) A condition in which the number of white blood cells circulating in the blood is abnormally low.

Macrovascular disease (mak″ro-vas′ku-lər dĭ-zēz′) Atherosclerosis of large and medium-size blood vessels.

Macroglossia (māk′rō-glô′sē-ə) Abnormally large tongue.

Megaloblast (′megələ-blast) A large, abnormally developed red blood cell typical of certain forms of anemia and associated with a deficiency of folic acid or vitamin B_{12}.

Menorrhagia (menə′rāj(ē)ə) Abnormally heavy bleeding during menstruation.

Microcyte (mi′kro-sīt) A red blood cell that is smaller than normal.

Microvascular disease (mi″kro-vas′ku-lər dĭ-zēz′) Damage to small blood vessels.

Myalgia (mi-al′jə) Muscle pain.

Neutropenia (noo″tro-pe′ne-ə) Decreased number of neutrophils in the blood.

Osteoporosis (os″te-o-pə-ro′sis) Abnormal rarefaction of bone.

Pancytopenia (pan″si-to-pe′ne-ə) A dramatic decrease in all types of circulating blood cells.

Parathormone (par″ə-thor′mōn) Parathyroid hormone.

Petechia (pə-te′ke-ə) (plural petechiae) A minute red spot on the skin or mucous membrane caused by escape of a small amount of blood.

Philadelphia chromosome (fih′luh-del″fee-uh kroh″muh-sohm) An abnormality of chromosome 22 in which part of chromosome 9 is transferred to chromosome 22.

Platelet (plāt′lət) Disk-shaped structure, also called a *thrombocyte,* found in the blood; it plays an important role in blood coagulation.

Polycythemia (pol″e-si-the′me-ə) Increase in the total red blood cell mass in the blood.

Polydipsia (pol″e-dip′se-ə) Chronic excessive thirst and intake of fluid.

Polyphagia (pòllee fáyjə) Increased appetite.

Polyuria (pälē′yoʔorēə) Excessive urination causing a profound loss of water and electrolytes.

Postprandial (pōs(t)′prandēəl) After a meal.

Purpura (pur′pu-rə) Blood disorders characterized by purplish or brownish-red discolorations caused by bleeding into the skin or tissues.

Receptor (re-sep′tər) A cell surface protein to which a specific molecule (e.g., a hormone) can bind; such binding leads to biochemical events.

Splenomegaly (sple″no-meg′ə-le) Enlargement of the spleen.

Thrombocyte (throm′bo-sit) A platelet.

Thrombocytopenia (throm″bo-si″to-pe′ne-ə) A decrease in the number of platelets in circulating blood.

Xerostomia (zēr″o-sto′me-ə) Dry mouth.

Many diseases that affect the body as a whole are associated with alterations of the oral mucosa, maxilla, and mandible. Systemic diseases can cause mucosal changes such as ulceration or mucosal bleeding. Generalized immunodeficiency can lead to the development of opportunistic diseases such as infection and neoplasia. Bone disease can affect the maxilla and mandible, and systemic disease can cause dental and periodontal changes. Drugs prescribed for a systemic disease can affect the oral tissues.

Local factors are frequently involved in manifestations of systemic disease in the oral mucosa. In some systemic diseases the mucosa is more easily injured; therefore mild irritation and chronic inflammation can cause lesions that would not occur without the presence of the systemic disease.

This chapter includes systemic diseases that have oral manifestations. Some overlap may occur among the diseases included in this chapter and those included in other chapters in this text. Included here are endocrine disorders, blood disorders (including those of red and white blood cells), disorders of **platelets**, and bleeding and clotting disorders. Also included are effects of drugs on the oral cavity. Oral changes can be similar for several different systemic diseases, and similar oral lesions can occur without the presence of systemic disease.

ENDOCRINE DISORDERS

The endocrine system consists of a group of integrated glands and cells that secrete **hormones.** The secretion of hormones by these glands is controlled by feedback mechanisms in which the amount of hormone circulating in blood triggers factors that control production. Diseases of this system can result from (1) conditions in which too much or too little hormone is produced and (2) from either dysfunction of the glands themselves or a problem in the mechanism that controls hormone production. Some of the endocrine gland diseases in which oral changes occur are included here.

Hyperpituitarism

Hyperpituitarism is excess hormone production by the anterior pituitary gland. It is caused most often by a benign tumor (**pituitary adenoma**) that produces growth hormone. If the increase in growth hormone production occurs during development before the closure of the long bones, **gigantism** results. Endocrine disturbances associated with genetic conditions such as McCune-Albright syndrome are responsible for close to 20% of the cases of gigantism. Treatment involves surgical removal or radiation of the pituitary adenoma.

Acromegaly is a rare condition that results when the hypersecretion occurs in adult life after closure of the long bones. The occurrence rate is about 65 patients per million. A pituitary adenoma is also thought to be the cause.

Clinical Features and Oral Manifestations

Gigantism includes excessive growth of the overall skeleton. Affected individuals can be more than 7 feet tall and weigh several hundred pounds. Acromegaly affects both men and women and most commonly occurs in the fourth decade of life. The onset is slow and insidious. Patients experience headaches, chronic fatigue, muscle and joint pain, poor vision, sensitivity to light, enlargement of the bones in the hands and feet, and

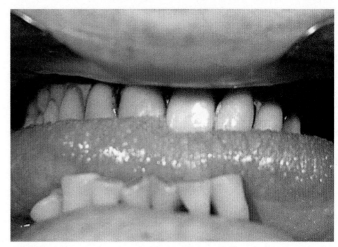

• **Figure 9.1** Enlarged tongue (macroglossia) in a patient with acromegaly.

an increase in rib size. The facial changes include enlargement of the maxilla and mandible, frontal bossing (an enlargement of the bones of the forehead), and enlargement of the nasal bones. An enlargement of the maxillary sinus also occurs, which causes a characteristically deep voice. The enlargement of the maxilla and mandible results in separation of teeth and malocclusion. Enlargement of the mandible results in mandibular prognathism. **Apertognathia** (anterior open bite) has been reported. Mucosal changes such as thickened lips and **macroglossia** (enlarged tongue) have also been described in patients with acromegaly (Fig. 9.1).

Diagnosis and Treatment

Laboratory tests may be performed to evaluate serum growth hormones by giving the patient an oral dose of glucose. Normally, growth hormone measured after intake of glucose would decrease. If the patient has acromegaly, the growth hormone will not decrease. Treatment for acromegaly involves surgical removal of the pituitary adenoma. The prognosis is good. Medical management may be attempted if surgery cannot be performed. Radiation therapy is also an option, but results are not as rapid or successful. In the untreated patient, other conditions such as diabetes, cardiomyopathy, hypertension, respiratory diseases, and colon cancer have been reported, increasing the patient's morbidity.

Hyperthyroidism (Thyrotoxicosis, Graves Disease)

Hyperthyroidism is a condition characterized by excessive production of thyroid hormone. It is 10 times more common in women than in men, and patients are typically diagnosed in their 30s or 40s. Hyperthyroidism has several different causes. The most common cause (60%–90%) is a condition called *Graves disease.* Graves disease is an autoimmune disorder in which antibodies called *thyroid-stimulating immunoglobulins* stimulate the thyroid cells, and as a result the thyroid gland enlarges and too much thyroid hormone is produced. This increase in hormone causes an increase in the patient's metabolism. In children hyperactivity is observed. Other causes of hyperthyroidism include hyperplasia of the gland, benign and malignant tumors of the thyroid, pituitary gland disease, and metastatic tumors.

Clinical Features and Oral Manifestations

The clinical features of hyperthyroidism include thyroid enlargement (goiter), rosy complexion, erythema of the palms, excessive sweating, fine hair, and softened nails. **Exophthalmos** (protrusion of the eyeballs) is a significant clinical characteristic and is often seen in patients with Graves disease. Weight loss, anxiety, weakness, restlessness, and cardiac problems (tachycardia) may be associated with this condition.

Hyperthyroidism in children may lead to premature exfoliation of deciduous teeth and premature eruption of permanent teeth. In adults **osteoporosis** may occur, which may affect alveolar bone. Dental caries and periodontal disease appear to develop and progress more rapidly in these patients than in other patients. Burning discomfort of the tongue has also been reported.

Diagnosis is made by evaluating thyroid hormones (T_4 and thyroid-stimulating hormone [TSH]) in circulating blood. In patients with hyperthyroidism, T_4 levels are elevated and TSH levels are usually depressed.

Treatment

Treatment of hyperthyroidism depends on the cause and may include surgery, medications to suppress thyroid activity, or the administration of radioactive iodine. Radioactive iodine is the most common treatment in adults. The treatment of hyperthyroidism is the most common cause of hypothyroidism. Clinical mismanagement of hyperthyroidism may lead to hypothyroidism and is thus described as iatrogenic or clinician-caused disease.

Hypothyroidism (Cretinism, Myxedema)

Hypothyroidism is characterized by decreased production of thyroid hormone by the thyroid gland. When hypothyroidism is present during infancy and childhood, it is called *cretinism.* Worldwide, congenital hypothyroidism is most often a result of endemic maternal iodine deficiency. The lack of iodine interferes with the development of the thyroid gland. In adults the condition is known as *myxedema.* Hypothyroidism has been classified as primary or secondary. In primary hypothyroidism the thyroid gland is abnormal. In secondary hypothyroidism, the pituitary gland does not produce sufficient TSH. Causes of hypoparathyroidism include developmental disturbances, autoimmune destruction of the thyroid gland (also known as Hashimoto thyroiditis), iodine deficiency, drugs, surgery, radiation and radioiodine thyroid treatment, and pituitary treatments for hyperthyroidism. In infants facial and oral changes include thickened lips, enlarged tongue, and failure of teeth to erupt. Adults with hypothyroidism may have dry skin, swelling of the face and extremities, weakness, fatigue, and an enlarged tongue (macroglossia). Individuals with hypothyroidism may have a slow heart rate and lower body temperature. Laboratory tests to determine the diagnosis of primary or secondary hypothyroidism include measurement of free thyroxine (T_4) and TSH levels. In primary hypothyroidism, T_4 levels are near normal or lower than normal, and TSH levels are high. In secondary hypothyroidism, both T_4 and TSH levels are usually lower than normal. Measurement of TSH levels differentiates secondary from primary hypothyroidism.

Treatment of hypothyroidism includes thyroid hormone replacement therapy; the most commonly prescribed is levothyroxine. Both adults and children respond well to thyroid replacement therapy. However, if the condition is not diagnosed and treated early in children, permanent damage to the central nervous system will result.

Hyperparathyroidism

Hyperparathyroidism results from excessive secretion of parathyroid hormone (**parathormone** [PTH]), which is secreted by the parathyroid glands. The four parathyroid glands are located near the thyroid gland. PTH plays an important role in calcium and phosphorus metabolism. Elevated blood levels of calcium (**hypercalcemia),** low blood levels of phosphorus (**hypophosphatemia),** and abnormal bone metabolism characterize primary hyperparathyroidism. Secondary hyperparathyroidism results when there is an overproduction of PTH in response to long-term decreased levels of serum calcium, often associated with chronic renal disease.

Primary hyperparathyroidism may be the result of hyperplasia of the parathyroid glands, a benign tumor of one or more of the parathyroid glands (parathyroid adenoma), or (less commonly) a malignant parathyroid tumor. Because of elevated serum calcium, these patients often have kidney stones. The disease is found in adults over 60 years of age and is far more common in women than in men.

Calcium is obtained mainly from dairy products and plays an important role in the contraction of all types of muscle. PTH maintains normal blood levels of calcium through its effects on the kidney, gastrointestinal tract, and bone. It increases the uptake of dietary calcium from the gastrointestinal tract and is able to move calcium from bone to circulating blood when necessary. The hormone appears to be able to remove calcium from bone through the action of osteoclasts.

Hyperparathyroidism that results from an abnormality of the parathyroid glands is called *primary hyperparathyroidism. Secondary hyperparathyroidism* occurs when calcium is abnormally excreted by the kidneys, and the parathyroid glands increase their production of PTH to maintain adequate blood levels of calcium. The most common cause of secondary hyperparathyroidism is kidney failure. Problems with absorption of nutrients and fat-soluble vitamins such as vitamin D through the gut or small intestine are also an important cause of secondary hyperparathyroidism.

Clinical Features and Oral Manifestations

The clinical manifestations of hyperparathyroidism are varied. Patients with mild cases can be asymptomatic. Joint pain or stiffness may be present. The disease can affect the kidneys, skeletal system, and gastrointestinal system. In severe disease lethargy, dementia, and coma can occur. Terms frequently used to describe systemic features of hyperparathyroidism include "stones, bones, and abdominal groans." "Stones" refers to kidney stones associated with primary hyperparathyroidism. "Bones" refers to resorption of the bones of the phalanges of fingers. "Abdominal groans" refers to the pain associated with duodenal ulcers.

The oral manifestations of hyperparathyroidism include changes in the bone of the mandible and maxilla. The chief oral manifestation is the appearance of well-defined unilocular or multilocular radiolucencies (Fig. 9.2A). Microscopically, these lesions appear indistinguishable from central (intraosseous) giant cell granulomas (described in Chapter 8) (Fig. 9.2B). Although rare, there have been reports of a few cases of peripheral giant cell granulomas (see Chapter 2) associated with hyperparathyroidism. Other radiographic changes that occur in secondary hyperparathyroidism include a generalized "ground-glass" appearance of the

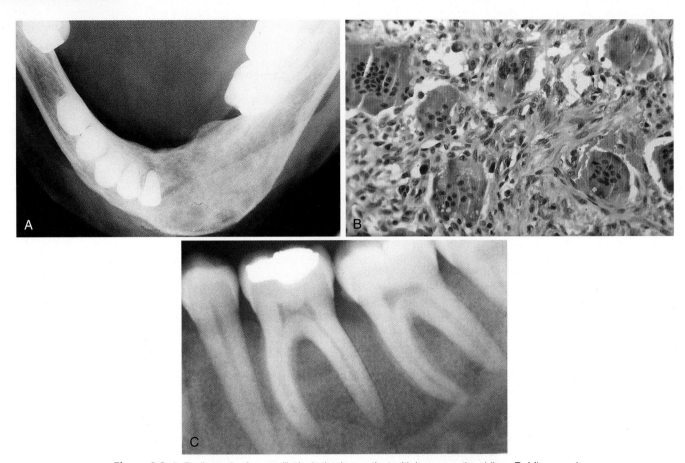

• **Figure 9.2** **A,** Radiograph of a mandibular lesion in a patient with hyperparathyroidism. **B,** Microscopic appearance of a jaw lesion occurring in a patient with hyperparathyroidism. The histologic appearance is identical to that of a central giant cell granuloma. **C,** This periapical radiograph reveals the "ground-glass" appearance of the trabeculae and loss of lamina dura in a patient with secondary hyperparathyroidism. (**A** courtesy Drs. Paul Freedman and Stanley Kerpel; **C,** from Neville BW, Damm DD, Allen CM, et al: *Oral and maxillofacial pathology*, ed 3, St. Louis, Saunders, 2009.)

trabeculae and loss of the lamina dura. Loosening of teeth can also occur (Fig. 9.2C).

Diagnosis and Treatment

The diagnosis of hyperparathyroidism involves the measurement of PTH blood levels and can also include serum calcium and phosphorus measurements. Treatment is directed at correcting the cause of the increased production of the hormone. Causes of increased production of hormone can include tumors, renal disease, and vitamin D deficiency. Bone lesions resolve when the hyperparathyroidism is treated successfully. In primary hyperparathyroidism, the functioning tumor must be surgically removed.

Diabetes Mellitus

Diabetes mellitus is an incurable disorder of carbohydrate (glucose) metabolism and is characterized by abnormally high blood glucose levels **(hyperglycemia),** which result from an absolute lack of the hormone **insulin** due to autoimmune destruction of pancreatic beta cells **(type 1);** or by a combination of peripheral resistance to insulin action and an inadequate secretory response by the pancreatic beta cells **(type 2).** Types 1 and 2 are classified as primary diabetes because these types do not develop secondarily to or are the result of another disease. Increased insulin

resistance, whereby the action of insulin is diminished in peripheral target tissues (e.g., skeletal muscle, fat cells), is often related to obesity.

Diabetes is appropriately defined as a syndrome because it has several components, including both acute (metabolic) and chronic (principally vascular) complications. This disorder of carbohydrate metabolism also leads to disorders of protein and fat metabolism. Normally, glucose signals the beta cells of the pancreas to make insulin. This hormone is then secreted directly into the bloodstream to facilitate the uptake of glucose into fat and skeletal muscle cells. In the presence of insulin, fat and skeletal muscle cells can use glucose as an energy source. When insulin is lacking, these cells are starved of energy. Without insulin to meet the body's demand for carbohydrate, tissues are broken down **(catabolism),** and weight loss occurs, as well as severe hyperglycemia that can lead to diabetic coma. Furthermore, the excessive production of ketone bodies from the breakdown of fatty tissue is a life-threatening condition and is a common metabolic disturbance in type 1 (insulin-dependent) diabetes. Ketone bodies, including acetone, can lower the pH of the blood **(ketoacidosis),** an acute condition that can lead to coma and death. White blood cell function is also affected in patients with diabetes mellitus. Phagocytic activity of macrophages is reduced, chemotaxis of neutrophils is delayed, and lymphocyte function (T lymphocytes) is adversely affected. These changes increase a patient's susceptibility to infection. In addition, collagen production is abnormal, thus affecting the healing process. With chronic hyperglycemia, collagen and other proteins become tagged with carbohydrate. The resulting advanced glycation end-products may also impair healing and contribute to the progression of periodontal disease. The precise cause of diabetes mellitus is unknown. Genetic and environmental factors have been implicated in its onset.

Diabetes mellitus is the most common endocrine disease in the United States with cases also increasing worldwide. According to the American Diabetes Association (ADA), diabetes (type 2) affects more than 29 million Americans, or nearly 10% of the population in the United States; nearly a third is currently unaware that they have hyperglycemia. Thus those individuals are at risk for developing the life-threatening complications of untreated diabetes. Approximately 1 million American children and adults have type 1 diabetes. The total costs (treatment of the disease and its complications) of diagnosed diabetes in the United States are approximately $245 billion.

A staggering 86 million adults in this country age 20 and older have impaired glucose tolerance, or "prediabetes," which is defined as elevated blood glucose that does not yet reach the criteria for the diagnosis of outright diabetes (see later). Without intervention, as many as 30% of individuals with impaired glucose tolerance will develop outright diabetes over 5 years with the additional risk factors of obesity and family history. Individuals with prediabetes also have a significant risk for cardiovascular disease. That risk may remain "concealed" until the patient ultimately develops more advanced clinical heart disease. Prediabetes is thus a wake-up call; it is not benign—it is a disease in its own right.

Compared with non-Hispanic whites, Native Americans, African Americans, and Hispanics are 1.5 to 2 times more likely to develop diabetes in their lifetime. In the United States diabetes is the leading cause of end-stage renal disease (renal failure), adult-onset blindness, and nontraumatic lower extremity amputations resulting from atherosclerosis. The World Health Organization (WHO) estimates that as many as 346 million people will have diabetes worldwide by the year 2030, with India and China being the largest contributors to the world's diabetic case load.

Diagnostic Criteria

Blood glucose is normally maintained in a very narrow reference range of 70 to 120 mg/dL (1 dL equals 100 mL); this is also known as *normal fasting blood glucose*. Blood glucose should return to fasting levels 2 hours after the completion of a meal (**postprandial**). According to the ADA and the WHO, the diagnostic criteria for overt or outright diabetes include any of the following:

1. A fasting blood glucose greater than or equal to 126 mg/dL.
2. A random blood glucose greater than or equal to 200 mg/dL in a symptomatic patient (the classic signs of hyperglycemia, the three Ps, as discussed later).
3. A 2-hour blood glucose greater than or equal to 200 mg/dL after drinking a glucose solution of 75 grams (oral glucose tolerance test, or OGTT). Patients who are not diabetic will "pass" the OGTT with blood glucose levels returning to normal reference range (70–120 mg/dL) after 2 hours.
4. A glycosylated hemoglobin (HbA$_{1c}$ or HgA$_{1C}$) level greater than or equal to 6.5% (glycosylated hemoglobin is further discussed later in the section on clinical management).

All of these tests, except the random blood glucose test in a patient with symptoms, need to *be repeated and confirmed on a separate day.*

Prediabetes

Prediabetes is defined with any of the following diagnostic criteria:

1. Fasting blood glucose between 100 and 125 mg/dL ("impaired fasting glucose")
2. Two-hour blood glucose between 140 and 199 mg/dL after the OGTT
3. Glycosylated hemoglobin level between 5.7% and 6.4%

Types of Diabetes

Insulin-Dependent Diabetes Mellitus, Pathology, and Clinical Management

Type 1 diabetes is called **insulin-dependent diabetes mellitus.** It may also be associated with other diseases of autoimmunity such as Addison disease, Graves disease, or autoimmune hyperthyroidism (most frequent) and pernicious anemia. Only 3% of all diabetic patients have this type of diabetes. Type 1 diabetes can occur at any age, but its time of onset is usually at a peak age of 20 years. The onset is abrupt due to the lack of insulin and can include the three Ps (i.e., the primary signs or classic triad of the metabolic derangements of type 1 diabetes): (1) **polydipsia** (excessive thirst and intake of fluid), (2) **polyuria** (excessive urination with electrolyte depletion), and (3) **polyphagia** (excessive appetite). Patients usually have a thin build.

Complications of Type 1 Diabetes. Complications can occur in up to 90% of individuals with type 1 diabetes within 20 years of diagnosis. These complications are due to damage of blood vessels from the largest to the smallest—the vascular system in diabetes takes the greatest beating. Difficulty in controlling blood glucose levels is a major problem for patients with type 1 diabetes. In recent years it has become increasingly evident that long-term rigorous control of blood glucose levels is important in minimizing the extent of chronic complications in patients with type 1 disease. This lack of control (chronic hyperglycemia) is closely linked with damage to the small blood vessels (**microvascular disease**) in diabetes and the complications with organ systems; these include, in particular, **the eyes (blindness), kidneys (end-stage kidney failure),** and **nerves (numbness, or *paresthesia*).** A patient with diabetes, for example, may have little or no feeling in the fingers or toes because of nerve damage. In such instances, the diabetes may lead to death of tissue, necessitating amputation of fingers or toes. However, it has also been shown conversely that blood glucose control works—small blood vessel disease may be prevented or its progression at least delayed with improved control. The physician determines a patient's blood glucose control (4-month period) with a glycosylated hemoglobin (HbA$_{1c}$ or HgA$_{1c}$) test. The lower the test result, the better is the control. An ideal target in type 1 diabetes is 7%. Aside from assessing blood glucose control, the HbA$_{1c}$ or HgA$_{1c}$ test result has also become another criterion for the diagnosis of diabetes in those patients who do not yet know they have the disease.

Disappointingly, the control of blood glucose alone does not tell the whole story because it does not prevent all the vascular complications in patients with diabetes. Unrelated to blood glucose control, **atherosclerosis of large and medium-size blood vessels (macrovascular disease)** in diabetes also affects, for example, the aorta and the coronary and cerebral arteries. In addition to control of blood glucose to avert microvascular disease, control of blood pressure and cholesterol may slow progression of macrovascular disease. Atherosclerosis has an earlier onset and is more extensive in patients with diabetes. The complications from atherosclerotic disease are as pernicious as malignancy. Involvement of the aorta can lead to weakening of the aortic wall (*abdominal aortic aneurysm*) with potential rupture, a condition that is invariably and rapidly fatal. Thrombi that form on atherosclerotic plaques within the aorta can also break off and travel downstream as emboli into the blood vessels of the lower extremities, leading to **gangrene and amputation of the legs or feet**. Atherosclerosis of the coronary arteries leads to **ischemia**, or a reduced supply of blood to the heart, and ultimately, *myocardial infarction* (MI) or heart attack—the most common cause of death in people with diabetes. Lastly, damage to the cerebral arteries can lead to a *stroke*, also called a *cerebrovascular accident* (CVA). Macrovascular disease is best minimized, however, with good control of serum cholesterol and blood pressure—this is generally true for patients with or without diabetes. Thus the concept of metabolic control in diabetes must be revisited and broadened because the control of blood glucose alone, although necessary, is not sufficient. A patient with diabetes must control not only blood sugar but also serum cholesterol and blood pressure to reduce the likelihood of vascular complications. Dentists and dental hygienists can thus better educate their patients about the control of diabetes and improve the quality of their patients' lives.

Rigorous control of glucose in type 1 diabetes is more likely achieved with multiple subcutaneous injections of insulin throughout the day to simulate physiologic conditions, rather than with a single daily injection. Multiple insulin injections, proper diet, exercise, and frequent determinations of blood glucose levels at home constitute the current approach to the management of the patient with type 1 diabetes. In some cases, oral hypoglycemic medications typically used in type 2 diabetes (see pharmacologic management of type 2 diabetes later) may be added as part of the medical management of patients with type 1 diabetes. These drugs may enhance the action of injected insulin. Multiple insulin injections as the mainstay of type 1 diabetes treatment can readily lead to low blood sugar (**hypoglycemia**); severe hypoglycemia (**insulin shock**) constitutes a medical emergency. The disease is controlled by replacement of the hormone insulin; however, insulin injections are not a cure for diabetes. All patients with type 1 diabetes remain dependent on insulin for their entire lives. Experimental approaches to restore insulin-producing cells in type 1 patients include the transplantation of pancreatic beta cells into the liver; alternatively, systemic stem cell infusion has the potential to halt the progression of diabetes, preserving the remaining pancreatic beta cells in patients in the early stages of the disease. If these approaches are successful, some patients may be spared from lifetime injections of insulin.

The Insulin Pump. An increasing number of patients with type 1 diabetes are receiving insulin pump therapy. This form of therapy is also part of the management of type 2 diabetes for those patients who take multiple insulin injections. Hence, the insulin pump is becoming more widely used for the clinical management of diabetes. The insulin pump is external and approximately the size of a pager; it delivers only rapidly acting insulin (e.g., NovoLog) through plastic tubing placed under the skin. The patient programs the pump to deliver small amounts of rapid-acting insulin on the hour over a 24-hour period (basal profile) according to the patient's metabolic needs. Thus the pump can maintain even more rigorous, predictable control of blood sugar levels than multiple insulin injections. Insulin dosage with the pump is also lower than with multiple insulin injections, making life-threatening hypoglycemia less frequent.

Very recent advances in technology now include external blood glucose sensors and transmitters that signal information to the insulin pump. The patient inserts the glucose sensor into the subcutaneous tissues. The sensor sends blood glucose information to the transmitter held in place with an adhesive patch on another area of the skin. The transmitter then sends the glucose data to the pump. The pump can be set to alert the patient (via an alarm) when the blood glucose is too low or too high. However, the patient must still deliver the insulin from the pump because the pump still lacks "a brain." Frequent blood sugar testing by the patient is still necessary. With further advances in pump technology, the sensor and transmitter working in synchrony may be able to prompt the pump if the blood sugar is too high to automatically deliver the right amount of insulin to match the blood sugar for that patient. Such an improvement in pump design would then "close the loop," and possibly represent the technological equivalent of a cure for diabetes. Alternatively, transplantation or stem cell infusions are biologic, experimental approaches to "close the loop."

The patient with diabetes who uses insulin pump therapy should carry a backup supply of syringes in case the pump fails to deliver insulin; such failure can lead to the rapid development of hyperglycemia and ketoacidosis, resulting in signs and symptoms of nausea, abdominal cramps, disorientation, and fatigue. It is also advisable to have a glucometer and test strips available in the dental operatory, as well as fast-acting carbohydrate to avert insulin shock. Lastly, monitoring of blood glucose is best accomplished several times a day with finger sticks (sterile lancets) to draw blood into a test strip. The blood sample is quite small, typically less than 1 μL. The strip is then inserted into and read by a glucometer within 5 seconds.

Non–Insulin-Dependent Diabetes Mellitus

Type 2 diabetes is also called **non–insulin-dependent diabetes mellitus.** Increased insulin resistance, rather than profound insulin deficiency, is characteristic of type 2 diabetes. Approximately 97% of all diabetic patients have type 2 diabetes. The onset of signs and symptoms is gradual and usually occurs in patients who are 35 to 40 years of age or older. When the metabolic rate starts to slow down with age, on comes the contributing factor of weight gain. However, there is now an epidemic of type 2 diabetes among children in major U.S. cities, particularly in minority neighborhoods; this epidemic has significant social, cultural, and ethical dimensions. Poor, high-crime neighborhoods in the inner cities restrict control of free space. People are less likely to get out and exercise, which may contribute to obesity. Hence, where you live may be an even more important determinant in developing type 2 diabetes than a person's genetic makeup. Fast-food companies also target their advertisements to the minority neighborhoods where less expensive but high-caloric food is a strong inducement, which is an ethically objectionable practice because it causes harm. Children are thus likely to succumb to pressures from other children and eat high-caloric foods. Studies have shown that second- and third-generation individuals whose parents were born in countries with a low diabetes rate ultimately approximate the diabetes rate in the United States. The Western diet is "obesogenic." The urban minority populations tragically bear the brunt of diabetes in the United States and suffer from its myriad life-threatening complications. Dentists and dental hygienists can play a major role in educating their patients about diabetes and oral health and, in doing so, advance public health.

Obesity is a common finding in many people with type 2 diabetes, and therefore this form of diabetes may be preventable. Obesity probably decreases the number of **receptors** for insulin binding in sensitive tissues such as fat and skeletal muscle, thereby leading to the development of the diabetic state. Hormones from fatty tissue (adipokines) may also contribute to insulin resistance. Complications are less common in this type of diabetes than in type 1 diabetes. Nonetheless, type 2 diabetes is definitely not benign. Poor or marginal control in type 2 diabetes can also lead to equally devastating complications as mentioned earlier for type 1 diabetes. The onset of type 2 diabetes among children is of extreme concern because life-threatening and debilitating complications may occur earlier in young adulthood at the active peak of life. Some patients achieve control of blood glucose levels with diet and weight reduction alone, whereas others require oral hypoglycemic agents to improve the secretion of "sluggish" insulin from the pancreas and binding of the secreted insulin to its target tissues. These medications thus also lower blood glucose levels but, unlike insulin, most are not given by injection. However, some patients with type 2 diabetes also require insulin injections to obtain improved control of blood glucose. Insulin can be effective and paradoxically lowers blood sugar even in those type 2 patients with insulin resistance.

Pharmacologic Management of Type 2 Diabetes. Unlike patients with type 1 diabetes (profound insulin deficiency), patients with type 2 diabetes mellitus are insulin resistant, often due to obesity. Serum levels of insulin in type 2 patients can vary widely (excessive, normal, or below normal). Over 100 oral and injectable medications combined (hypoglycemic drugs) are now marketed to treat type 2 diabetes in addition to insulin. These medications target different pathways to control blood glucose. Drug development has been explosive. These medications and their actions include but are not necessarily limited to decreasing the production of glucose by the liver (biguanides); stimulating the release of insulin from sluggish pancreatic beta cells (sulfonyl-ureas); improving skeletal and fatty tissue response to insulin (thiazolidinediones); incretin mimetics that mimic the action of a hormone called *glucagon-like peptide;* and more recently, newly developed and approved drugs such as Farxiga, Jardiance, and Onglyza. These newer drugs are taken by mouth and decrease blood glucose by increasing urinary glucose excretion (selective

sodium-glucose cotransporter-2 inhibitors). Along with diet control and exercise, the combinations of drugs and their mechanisms of action will likely lead to improved care with even more treatment options for patients with type 2 diabetes. Website references at the end of this chapter include a more in-depth and updated presentation on diabetes drugs.

Gestational Diabetes

Unlike type 1 and type 2 diabetes, gestational diabetes represents a separate classification of diabetes. It can occur during pregnancy (2%–10% of cases) and disappears after it. For most women, it does not cause noticeable symptoms. However, screening for gestational diabetes is a recommended and routine part of pre-natal care. Gestational diabetes is a disease of insulin resistance likely resulting from the antagonistic effects of the hormones progesterone and cortisol, and it follows the pattern of type 2 diabetes. The birth weight of the child is typically greater than normal, resulting in a large baby (*fetal macrosomia*). Gestational diabetes is particularly significant because mothers have a much higher risk of developing type 2 diabetes later in life, as do their babies.

Clinical Features and Oral Manifestations of Diabetes

The vascular system is the most severely affected system in diabetes, leading to a myriad of devastating systemic complications as mentioned previously. Decreased resistance to infection is seen, particularly in uncontrolled diabetes. Skin infections, especially furuncles (boils), urinary tract infections, and tuberculosis, are also common.

A skin disorder called *acanthosis nigricans* has been reported to be associated with type 2 diabetes mellitus and has been suggested to be a useful clinical indicator in screening for type 2 diabetes. Obesity in children and adults appears to increase the risk of development of this skin condition. Acanthosis nigricans is characterized by hyperpigmented, velvety-textured plaques that appear symmetrically distributed in folds and creases of the body. Acanthosis nigricans affecting the neck (Fig. 9.3A) and hands (Fig. 9.3B) may be identified by the dental hygienist during the physical/clinical evaluation of a patient.

The oral complications of diabetes are most severe when blood glucose levels are not controlled. In some patients control is

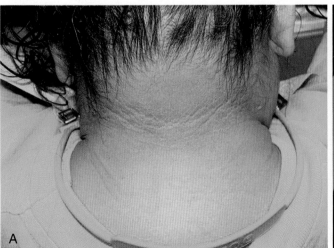
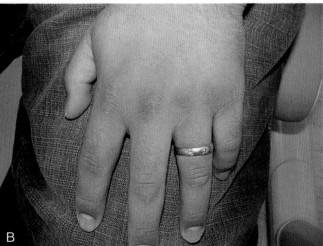

• **Figure 9.3 A,** Acanthosis nigricans affecting the back of the neck. **B,** Acanthosis nigricans affecting the hand. (Courtesy Lana Crawford.)

difficult, even with careful monitoring of these levels and insulin injections. These patients are said to have *brittle diabetes* and may benefit from recent advances in insulin pump therapy.

Increased colonization of the oral mucosa by *Candida albicans* and an increased prevalence of oral candidiasis have been reported in patients with diabetes mellitus, as has mucormycosis, a rare fungal infection that affects the palate and maxillary sinuses. These infections generally are seen in poorly controlled or uncontrolled diabetes mellitus. (Both oral candidiasis and mucormycosis are described in Chapter 4.) The presence of such fungal infections is indicative of the compromised innate and acquired immune responses that occur in diabetes mellitus.

Bilateral, asymptomatic parotid gland enlargement occurs in some patients; this results from either a deposition of fat or hypertrophy of the salivary gland tissue.

Xerostomia (dry mouth) is usually associated with uncontrolled diabetes mellitus. Dehydration of the oral tissues can result, increasing the risk of the development of oral candidiasis and dental caries, and may diminish taste sensation. Altered subgingival flora has been described in diabetes and may be the result of immunologic or salivary changes. Other significant oral findings include burning mouth syndrome, which may or may not be related to xerostomia. Burning mouth or tongue has been reported to occur in undiagnosed cases of type 2 diabetes. These may mostly resolve after medical diagnosis of the diabetes and subsequent treatment toward improving blood sugar control. Xerostomia can be a physically and psychologically debilitating condition.

Patients with diabetes mellitus have an accentuated response to plaque. The gingiva can be hyperplastic and erythematous, and acute and fulminating gingival abscesses can occur. Excessive periodontal bone loss, tooth mobility, and early tooth loss can also be associated with diabetes mellitus (Fig. 9.4). Periodontal disease is considered to be a significant complication of diabetes, and it also aggravates the control of diabetes—it is a destructive two-way relationship. Slow wound healing and increased susceptibility to infection occur as a result of the immunologic changes and defective collagen production. Periodontal disease is also a significant prognostic, or predictive, clinical marker for diabetes in those patients who have not yet developed it. Individuals who belong to certain ethnic groups in the United States—for example, Native Americans, African Americans, and Hispanic Americans—who are obese have a significant risk for developing type 2 diabetes. Periodontal disease in those individuals, however, should necessitate immediate referral to physicians or nurse practitioners for follow-up and diagnosis of diabetes before any dental treatment is initiated. In addition, if the patient is diabetic and not diagnosed and the disease is therefore not controlled, the dental clinician will never achieve control of periodontal conditions.

The patient with diabetes who is receiving good medical management and whose glucose levels are controlled can receive any indicated dental treatment. Early identification of oral infections is important. Infection aggravates diabetes because it often results in the loss of blood glucose control, thus creating a vicious cycle because susceptibility to infection is increased. Therefore elimination of infection is extremely important in patients with diabetes. Antibiotic medication, calculus and plaque removal, effective oral hygiene care, and adequate nutrition are especially important in the management of the patient with diabetes. One final point deserves mention here. People with well-controlled diabetes of either type can lead long, productive lives. However,

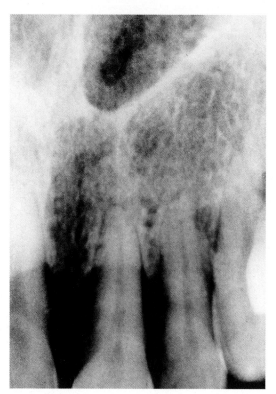

• **Figure 9.4** Periapical radiograph of a patient with diabetes mellitus shows severe alveolar bone loss.

diabetes control is not an "in-between." A patient either controls his or her diabetes or does not—there is also no such thing as "mild" diabetes. In the absence of good control, diabetes and its myriad complications are relentless and destructive, leading to the failure of multiple organ systems.

Good control of diabetes represents a synthesis of effort between the physician, nurse, nutritionist, dentist, and dental hygienist. It is truly a team effort. The dental hygienist is at the vanguard in the recognition, treatment, and long-term management of oral diseases. Periodontal disease in the setting of diabetes is perhaps the prototype for clinical management. The implication is powerful: the dental hygienist may reduce morbidity and mortality from diabetes through the proper treatment of periodontal disease, counseling, and education of patients. The dental hygienist may be the first to recognize the clinical manifestations of undiagnosed diabetes, particularly in those cases where treatment of periodontal disease remains refractory.

Addison Disease (Primary Hypoadrenocorticism)

Addison disease, also known as **primary hypoadrenocorticism** and **primary adrenal insufficiency,** is characterized by an insufficient production of glucocorticoid (cortisol) and mineralocorticoid (aldosterone) hormones that are normally produced by the cortex of the adrenal gland. The predominant cause of Addison disease in the United States and Europe is considered to be destruction of the adrenal gland due to an autoimmune disease. Circulating autoantibodies are found in most patients with Addison disease, and as with other autoimmune diseases, many patients with Addison disease have other coexisting autoimmune diseases. A malignant tumor and infections such as

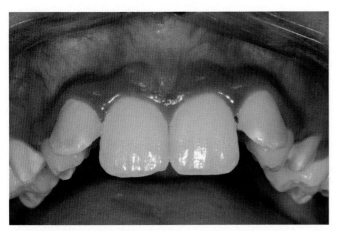

• **Figure 9.5** Diffuse pigmentation of the maxillary facial gingiva in a patient with Addison disease. (Courtesy Dr. John Kalmar.)

tuberculosis, deep fungal infections, and HIV infection have also been reported to cause Addison disease due to destruction of the adrenal gland.

Clinical Features and Oral Manifestations

Clinical features of Addison disease do not appear until 90% of the adrenal gland is destroyed. The onset of disease is subtle and includes increasing depression, general weakness, and low blood pressure. Without treatment, these features continue to worsen. As a result of the decrease in aldosterone, patients develop low levels of sodium in the blood (**hyponatremia**) resulting in gastro-intestinal symptoms, weight loss, nausea and vomiting, and a craving for salt. Due to the decreased production of adrenal ste-roids, the pituitary gland increases its production of adrenocorti-cotropic hormone (ACTH), which would normally increase the production of adrenal steroids. This hormone is similar to melanin-stimulating hormone and causes stimulation of melano-cytes. Consequently, brown pigmentation (bronzing) of the skin occurs, and melanotic macules can develop on the oral mucosa (Fig. 9.5). These diffuse oral melanotic macules resemble physi-ologic pigmentation; however, they differ in that they are of recent onset. They may precede the skin pigmentation and be the first sign of the disease.

Treatment

Treatment of Addison disease involves corticosteroid replacement therapy.

Hypercortisolism (Cushing Syndrome)

Hypercortisolism, or Cushing syndrome, is caused by a sustained increase in glucocorticoid levels. The most common cause is long-term corticosteroid therapy for autoimmune disease and organ transplantation. A pituitary adenoma or adrenal tumor can also result in increased glucocorticoid production. The term *Cushing disease* is applied when a pituitary adenoma is the cause. This is quite rare and usually occurs in young women.

Clinical Features and Oral Manifestations

Clinically, the signs of Cushing syndrome develop slowly. Weight gain is the most significant and obvious clinical feature. Accumulation of fat is responsible for most of the clinical signs

of Cushing syndrome. This includes a very rounded facial appearance ("moon" facies). Other signs and symptoms include hypertension, hyperglycemia, mood alterations, and a decreased ability to respond to stress. Cortisol production by the adrenal gland is a normal mechanism of responding to stress. In patients with Cushing syndrome there is interference with the feedback mechanism that causes the pituitary gland to release ACTH so the patient cannot respond normally to stress. For stressful dental treatment, an increase in the patient's corticosteroid therapy may be necessary. If clinical features suggest hypercortisolism, the patient should be referred to an endocrinologist to diag-nose and manage the condition. Because most cases are caused by corticosteroid therapy, the lowest possible dose should be prescribed.

BLOOD DISORDERS

The **complete blood count (CBC)** is important in the diagnosis of blood disorders. The CBC is a series of tests that examine the red blood cells, white blood cells, and platelets. It provides information about the number of each type of cell, the ratio of types of cells, and the appearance of the cells. The infor-mation included in a CBC and normal values are listed in Box 9.1.

• **BOX 9.1 Complete Blood Count: Normal Adult Values**

Red Blood Cells

Count: The total number of red blood cells (RBCs) per mm³ of whole blood
  Males: $4.7–6.1 \times 10^6$
  Females: $4.2–5.4 \times 10^6$
Hemoglobin: The amount of hemoglobin contained in 100 mL of whole blood
  Males: 13.8–17.2 gm/deciliter (dL)
  Females: 12.1–15.1 gm/deciliter (dL)
Hematocrit: The volume of packed RBCs in a sample of whole blood
  Males: 40.7%–50.3%
  Females: 36.1%–44.3%
Indices
  Mean corpuscular (cell) volume: Describes the average size of an individual RBC: 80–95 femtoliter (fm)
  Mean corpuscular (cell) hemoglobin: Indicates the amount of hemoglobin present in an RBC by weight: 27–31 picograms/cell (pg/cell)
  Mean corpuscular (cell) hemoglobin concentration: Indicates the proportion of each cell occupied by hemoglobin: 32–36 gm/deciliter (dL)

White Blood Cells

Count: 4500–10,000 cells/microliter of whole blood
Differential count: The number of each type of white blood cell (WBC) expressed as a percentage of the total number of WBCs:

Mature neutrophils (granulocytes)	40%–60%
Immature neutrophils (bands)	0%–3%
Lymphocytes	20%–40%
Monocytes	2%–8%
Basophils	0.5%–1%
Eosinophils	1%–4%

From www.nlm.nih.gov/medlineplus/ency/article/003642.htm and www.nlm.nih.gov/medlineplus/ency/article/003657.htm

Disorders of Red Blood Cells and Hemoglobin

Anemia

Anemia is defined as a reduction in the oxygen-carrying capacity of the blood that in most cases is related to a decrease in the number of circulating red blood cells. There are many different types and causes of anemia.

Nutritional anemias occur when a substance necessary for the normal development of red blood cells is in scant supply in the bone marrow. The most common deficiencies are of iron, folic acid, or vitamin B_{12}. These deficiencies can occur when the intake of the nutrient is insufficient or when disorders of absorption prevent its uptake. Anemia can also occur when suppression of the bone marrow stem cells takes place, resulting in an inability of the bone marrow to produce red blood cells.

Oral manifestations are similar for all types of anemia and include skin and mucosal pallor, angular cheilitis, erythema and atrophy of the oral mucosa, and loss of filiform and fungiform papillae on the dorsum of the tongue. Circumvallate papillae and foliate papillae are not affected.

Iron Deficiency Anemia

Iron deficiency anemia occurs when an insufficient amount of iron is supplied to the bone marrow for red blood cell development. It is the most common cause of anemia in the United States. This type of anemia can occur as a result of a deficiency of iron intake, excessive blood loss from heavy menstrual bleeding (**menorrhagia**) or chronic gastrointestinal bleeding, poor iron absorption, or an increased requirement for iron, as in pregnancy or infancy.

Plummer-Vinson syndrome is rare and can develop as a result of long-standing iron deficiency anemia. It most commonly occurs in Northern European and Scandinavian women. This syndrome includes **dysphagia** (difficulty swallowing), glossitis (inflammation of the tongue, causing a burning sensation), angular cheilitis, atrophy of the papilla on the dorsal tongue, atrophy of the upper alimentary tract, and a predisposition to the development of esophageal and oral cancer. In Plummer-Vinson syndrome evaluation of the esophagus is performed by endoscopy or esophageal barium, which will help to identify esophageal webs. These abnormal bands of tissue in the esophagus contribute to the diagnosis. Patients with Plummer-Vinson syndrome should be evaluated for oral and esophageal cancer because of their increased risk of developing these malignancies. Treatment of Plummer-Vinson syndrome usually involves increasing dietary iron.

Clinical Features and Oral Manifestations

Iron deficiency anemia is most often asymptomatic. When significant enough to show systemic symptoms, patients experience weakness (tiring easily), fatigue, low energy, shortness of breath, and sometimes cardiac palpitations. Oral mucosal signs in severe cases include angular cheilitis; pallor of the oral tissues; and an erythematous, depapillated, smooth, painful, burning tongue (Fig. 9.6). The changes in the oral mucosa occur as a result of a lack of nutrients to the epithelium. The filiform papillae on the dorsum of the tongue disappear first because they have the highest metabolic requirements. Disappearance of the fungiform papillae can also occur in chronic and severe cases. Some researchers have

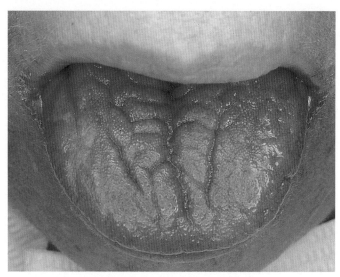

• **Figure 9.6** Iron deficiency anemia. The tongue is devoid of filiform papillae. Angular cheilitis was also present in this patient.

suggested that iron deficiency anemia places the patient at risk for oral candidiasis, which exacerbates angular cheilitis and depapillation of the tongue.

Diagnosis and Treatment

The diagnosis of iron deficiency anemia is made by laboratory tests, which show a low hemoglobin content of red blood cells, a reduced **hematocrit** (the volume of red blood cells in blood) value, and reduced serum iron level. Iron is needed for hemoglobin synthesis; therefore in iron deficiency anemia the red blood cells appear smaller than normal (microcytic) and lighter in color than normal (**hypochromic**). Increasing the intake of iron is the treatment for iron deficiency anemia; dietary supplements, particularly oral ferrous sulfate, are usually used. The oral lesions resolve when the deficiency is corrected.

Pernicious Anemia

Pernicious anemia is a vitamin B_{12} deficiency that is caused by a deficiency of intrinsic factor, a substance secreted by the parietal cells of the stomach. Intrinsic factor is necessary for the absorption of vitamin B_{12}. Normally vitamin B_{12} is transported across the intestinal mucosa by intrinsic factor. An autoimmune mechanism is the most likely cause of this type of pernicious anemia. Antibodies to components of gastric mucosa have been identified in patients with pernicious anemia. Vitamin B_{12} is needed for DNA synthesis; when it is lacking, the development of rapidly dividing cells such as bone marrow cells and epithelial cells is affected.

Other causes of vitamin B_{12} deficiency that involve an inability to absorb vitamin B_{12} include surgical removal of the stomach (**gastrectomy**), gastric cancer, or gastritis. The systemic and oral manifestations and treatment of these vitamin B_{12} deficiencies are the same as pernicious anemia.

Clinical Features and Oral Manifestations

The systemic signs and symptoms of pernicious anemia are those caused by vitamin B_{12} deficiency. These include weakness, pallor, fatigue, headache, shortness of breath on exertion, nausea, dizziness, diarrhea, abdominal pain, loss of appetite, and weight loss. Neurologic changes (such as severe paresthesia or tingling) may

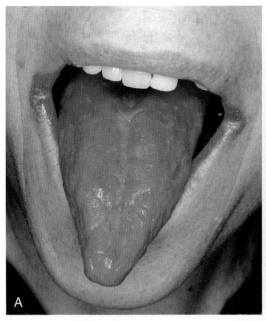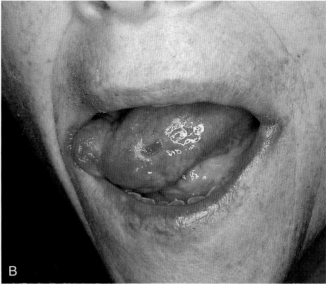

• **Figure 9.7** Pernicious anemia. **A,** Angular cheilitis and depapillation of the tongue in a patient with pernicious anemia. **B,** The mucosa becomes atrophic in pernicious anemia and easily ulcerated. Note ulcer on left lateral aspect of tongue.

also occur in patients with pernicious anemia because vitamin B_{12} helps to maintain the myelin needed for integrity of the nervous system. Psychiatric issues such as depression, dementia, and schizophrenia-like symptoms have been reported in patients with pernicious anemia.

Oral manifestations of pernicious anemia include angular cheilitis; mucosal pallor; painful, atrophic, and erythematous mucosa; mucosal ulceration; loss of papillae on the dorsum of the tongue; and burning and painful tongue (Fig. 9.7). Tongue changes have been reported in up to 60% of patients with pernicious anemia.

Diagnosis and Treatment

The diagnosis of pernicious anemia is made by laboratory testing. The diagnostic features include low serum vitamin B_{12} levels and gastric achlorhydria (lack of hydrochloric acid). Pernicious anemia is a megaloblastic anemia. *Megaloblastic anemia* is characterized by red blood cells that are immature, abnormally large, and have nuclei (**megaloblasts**). Immature neutrophils and platelets are also seen in both the bone marrow and the circulating blood. The Schilling test, a complex test that detects an inability to absorb an oral dose of vitamin B_{12}, has been used to diagnose pernicious anemia. Another test used more frequently today that is specific for pernicious anemia is one that identifies the presence of serum antibodies directed against intrinsic factor. Patients with pernicious anemia cannot absorb vitamin B_{12} through the intestinal wall. Therefore treatment consists of monthly injections of cyanocobalamin (a synthesized form of vitamin B_{12}). The oral mucosa improves in time, but the papillae on the dorsum of the tongue may not regenerate completely. There is an increased risk of gastric cancer in patients with pernicious anemia.

Folic Acid and Vitamin B_{12} Deficiency Anemia

Dietary deficiencies of **folic acid** and **vitamin B_{12}** can result in anemia and can occur in association with malnutrition and increased metabolic requirements. Individuals on vegetarian and vegan diets may also develop vitamin B_{12} deficiency. Malnutrition and associated vitamin B_{12} deficiency occur in association with alcoholism. Pregnant women are at increased risk for folic acid deficiency, and dietary supplementation in pregnancy is routine. Folic acid and vitamin B_{12} are essential for DNA synthesis. Deficiency of folic acid in pregnancy is associated with developmental neural tube abnormalities.

Oral Manifestations

The oral manifestations are indistinguishable from those of pernicious anemia.

Diagnosis and Treatment

The diagnosis of these anemias is based on laboratory test results that include serum assays of folic acid and vitamin B_{12}. These are also megaloblastic anemias. Thus, as in pernicious anemia, the red blood cells are immature, abnormally large, and nucleated (megaloblasts). Treatment involves dietary supplements.

Thalassemia

Thalassemia, also called *Mediterranean* or *Cooley anemia,* is the name of a group of inherited disorders of hemoglobin synthesis (see Chapter 6). It has an autosomal inheritance pattern and both heterozygous and homozygous forms; no predilection for either sex is seen. The heterozygous form, in which only one gene at a locus is involved, is called *thalassemia minor* and can be asymptomatic or only mildly symptomatic. The homozygous form, in which the genes on both chromosomes are involved, is called *thalassemia major* and is associated with severe hemolytic anemia, which results from damage to the red blood cell membranes and destruction of the red blood cells. Most cases of thalassemia occur in the Mediterranean region. It is much rarer in Northern Europe and the United States. There is evidence that thalassemia protects against malaria.

Clinical Features and Oral Manifestations

The severe form of the disease begins within the first year of life. Thalassemia is characterized by the defective production of hemoglobin; red blood cells produced are fragile and survive only a few days in circulation. The unstable hemoglobin causes a mild-to-moderate hemolytic and hypochromic anemia. The child has a yellowish skin pallor, fever, malaise, and weakness. An enlarged liver and spleen are common. The characteristic facies includes prominent cheekbones, depression of the bridge of the nose, an unusual prominence of the premaxilla, and protrusion or flaring of the maxillary anterior teeth. Intraoral radiographs show a peculiar trabecular pattern, showing reduced trabeculation of the maxilla and mandible because of the increase in hematopoiesis. There is a prominence of some trabeculae and a blurring and disappearance of others, resulting in a "salt and pepper" effect. Thinning of the lamina dura and circular radiolucencies in the alveolar bone have also been described. Lateral skull radiographs may demonstrate the characteristic "hair-on-end" appearance.

Treatment

Treatment of thalassemia major requires regular transfusions. This has been successful in reducing the effects of ineffective hematopoiesis and the consequential bone destruction, but results in iron overload (**hemochromatosis**) that can result in heart failure. Major advances using iron-chelating agents are now available to combat this iron overload. Improved prognosis for patients with thalassemia has resulted from advances in treatment.

Sickle Cell Anemia

Sickle cell anemia is the most common inherited disorder of red blood cells. It is found predominantly in black individuals and those of Mediterranean or Asian origin. Persons who are heterozygous for the disease are carriers and are generally asymptomatic. This is called *sickle cell trait.* Those who are homozygous are much more severely affected. This is called *sickle cell disease.* The disease can present as early as 6 months of age, and its signs and symptoms are evident before 30 years of age. Newborn screening identifies this condition early and helps prevent destructive consequence of the disease. Sickle cell anemia involves an abnormal type of hemoglobin in red blood cells that results from the mutation of a single amino acid in the hemoglobin structure. Because of this abnormal hemoglobin, the cells develop a sickle shape in the presence of decreased oxygen; hence the name *sickle cell anemia.* Exercise, exertion, administration of a general anesthetic, pregnancy, or even sleep can trigger a sickling of the red blood cells. Because of the change in their shape, the red blood cells are no longer able to pass through small blood vessels. The sickled red blood cells are destroyed more rapidly than normal, resulting in anemia and occlusion of the microvasculature circulation, which results in tissue ischemia and infarction. The multiple problems associated with sickle cell disease include an increased susceptibility to infection, vaso-occlusion of the pulmonary microvasculature, stroke, and cardiac failure.

Clinical Features and Oral Manifestations

Pain is a hallmark feature of sickle cell anemia. The patient with sickle cell anemia experiences weakness, shortness of breath,

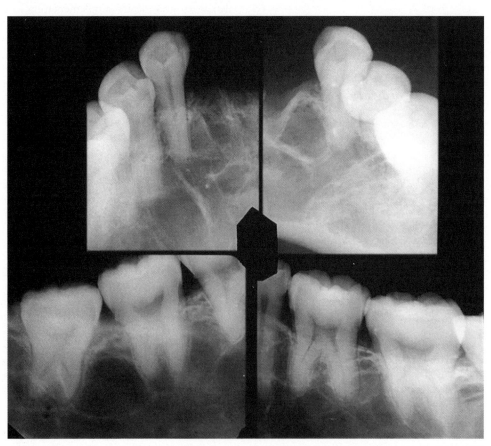

• **Figure 9.8** Sickle cell anemia. Radiograph shows abnormal trabeculation. (Courtesy Dr. Edward V. Zegarelli.)

fatigue, joint pain, and nausea. Two severe systemic characteristics of sickle cell anemia include **sickle cell crisis** in which severe sickling of erythrocytes occurs, and acute chest syndrome in which there is pulmonary involvement. Abnormalities in kidney function, the eyes, the cardiovascular system, and the central nervous system have all been reported. All organs and tissues of the body can be affected by sickle cell anemia. Oral manifestations are seen on dental radiographs (Fig. 9.8). As a result of increased hematopoiesis, a loss of trabeculation takes place, with the appearance of large, irregular marrow spaces. This change is most prominent in the alveolar bone. Changes in the skull have been described as a "hair-on-end" pattern because the trabeculae radiate outward.

Diagnosis and Treatment

The sickle-shaped cells may be seen on a blood smear (Fig. 9.9). The number of red blood cells is usually low, as is the hemoglobin content. Management of sickle cell disease includes administration of hydroxyurea to prevent complications from microvasculature occlusion. Treatment also includes blood transfusions or removal of the abnormal red blood cells and transfusion replacement with normal red blood cells. Because this may result in iron overload and the need for the administration of iron-chelating agents, transfusions are generally reserved for life-threatening complications. Antibiotics are important in managing infection. Sickle cell anemia can result in profound changes of the heart, such as enlargement, and lead to cardiac failure.

Aplastic Anemia

In **aplastic anemia** patients experience a dramatic decrease in all types of circulating blood cells **(pancytopenia)** because of a severe depression of bone marrow activity. Because all blood cells are produced from stem cells in the bone marrow (Fig. 9.10), aplastic anemia is therefore a life-threatening blood disorder. The cause of primary aplastic anemia is unknown. In secondary aplastic anemia the bone marrow failure is a result of a drug or chemical agent. Chemotherapy, radioactive isotopes, radium, and radiant energy have been associated with the development of aplastic anemia. Primary aplastic anemia occurs most frequently in young adults.

Clinical Features and Oral Manifestations

Systemic and oral manifestations are related to the generalized decrease in red and white blood cells and platelets and include infection, spontaneous bleeding, **petechiae,** and purpuric spots (Fig. 9.11). Systemically, because of the decreased oxygen in the blood, patients experience fatigue, weakness, and tachycardia; low platelet counts are responsible for significant bruising (i.e.,

hematomas) and **ecchymoses**. Retinal and cerebral hemorrhages have been reported. Low white blood cell counts (neutropenia) predispose the patient to infections that are often the cause of death. Oral manifestations include gingival hemorrhage, petechiae, and ecchymoses. Anemia results in pallor of the oral mucosa, and ulceration may be the result of infection.

Diagnosis and Treatment

Diagnosis is made on the basis of laboratory test results. In both forms of aplastic anemia a generalized decrease in circulating blood cells occurs. In addition to anemia, **leukopenia** (a decrease in white blood cells) and **thrombocytopenia** (a decrease in platelets) occur. White blood cells are essential in the defense against infection, and platelets are essential in the clotting of blood. Primary aplastic anemia is usually progressive and fatal. Treatment of secondary aplastic anemia involves removing the cause. Antibiotics are given to treat infections. Transfusions, bone marrow transplantation, and immunosuppressive therapy are all used to manage patients with aplastic anemia.

Polycythemia

Polycythemia is characterized by an increase in the number of circulating red blood cells. This increase can be either absolute or relative. Normal red blood cell production is carefully regulated and involves both the precursor cells in the bone marrow and the hormone erythropoietin, which is produced by the kidney.

Types of Polycythemia

The three forms of polycythemia are (1) polycythemia vera (primary polycythemia), (2) secondary polycythemia, and (3) relative polycythemia.

Polycythemia Vera (Primary Polycythemia)

In polycythemia vera a neoplastic proliferation of bone marrow stem cells results in an abnormally high number of circulating red blood cells. The production of red blood cells is uncontrolled. The cause of this disorder is unknown. It is somewhat more common in men than in women, and the age of onset is usually between 40 and 60 years. It is generally seen in white individuals and is extremely rare in black individuals. The symptoms of polycythemia vera include headache, dizziness, and itching of the skin (pruritus). The increase in red blood cells leads to impaired blood flow, vascular stasis, and poor circulation. The formation of thrombi can cause a disruption of the blood supply to the brain, heart, or peripheral vessels. A decrease in platelets (thrombocytopenia) can occur because of the disruption of the marrow from which they are derived.

Secondary Polycythemia

In secondary polycythemia the increase in red blood cells is caused by a physiologic response to decreased oxygen. A decrease in oxygen in the blood triggers an increase in erythropoietin by the kidneys, which results in increased production of red blood cells. A number of factors can cause a decrease in oxygen, including pulmonary disease, heart disease, living at high altitudes, and an elevation in carbon monoxide. The increase in carbon monoxide has been associated with tobacco smoking.

Relative Polycythemia

Relative polycythemia is caused by a decreased plasma volume and not an increase in red blood cells. In acute forms the cause is

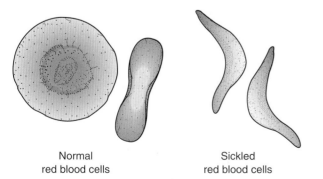

Normal
red blood cells

Sickled
red blood cells

• **Figure 9.9** Sickled red blood cells compared with normal red blood cells.

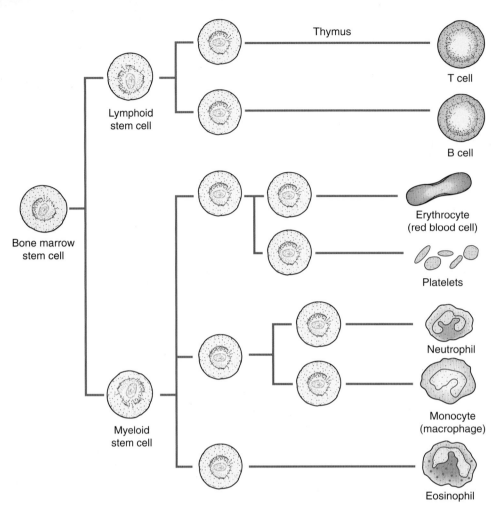

• **Figure 9.10** Blood cells are derived from stem cells in the bone marrow.

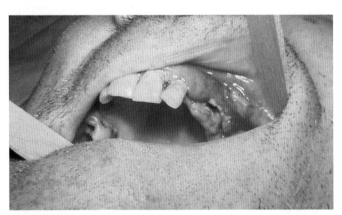

• **Figure 9.11** Aplastic anemia. Severe oral infection occurred after extraction of teeth in this patient with aplastic anemia. (Courtesy Dr. Harry Lumerman.)

usually easily recognized. Causes of acute relative polycythemia include diuretic use, vomiting, diarrhea, or excessive sweating. A chronic form of relative polycythemia has been called *stress polycythemia*. Most patients with this type of polycythemia are middle-age white men who are under physiologic stress, mildly overweight, hypertensive, and heavy smokers. The risk of CVA (stroke) and MI (heart attack) is increased in these patients.

Clinical Features and Oral Manifestations

The oral mucosa in patients with polycythemia may appear deep red to purple, and the gingiva may be edematous. The mucosal erythema may resemble erythematous candidiasis. The gingiva may bleed easily, and submucosal petechiae, **ecchymoses,** and **hematoma** formation can be present. There can be excessive bleeding after oral surgical procedures. Abnormalities of the oral mucosa result from an increase in circulating red blood cells, impaired blood flow, and thrombocytopenia.

Diagnosis and Treatment

Diagnosis of the various forms of polycythemia involves laboratory testing and measurement of the hemoglobin content and the hematocrit. Treatment is related to the type of polycythemia and may include removal of causative factors, chemotherapy, and phlebotomy ([bloodletting] removing up to 500 mL of blood each day). Oral lesions generally do not require local treatment; however, patients tend to have increased bleeding after oral surgery.

Disorders of White Blood Cells

Three groups of white blood cells are found in the circulation: granulocytes, lymphocytes, and monocytes. The three types of granulocytes are polymorphonuclear leukocytes (neutrophils), eosinophils, and basophils. The primary function of the neutrophils is to defend the body against foreign invaders such as bacteria, viruses, and fungi (described in Chapter 4). These cells are produced primarily in the bone marrow and are released into the circulating blood (see Fig. 9.10). Their response to infection is known as the **inflammatory response** (see Chapter 2).

Agranulocytosis

In **agranulocytosis** a significant reduction in circulating neutrophils **(leukopenia)** occurs, which has serious consequences. Any of the white blood cells can be involved, but leukopenia most commonly involves the neutrophils. A reduction in the number of circulating neutrophils is called **neutropenia.**

Agranulocytosis can result from either a reduced production of neutrophils or an accelerated destruction of neutrophils. Primary and secondary forms of agranulocytosis have been described. The cause of the primary form is unknown; it may be an immunologic disorder. The secondary form of agranulocytosis is most commonly produced by chemotherapeutic drugs for cancer chemotherapy and other immunologic reactions. Secondary agranulocytosis is most commonly seen in women.

Clinical Features and Oral Manifestations

After ingesting the offending drug, clinically patients experience a sudden onset of high fever, chills, jaundice (**icterus**), weakness, and sore throat. Orally the most characteristic feature is the presence of ulcerations and infection. Necrotizing ulcerations of the buccal mucosa, tongue, and palate resemble necrotizing ulcerative gingivitis; excessive bleeding from the gingiva and rapid destruction of the supporting tissue of the teeth have been described. Regional lymphadenopathy can accompany the oral problems.

Diagnosis and Treatment

The diagnosis is made by laboratory testing. The white blood cell count, which is normally 4500 to 10,000 cells/microliter, is dramatically reduced to less than 1000 cells/microliter. Treatment includes transfusions; antibiotics to control infection; and, in the secondary form, removal of the causative drug. Infections can become overwhelming and cause death. All surgical procedures, including dental hygiene procedures, are contraindicated.

Cyclic Neutropenia

Cyclic neutropenia is a rare form of agranulocytosis. A severe depression of neutrophils occurs at periodic intervals. It is inherited as an autosomal-dominant condition and is also described in Chapter 6. The main cause of cyclic neutropenia is a mutation of the gene *ELA-2*. This disorder is characterized by cycles every 21 to 27 days, when there is a sharp decrease in the neutrophil count that lasts 2 to 3 days.

Clinical Features and Oral Manifestations

The clinical manifestations of cyclic neutropenia are related to the decrease in neutrophils. Oral manifestations consist of severe ulcerative gingivitis or gingivostomatitis (see Fig. 6.15). In addition to the gingiva, areas of ulceration can occur on the tongue and surfaces of the oral mucosa. The ulcers are of variable size and have a craterlike appearance. They are very painful and have a bleeding base. In general, the oral lesions are infected secondarily. When neutrophils return to normal, the oral lesions tend to improve. Systemic manifestations include fever, malaise, sore throat, and occasional cutaneous and gastrointestinal infections.

Diagnosis and Treatment

Diagnosis of cyclic neutropenia is made by repeated CBCs. The test is done three times a week for 8 weeks.

Patients with cyclic neutropenia are usually managed by first determining the frequency of the cycles through periodic neutrophil counts and then instituting preventive antibiotic therapy to protect against secondary opportunistic infections. Over time, episodes of neutropenia and associated ulcerative gingivitis lead to severe periodontal disease, with loss of alveolar bone, tooth mobility, and exfoliation of teeth. Corticosteroid therapy is used to attempt to decrease the frequency of recurrent neutropenia. Supplements help maintain adequate nutrition. Dental hygiene treatment should be initiated when the circulating neutrophil count is normal to reduce the risk of complications such as gingival hemorrhage and secondary infection. Frequent dental hygiene appointments for removal of local irritants and maintenance of optimal oral hygiene reduce the risk of opportunistic infections in patients with cyclic neutropenia.

Leukemia

Leukemias are malignant neoplasms of the hematopoietic (blood-forming) stem cells. They are disorders that primarily originate in the stem cells of the bone marrow. The most dramatic feature of leukemias is the excessive number of abnormal white blood cells in the circulating blood. The pathogenesis is not clear. Environmental and genetic factors have been associated with the development of leukemia. Current investigations are focusing on oncogenic viruses (see Chapter 7). Many different types of leukemia exist. They are classified on the basis of the cell type involved and the maturity of the neoplastic cells (Box 9.2). Leukemias are described in this chapter with other abnormalities of the blood. They also have been included in Chapter 7, together with other white blood cell neoplasms. Many different types of leukemia are known; this text gives only an overview of the two general categories, acute and chronic, with a focus on the oral manifestations. Oral lesions are most common in acute leukemias but may also occur in chronic forms.

Acute Leukemias

Acute leukemias are characterized by the presence of very immature cells (blast cells) and by a rapidly fatal course if not treated. They can involve immature lymphocytes (acute lymphoblastic leukemia) or immature granulocytes (acute myelogenous or myeloid leukemia). Acute lymphoblastic leukemia primarily affects children and young adults and has a good prognosis. Acute myeloblastic leukemia involves adolescents and young adults (age range, 15 to 39 years), and the prognosis is not as good. The onset of acute leukemia is sudden and dramatic.

• BOX 9.2 Classification of Leukemias

Acute Leukemias	Chronic Leukemias
Acute lymphoblastic (lymphocytes) leukemia	Chronic lymphocytic leukemia
Acute nonlymphoblastic leukemia (granulocytes, monocytes, erythrocytes)	Chronic myelogenous (myeloid, granulocytic) leukemia

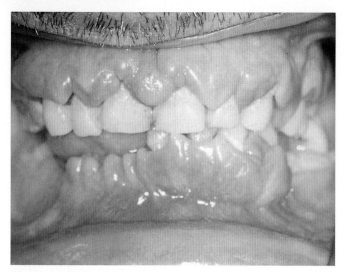

• **Figure 9.12** Generalized gingival hyperplasia in a patient with leukemia. (Courtesy Dr. Edward V. Zegarelli.)

Clinical Features and Oral Manifestations

Clinically, patients experience weakness, fever, enlargement of lymph nodes, bleeding, and spontaneous bruising. The lymph node enlargement can include cervical lymphadenopathy (enlargement of the lymph nodes in the neck) and is typically seen earlier in the course of disease, with the leukemias that involve immature lymphocytes. A general loss of cells produced by the bone marrow occurs. The fatigue results mainly from anemia, the fever from infection, and the bleeding from a decrease in platelets (thrombocytopenia). In advanced disease enlargement of the spleen **(splenomegaly)** and liver **(hepatomegaly)** occurs when these organs are infiltrated by the leukemic cells.

Oral manifestations can include gingival enlargement (which can be severe) caused by infiltration of leukemic cells (Fig. 9.12) and oral infections (including necrotizing ulcerative gingivitis) because the white blood cells are not functioning. In addition, if a decrease in platelets occurs, spontaneous gingival bleeding, petechiae, and ecchymoses may be present. Toothache as the result of invasion of the pulp by leukemic cells has been reported.

Diagnosis and Treatment

In acute leukemia laboratory findings include an elevated white blood cell count with the presence of many immature cells, anemia, and a low platelet count. In young children with acute lymphocytic leukemia, the prognosis with treatment is very good. In adolescents and adults with acute myelogenous (myeloid) leukemia, the prognosis is poor. Remissions occur with chemotherapy, and then relapses occur. Bone marrow transplantation is a treatment for this form of leukemia. Supportive care includes antibiotics to prevent infection and nutritional supplements to maintain adequate nutrition.

Chronic Leukemias

Several different types of chronic leukemia exist. They are all characterized by a slow onset, and they all primarily affect adults. The disease can be present for months before a diagnosis is made, and occasionally the diagnosis is made during a routine physical examination based on laboratory testing. One of the forms of chronic leukemia, *chronic myeloid leukemia*, is associated with a distinctive chromosomal abnormality, the **Philadelphia chromosome**. Another form of chronic leukemia, *chronic lymphocytic leukemia*, is the most common form and accounts for about one quarter of the total cases of leukemia. It may be asymptomatic for a long time. About half the patients with this type of leukemia have abnormal karyotypes; however, the abnormality is different from the Philadelphia chromosome.

Clinical Features and Oral Manifestations

The clinical onset is slow. The symptoms are nonspecific and include easy fatigability, weakness, weight loss, and anorexia. Oral manifestations include pallor of the lips and gingiva, gingival enlargement, petechiae and ecchymoses, gingival bleeding, and atypical periodontal disease. Cervical lymphadenopathy may be an early manifestation of chronic leukemia.

Diagnosis and Treatment

The normal white blood cell count is 4000 to 11,000/mm^3. The white blood cell count in leukemia can increase to 500,000/mm^3, and most of the total cells can be leukemia cells. Remissions occur with chemotherapy. High doses of chemotherapy over a short time is called *induction chemotherapy*. This type of therapy results in multiple unpleasant side effects for the patient. Cryotherapy (sucking on crushed ice during the administrations of intravenous chemotherapy) decreases the oral ulceration. After induction chemotherapy, once remission has started, low-dose chemotherapy over a longer period, referred to as *maintenance chemotherapy*, is the standard protocol. Bone marrow transplantation is used to treat both chronic and acute leukemia.

Celiac Disease

Celiac disease (celiac sprue, gluten-sensitive enteropathy) is a chronic disorder associated with sensitivity to dietary gluten, a protein found in wheat and wheat products. The ingestion of gluten results in injury to the intestinal mucosa. Malabsorption of other nutrients such as vitamin B$_{12}$ and folic acid occurs because of mucosal injury, and anemia develops as a result.

Clinical Features and Oral Manifestations

Oral manifestations are the same as those that occur in anemia due to other causes. These include a painful burning tongue (glossitis), atrophy of the papillae of the tongue, and ulceration of the oral mucosa. Systemic symptoms include diarrhea, nervousness, and paresthesia of the extremities.

Diagnosis and Treatment

Patients should adhere to a gluten-free diet. Oral manifestations resolve when the systemic disease is under control.

BLEEDING DISORDERS

Hemostasis

Patients with bleeding disorders can have one of a number of different defects.

Hemostasis (the cessation of bleeding) is a complex process that involves a number of events (Fig. 9.13). When a blood vessel is damaged, marked constriction of the vessel (vasoconstriction) occurs in an attempt to stop the flow of blood. Platelets **(thrombocytes)** that are produced by the bone marrow and circulating

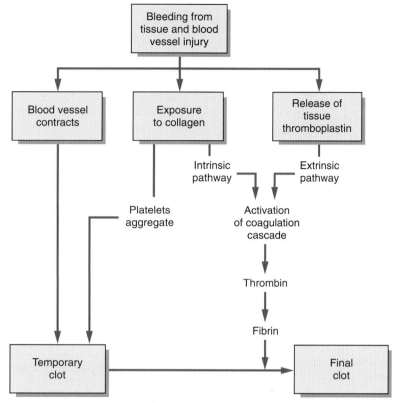

• **Figure 9.13** Hemostasis.

in blood adhere to the damaged surface and aggregate to form a temporary clot. To stop the bleeding permanently, it is necessary for **fibrin** to be produced. Fibrin tightly binds the aggregating platelets to form a clot. A cascade of circulating plasma proteins that are made almost exclusively in the liver and called *clotting factors* or *coagulation factors* is necessary to convert the precursor fibrinogen to fibrin (Table 9.1 and Fig. 9.13).

Finally, anticlotting mechanisms are activated to prevent the spread of more clots and to allow the clot to dissolve so that the damaged vessel can be repaired. This complexity is necessary to prevent inappropriate clotting. Successful hemostasis depends on the walls of the blood vessels, adequate numbers of functioning platelets, and adequate levels of properly functioning clotting factors.

Defects in hemostasis are caused by abnormalities of either platelets or coagulation factors. These defects can be diagnosed with a few laboratory tests (Table 9.2). Normal values may differ according to the specific test used and the individual laboratory.

Platelet Count

The **platelet count** is usually included in a CBC. The platelet count provides a quantitative or numeric evaluation of platelets. A normal platelet count should be 200,000 to 400,000/mm^3. A platelet count less than 100,000/mm^3 is considered thrombocytopenia. Spontaneous gingival bleeding can occur when a patient's platelet count is less than 20,000/mm^3. In addition, a physician can request specific clotting factor assays, which can also be performed in patients with suspected or known clotting factor deficiencies. Nearly all bleeding disorders are caused by abnormalities

TABLE 9.1	Factors Involved in Coagulation*
Factor Name	**Name**
I	Fibrinogen
II	Prothrombin
III	Tissue factor
IV	Calcium ions
V	Proaccelerin
VII	Proconvertin
VIII	Antihemophilic factor, plasma thromboplastinogen
IX	Plasma thromboplastin
X	Stuart factor
XI	Plasma thromboplastin antecedent
XII	Hageman factor
XIII	Fibrin-stabilizing factor

*Factors are numbered in the order in which they were discovered and not in the order in which they function. (No factor VI is included.)

TABLE 9.2	Laboratory Tests for Hemostasis	
Test	**Normal Values**
Platelet count (number of platelets)	200,000–400,000/mm³
Bleeding time (platelet function) (test is not easily available any longer)	1–6 min*
Prothrombin time (fibrin clot formation—extrinsic pathway)	11–16 seconds*
Partial thromboplastin time (fibrin clot formation—intrinsic pathway)	25–40 seconds*

*Normal values may differ according to the specific test used and the individual laboratory.

of either platelets or clotting factors. Rarely, bleeding disorders result from capillary fragility or weakness of the blood vessel walls.

Bleeding Time

The **bleeding time** provides an assessment of the adequacy of platelet function, not platelet number. The test measures how long it takes a standardized skin incision to stop bleeding by the formation of a temporary hemostatic plug or clot. The normal range of bleeding time depends on the way the test is performed, but is usually between 1 and 6 minutes. The bleeding time is prolonged—longer than 5 to 10 minutes—in patients with platelet abnormalities. Aspirin can also prolong the bleeding time but has no effect on the platelet count. It is now difficult to get bleeding time results because this test is no longer easily available.

Prothrombin Time

The **prothrombin time (PT)** measures the patient's ability to form a clot. It is performed by measuring the time it takes for a clot to form when calcium and a tissue factor are added to the patient's plasma. A normal PT is usually between 11 and 16 seconds. The value is usually compared with a normal control, which is generated daily by the laboratory, using standardized plasma. A prolonged or greater-than-normal PT can be associated with postoperative bleeding because of abnormal clot formation. A prolonged PT is usually not associated with bleeding unless it is longer than 1.5 times the control. Most often physicians use PT to monitor anticoagulant therapy (as in Coumadin [warfarin sodium]) for preventing MI. A more accurate determination of PT is the **international normalized ratio (INR)**, an expression of the ratio of PT to thromboplastin activity. The INR is more accurate because it is standardized from laboratory to laboratory. The normal range for an individual not on warfarin is 0.8 to 1.1. Patients receiving anticoagulants such as warfarin (Coumadin) may be maintained on INR values of 2 to 3. An INR cannot be used to assess bleeding for the new anticoagulants such as clopidogrel, which affect platelets rather than coagulation factors. This is also true for acetylsalicylic acid (aspirin).

Partial Thromboplastin Time

The **partial thromboplastin time (PTT)** also measures the effectiveness of clot formation. Two different pathways exist by which clot formation occurs. PT measures one of these, and PTT

measures the other. The test is performed by measuring the time it takes for a clot to form after the addition of kaolin, a surface-activating factor, and cephalin, a substitute platelet factor, to the patient's plasma. A normal PTT is usually 25 to 40 seconds. Prolongation of the PTT to 45 to 50 seconds can be associated with mild bleeding problems. With further prolongation (more than 50 s) severe bleeding can occur. PTT is also used by physicians to monitor heparin therapy, which is commonly used for kidney hemodialysis in patients with renal failure.

Purpura

Purpura is a reddish-blue or purplish discoloration of the skin or mucosa that results from spontaneous extravasation of blood. It can be caused by a defect or deficiency in blood platelets or an increase in capillary fragility. A significant oral clinical finding is the oozing of blood at the gingival margins in several sites without the presence of gingivitis or inflammation. Areas of submucosal bleeding range in size from **petechiae** (1–2 mm) to **ecchymoses**, which are much larger. A **purpura** is sometimes used for an area of submucosal bleeding that is larger than petechiae but smaller than an ecchymosis. Bleeding into the tissue that causes swelling or a blister is called a **hematoma.**

Thrombocytopenic Purpura

Thrombocytopenic purpura is a bleeding disorder that results from a severe reduction in circulating platelets. The normal platelet level is 200,000 to 400,000/mm³ of blood. Spontaneous bleeding occurs when platelet levels fall to less than 20,000/mm³. When the cause is unknown, the condition is called **idiopathic thrombocytopenic purpura.** An autoimmune type of process has been identified for thrombocytopenia; therefore it is sometimes called *immune thrombocytopenia.* The condition can also be secondary to an existing disease or condition. **Secondary thrombocytopenic purpura** is often associated with drugs, including those used for cancer chemotherapy. The idiopathic or primary form is usually seen in young patients, with the greatest incidence occurring before the age of 10 years. No age predilection for the secondary type and no sex predilection for either type are seen.

Clinical Features and Oral Manifestations

Clinically, spontaneous purpuric or hemorrhagic lesions of the skin develop that can vary in size and severity. In addition, these patients bruise easily, can have blood in the urine (**hematuria**), and have frequent nosebleeds (**epistaxis**). Oral manifestations include spontaneous gingival bleeding, **petechiae**, and clusters of petechiae or purpuric spots. **Ecchymoses** may also develop.

Diagnosis and Treatment

Laboratory tests show a significant decrease in platelets. Bleeding time can be prolonged to 1 hour or more, and the capillary fragility test result is positive. Treatment depends on the cause and includes transfusions, corticosteroids, and splenectomy. Any dental surgical procedure, including scaling, is contraindicated until laboratory test results confirm sufficient improvement in the patient's bleeding problem.

Nonthrombocytopenic Purpura

Nonthrombocytopenic purpuras are bleeding disorders that can result from either a defect in the capillary walls or disorders of platelet function. Vascular wall alterations occur in vitamin C deficiency and infections and can also result from chemicals and allergy. Many factors can cause disorders of platelet function, including drugs, allergy, and autoimmune disease. By far the most common reason for a prolonged bleeding time is the ingestion of drugs that affect platelet function. Ingestion of small doses of aspirin (0.3–1.5 g) produces an impairment of platelet function for 7 to 10 days. Nonsteroidal antiinflammatory drugs (e.g., ibuprofen, naproxen, indomethacin) can also adversely affect platelet function. Patients with kidney failure and those with leukemia can have impaired platelet function. **von Willebrand disease** is one of the most common inherited disorders of bleeding in humans. In most cases, it is transmitted as an autosomal-dominant disorder of platelet function. In addition, several autosomal-recessive variants have been identified. Both men and women may be affected with this disorder.

Clinical Features and Oral Manifestations

The oral and systemic manifestations in nonthrombocytopenic purpura are the same as those that occur in thrombocytopenic purpura and include spontaneous gingival bleeding, **petechiae, ecchymoses,** and hemorrhagic blisters.

Diagnosis and Treatment

The platelet count is normal in nonthrombocytopenic purpura. The bleeding time is prolonged. Treatment includes systemic corticosteroids, splenectomy, and permanent or temporary discontinuation of the causative agent.

Hemophilia

Hemophilia is an inherited disorder of blood **coagulation** that results in severely prolonged clotting time. The problem results from a deficiency of one of the plasma proteins involved in the coagulation cascade that is necessary for the conversion of fibrinogen to fibrin (Fig. 9.14).

Types of Hemophilia

The two most common types of hemophilia are type A and type B. These types of hemophilia are inherited as X-linked recessive traits and therefore are transmitted through a female carrier and affect males and homozygous females. Males with the abnormal gene have a severe coagulation defect. In the female carrier some of the cancelled X chromosomes have the abnormal gene and others have the normal one. Although female carriers of the gene for hemophilia do not have as severe a problem as males, they tend to have a mildly prolonged coagulation time.

Hemophilia A is the classic and most common type and is caused by a deficiency of the clotting factor called *plasma thromboplastinogen* or *factor VIII*. This deficiency is characterized by severe hemorrhage after even mild-to-moderate injury or surgery. Hemophilia B, or *Christmas disease,* is less common, and the clotting defect is in *plasma thromboplastin* or *factor IX*. In hemophilia A and B, blood does not coagulate because of the low or almost nonexistent levels of factor VIII or IX in circulating blood. Patients with this condition bleed more than usual after extraction of teeth or scaling and curettage.

Another clotting disorder is called *von Willebrand disease.* von Willebrand disease is the most common of the inherited bleeding disorders. It is transmitted as both autosomal-dominant and autosomal-recessive patterns. It is characterized by a deficiency of a plasma glycoprotein (*von Willebrand factor*) that aids in platelet adhesion. Although some patients with von Willebrand disease may have severe symptoms, most are asymptomatic and the condition is clinically insignificant.

Clinical Features and Oral Manifestations

The oral manifestations of hemophilia include spontaneous gingival bleeding and ecchymoses. Males with hemophilia A or B are at risk of hemorrhage after oral surgery procedures and scaling. Female carriers tend to bleed more than usual after extraction of teeth or scaling and curettage. Plans for controlling bleeding must

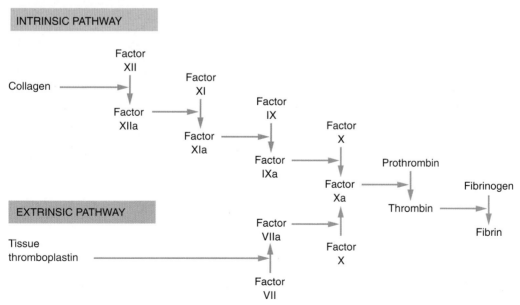

• **Figure 9.14** Coagulation cascade. Coagulation factors remain inactive until needed. As each coagulation factor becomes activated (a), it is responsible for the activation of another factor until all have been activated and the final clot is formed. The two pathways by which this cascade is activated are the intrinsic and extrinsic pathways.

be established before any dental hygiene care or oral surgery is initiated. Doses of clotting factor may be required to control bleeding after tooth extraction.

Diagnosis and Treatment

The PT in patients with hemophilia is normal, and the PTT is prolonged. Diagnosis involves identifying the missing factor, and treatment involves replacing it.

ORAL MANIFESTATIONS OF THERAPY FOR ORAL CANCER

Oral cancer can be treated by surgery, radiation therapy, chemotherapy, or any combination of the three. Radiation therapy and chemotherapy can result in the development of several different oral manifestations.

Radiation Therapy

During **radiation therapy** the patient often experiences mucositis (Fig. 9.15A-B), which begins about the second week of therapy and subsides a few weeks after its completion. The mucositis is painful and appears as erythematous and ulcerated mucosa. Difficulty in eating, pain on swallowing, and loss of taste can occur as a result of the mucositis. If the radiation affects the major salivary glands, irreversible salivary gland destruction can occur, resulting in severe xerostomia. As a result, the mucosal tissues are easily irritated, and the patient is prone to the development of radiation caries (Fig. 9.16) and oral candidiasis (see Chapter 3). Pilocarpine hydrochloride taken during the course of radiation treatment has been reported to decrease the severity of radiation-induced xerostomia. A patient who has received radiation therapy for oral cancer is also at risk for the development of **osteoradionecrosis** (necrosis of bone from radiation therapy) because of the decreased blood supply to the bone after radiation therapy. Osteoradionecrosis develops in the mandible more frequently than in the maxilla, and the risk for its development does not decrease with time.

Patients for whom head and neck radiation is planned should have an oral evaluation before the initiation of radiation therapy. Potential sources of oral infection should be eliminated, and teeth for which the prognosis is questionable should be removed. The role of the dental hygienist in the management of patients receiving head and neck radiation treatment expected to result in xerostomia (Fig. 9-15C) involves fluoride application both by the dental hygienist and the patient, patient education in oral hygiene care, and frequent follow-up appointments to ensure patient compliance.

Saliva substitutes can be used by the patient for symptomatic relief of xerostomia.

Chemotherapy

The complications of cancer **chemotherapy** are predictable and differ for the various types of chemotherapy used. Mucositis and oral ulceration are frequent complications because drugs used for cancer chemotherapy affect rapidly dividing cells and therefore the basal cells of the epithelium. The epithelium becomes atrophic and ulcerated with minor irritation. Cells of the bone marrow are also affected; therefore a decrease in all blood cells (red blood cells,

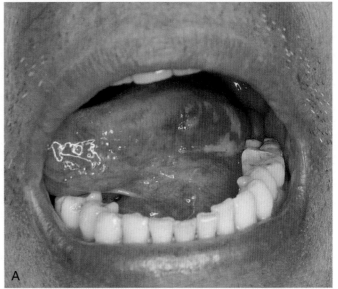

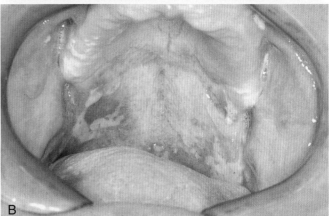

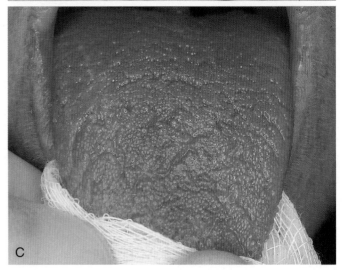

• **Figure 9.15** A and B, Radiation mucositis. C, Postradiation xerostomia.

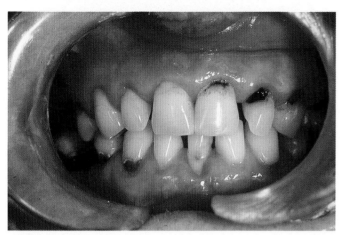

• **Figure 9.16** Clinical appearance of radiation caries. (Courtesy Dr. Jonathan A. Ship.)

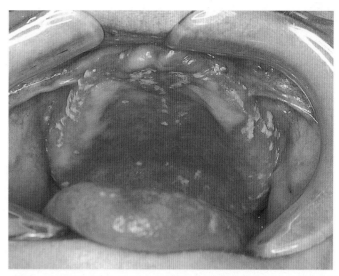

• **Figure 9.18** Candidiasis in a patient taking prednisone for rheumatoid arthritis.

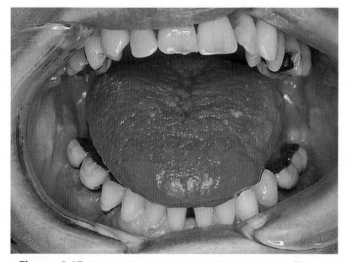

• **Figure 9.17** Xerostomia caused by chlorpromazine (Thorazine) administration.

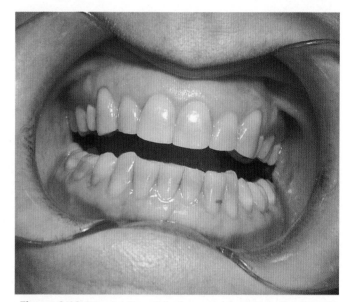

• **Figure 9.19** Discoloration of teeth caused by tetracycline ingestion when teeth are forming.

white blood cells, and platelets) can result. The patient can experience anemia because of a decrease in red blood cells, is at increased risk for opportunistic infections (e.g., candidiasis) because of a decrease in white blood cells, and is at increased risk for bleeding problems because of a decrease in the number of platelets.

Before the initiation of cancer chemotherapy, the patient should receive an oral evaluation to identify and eliminate any source of oral infection that may exacerbate during the course of chemotherapy.

EFFECTS OF DRUGS ON THE ORAL CAVITY

Many drugs can cause changes in the oral tissues. Xerostomia can be caused by drugs used to control blood pressure. Antianxiety medications, antipsychotic medications, and antihistamines can also cause xerostomia (Fig. 9.17). Drugs such as prednisone that suppress the immune system can increase the risk of candidiasis and other oral infections (Fig. 9.18). Antibiotics can also increase

the risk of candidiasis. Tetracycline taken when teeth are forming can cause tooth discoloration (Fig. 9.19). Phenytoin (Dilantin) and nifedipine (Procardia) can cause gingival enlargement (Fig. 9.20). Cyclosporine, an immunosuppressant drug used to prevent rejection of transplanted organs, can also cause gingival enlargement.

The complete medical history should include a listing of the medications taken by a patient and is useful in establishing the diagnosis of drug-induced oral lesions.

Medication-Related Osteonecrosis of the Jaw

Medication-related osteonecrosis of the jaw (MRONJ) is a clinical diagnosis based on history and physical examination; radiographic findings are nonspecific. This condition was first identified as a

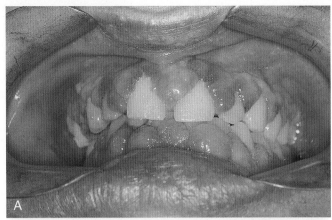

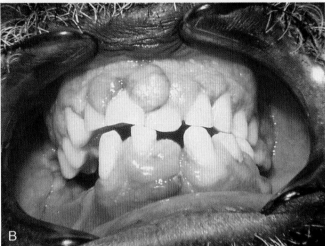

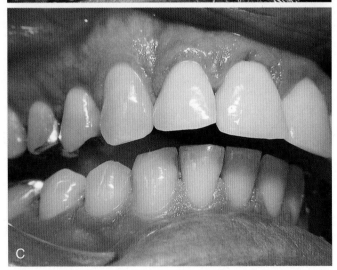

• **Figure 9.20** Drug-induced gingival enlargement. **A,** Gingival enlarge-ment caused by phenytoin (Dilantin). **B and C,** Gingival enlargement caused by nifedipine (Procardia). (**A** courtesy Dr. Edward V. Zegarelli; **B and C** courtesy Dr. Victor M. Sternberg.)

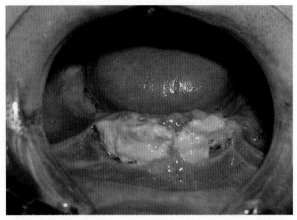

• **Figure 9.21** Osteonecrosis associated with bisphosphonate therapy involving the mandible.

complication of bisphosphonate therapy. According to the American Association of Oral and Maxillofacial Surgeons guidelines, patients may be considered to have MRONJ if all of the following clinical characteristics are present:

• Current or previous treatment with an antiresorptive or anti-angiogenic agent
• Exposed bone or bone that can be probed through an intraoral or extraoral fistula in the maxillofacial region that has persisted for longer than 8 weeks (Fig. 9.21)
• No history of radiation therapy to the jaws.

The risk of MRONJ for patients with cancer ranges from 0% to 6.7%, and the risk for patients with osteoporosis is less than 0.1%. Although it has now been over a decade since the first report of osteonecrosis associated with bisphosphonate medication, the pathophysiology has not been determined. There are many hypotheses to explain the pathogenesis of MRONJ, including oversuppression of bone remodeling, direct bone toxicity, inhibition of angiogenesis, inhibition of oral epithelium, microtrauma, infection/biofilm, inflammation, impaired host defense, vitamin D deficiency, and genetic predisposition. Risk factors for MRONJ may be classified as local, systemic, and drug related. Local risk factors include dental extraction, periodontal disease, dental infection or inflammation, poor oral hygiene, ill-fitting dentures, smoking, and anatomy (i.e., mylohyoid ridge, prominent exostosis). MRONJ lesions occur more commonly in the mandible than in the maxilla (2 : 1) and more frequently in the posterior lingual mandible, possibly due to the thin nonkeratinized mucosa, decreased vascularity, prominent exostosis, trauma, and accumulation of debris. Systemic risk factors include malignancy, smoking, obesity, diabetes, anemia, vitamin D deficiency, and genetic polymorphisms. Drug-related risk factors include duration and type of antiresorptive therapy, cancer chemotherapy, and corticosteroid therapy. Patients at risk for MRONJ should be educated as to the importance of maintaining meticulous oral hygiene and 3-month dental recare visits. Preventive strategies include a comprehensive oral examination, radiographic evaluation, oral hygiene instruction, and education regarding dental care.

Selected References

Books

de Leeuw R, Klasser GD, editors: *Orofacial pain, guidelines for assessment, diagnosis and management*, ed 5, Chicago, 2013, Quintessence Publishing Co, Inc.

Glick M, editor: *Burket's oral medicine*, ed 12, Hamilton, 2015, BC Dekker.

Kumar V, Abbas AK, Aster JC: *Robbins and Cotran pathologic basis of disease*, ed 9, Philadelphia, 2015, Elsevier.

Little JW, Falace D, Miller C, et al: *Dental management of the medically compromised patient*, ed 8, St. Louis, 2012, Mosby.

Longo D, Jameson J, Loscalzo J, et al: *Harrison's principles of internal medicine*, ed 19, New York, 2015, The McGraw-Hill Companies.

Neville BW, Damm DD, Allen CM, et al: *Oral and maxillofacial pathology*, ed 4, St. Louis, 2016, Elsevier.

Okeson JP: *Bell's oral & facial pain*, ed 7, Chicago, 2014, Quintessence Publishing Co, Inc.

Regezi JA, Sciubba JJ, Jordan RCK: *Oral pathology: clinical-pathologic correlations*, ed 7, Philadelphia, 2017, Elsevier.

Wynn RL, Meiller TF, Crossley HL: *Drug information handbook for dentistry*, ed 22, Hudson, 2016-2017, Lexi-Comp.

Journal Articles

Avcu N, Avcu F, Beyan C, et al: The relationship between gastric-oral *Helicobacter pylori* and oral hygiene in patients with vitamin B_{12}-deficiency anemia, *Oral Surg Oral Med Oral Pathol Oral Radiol Endod* 92:166, 2001.

Centers for Disease Control and Prevention: Iron deficiency—United States, 1999-2000, *MMWR Morb Mortal Wkly Rep* 51:89, 2002.

Chávez EM, Borrell LN, Taylor GW, et al: A longitudinal analysis of salivary flow in control subjects and older adults with type 2 diabetes, *Oral Surg Oral Med Oral Pathol Oral Radiol Endod* 91:166, 2001.

Collin HL, Niskanen L, Uusitupa M, et al: Oral symptoms and signs in elderly patients with type 2 diabetes mellitus, *Oral Surg Oral Med Oral Pathol Oral Radiol Endod* 90:299, 2000.

Couri CE, Voltarelli JC: Stem cell therapy for type 1 diabetes mellitus: a review of recent clinical trials, *Diabetol Metab Syndr* 1:19, 2009.

Dodson T: The frequency of medication-related osteonecrosis of the jaw and its associated risk factors, *Oral Maxillofac Surg Clin North Am* 27:509–516, 2015.

Fletcher PD, Scopp IV, Hersh RA: Oral manifestations of secondary hyperparathyroidism related to long-term hemodialysis therapy, *Oral Surg Oral Med Oral Pathol* 43:218, 1977.

Garg AK, Malo M: Manifestations and treatment of xerostomia and associated oral effects secondary to head and neck radiation therapy, *J Am Dent Assoc* 128:1128, 1997.

Hardin DS: Screening for type 2 diabetes in children with acanthosis nigricans, *Diabetes Educ* 32:547, 2006.

Hess LM, Jeter JM, Benham-Hutchins M, et al: Factors associated with osteonecrosis of the jaw among bisphosphonate users, *Am J Med* 121:475, 2008.

Husebye ES, Allolio B, Arlt W, et al: Consensus statement on the diagnosis, treatment and follow-up of patients with primary adrenal insufficiency, *J Intern Med* 275:104, 2014.

Inokuchi T, Sano K, Kamingo M: Osteoradionecrosis of the sphenoid and temporal bones in a patient with maxillary sinus carcinoma: a case report, *Oral Surg Oral Med Oral Pathol* 70:278, 1990.

Kanter J, Kruse-Jarres R: Management of sickle cell disease from childhood through adulthood, *Blood Rev* 27:279, 2013.

Khan A, Morrison A, Hanley D, et al: Diagnosis and management of osteonecrosis of the jaw: a systematic review and inernational consensus, *J Bone Miner Res* 30:3–23, 2015.

Khocht A, Schneider LC: Periodontal management of gingival overgrowth in the heart transplant patient: a case report, *J Periodontol* 68:1140, 1997.

Kong AS, Williams RL, Smith M, et al; RIOS Net Clinicians: Acanthosis nigricans and diabetes risk factors: prevalence in young persons seen in southwestern US primary care practices, *Ann Fam Med* 5:202, 2007.

McDonough RJ, Nelson CL: Clinical implications of factor XII deficiency, *Oral Surg Oral Med Oral Pathol* 68:264, 1989.

Miranda J, et al: Prevalence and risk of gingival enlargement in patients treated with nifedipine, *J Periodontol* 72:605, 2001.

Moore PA, Guggenheimer J, Etzel KR, et al: Type 1 diabetes mellitus, xerostomia and salivary flow rates, *Oral Surg Oral Med Oral Pathol Oral Radiol Endod* 92:281, 2001.

Moore PA, Weyant RJ, Etzel KR, et al: Type 1 diabetes mellitus and oral health: assessment of coronal and root caries, *Community Dent Oral Epidemiol* 29:183, 2001.

Ohishi M, Oobu K, Miyanoshita Y, et al: Acute gingival necrosis caused by drug-induced agranulocytosis, *Oral Surg Oral Med Oral Pathol* 66:194, 1988.

Redding SW, Luce EB, Boren MW: Oral herpes simplex virus infection in patients receiving head and neck radiation, *Oral Surg Oral Med Oral Pathol* 69:578, 1990.

Rodrigo A, Brandão N, de Carvalho JF: Diagnosis and classification of Addison's disease (autoimmune adrenalitis), *Autoimmun Rev* 13:408, 2014.

Ruggiero S, Dodson T, Fantasia J, et al: AAOMS Position Paper: Medication-Related Osteonecrosis of the Jaw – 2014 Update, *J Oral Maxillofac Surg* 72:1938–1956, 2014.

Ruggiero SL, Drew SJ: Osteonecrosis of the jaws and bisphosphonate therapy, *J Dent Res* 86:1013, 2007.

Sankaran VG, Nathan DG: Thalassemia: an overview of 50 years of clinical research, *Hematol Oncol Clin North Am* 24(6):1005, 2010.

Shanshan L, Paige LW, Douglass CW: JADA continuing education: development of a clinical guideline to predict undiagnosed diabetes in dental patients, *J Am Dent Assoc* 142:28, 2011.

Sreebny LM, Valdini A, Yu A: Xerostomia. II. Relationship to nonoral symptoms, drugs and diseases, *Oral Surg Oral Med Oral Pathol* 68:419, 1989.

Teeuw NJ, Gerdes VE, Loos BG: Effect of periodontal treatment in glycemic control of diabetic patients: a systematic review and meta-analysis, *Diabetes Care* 33:421, 2010.

Vernillo AT: Dental considerations for the treatment of patients with diabetes mellitus, *J Am Dent Assoc* 134:24S, 2003.

Wahlin YB: Effects of chlorhexidine mouth rinse on oral health in patients with acute leukemia, *Oral Surg Oral Med Oral Pathol* 68:279, 1989.

Wu J, Fantasia JE, Kaplan R: Oral manifestations of acute myelomonocytic leukemia: a case report and review of the classification of leukemias, *J Periodontol* 73:664, 2002.

Newspaper Articles

Kleinfield NR: Diabetes and its awful toll quietly emerge as a crisis. *The New York Times*, January 9, 2006, pp. A1, A18–A19.

Kleinfield NR: Living at an epicenter of diabetes: defiance and despair. *The New York Times*, January 10, 2006, pp. A1, A20–A21.

Santora M: East meets West, adding pounds and peril. *The New York Times*, January 12, 2006, pp. A1, A22–A23.

Urbina I: In the treatment of diabetes, success often does not pay. *The New York Times*, January 11, 2006, pp. A1, A22–A23.

Websites

American Diabetes Association Statistics about Diabetes. Available at: http://www.diabetes.org/diabetes-basics/statistics/.

Barclay L: HbA1c may be useful for diabetes screening, diagnosis in routine clinical practice, Medscape Today News, January 22, 2010. Available at: http://www.medscape.com/viewarticle/715565.

Mayo Clinic: Gestational diabetes. Available at: http://www.mayoclinic.com/health/gestational-diabetes/DS00316/DSECTION=symptoms.

Minimed Insulin Pump Therapy/Medtronic Diabetes. Available at: www.medtronicdiabetes.com/home.

WebMD: Diabetes drugs. Available at: www.webmd.com/diabetes/diabetes-medications.

Review Questions

1. Hyperpituitarism results from an excessive production of growth hormone. Which of the following most often causes it?
   a. Pituitary adenoma
   b. Pituitary sarcoma
   c. Carcinoma in situ
   d. Ameloblastoma

2. Hyperthyroidism in children can lead to:
   a. Partial anodontia
   b. Amelogenesis imperfecta
   c. Ankylosis
   d. Early exfoliation of the deciduous dentition and early eruption of the permanent teeth

3. Hypercalcemia, hypophosphatemia, and abnormal bone metabolism are characteristic of which of the following conditions?
   a. Hyperthyroidism
   b. Hypothyroidism
   c. Hyperparathyroidism
   d. Hyperpituitarism

4. All of the following are typically acute metabolic complications of uncontrolled diabetes mellitus except one. Which one is the exception?
   a. Electrolyte depletion
   b. Myocardial infarction
   c. Polyphagia
   d. Polydipsia

5. Polydipsia, polyuria, and polyphagia are all typically characteristic of which of the following?
   a. Hyperparathyroidism
   b. Hyperthyroidism
   c. Type 1 diabetes mellitus
   d. Addison disease

6. Which of the following is *not* true of type 2 diabetes mellitus?
   a. Those with it have increased insulin resistance.
   b. It typically occurs at 40 years of age or older.
   c. It represents approximately 3% of primary diabetes cases.
   d. Glucose control can be achieved without daily insulin injections.

7. Which of the following oral complications is *not* typically associated with diabetes mellitus?
   a. Candidiasis
   b. Xerostomia
   c. Periodontal bone loss
   d. Excessive bleeding

8. Which one of the following is *false* concerning Addison disease?
   a. It is also known as primary adrenal cortical insufficiency.
   b. There may be bronzing of the skin.
   c. It may be caused by a malignant tumor that destroys the adrenal gland.
   d. The patient may experience pathologic fracture.

9. Which of the following statements is *false* regarding diabetes mellitus?
   a. Candidiasis may be indicative of compromised immunity in a patient with diabetes.
   b. Rigorous control of blood glucose may delay progression of coronary artery disease.
   c. Microvascular disease typically affects eyes, kidneys, and nerves.
   d. Diabetes mellitus is a syndrome.

10. Which one of the following is *not* a cause of iron deficiency anemia?
    a. Chronic blood loss
    b. A deficiency of iron intake
    c. An increased requirement for iron
    d. Normal bone marrow function

11. Thalassemia major is:
    a. Caused by a nutritional deficiency
    b. The same as celiac sprue
    c. An autoimmune condition
    d. Associated with a severe hemolytic anemia

12. Achlorhydria, failure to absorb vitamin B_{12}, and megaloblastic anemia are characteristic features of which of the following?
    a. Pernicious anemia
    b. Thalassemia
    c. Sickle cell anemia
    d. Thrombocytopenic purpura

13. Which one of the following is *not* a characteristic of sickle cell anemia?
    a. It is an inherited blood disorder found predominantly in blacks.
    b. It occurs as a result of an abnormal type of hemoglobin and decreased oxygen in the red blood cells.
    c. The individual with sickle cell anemia can experience weakness, fatigue, and joint pain.
    d. Red blood cells are circular in shape.

14. Which of the following is characterized by a decrease in platelets?
    a. Celiac disease
    b. Thrombocytopenia
    c. Thalassemia
    d. Plummer-Vinson syndrome

15. Secondary aplastic anemia can be caused by:
    a. Chemotherapy
    b. Dental radiographs
    c. A genetic disorder
    d. An autoimmune factor

16. Which of the following is characterized by an abnormal increase in circulating red blood cells?
    a. Leukopenia
    b. Polydipsia
    c. Thrombocytopenia
    d. Polycythemia

17. Leukopenia most often involves which cell type?
    a. Eosinophils
    b. Neutrophils
    c. Basophils
    d. Erythrocytes

18. If a patient's white blood cell count is 1000 cells/microliter, the patient has:
    a. Leukopenia
    b. Thrombocytopenia
    c. Hemophilia
    d. Cyclic neutropenia

19. Excessive numbers of abnormal white blood cells are characteristic of:
    a. Agranulocytosis
    b. Leukopenia
    c. Cyclic neutropenia
    d. Leukemia

20. Normal bleeding time is usually between:
    a. 1 and 6 minutes
    b. 2 and 3 minutes
    c. 15 and 45 seconds
    d. 10 and 15 minutes

21. The normal prothrombin time is:
    a. 2 to 5 minutes
    b. 11 to 16 seconds
    c. 10 to 15 minutes
    d. 1 to 6 seconds

22. The International Normalized Ratio is all of the following *except one*. Which one is the exception?
    a. An expression of the ratio of prothrombin time to thromboplastin activity
    b. More accurate than the prothrombin time because it is standardized from laboratory to laboratory
    c. A test used to determine the patient's ability to form a clot
    d. A test used to assess the patient's platelet number

23. Which of the following is the normal INR range for an individual *not* on warfarin?
    a. 0.8 to 12.0
    b. 3.0 to 4.0
    c. 0.8 to 1.1
    d. 5.0 to 6.0

24. Symptoms of leukemia can be similar to those found in:
    a. Hepatitis
    b. Amelogenesis imperfecta
    c. Nonthrombocytopenic purpura
    d. Infectious mononucleosis

25. All of the following are characteristic of primary hyperparathyroidism except one. Which one is the exception?
    a. Osteoclastic resorption
    b. Excessive production of parathyroid hormone
    c. Cotton-wool radiographic appearance
    d. Increased serum calcium

26. Osteonecrosis of the jaw is associated with:
    a. Antipsychotic medications
    b. Tetracycline
    c. Phenytoin
    d. Bisphosphonates

27. Which of the following is *not true* about the insulin pump?
    a. It uses only long-acting or slow-acting insulin.
    b. The patient must still test blood sugar several times daily.
    c. Rapid onset of ketoacidosis may occur with pump failure.
    d. Insulin dosage may be less than with syringe delivery.

28. Which of the following does *not* apply to the glycosylated hemoglobin (HbA$_{1c}$) test?
    a. It measures glucose control over a 4-month period.
    b. It is one of several criteria used for the diagnosis of diabetes.
    c. The lower the value, the better the glucose control.
    d. It is used only in the management of type 1 diabetes.

29. All of the following conditions are associated with type 1 diabetes mellitus *except one*. Which one is the exception?
    a. Addison disease
    b. Hyperpituitarism
    c. Graves disease
    d. Pernicious anemia

30. Which of the following is *false* concerning periodontal disease and its relationship to diabetes mellitus?
    a. It aggravates diabetic control.
    b. It has prognostic or predictive value for the diagnosis of type 2 diabetes in certain ethnic groups.
    c. Patients who do not respond to periodontal therapy may have undiagnosed diabetes.
    d. Good oral hygiene will resolve all gingival conditions.

31. Which of the following is *false* concerning gestational diabetes?
    a. It occurs in the majority of women during pregnancy.
    b. It follows the pattern of insulin resistance.
    c. The hormones progesterone and cortisol may play a role in its development.
    d. There is an increased risk for the mother to develop type 2 diabetes later in life.

32. In leukemia, which type of therapy can have the most significant side effects for the patient?
    a. Induction chemotherapy
    b. Maintenance chemotherapy
    c. Radiation to central nervous system
    d. Drugs and radiation

33. Which patient group is most likely to get sickle cell anemia?
    a. Whites
    b. Blacks
    c. Indians
    d. Europeans

34. Acanthosis nigricans is a skin disorder associated with which condition?
a. Anemia
b. Hyperthyroidism
c. Type 2 diabetes
d. Addison disease

35. Patients with Addison disease crave which one of the following due to hyponatremia?
a. Natural vitamins
b. Sugar
c. Dairy products
d. Salt

36. Which one of the following is an inherited disorder of hemoglobin synthesis?
a. Iron deficiency anemia
b. Pernicious anemia
c. Cooley anemia
d. Nutritional anemia

37. According to the World Health Organization, which two countries will contribute the largest number of diabetes cases worldwide by the year 2030?
a. The United States and Brazil
b. India and China
c. Sweden and Finland
d. Denmark and Germany

38. Approximately what percentage of patients with prediabetes will likely develop outright clinical diabetes given their additional risk factors of obesity and family history?
a. 5%
b. 25%
c. 50%
d. 75%

39. Type 1 and type 2 diabetes mellitus typically have which of the following in common?
a. Autoimmune-mediated disease
b. Insulin resistance
c. Chronic hyperglycemia
d. Time of onset

40. In the management of type 2 diabetes mellitus, which classification of newly developed drugs decreases blood glucose by increasing the excretion of urinary glucose?
a. Sulfonylureas
b. Biguanides
c. SGLT2
d. Incretin mimetics

Chapter 9 Synopsis

Condition/Disease	Cause	Age/Race/Sex	Location
Hyperpituitarism	Excess growth hormone produced by the pituitary gland Most commonly caused by a pituitary adenoma	Children: gigantism Adults (most commonly in fourth decade): acromegaly	Generalized bone involvement Affects only certain bones
Hyperthyroidism (Graves disease)	Excessive production of thyroid hormone	Children and adults	Systemic disease

N/A, Not applicable.
*Not covered in text.

41. All of the following are typical oral complications of diabetes *except one*. Which one is the exception?
    a. Squamous cell carcinoma
    b. Candidiasis
    c. Dental caries
    d. Periodontal disease

42. All of the following occur in the uncontrolled diabetic state *except one*. Which one is the exception?
    a. Reduction in the phagocytic activity of macrophages
    b. Delay in chemotaxis of neutrophils
    c. Ketoacidosis
    d. Preservation of body mass

43. All of the following are complications from macrovascular disease in diabetes mellitus *except one*. Which one is the exception?
    a. Abdominal aortic aneurysm
    b. Cerebrovascular accident
    c. Myocardial infarction
    d. Damage to nerves with impairment of sensation

44. Exophthalmos is a characteristic feature in which one of the following?
    a. Hypothyroidism
    b. Acromegaly
    c. Graves disease
    d. Myxedema

45. The most common cause of secondary hyperparathyroidism is:
    a. Abnormal parathyroid glands
    b. Kidney failure
    c. Hyperplasia of the parathyroid gland
    d. A malignant parathyroid tumor

46. Cushing syndrome is caused by an increase in:
    a. Vitamin D
    b. Cortisol
    c. Malignant tumors
    d. ACTH

Clinical Features	Radiographic Features	Microscopic Features	Treatment	Diagnostic Process
Excessive growth of the skeleton overall Enlargement of the hands and feet Increase in rib size Enlargement of the mandible, maxilla, and maxillary sinus Separation of teeth with malocclusion Frontal bossing and enlargement of nasal bones	*	N/A	May involve pituitary gland surgery	Laboratory
Rosy complexion, erythema of the palms, excessive sweating, fine hair and softened nails, exophthalmos Anxiety, weakness, restlessness, cardiac problems Children: premature exfoliation of deciduous teeth and premature eruption of permanent teeth Adults: osteoporosis; dental caries, and periodontal disease appear to progress rapidly	*	*	Suppression of thyroid activity May involve surgery, medication, radioactive iodine	Laboratory

Continued

Chapter 9 Synopsis—cont'd

Condition/Disease	Cause	Age/Race/Sex	Location
Hypothyroidism	Decreased production of thyroid hormone	Children: cretinism	Systemic disease
Hyperparathyroidism	Excessive secretion of parathyroid hormone Primary: may be caused by hyperplasia or tumor of the parathyroid glands Secondary: causes include renal disease and vitamin D deficiency	Usually adults	Systemic disease
Diabetes mellitus	Abnormally high blood glucose levels resulting from lack of the hormone insulin	Type 1 (IDDM): peak age of onset, 20 yr Type 2 (NIDDM): 40 yr or older	Systemic disease
Addison disease	Insufficient production of adrenal steroids, caused by: • Malignant tumor of the adrenal gland • Infection (e.g., tuberculosis) • Often undetermined; possibly autoimmune disease	*	Systemic disease
Iron deficiency anemia	Nutritional deficiency of iron intake Blood loss Increased demand for iron Poor absorption of iron	Any age, race, sex	Systemic disease
Plummer-Vinson syndrome	Chronic iron deficiency	Usually adults	Systemic disease
Pernicious anemia	Deficiency of intrinsic factor (produced by parietal cells of the stomach) Autoimmune mechanism most likely	Usually adults	Systemic disease
Folic acid and vitamin B_{12} deficiencies	Malnutrition Increased metabolic requirements	Usually adults	Systemic disease

N/A, Not applicable.
*Not covered in text.

Clinical Features	Radiographic Features	Microscopic Features	Treatment	Diagnostic Process
Children: thickened lips, enlarged tongue, delayed eruption of teeth Adults: enlarged tongue	Delayed eruption pattern may be observed	*	*	*
Joint pain or stiffness, lethargy Loosening of teeth	Well-circumscribed bone lesions, changes in trabeculation, partial loss of lamina dura	Bone lesions—indistinguishable from central giant cell lesion	Dependent on cause	Laboratory
Accelerated atherosclerosis resulting in impaired circulation of blood Increased risk of ulceration, gangrene of the feet, high blood pressure, kidney failure, and stroke Acanthosis nigricans Eye damage and blindness Neurologic complaints Decreased resistance to infection, including oral candidiasis Slow wound healing Bilateral salivary gland enlargement Xerostomia (usually with uncontrolled diabetes) Accentuated response to dental plaque	Increased severity of periodontal bone loss	N/A	Control of blood glucose with insulin injections, oral hypoglycemic agents, and diet	Laboratory
Brown pigmentation of the skin (bronzing) and oral melanotic macules	N/A	*	Steroid replacement therapy	Laboratory
Weakness, fatigue, low energy, shortness of breath Oral: angular cheilitis, papillary atrophy of the tongue with burning sensation, pallor of oral mucosa	N/A	Microcytic, hypochromic red blood cells	Treatment of underlying cause Increased iron intake	Laboratory
Same features as iron deficiency with increased risk of esophageal and oral cancer	N/A	Microcytic, hypochromic red blood cells	Treatment of underlying cause Increased iron intake	Laboratory
Weakness, fatigue, skin pallor, nausea, dizziness, diarrhea, abdominal pain, loss of appetite, weight loss Oral: angular cheilitis; pallor; painful, erythematous, and depapillated tongue; mucosal ulceration	N/A	Abnormally large red blood cells (megaloblastic anemia)	Vitamin B$_{12}$ by injection	Laboratory
Weakness, fatigue, skin pallor, nausea, dizziness, diarrhea, abdominal pain, loss of appetite, weight loss Oral: angular cheilitis; pallor; painful, erythematous, and depapillated tongue; oral ulcers	N/A	Abnormally large red blood cells (megaloblastic anemia)	Dietary supplements, if nutritional	Laboratory

Continued

Chapter 9 Synopsis—cont'd

Condition/Disease	Cause	Age/Race/Sex	Location
Thalassemia: • Thalassemia major • Thalassemia minor	Inherited disorder (autosomal pattern; minor: heterozygous, major: homozygous) Disorder of hemoglobin synthesis	Begins in early childhood	Systemic disease Thalassemia major: severe symptoms Thalassemia minor: asymptomatic or mildly symptomatic
Sickle cell anemia Sickle cell trait	Inherited disorder (sickle cell anemia: homozygous; sickle cell trait: heterozygous) Abnormal hemoglobin in red blood cells	Before age 30 yr Mostly in black individuals and those of Mediterranean origin Women > men	Systemic disease
Aplastic anemia	Decrease in all circulating blood cell types because of severe depression of bone marrow activity Primary: cause unknown Secondary: drug or chemical agent	Primary: young adults Secondary: any age	Systemic disease
Polycythemia: • Polycythemia vera (primary polycythemia) • Secondary polycythemia • Relative polycythemia	Polycythemia vera: abnormal increase in circulating red blood cells (neoplasia); cause unknown Secondary polycythemia: physiologic response to decreased oxygen Relative polycythemia: decreased plasma volume, not an increase in red blood cells; diuretic use, vomiting, diarrhea, or excessive sweating	Usually adults	Systemic disease
Agranulocytosis	Marked reduction in circulating neutrophils (neutropenia) Primary: may be immunologic Secondary: drugs and other chemicals	Secondary agranulocytosis F>M	Systemic disease
Cyclic neutropenia	Autosomal-dominant gene *ELA-2,* 19p13.3	From birth M = F	Oral mucosa and periodontium
Leukemias	Neoplastic Oncogenic viruses suggested	Children (acute lymphoblastic) Adolescents and young adults (acute myelogenous) Adults (chronic)	Systemic disease

N/A, Not applicable.
*Not covered in text.

Clinical Features	Radiographic Features	Microscopic Features	Treatment	Diagnostic Process
Yellowish skin pallor, fever, malaise, weakness, enlarged liver and spleen Facies: prominent cheekbones, depression of the bridge of the nose, prominent premaxilla, protrusion or flaring of the maxillary anterior teeth	Atypical trabecular pattern ("salt and pepper" effect) Thinning of the lamina dura Circular Radiolucencies in the alveolar bone also described	*	Experimental	Clinical Laboratory
Weakness, shortness of breath, fatigue, joint pain, nausea	Loss of trabeculation with large, irregular marrow spaces	Sickle-shaped red blood cells on blood smear	Symptomatic and supportive oxygen, intravenous and oral fluids	Laboratory
Infection, spontaneous bleeding, petechiae and purpuric spots	N/A	N/A	Primary: experimental, poor prognosis Secondary: removal of cause	Laboratory
Oral mucosa may appear deep red to purple Gingiva may be edematous and bleed easily Petechiae, ecchymoses, and hematoma formation can be present	N/A	N/A	Secondary and relative polycythemia: management of causative factors	Laboratory
Sudden onset of fever, chills, jaundice, weakness, and sore throat Oral infection with rapid periodontal destruction Gingival bleeding	N/A	N/A	Transfusions Antibiotics to control infection Removal of causative agent if identified	Laboratory
Gingivitis, periodontitis, ulcers, hemorrhage	Alveolar bone loss, pocket formation	Cyclic diminished neutrophils in peripheral blood	Root planing, scaling, antibiotics G-CSF	Clinical and blood studies
Acute: sudden onset of symptoms; weakness, fever, lymph node enlargement, bleeding, enlarged liver and spleen; gingival enlargement because of infiltration of leukemic cells, oral infections, spontaneous gingival bleeding, petechiae, and ecchymoses Chronic: slow onset of symptoms; easy fatigability, weakness, weight loss, anorexia; pallor of the lips and gingiva, gingival enlargement, petechiae, ecchymoses, gingival bleeding, and atypical periodontal disease	N/A	*	Acute: chemotherapy, bone marrow transplantation Chronic: induction and maintenance chemotherapy, bone marrow transplantation	Laboratory

Continued

Chapter 9 Synopsis—cont'd

Condition/Disease	Cause	Age/Race/Sex	Location
Celiac disease	Sensitivity to dietary gluten resulting in injury to the intestinal mucosa and subsequent anemia	N/A	Systemic disease
Thrombocytopenic purpura: • Idiopathic (primary and autoimmune) types • Secondary type	Severe reduction in circulating platelets Idiopathic: cause unknown Autoimmune: drugs, often chemotherapeutic agents	Primary and autoimmune types: usually children and young adults No age predilection for secondary type	Systemic disease
Hemophilia: • Type A • Type B (Christmas disease)	Inherited (X-linked) • Type A: factor VIII deficiency • Type B: factor IX deficiency	Identified in childhood Affects boys	Systemic disease
Bisphosphonate-associated osteonecrosis	Bisphosphonate therapy for osteoporosis, multiple myeloma, metastatic carcinoma of the breast and prostate, and Paget disease of bone	N/A	Maxilla and mandible

N/A, Not applicable.
*Not covered in text.

Clinical Features	Radiographic Features	Microscopic Features	Treatment	Diagnostic Process
Same clinical features as for anemias; diarrhea, nervousness, and paresthesia of the extremities	N/A	*	Adherence to gluten-free diet	*
Spontaneous hemorrhagic lesions of the skin and/or mucosa Gingival bleeding Frequent nosebleeds Blood in urine (hematuria)	N/A	N/A	Transfusions, systemic corticosteroids, splenectomy Discontinuation of causative agent	Laboratory
Spontaneous bleeding, petechiae, ecchymoses Risk of hemorrhage after oral surgery and dental hygiene procedures	N/A	N/A	Replacement of missing clotting factors	Laboratory
Exposed bone persisting more than 8 wk in a patient taking bisphosphonate medication	*	*	*	Clinical Microscopic (rule out metastatic disease)

10

Orofacial Pain and Temporomandibular Disorders

OLGA A.C. IBSEN, KENNETH E. FLEISHER, AND JOAN ANDERSEN PHELAN

OBJECTIVES

After studying this chapter, the student will be able to:

1. Define each of the words in the vocabulary list for this chapter.
2. Describe the clinical features, oral manifestations, diagnosis, and treatment of burning mouth disorder.
3. Describe the clinical features, diagnosis, and treatment of trigeminal neuralgia.
4. Describe the clinical features, diagnosis, and management of Bell's palsy (idiopathic facial paralysis).
5. Do the following related to the anatomy of the temporomandibular joint:
   - Label the following on a diagram of the temporomandibular joint: glenoid (mandibular) fossa of the temporal bone, articular disk, mandibular condyle, joint capsule, and superior belly of the lateral pterygoid muscle.
   - State the function of the muscles of mastication.
6. Name and explain the various factors on which normal function of the temporomandibular joint depends.
7. Do the following related to temporomandibular disorders:
   - Describe the epidemiology of temporomandibular disorders.
   - Discuss the pathophysiology of temporomandibular disorders.
   - List at least five causes of orofacial pain *not* including dental conditions and temporomandibular disorders.

- State three factors that have been implicated in the cause of temporomandibular disorders and three questions that would be appropriate to ask of a patient suspected of having a temporomandibular disorder.
- List at least two symptoms that are suggestive of temporomandibular dysfunction.
- Describe what is involved in a comprehensive examination of a patient in relation to temporomandibular disorders.
- List three imaging techniques useful for evaluating the temporomandibular joint and describe the rationale for each one.
8. List and describe the five types of temporomandibular disorders.
9. Do the following related to the treatment of temporomandibular disorders:
   - Discuss the treatment goals for myofascial pain and dysfunction, internal derangement, and arthritis of the temporomandibular joint.
   - List and describe the two main categories of treatment for temporomandibular disorders.

❖ Vocabulary

Arthrocentesis (ahr″thro-sen-te′sis) Surgical puncture of a joint followed by lavage of the joint space.

Arthrography (ahr-throg′rə-fe) Radiography of a joint after injection of opaque contrast material.

Arthroscopy (ahr-thros′kə-pe) Method for evaluating and manipulating a joint via the insertion of a camera and instruments.

Articulation (ahr-tik″u-la′shən) Joint.

Auscultation (aws″kəl-ta′shən) Listening to sounds within the body using a stethoscope.

Avascular (avas′kyələr) Does not contain blood vessels.

Crepitus (krep′ĭ-təs) Dry, crackling sound.

Douloureux (dooloo-roe′) From the French meaning *painful tic or twitch.*

Dysgeusia (dɪsˈgjuːziə) A distortion of the sense of taste.

Hyperacusia (hī′pər-ə-kōō′sĭe) An increased sensitivity to normal environmental sound.

Iatrogenic (i-at″ro-jen′ik) Induced inadvertently by a medical or dental care provider or by medical treatment or a diagnostic procedure.

Idiopathic (id′e-ə-path″ik) Relating to a disease or condition for which the cause is unknown.

Magnetic resonance imaging (mag-net′ik rez′o-nəns im′ə-jing) MRI; noninvasive diagnostic technique that uses radio waves to produce computerized images of internal body tissues.

Palpation (pal-pa′shən) Physical examination, using pressure of the hand or fingers.

Paresthesia (par′esthee′zhə) An abnormal sensation of tingling or numbness.

Sign (sīn) Objective evidence of disease that can be observed by a health care provider rather than by the patient.

Stomatodynia (sto″mə-tə-din′e-ə) Burning mouth.

Symptom (simp′təm) Subjective evidence of disease or a physical disorder that is observed by the patient.

"Trigger point" A specific area on the face in which a touch or temperature change can trigger an episode of trigeminal neuralgia.

Trismus (triz′məs) Inability to fully open the mouth.

OROFACIAL PAIN

Burning Mouth Disorder (Burning Mouth Syndrome)

Burning mouth disorder, also called burning mouth syndrome, is characterized by an unexplained and usually continuous burning sensation of the oral soft tissues. The condition is also known as **stomatodynia** (*stomato,* mouth; *dynia,* burning). The term *burning mouth disorder* has recently replaced burning mouth syndrome because this condition does not fit the definition of a syndrome. Idiopathic burning mouth disorder is used to describe the condition when there is no identifiable local, systemic, or laboratory findings to explain the burning discomfort. Secondary burning mouth disorder describes the condition when it is associated with local or systemic factors, including those listed in Box 10.1.

> ### • BOX 10.1   Local and Systemic Factors Reportedly Associated With Burning Mouth Disorder
>
> **Local Factors**
> - Xerostomia
> - Chronic mouth breathing
> - Chronic tongue-thrust habit
> - Chronic mechanical trauma
> - Referred pain from teeth or tonsils
> - Trigeminal neuralgia
> - Atypical facial pain or neuralgia
> - Angioedema (angioneurotic edema)
> - Oral candidiasis
> - Temporomandibular dysfunction
> - Oral submucous fibrosis
> - Fusospirochetal infection
> - Contact stomatitis (allergy)
> - Trauma to lingual nerve
>
> **Systemic Factors**
> - Vitamin B deficiency
>   - Vitamin B1 or B2 deficiency
>   - Pernicious anemia (B12)
> - Pellagra (niacin deficiency)
> - Folic acid deficiency
> - Diabetes mellitus
> - Chronic gastritis or regurgitation
> - Chronic gastric hypoacidity
> - Hypothyroidism
> - Mercurialism
> - Estrogen deficiency
> - Anxiety, stress, and depression
> - Parkinson disease
> - AIDS
>
> *From Neville BW, Damm DD, Allen CM, et al: Oral and maxillofacial pathology, ed 4, St Louis, Elsevier, 2016.*

The etiology of **idiopathic** burning mouth disorder is not understood, but it is most likely a neuropathic etiology. There is a clear 6 : 1 predilection for women, mostly of perimenopausal or postmenopausal age, which suggests that hormonal changes may be involved in the etiology. The association between depression and psychological disturbances and burning mouth disorder is controversial. It is not clear whether pain is responsible for the psychological disorders or if the psychological disorder is an etiologic factor.

Clinical Features and Oral Manifestations

With idiopathic burning mouth disorder, the onset of discomfort is usually spontaneous, without any responsible initiating events. Patients complain of a burning and painful tongue and a hard palate and lips. The dorsal anterior and middle third of the tongue are specifically affected. Most patients report that the burning discomfort is minimal upon awakening in the morning, gradually increases during the day, and is most intense in the evening. In one reported study, two thirds of patients reported an altered taste sensation (**dysgeusia**). A change in taste, stress, or depression exacerbates burning mouth disorder. Patients often complain of a feeling of mouth dryness.

Treatment and Prognosis

For patients with burning mouth symptoms, evaluation involves a careful workup to identify any local or systemic identifiable causes of the burning. Many patients complain of mouth dryness. Local causes include oral candidiasis and xerostomia. Burning discomfort due to oral candidiasis would be expected to respond to antifungal therapy. Stimulation of salivary flow for patients with **hyposalivation** (measured low salivary flow) may decrease the burning symptoms. Laboratory testing may identify undiagnosed systemic diseases such as anemia and diabetes mellitus. Antianxiety medications, anticonvulsants, and antidepressants are often prescribed for the treatment of burning mouth disorder. There is evidence that the antioxidant alpha lipoic acid has resulted in symptomatic improvement for some patients. Topical clonazepam rinses and systemic clonazepam have also been successful for some patients. In addition, an herbal compound called Catuama has been reported to have some successful results. Sometimes the condition resolves on its own over time.

Trigeminal Neuralgia (Tic Douloureux)

Trigeminal neuralgia *(tic douloureux)* is a well-known pathologic condition involving the fifth cranial nerve, also called the trigeminal nerve. Trigeminal neuralgia is characterized by a unilateral sharp, shooting, knifelike, or electric shock–type pain. The maxillary division of the trigeminal nerve is most often affected, followed by the mandibular branch. Only about 4% of cases have been associated with the ophthalmic division.

Clinical Features and Oral Manifestations

Although usually unilateral, trigeminal neuralgia can be bilateral. Initially, the patient may experience a dull ache or burning sensation referred to as **pretrigeminal neuralgia**. These early symptoms have been described in up to 20% of patients who are eventually diagnosed with trigeminal neuralgia. This pretrigeminal phase can last for months to years. Approximately 50% of patients have specific **"trigger points,"** or zones on the face in which a touch or temperature change can trigger an episode of trigeminal neuralgia. A "trigger point" is a small area in the nasolabial fold, skin, or mucosa innervated by the trigeminal nerve. The pain lasts less than 2 minutes, but the patient experiences recurrent episodes of sharp, shooting, and excruciating pain. The pain is so severe that suicide has been reported to be associated with trigeminal neuralgia. The term **douloureux** (French for "painful twitch") has been used to describe the shooting, "painful jerking" that the patient experiences during an episode, thus the term *tic* (a habitual spasmodic contraction of the muscles) *douloureux*. After an episode of pain under 2 minutes, there is a refractory period in which a trigger cannot bring about pain. The identification of this refractory period can be very helpful in the diagnosis of trigeminal neuralgia.

The etiology of trigeminal neuralgia is unknown. It is more common in females than in males, and there is a predilection for patients in their mid fifties to seventies. If diagnosed in younger patients, a systemic illness such as multiple sclerosis should be suspected. In younger patients, the pain is often bilateral.

Diagnosis

The diagnosis of trigeminal neuralgia is based on the history and onset of the pain and its associated clinical symptoms. Radiographic findings are noncontributory. CT scans and MRIs are performed to rule out other pathologic conditions. In trigeminal neuralgia, sensory loss is not detected clinically on physical examination. If sensory loss or facial weakness is observed, the patient should be evaluated for a central nervous system tumor.

Treatment and Prognosis

Opioids do not control the pain of trigeminal neuralgia. The anticonvulsant drug carbamazepine (Tegretol) is most often used and has been shown to be most effective, especially in pretrigeminal neuralgia. Other anticonvulsant drugs such as phenytoin, oxycarbazepine, and gabapentin are used in combination with baclofen, a skeletal muscle relaxant. The injection of alcohol or glycerol into the trigeminal ganglion can be helpful but does not eliminate the condition. Some surgical interventions exist but carry the risk of **paresthesia**. One of the newest procedures used for treating trigeminal neuralgia, gamma radiosurgery, has shown promising results.

Bell's Palsy (Idiopathic Facial Paralysis, Idiopathic Seventh Nerve Paralysis)

Bell's palsy (*idiopathic facial paralysis, idiopathic seventh nerve paralysis*) is an acute, self-limiting loss of muscle control on one side of the face. Bell's palsy is a clinical diagnosis that is made after excluding other causes of facial paralysis through diagnostic procedures that include patient history, physical examination, and laboratory and imaging studies. The condition is named after Sir Charles Bell, who described the anatomy of the facial nerve in 1821.

The cause of Bell's palsy remains unclear. Reactivation of the herpes simplex or herpes zoster virus has been suggested, as well as damage to the facial nerve from ischemia and edema. Hereditary factors have also been implicated. Patients with diabetes mellitus, hypertension, immunodeficiency, upper respiratory viral infection, and pregnancy are at greater risk for developing Bell's palsy.

Clinical Features and Oral Manifestations

Bell's palsy occurs in people of all ages, with the greatest incidence between 15 and 45 years of age. Women are affected more frequently than men. The condition is characterized by an abrupt loss of muscular control on one side of the face. The clinical presentation reflects the anatomic distribution of the seventh cranial (facial) nerve. The individual is unable to smile, close the eye, or raise the eyebrow on the affected side of the face. The paralysis may take several hours to become complete, and the facial weakness tends to reach its peak within 72 hours. The corner of the mouth usually droops, causing saliva to drool. Speech is affected, and taste may be abnormal. These features are often accompanied by neck, mastoid, or ear pain; dysgeusia; **hyperacusis;** or altered facial sensation.

Diagnosis

Bell's palsy is a clinical diagnosis. Laboratory tests and imaging are used to rule out an etiology for the paralysis, but such tests are usually not helpful unless the history and clinical features suggest an etiology for the facial paralysis. Possible causes of facial paralysis such as uveoparotid fever (a form of sarcoidosis), Lyme disease, other infectious diseases, autoimmune disease, neoplasia, and trauma need to be ruled out.

Treatment and Prognosis

A variety of treatments are used in the management of Bell's palsy, including systemic corticosteroids, antiviral therapy, physical therapy, and hyperbaric oxygen therapy. Eye protection is essential to prevent eye damage. Such protection includes artificial tears, topical ocular antibiotics and, possibly, taping the eye shut.

Facial paralysis usually begins to regress slowly and spontaneously within 1 to 2 months. For most patients, the paralysis completely resolves within 6 months. Symptoms that remain after 1 year will likely remain indefinitely. For most of these patients, the residual sequelae are mild to moderate.

TEMPOROMANDIBULAR DISORDERS

Knowledge of the anatomy and function of the temporomandibular joint (TMJ) enables the dental hygienist to understand the disorders that affect the joint. Disorders of the TMJ include myofascial pain and dysfunction (MPD), internal derangements (ID), osteoarthritis, and rheumatoid arthritis. Benign and malignant tumors can also affect the TMJ.

Anatomy of the Temporomandibular Joint

The TMJ is the **articulation** between the condyle of the mandible and the glenoid (mandibular) fossa of the temporal bone (Fig. 10.1). It is a highly specialized joint that differs from other joints because of the fibrocartilage that covers the bony articulating

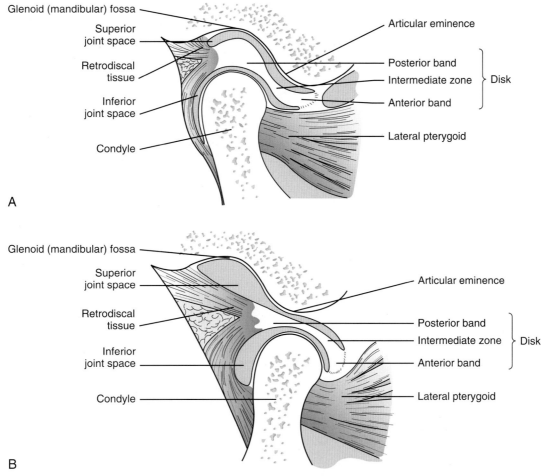

Glenoid (mandibular) fossa
Superior joint space
Retrodiscal tissue
Inferior joint space
Condyle
Articular eminence
Posterior band
Intermediate zone } Disk
Anterior band
Lateral pterygoid

A

Glenoid (mandibular) fossa
Superior joint space
Retrodiscal tissue
Inferior joint space
Condyle
Articular eminence
Posterior band
Intermediate zone } Disk
Anterior band
Lateral pterygoid

B

• **Figure 10.1** Lateral views of the temporomandibular joint. **A,** Jaw closed. **B,** Jaw open. (From Kaplan AS, Assael LA: *Temporomandibular disorders*, Philadelphia, Saunders, 1991.)

surfaces, its ginglymoarthrodial (rotational and translational) movement, the fact that its function and overall health are dictated by jaw movement, and its dependence on the contralateral joint. An articular disk is interposed in the space between the temporal bone and the mandible. This disk divides the space into an upper compartment (superior joint space) and a lower compartment (inferior joint space) (see Fig. 10.1).

Translational movements occur in the upper compartment, whereas the lower compartment functions primarily as the hinge or rotational component. The superior and inferior spaces contain **synovial fluid,** which is produced by the **synovial membrane** that lines the joint. The synovial fluid provides nourishment and lubrication of the avascular structures. The articular disk is attached to the lateral and medial aspects of the condyle, to the superior belly of the lateral pterygoid muscle, and to the joint capsule (see Fig. 10.1). The articular disk and the bony surfaces are **avascular** (i.e., they do not contain blood vessels) and devoid of nerve fibers. The joint is further surrounded and protected by the fibrous connective tissue joint capsule. The primary innervation of the TMJ capsule and disk attachments is from the auriculotemporal nerve, with secondary innervation from the deep temporal and masseteric nerves. The function of the disk is to separate the forces resulting from rotation and translation, absorb

shock, improve the fit between bony surfaces, protect the edges of the articulating surfaces, distribute weight over a larger area, and spread the lubricating synovial fluid.

Understanding the location and action of the **muscles of mastication** is important in the evaluation of disorders affecting the TMJ. **Palpation** of these muscles during a clinical evaluation is done to determine whether muscle spasm or dysfunctional muscle activity is occurring. The muscles of mastication comprise major muscles about the facial region that govern the movement of the mandible. They include the masseter, temporalis, medial pterygoid, lateral pterygoid, anterior digastric, and mylohyoid (suprahyoids) (Figs. 10.2 to 10.4). The function of these muscles is to create the mandibular envelope of motion. Three of these muscles—the masseter, medial pterygoid, and temporalis—are elevator muscles that, when activated, close the mandible. The opening, or depressor, function is accomplished mainly by the lateral pterygoid muscle with some help from the anterior digastric muscle. Studies have shown that the two components of the lateral pterygoid muscle are active at different times in the functioning of the mandible (see Fig. 10.4). The superior portion of the muscle seats the articular disk on the eminence of the articulating surface. The inferior belly is attached to the mandibular condyle and functions during mouth opening.

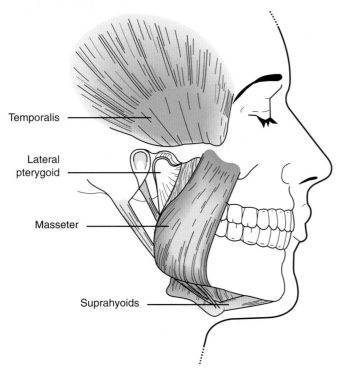

• **Figure 10.2** Muscles of mastication: the temporalis, lateral pterygoid, masseter, and suprahyoid. (From Kaplan AS, Assael LA: *Temporomandibular disorders,* Philadelphia, Saunders, 1991.)

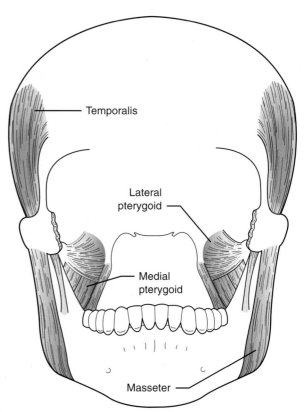

• **Figure 10.4** Muscles of mastication. Illustrated are the four paired muscles of mastication: the masseter, temporalis, medial pterygoid, and lateral pterygoid. (From Kaplan AS, Assael LA: *Temporomandibular disorders,* Philadelphia, Saunders, 1991.)

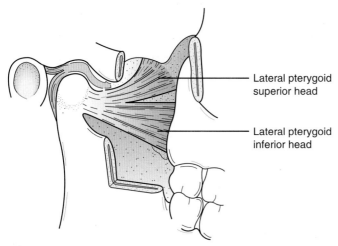

• **Figure 10.3** Muscles of mastication. The two distinct heads of the lateral pterygoid muscle are illustrated. (From Kaplan AS, Assael LA: *Temporomandibular disorders,* Philadelphia, Saunders, 1991.)

Normal Function of the Temporomandibular Joint

The harmonious function of the TMJ depends on various factors. The anatomic relationship of the condyle–disk complex governs the smooth functioning of the mandible. This articulation, along with the muscles of mastication, provides the movement of the mandible. The muscles of mastication are the machinery that powers mandibular movement; the anatomic joint structures such as the condyle, articular eminence, and disk act as the gears or bearings of the jaw.

In **normal joint function** the jaw begins at a rest position of maximal occlusal contact. In this position the mandibular condyle rests within the glenoid (mandibular) fossa, with the articular disk situated between the condyle, roof of the glenoid (mandibular) fossa, and articular eminence (see Fig. 10.1A-B). The first phase of opening is characterized by a rotational (hinge) movement of the condyle, followed by anterior translation (sliding movement) to approximately the anterior peak of the articular eminence. During translation the disk assumes a more posterior position in relation to the condyle. The inferior and superior joint spaces assume different configurations during each of these movements.

Temporomandibular Disorders

Epidemiology of Temporomandibular Disorders

Temporomandibular disorders (TMDs) are caused by abnormalities in the functioning of the TMJ or associated structures. TMDs, which have been a clinical and diagnostic challenge in dentistry for many years, are reported to affect up to 36 million adults in the United States. Hippocrates documented jaw dysfunction problems as early as the fifth century BC. However, it was not until 1934 that James Costen, an otolaryngologist, described a group of symptoms centered around the jaw and ear. Costen syndrome included such symptoms as impaired hearing, ear pain, tinnitus, dizziness, burning in the throat and tongue, headache, and trismus. Although most, if not all, of Costen's explanations have been refuted, the dental profession's interest was stimulated by his view that malocclusion plays a pivotal role in this condition. The 1980s were marked by a growing interest in TMDs, facilitated by advances in pain neurophysiology, multicenter research, the American Academy of Craniomandibular Disorders (later to become the American Academy of Orofacial Pain), the American Dental Association, and pivotal work published in 1986 by Sanders for the treatment of closed lock by arthroscopy.

Although up to 75% of the adult population has at least one sign, with 33% having at least one symptom, most studies suggest that clinically significant TMD-related jaw pain, dysfunction, or both affects 10% to 16% of the adult population. The majority of patients with TMDs are females aged between 20 and 40 years, and some researchers suggest that female sex hormones may have a role in the pathogenesis. Furthermore, TMDs are often associated with comorbid conditions such as depression, rheumatoid arthritis, chronic fatigue syndrome, chronic headache, fibromyalgia, sleep disturbances, and irritable bowel syndrome.

Pathophysiology of Temporomandibular Disorders

The precise cause of TMDs remains controversial and is often considered multifactorial. Trauma, which overloads the masticatory system, has been suggested as the most likely cause of TMDs. Trauma affecting the TMJ is classified as *direct* (assault), *indirect* (whiplash injury), or secondary to *parafunctional habits* (clenching, bruxism). In addition, psychosocial factors such as stress have been implicated in masticatory muscle pain. The relationship between TMDs and dentofacial deformity is controversial. Numerous studies continue to dispute the significance of occlusal relationships, and there is little evidence that malocclusion, loss of teeth, loss of vertical dimension, or occlusal instability is the primary cause of TMDs, although these conditions should be addressed to achieve optimal dental occlusion and masticatory function. Nor is there sufficient evidence to suggest that oral surgery procedures (e.g., extraction of third molars) can cause TMDs. TMJ disorders may also be the result of disorders in growth and development, as seen in condylar hyperplasia or hypoplasia. The most common systemic conditions that may affect the TMJ are rheumatoid arthritis and juvenile rheumatoid arthritis; less common systemic diseases include Sjögren syndrome, ankylosing spondylitis, psoriatic arthritis, reactive arthritis (Reiter syndrome), systemic lupus erythematosus, scleroderma, mixed connective tissue disease, calcium pyrophosphate deposition disease, and gout. **Iatrogenic** causes (resulting from the action of a health care provider) of TMDs include the indiscriminate use of corticosteroid injection into the joint.

Evaluation of Temporomandibular Disorders

Temporomandibular dysfunction can be caused by disorders of the muscles of mastication or internal derangements of the components of the joint. The "gold standard" for evaluating patients with potential TMDs and establishing a differential diagnosis involves a comprehensive history (i.e., chief complaint, history of the chief complaint, dental and medical history), a thorough clinical examination, and a panoramic radiograph to detect dental, periodontal, or other potential problems. Although dental hygienists do not generally perform comprehensive TMD examinations, they may participate in diagnostic procedures and should recognize risk factors, signs, and symptoms of TMDs to facilitate the

appropriate referral. Understanding TMDs is clinically significant for the dental hygienist, as these conditions may affect patient management (e.g., reduced mouth opening, shorter appointment times, pain control). Three cardinal features suggest a TMD: orofacial pain, joint noise, and restricted jaw function.

History

A history of aberrant growth, previous injuries, illnesses, musculoskeletal complaints, and possible emotional disturbances is an important consideration in the evaluation of patients with TMDs. The patient history specific to TMDs includes questions regarding the following:
- Medical/dental history
- Precipitating events (mastication, spontaneous, yawning, trauma)
- Circumstances that exacerbate or diminish symptoms
- Onset of symptoms (sudden, gradual)
- Joint symptoms (clicking, popping)
- Pain (localized or diffuse; quality such as sharp, dull, burning, aching)
- Problems with mastication
- Trismus
- Malocclusion
- Parafunctional habits (bruxing, clenching, chronic gum chewing)
- Dental symptoms
- Extensive dental or orthodontic treatment
- History of surgical treatment of the jaws

Clicking and popping most commonly reflect disk displacement with reduction and occur in approximately 33% of asymptomatic patients. They are of little clinical consequence in the absence of pain or other symptoms relating to the TMJ, as there is controversy concerning whether these noises represent an adaptive response (i.e., normal variant) or an early symptom of progression to disk displacement without reduction. The incidence of orofacial pain among the adult population has been reported to be 26%, and the differential diagnosis includes TMDs, odontogenic pain (e.g., pericoronitis, caries, cracked tooth syndrome, infection, pulpalgia), mucosal disorders, burning mouth disorder, headache, neuralgia (e.g., trigeminal neuralgia), fibromyalgia, otitis media, sinus infection, cervical spine pain, salivary gland pathology, and tumor (e.g., TMJ, intracranial). Therefore referral to a medical specialist (e.g., otolaryngologist, neurologist) may be necessary if the patient's signs and/or symptoms are unclear or suggest the presence of other pathology or conditions. Etiologies of **trismus** other than TMDs include odontogenic infection, oral surgery procedures, local anesthetic during dental treatment (e.g., inferior alveolar nerve block, posterior maxillary infiltration), tumors, facial bone fractures, radiation therapy, and medications (e.g., phenothiazine).

Clinical Examination

A comprehensive examination of a patient in relation to TMJ disorders includes an examination of the joint, muscles of mastication (e.g., masseter, temporalis, medial and lateral pterygoid muscles), oral cavity, and cervical spine. Joint examination involves **auscultation** (using a stethoscope) and palpation. The clinician relates joint noises such as clicking, **crepitus** (crackling), or popping to the mandibular movement cycle. Tenderness over the lateral pole of the condyle suggests **capsulitis**. The muscles of mastication are palpated to determine tenderness. The lateral pterygoid muscle cannot be reliably palpated, and the superior

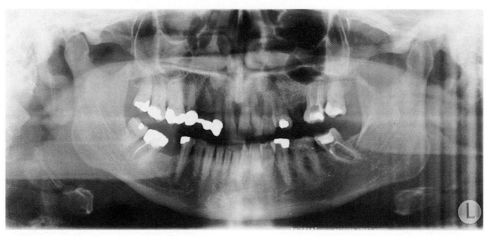

• **Figure 10.5** Panoramic radiograph of a patient with temporomandibular dysfunction and normal anatomy of the mandibular condyles.

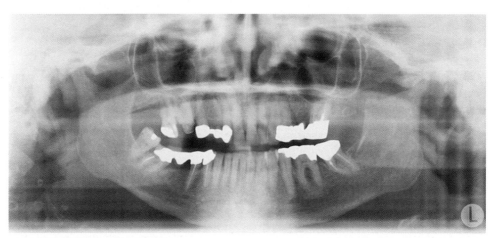

• **Figure 10.6** Panoramic radiograph shows resorption of both the right and the left condyles. In this patient degenerative arthritis followed bilateral surgery of the temporomandibular joint. The left coronoid process was removed during surgery.

head can be assessed by asking the patient to bite on tongue blades placed bilaterally over the posterior teeth. The inferior head of the lateral pterygoid muscle can be examined for symptoms by asking the patient to protrude and laterally move the mandible against resistance. In addition to a thorough oral examination, the patient is asked to move the mandible in a normal rotation (hinge) and translatory (forward slide) cycle. Although maximal mouth opening tends to decrease with age, it is generally considered restricted only if it is less than 40 mm. *Deviation* (shifting of the mandible to one side before returning to midline) and *deflection* (shifting of the mandible to one side, with no return to midline) to the right or left side are also observed on maximal interincisal opening. The patient's ability to manipulate the mandible into right and left lateral excursions is also noted. Assisted mouth opening beyond the patient's maximal opening should be attempted to determine additional range of motion and to palpate "end-feel." Muscle restrictions are associated with a soft end-feel, and the range of motion can be increased by 5 mm, unlike disk displacement without reduction, in which assisted opening is less than 5 mm with a firm end-feel. Finally, anesthetic injections (e.g., auriculotemporal nerve block, local infiltration) may be useful to distinguish between arthrogenous (joint-related), myogenous (muscle-related), and odontogenic (dental) pain. Signs of

parafunctional habits such as ridging of the buccal mucosa on the inside of the cheeks or abnormal dental attrition should be documented.

Imaging

Radiographic studies may be helpful in determining the cause of the patient's pain or dysfunction. Several different types of radiographs and views are obtained to determine the shape of the condyle and whether evidence of degenerative joint disease exists (Figs. 10.5 and 10.6). Radiographic evaluation of patients with TMDs typically includes panoramic or transcranial imaging. These radiographs are limited to identifying gross changes in bone, which are often not seen until a significant volume of destruction or alteration in bone mineral content has occurred. Tomography may provide greater accuracy in assessing condylar position and range of mobility.

Several specialized imaging studies that are useful in the diagnosis of TMDs have become available. Computerized tomography (CT) and cone-beam CT are most accurate for identifying bone abnormalities such as osteophytes, condylar erosion, fractures, ankylosis, and condylar hyperplasia. In-office cone-beam CT is advantageous because of its accessibility, higher spatial resolution, reduced radiation exposure, and faster imaging, and it is

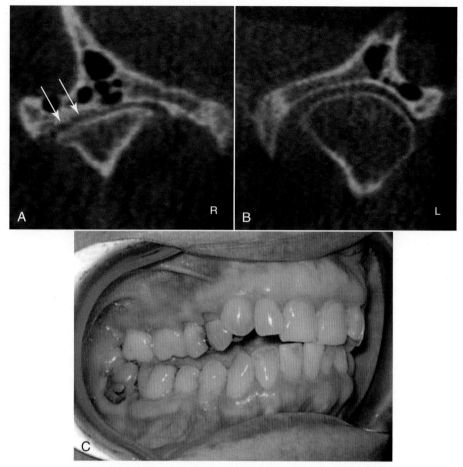

• **Figure 10.7 A** and **B,** Cone-beam computed tomography illustrating degenerative joint changes in the right temporomandibular joint (TMJ) and normal left TMJ anatomy. There is flattening of the right condyle and erosive changes in the glenoid (mandibular) fossa (*arrows*). **C,** Malocclusion consisting of a prematurity of the right maxillary and mandibular second molars due to reduced vertical dimension of the right condyle and glenoid (mandibular) fossa.

less expensive compared with conventional CT (Fig. 10.7). **Magnetic resonance imaging (MRI)** is mandatory for examining disk position, function, and morphology and the presence of joint effusions (inflammatory changes) (Fig. 10.8). MRI is advantageous because no ionizing radiation is used. **Arthrography,** which uses a radiopaque contrast agent that is injected into the joint, may be useful when MRI is not tolerated and information regarding the position and morphology of the disk is required.

Types of Temporomandibular Disorders

TMDs can be classified according to structural and functional changes (Box 10.2).

Masticatory Muscle Disorder

Myofascial Pain and Dysfunction

MPD comprises at least 50% of all TMDs and most commonly involves the masseter muscle. Pain is often described as dull or achy, diffuse and cyclic, frequently worse in the morning, particularly in patients who clench or grind their teeth during sleep. It is characterized as dysfunctional muscle hyperactivity with regional pain, tenderness of the affected muscles (i.e., trigger points), and variable amounts of reduced opening and complaints of

---

• BOX 10.2 TMD Classification

Masticatory Muscle Disorder
- Myofascial pain and dysfunction

Internal Derangement (Disk Derangement)
- Disk displacement with reduction
- Disk displacement without reduction
- Disk perforation

Arthritis
- Inflammatory: rheumatoid arthritis
- Noninflammatory: osteoarthritis (degenerative joint disease)

TMJ Mobility Disorders
- Hypermobility: subluxation, dislocation
- Hypomobility: ankylosis

Neoplasia
- Benign
- Malignant

TMD, temporomandibular disorder; TMJ, temporomandibular joint.

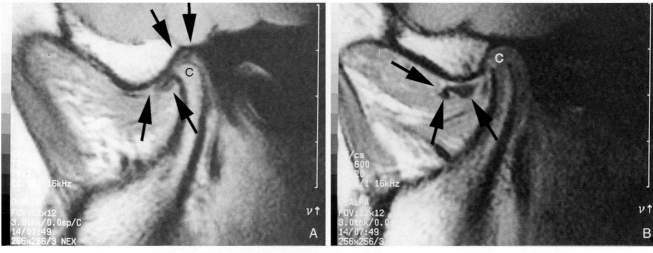

• **Figure 10.8** **A,** Magnetic resonance imaging (MRI) scan of the right temporomandibular joint shows the normal position of the disk. Arrows point to the disk. **B,** MRI scan of the left temporomandibular joint in the same patient shows displacement of the disk. **C,** Condyle.

malocclusion. The direction of deflection depends on the location of the involved muscle.

Internal Derangement

Internal derangement or **disk derangement** is defined as an abnormal positional relationship of the disk (meniscus) relative to the mandibular condyle and the articular eminence. Patients often present with continuous sharp, sudden pain localized to the TMJ that is exacerbated by jaw movement. In some cases the disk is displaced anteriorly and returns to its normal position on opening of the mouth or movement away from the affected side (disk displacement with reduction). In another form of disk displacement the displaced disk acts as an obstacle to the sliding condyle. In this type of displacement patients complain of problems such as intermittent locking of the jaw; a sudden onset of limited mouth opening, usually associated with cessation of joint sounds; deflection of the mandible to the affected (ipsilateral) side; and restricted lateral excursive movements away from the affected side (disk displacement without reduction). Patients may also complain of morning "stiffness" in their jaw. Disk displacement has been categorized according to a widely accepted staging system developed by Wilkes that is based on clinical and radiographic changes (Table 10.1). A study in which TMJ loading was provoked by gum chewing in patients with disk displacement without reduction increased the risk of nonreducing disk displacement.

Arthritis

Arthritis is defined as inflammation of a joint and is classified as either **osteoarthritis** or **rheumatoid arthritis.** Osteoarthritis, also referred to as *degenerative joint disease,* is the most common disease affecting the TMJ. Dysfunctional articular remodeling, due to either decreased adaptive capacity of the articulating structures or excessive or sustained physical stress that exceeds the normal adaptive capacity, leads to degenerative changes. Although it may be associated with disk displacement or disk perforation, the precise relationship is unclear. It may be clinically silent, and progression cannot be reliably determined. Patients may have pain symptoms that are worse in the evening, as well as limited opening, muscle splinting, and crepitus of the TMJ. Rheumatoid arthritis

TABLE 10.1	Wilkes Classification
Stage	**Description**
I	Early reducing disk displacement
II	Late reducing disk displacement
III	Acute or subacute nonreducing disk displacement
IV	Chronic nonreducing disk displacement
V	Chronic nonreducing disk displacement with osteoarthritis

Data from Wilkes C: Internal derangements of the temporomandibular joint: pathological variations. *Arch Otolaryngol Head Neck Surg* 115:469, 1989.

is an inflammatory autoimmune disorder of the joints. Approximately 50% to 75% of patients with rheumatoid arthritis have involvement of the TMJ during the course of the disease. In rheumatoid arthritis, patients may complain of pain that is worse in the morning, limited opening, occlusal changes, and preauricular edema and tenderness. Intraarticular corticosteroid injections have been reported to improve pain and other symptoms for children with juvenile idiopathic arthritis.

TMJ Mobility Disorders

Hypermobility Disorders

Hypermobility disorders include **dislocation** and **subluxation.** *Dislocation* occurs when one or both of the condyles translate anteriorly to the articular eminence, resulting in an open lock that the patient cannot reduce. It may occur spontaneously or after opening the mouth widely, such as when yawing, eating, or during a dental procedure. Dislocation should be reduced immediately by applying downward and posterior pressure on the mandible to relocate the condyle within the glenoid (mandibular) fossa. Prolonged or chronic dislocation may require muscle relaxants or general anesthesia. *Subluxation* refers to hypermobility in which the patient is able to relocate the mandible back into the glenoid (mandibular) fossa.

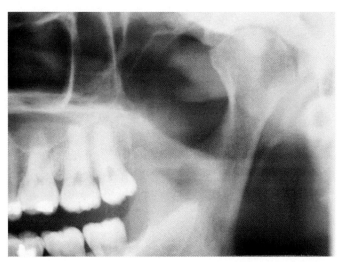

• **Figure 10.9** Panoramic radiograph of an osteochondroma of the mandibular condyle. (Courtesy Dr. David L. Hirsch.)

Ankylosis

Ankylosis of the TMJ is defined as immobility of the condyle because of fibrous or bony union between the articulating structures of the joint. Ankylosis can be classified by tissue type (fibrous, bony), location (intraarticular, extraarticular), and extent of fusion (complete, incomplete). Joint infection, usually after trauma, accounts for 50% of all TMJ ankylosis cases, but 30% result from trauma without infection. Fibrotic intraarticular ankylosis is the most common type seen in the TMJ. Trauma-induced hemorrhage (hemarthrosis) is a common cause of this type of ankylosis. Children are more prone to ankylosis because of greater osteogenic potential and less development of the joint meniscus.

Neoplasia

Tumors arising in the TMJ are rare. The most common benign tumors that arise in the condyle include the osteochondroma (Fig. 10.9), osteoblastoma, chondroblastoma, and osteoma. Synovial chondromatosis is the most common benign neoplasm of the synovium and is characterized by the development of metaplastic, highly cellular, cartilaginous foci in the synovial membrane that results in degenerative changes consistent with osteoarthritis, and by swelling, pain, and limitation of movement. Radiographic findings are variable and may include loose radiopaque bodies in the TMJ, degenerative changes of the articular surfaces, and variable widening or loss of joint space. Osteosarcoma (see Chapter 7) is one of the most frequently occurring malignant bone tumors. Approximately 6% to 8% of all osteosarcomas occur in the jaws. It is unusual for osteosarcoma to originate in the TMJ.

Treatment of Temporomandibular Disorders

Nonsurgical Treatment

Treatment goals for MPD, internal derangement, and arthritis of the TMJ include the following:
- Improving joint function (i.e., range of motion)
- Reducing pain
- Preventing further joint damage (i.e., reducing mechanical stress and inflammation)

Treatment typically begins with nonsurgical modalities. The first phase of nonsurgical treatment includes pharmacologic therapy, heat/ice packs, physical therapy, soft mechanical diet, stretch therapy, and exercise therapy. Passive jaw exercises are effective to improve pain and mobility for MPD, but are contraindicated with severely displaced disks. The local application of heat or ice will increase circulation and relax muscles. It may seem paradoxical that both heat and ice can be used for the same purpose, but localized vasodilation occurs in response to both, in the body's attempt to return the area to its normal temperature. Although patients may benefit from occlusal adjustment, this has not been found to prevent or improve TMD symptoms. Despite numerous studies that have demonstrated the usefulness of acupuncture, its efficacy is considered equivocal.

Medications are used to control pain and inflammation. Traditional nonsteroidal antiinflammatory drugs (NSAIDs) are often used in the acute stage. Cyclooxygenase-2 selective inhibitors (coxibs or COX-2 inhibitors) are the newest types of NSAIDs and may be considered for patients at high risk for gastrointestinal bleeding and who do not respond to traditional NSAIDs. Caution is recommended with the chronic use of either type of NSAID because of possible cardiovascular complications. Tramadol, when used with acetaminophen, is more effective than NSAIDs for reducing musculoskeletal pain, but should be restricted to short-term use because of the potential for habituation and dependence. Tricyclic antidepressants and serotonin and norepinephrine reuptake inhibitors have shown the greatest benefit in patients with chronic pain, probably due to their analgesic and antidepressant actions. Although these drugs may be considered for chronic muscle pain, side effects include nausea, sedation, psychomotor impairment, xerostomia, and constipation. Muscle relaxants, botulinum toxin, and antianxiety agents can be used to reduce muscle hypertonicity. Intramuscular botulinum toxin-A may also reduce stress on the TMJ and may be considered for patients with myofascial pain who cannot be treated effectively with conservative modalities. Data are emerging that intraarticular injection with sodium hyaluronate, which is normally produced by synovial cells, will facilitate joint lubrication and restore joint stabilization for patients with positional disk abnormalities.

If a patient fails to improve or worsens after approximately 1 to 2 months of conservative nonsurgical management, the second phase, which involves the use of occlusal appliances, may be initiated. **Stabilization appliances** function by relaxing muscles, protecting the dentition, stabilizing and protecting the joint, redistributing occlusal forces, providing biofeedback by making patients aware of bruxing habits, or relieving the load on the disk to allow repair of damaged retrodiscal tissues. Reduction of TMJ pain and not sounds (e.g., clicking, popping, crepitus) is the primary objective for oral appliance therapy. **Anterior repositioning appliances** are indicated for patients with painful clicking or frequent locking, but should be carefully monitored and used part-time because of possible irreversible changes to the occlusion.

Psychosocial (e.g., stress, coping abilities) and environmental factors (e.g., ethnicity, culture) may negatively affect the prognosis for orofacial muscle pain, and early cognitive-behavioral intervention (e.g., education, biofeedback, relaxation training, stress management) may improve outcomes.

Surgical Treatment

Patients with TMDs other than MPD may be considered for surgical treatment if they do not respond to nonsurgical therapy and continue to suffer from pain and functional impairment because of interferences in TMJ function. Various surgical techniques are used to treat TMDs. **Arthrocentesis** is a minimally invasive procedure that involves lavaging the joint through a needle to address three common symptoms of the TMJ associated with closed lock: limited opening, pain, and dysfunction. The rationale is to release the disk and adhesions, reduce the viscosity of the synovial fluid, and wash out inflammatory mediators. The success rate for arthrocentesis has been reported to be 83%. The use of platelet-rich plasma injections during arthrocentesis may improve reparative remodeling of the TMJ. **Arthroscopy** is a minimally invasive closed joint procedure that allows direct visualization and manipulation of the joint. **Open joint surgery** (i.e., arthrotomy) is a broad term encompassing all procedures allowing direct access to the TMJ and generally used to improve the disk–condyle relationship. Such procedures include disk manipulation (i.e., diskoplasty, disk repositioning, disk replacement, diskectomy), condylar repositioning (i.e., condylotomy), recontouring of the articular surfaces of the condyle and glenoid (mandibular) fossa (i.e., gap arthroplasty), and total joint reconstruction using a prosthetic device or autogenous graft. Eminectomy is performed for recurrent mandibular hypermobility/subluxation and involves removal of the articular eminence of the temporal bone, which blocks the path of the condyle when closing. The chronic nature associated with rheumatoid arthritis is especially challenging, and management strategies are focused on prevention and repair.

Multidisciplinary Management

Temporomandibular disorders remain a frequent cause of visits to primary care physicians and general dentists. Additional considerations for patients with oral, facial, and head and neck pain may necessitate referral to medical and dental specialists. This management strategy is especially relevant for patients with headaches, which may be exacerbated by TMDs.

Selected References

Books

Greenberg M, Glick M, Ship J: *Burket's oral medicine*, ed 11, Hamilton, 2008, BC Decker.

Hupp J, Ellis E, Tucker M: *Contemporary oral and maxillofacial surgery*, ed 6, St. Louis, 2014, Elsevier.

Okeson J: *Management of temporomandibular disorders and occlusion*, ed 7, St. Louis, 2013, Elsevier.

Journal Articles

Aggarwal V, Tickle M, Javidi H, et al: Reviewing the evidence: can cognitive behavioral therapy improve outcomes for patients with chronic orofacial pain?, *J Orofac Pain* 24:163, 2010.

Al-Belasy F, Dolwick M: Arthrocentesis for the treatment of temporomandibular joint closed lock: a review article, *Int J Oral Maxillofac Surg* 36:773, 2007.

Al-Din AS, Mirr R, Davey R, et al: Trigeminal cephalgias and facial pain syndromes associated with autonomic dysfunction, *Cephalalgia* 25(8):605, 2005.

Benoliel R, Sharav Y: Chronic orofacial pain, *Curr Pain Headache Rep* 14:33, 2010.

Burchiel KJ, Slavin KV: On the natural history of trigeminal neuralgia, *Neurosurgery* 46:152, 2000.

Clark G: Classification, causation and treatment of masticatory myogenous pain and dysfunction, *Oral Maxillofac Surg Clin North Am* 20:147, 2008.

Conti P, dos Santos C, Kogawa E, et al: The treatment of painful temporomandibular joint clicking with oral splints: a randomized clinical trial, *J Am Dent Assoc* 137:1108, 2006.

de Bont L, Dijkgraaf L, Stegenga B: Epidemiology and natural progression of articular temporomandibular disorders, *Oral Surg Oral Med Oral Pathol Oral Radiol Endod* 83:72, 1997.

DeMoraes M, do Amaral Bezerra BA, da Rocha Neto PC, et al: Randomized trials for the treatment of burning mouth syndrome: an evidence-based review of the literature, *Oral Surg Oral Med Oral Pathol Oral Radiol Endod* 117:e221, 2014.

Dimitroulis G: Temporomandibular disorders: a clinical update, *BMJ* 317:190, 1998.

Dimitroulis G: The prevalence of osteoarthrosis in cases of advanced internal derangement of the temporomandibular joint: a clinical, surgical and histologic study, *Int J Oral Maxillofac Surg* 34:345, 2005.

Dworkin S, Huggins K, LeResche L, et al: Epidemiology of signs and symptoms in temporomandibular disorders: clinical signs in cases and controls, *J Am Dent Assoc* 120:273, 1990.

Eviston TJ, Croxson GR, Kennedy PGE, et al: Bell's palsy: aetiology, clinical features and multidisciplinary care, *J Neurol Neurosurg Psychiatry* 86:1356, 2015.

Gatchel R, Wright-Stowell A, Wildenstein L, et al: Efficacy of an early intervention for patients with acute temporomandibular disorder–related pain, *J Am Dent Assoc* 137:339, 2006.

Hoffman R, Kotchen J, Kotchen T, et al: Temporomandibular disorders and associated clinical comorbidities, *Clin J Pain* 27:268, 2011.

Horowitz M, Horowitz M, Ochs M, et al: Trigeminal neuralgia: glossopharyngeal neuralgia: two orofacial pain syndromes encountered by dentists, *J Am Dent Assoc* 135:1427, 2004.

Humphrey S, Lindroth J, Carlson C: Routine dental care in patients with temporomandibular disorders, *J Orofac Pain* 16:129, 2002.

Ingawale S, Goswami T: Temporomandibular joint: disorders, treatments, and biomechanics, *Ann Biomed Eng* 37:976, 2009.

Israel H, Syrop S: The important role of motion in the rehabilitation of patients with mandibular hypomobility: a review of the literature, *J Craniomandibular Pract* 15:74, 1993.

Kahn OA: Gabapentin relieves trigeminal neuralgia in multiple sclerosis patients, *Neurology* 51:611, 1998.

Klasser GD, Fischer DJ, Epstein JB: Burning mouth syndrome: recognition, understanding, and management, *Oral Maxillofac Surg Clin North Am* 20(2):255, 2008.

Kilic S, Gungormus M, Sumbullu M: Is arthrocentesis plus platelet-rich plasma superior to arthrocentesis alone in the treatment of temporomandibular joint osteoarthritis? A ramdomized clinical trial, *J Oral Maxillofac Surg* 73:1473–1483, 2015.

LeResche L: Epidemiology of temporomandibular disorders: implications for the investigation of etiologic factors, *Crit Rev Oral Biol Med* 8:291, 1997.

McNeill C: History of evolution of TMD concepts, *Oral Surg Oral Med Oral Pathol Oral Radiol Endod* 83:51, 1997.

Mendak-Ziółko M, Konopka T, Bogucki ZA: Evaluation of select neurophysiological, clinical and psychological tests for burning mouth syndrome, *Oral Surg Oral Med Oral Pathol Oral Radiol* 114(3):325, 2012.

Palmason S, Stock S, Woo SB, et al: Topical clonazepam solution for the treatment of burning mouth syndrome, *Oral Surg Oral Med Oral Pathol Oral Radiol* 116(3):e200, 2013.

Poon R, Su N, Ching V, et al: Salivary flows in patients with burning mouth syndrome, *Oral Surg Oral Med Oral Pathol Oral Radiol* 117(5):e358, 2014.

Sanders B: Arthroscopic surgery of the temporomandibular joint: treatment of internal derangement with persistent closed lock, *Oral Surg Oral Med Oral Pathol* 62:361, 1986.

Scrivani SJ, Keith DA, Kaban LB: Temporomandibular disorders, *N Engl J Med* 359:2693, 2008.

Spanemberg JC, Cherubini K, de Figueiredo MA, et al: Effect of an herbal compound for treatment of burning mouth syndrome: randomized, controlled, double-blind clinical trial, *Oral Surg Oral Med Oral Pathol Oral Radiol* 113:373, 2012.

Vakaria K, Vakharia K: Bell's palsy, *Facial Plast Surg Clin North Am* 4:1, 2016.

Wilkes C: Internal derangement of the temporomandibular joint: pathological variations, *Arch Otolaryngol Head Neck Surg* 115:469, 1989.

Review Questions

1. All of the following are possible explanations for burning mouth disorder except one. Which one is the exception?
   a. Neuropathic etiology
   b. Anemia
   c. Sensory nerve damage
   d. Allergic reaction

2. Which one of the following is important in the initial diagnosis of idiopathic burning mouth disorder?
   a. Biopsy and histopathologic examination
   b. Blood tests
   c. Psychological testing
   d. Nerve conduction tests

3. Which one of the following is a significant part of the historical diagnosis for burning mouth disorder?
   a. Postmenopausal women
   b. Men over 60
   c. Women with sickle cell anemia
   d. Patients undergoing psychotherapy

4. All of the following drugs are helpful in treating trigeminal neuralgia except one. Which one is the exception?
   a. Gabapentin
   b. Carbamazepine
   c. Percocet
   d. Phenytoin

5. Which systemic illness is most often seen in younger patients with trigeminal neuralgia?
   a. Colitis
   b. Multiple sclerosis
   c. Lung disease
   d. Cardiac disease

6. The pain in trigeminal neuralgia has been described as:
   a. Dull ache
   b. Throbbing
   c. Electric shock–like
   d. Slight burning

7. Which of the following characteristics of trigeminal neuralgia is most helpful in establishing the diagnosis?
   a. Branch of the nerve affected
   b. Description of pain
   c. Identification of the refractory period
   d. Identification of the trigger point

8. The symptoms in pretrigeminal neuralgia:
   a. Are the same as trigeminal neuralgia
   b. Cause facial paralysis
   c. Are a dull ache and burning pain
   d. Last only 1 week

9. Bell's palsy is a disorder involving the:
   a. Trigeminal nerve
   b. Parotid gland
   c. Facial nerve
   d. Temporomandibular joint

10. All of the following statements are correct for Bell's palsy except one. Which one is the exception?
    a. The condition develops rapidly.
    b. The condition usually resolves within 1 to 2 months.
    c. Most patients experience complete resolution.
    d. It is characterized by paralysis of the bilateral facial muscles.

11. Disorders of the articulation between the mandible and maxilla are called:
    a. Synovial hyperplasias
    b. Mandibulomaxillary dysfunction
    c. Temporomandibular disorders
    d. Mandibular dysfunction

12. Using a stethoscope to listen to abnormal noises in the temporomandibular joint is called:
    a. Audiology
    b. Auscultation
    c. Arthrography
    d. Crepitus

13. Which of the following is the most important aspect of the management of temporomandibular disorders?
    a. Palpation of the muscles of mastication
    b. Using a nonsurgical approach
    c. Adjusting the occlusion
    d. Establishing an accurate diagnosis

14. Translational movements of the temporomandibular movements are:
    a. Hinge movements
    b. Sliding movements
    c. Rotational movements
    d. Used only for diagnosis

15. Which of the following is considered a parafunctional habit?
a. Palpation
b. Mastication
c. Bruxing
d. Trauma

16. All of the following are considered functions of the articular disk *except:*
a. Shock absorption
b. Sensory innervation
c. Dissipation of synovial fluid
d. Facilitation of rotation and translation

17. Which of the following is a symptom of a temporomandibular disorder?
a. Pain
b. Malocclusion
c. A history of surgical treatment of the jaws
d. Occlusal adjustment

18. Which of the following comprises at least 50% of all temporomandibular disorders?
a. Hypermobility
b. Myofascial pain and dysfunction
c. Internal disk derangements
d. Osteoarthritis

19. Immobility of the temporomandibular joint because of fibrous or bony union between the articulating structures of the joint is called:
a. Hypermobility
b. Ankylosis
c. Disk displacement
d. Osteoarthritis

20. Which of the following is *not* a form of surgical treatment used for temporomandibular disorders?
a. Arthrocentesis
b. Condylotomy
c. Joint reconstruction
d. Occlusal appliance

21. Which of the following is the most common benign tumor of the synovium of the temporomandibular joint?
a. Osteoblastoma
b. Osteochondroma
c. Chondroblastoma
d. Synovial chondromatosis

22. Which of the following diagnostic modalities should be used for patients suspected of osteoarthritis of the temporomandibular joint?
a. Cone-beam computed tomography
b. Magnetic resonance tomography
c. Local anesthesia injected into the joint
d. Arthrography

23. Which of the following muscles *cannot* be palpated on clinical examination?
a. Medial pterygoid
b. Lateral pterygoid
c. Masseter
d. Temporalis

24. The primary goals for management of temporomandibular disorders include all of the following *except:*
a. Improving oral function
b. Reducing pain
c. Preventing further joint damage
d. Improving oral health

25. Which management would you recommend to a patient who complains of chronic subluxation?
a. Arthrocentesis
b. Eminectomy
c. Appliance therapy
d. Nonsteroidal antiinflammatory drugs (NSAIDs)

26. How may dental hygiene management be modified for a patient with myofascial pain and dysfunction?
    a. Shorter appointments
    b. Jaw exercises before and after the appointment
    c. Pain management with nitrous oxide analgesia
    d. All of the above

27. Which of the following therapies would you recommend to a patient diagnosed with myofascial pain and dysfunction and who did not respond to a 2-month course of soft diet, oral appliance therapy, and hot/cold compresses?
    a. Continue the present therapy for another 2 months
    b. Occlusal adjustment
    c. TMJ arthrotomy
    d. Physical therapy

28. Which condition is associated with crepitus?
    a. Disk displacement with reduction
    b. Disk displacement without reduction
    c. Degenerative joint disease
    d. Myofascial pain and dysfunction

29. Which nerve is primarily responsible for innervating the temporomandibular joint?
    a. Deep temporal nerve
    b. Great occipital nerve
    c. Masseteric nerve
    d. Auriculotemporal nerve

30. All of the following are mandatory for evaluating a patient suspected of disk displacement without reduction *except:*
    a. Panoramic radiographic examination
    b. Medical history
    c. History of symptoms
    d. Medical consultation

31. Disorders in growth and development that may result in temporomandibular disorders (TMDs) include:
    a. Rheumatoid arthritis
    b. Ankylosing spondylitis
    c. Scleroderma
    d. Condylar hyperplasia and hypoplasia

32. All of the following are clinical features that suggest a temporomandibular disorder except:
    a. Orofacial pain
    b. Joint noise
    c. Missing teeth
    d. Restricted jaw function

33. The most common disease affecting the temporomandibular joint is:
    a. Rheumatoid arthritis
    b. Osteoarthritis
    c. Osteosarcoma
    d. Reactive arthritis

34. The presence of muscle spasm or dysfunctional muscle activity is determined by:
    a. Auscultation
    b. Radiologic imaging
    c. Palpation
    d. Patient history

35. The fluid that fills the temporomandibular joint upper and lower compartments is:
    a. Transudate
    b. Serum
    c. Synovial fluid
    d. Blood plasma

Chapter 10 Synopsis

Condition/Disease	Cause	Age/Race/Sex	Location

Burning mouth disorder	Idiopathic
	  Neuropathic
	Local
	  Xerostomia
	  Trigeminal neuralgia
	  Angioedema
	  TMD
	  Oral candidiasis
	  Mouth breathing
	Systemic
	  Vitamin B deficiency
	  Anemia
	  Diabetes mellitus
	  Hypothyroidism
	  Stress/depression
	  Estrogen deficiency
		6:1 Female (perimenopausal or postmenopausal age)	Tongue, lips, and hard palate

Trigeminal neuralgia (tic douloureux)	Unknown	Female predilection Age 50-70 yr In younger patients, suspect systemic illness such as multiple sclerosis	5th cranial nerve Maxillary division most often affected
Bell's palsy	Unclear Reactivation of herpes simplex or herpes zoster virus Damage to facial nerve Patients at risk include those with diabetes mellitus, hypertension, immunodeficiency, URI, pregnancy	15-45 yr	7th facial nerve

Temporomandibular disorder (TMD)	Abnormalities in functioning of the TMJ or associated structures
	Multifactorial trauma
	Comorbid conditions
	  Depression
	  Rheumatoid arthritis
	  Chronic fatigue syndrome
	  Chronic headache
	  Fibromyalgia
	  Sleep disturbances
	  Irritable bowel syndrome
	Disorders in growth and development
	Systemic condition
	  Rheumatoid arthritis
		10% to 16% of adult population
		Females 20-40 yr
			TMJ
			Muscles of mastication

N/A, Not applicable.

Clinical Features	Radiographic Features	Microscopic Features	Treatment	Diagnostic Process
Burning and painful tongue, lips, and hard palate Xerostomia Dysgeusia Candidiasis	N/A	N/A	Antianxiety medication Anticonvulsants Antidepressants Topical clonazepam rinse Systemic clonazepam Catuama Antioxidant alpha lipoic acid	Clinical Historical Laboratory (usually performed to determine anemia or diabetes mellitus)

Unilateral shooting, knifelike pain
"Trigger points"
Pretrigeminal neuralgia: patient experiences a dull ache or burning sensation
Sensory loss not detected on clinical examination
	CT scans and MRIs sometimes performed to rule out other pathology	N/A	Carbamazepine (Tegretol)
			Anticonvulsant drugs
			  Phenytoin
			  Gabapentin
			Muscle relaxants
			  Baclofen (usually used in combination with anticonvulsant drugs)
			Gamma radiosurgery
				Clinical
				Historical

Abrupt unilateral loss of muscle control on one side of the face Inability of patient to smile, close eye, raise eyebrow Paralysis Drooping corner of mouth Slurred speech Dysgeusia	Sometimes used to rule out the etiology for paralysis	Sometimes used to rule out the etiology for paralysis	Systemic corticosteroids Antiviral therapy Physical therapy Eye protection (essential) Facial paralysis usually regresses in 1-2 months and completely in 6 months	Clinical Historical

Pain
Dysfunction
	Panoramic radiograph
	Computed tomography (CT)
	Cone beam CT
	MRI
	Arthrography
		N/A	Nonsurgical treatment
			  Medication
			  Physical therapy
			  Exercise/stretch therapy
			  Soft diet
			  Heat/ice therapy
			  Appliances
			Surgical treatment
			  Arthrocentesis
			  Arthroscopy
			  Open joint surgery
				Radiographic
				Historical
				Clinical
				(All three play a significant role)

Answers

Chapter 1

1. C	8. C	15. A	22. D	29. B	36. D
2. D	9. A	16. A	23. B	30. C	37. B
3. C	10. C	17. D	24. D	31. A	38. B
4. B	11. A	18. A	25. B	32. C	
5. D	12. B	19. C	26. D	33. C	
6. A	13. D	20. C	27. D	34. D	
7. B	14. B	21. A	28. A	35. C	

Chapter 2

1. B	14. D	27. C	40. D	53. D	66. C
2. B	15. B	28. B	41. C	54. B	67. C
3. D	16. D	29. C	42. B	55. B	68. B
4. C	17. B	30. D	43. C	56. C	69. B
5. C	18. B	31. D	44. B	57. C	70. B
6. A	19. A	32. A	45. B	58. C	71. D
7. D	20. B	33. C	46. A	59. B	72. D
8. A	21. C	34. A	47. C	60. A	73. B
9. A	22. B	35. D	48. C	61. B	74. A
10. D	23. B	36. A	49. B	62. B	75. A
11. C	24. A	37. D	50. D	63. C	
12. A	25. B	38. B	51. D	64. D	
13. C	26. B	39. A	52. C	65. A	

Chapter 3

1. C	10. A	19. D	28. A	37. C	46. C
2. B	11. A	20. B	29. B	38. B	47. B
3. D	12. C	21. B	30. D	39. B	48. C
4. D	13. B	22. C	31. A	40. A	49. B
5. D	14. C	23. D	32. C	41. D	50. A
6. C	15. B	24. C	33. D	42. C	51. D
7. D	16. D	25. C	34. A	43. D	52. A
8. A	17. B	26. B	35. D	44. D	
9. B	18. D	27. B	36. B	45. D	

Chapter 4

1. B	8. C	15. D	22. C	29. D	36. C
2. B	9. D	16. B	23. D	30. D	37. B
3. B	10. B	17. D	24. B	31. B	38. B
4. B	11. C	18. D	25. A	32. A	39. C
5. B	12. D	19. B	26. D	33. C	
6. C	13. C	20. B	27. C	34. A	
7. B	14. C	21. C	28. C	35. C	

Chapter 5

1. C	11. A	21. B	31. B	41. D	51. B
2. A	12. B	22. B	32. A	42. C	52. B
3. D	13. A	23. C	33. D	43. C	53. D
4. C	14. B	24. D	34. A	44. C	54. B
5. A	15. D	25. D	35. B	45. D	55. C
6. B	16. C	26. A	36. D	46. C	56. B
7. B	17. D	27. D	37. C	47. B	57. C
8. C	18. C	28. A	38. C	48. B	58. B
9. D	19. C	29. B	39. A	49. B	59. B
10. C	20. A	30. B	40. B	50. B	60. D

Chapter 6

1. C	9. D	17. D	25. C	33. B	41. D
2. D	10. B	18. D	26. B	34. C	42. B
3. C	11. C	19. A	27. A	35. C	43. D
4. A	12. D	20. C	28. B	36. A	
5. C	13. B	21. A	29. C	37. A	
6. D	14. D	22. B	30. D	38. C	
7. C	15. B	23. C	31. C	39. A	
8. B	16. C	24. B	32. B	40. A	

Chapter 7

1. C	13. A	25. A	37. A	49. A	61. B
2. A	14. D	26. C	38. C	50. D	62. D
3. C	15. B	27. B	39. B	51. B	63. C
4. C	16. B	28. B	40. C	52. D	64. A
5. D	17. A	29. D	41. A	53. C	65. B
6. B	18. B	30. B	42. A	54. D	66. C
7. C	19. C	31. D	43. C	55. A	67. B
8. D	20. A	32. A	44. B	56. B	68. B
9. A	21. B	33. C	45. D	57. D	
10. C	22. A	34. B	46. B	58. C	
11. D	23. C	35. C	47. D	59. C	
12. C	24. C	36. B	48. A	60. C	

Chapter 8

1. B	9. C	17. B	25. A	33. D	41. C
2. D	10. D	18. A	26. D	34. A	42. B
3. C	11. B	19. B	27. B	35. B	43. A
4. D	12. A	20. D	28. C	36. D	
5. A	13. B	21. B	29. A	37. D	
6. A	14. B	22. D	30. B	38. D	
7. C	15. D	23. D	31. C	39. D	
8. A	16. A	24. D	32. D	40. A	

Chapter 9

1. A	9. B	17. B	25. C	33. B	41. A
2. D	10. D	18. A	26. D	34. C	42. D
3. C	11. D	19. D	27. A	35. D	43. D
4. B	12. A	20. A	28. D	36. C	44. C
5. C	13. D	21. B	29. B	37. B	45. B
6. C	14. B	22. D	30. D	38. B	46. B
7. D	15. A	23. C	31. A	39. C	
8. D	16. D	24. D	32. A	40. C	

Chapter 10

1. D	**7.** C	**13.** D	**19.** B	**25.** B	**31.** D
2. B	**8.** C	**14.** B	**20.** D	**26.** D	**32.** C
3. A	**9.** C	**15.** C	**21.** B	**27.** D	**33.** B
4. C	**10.** D	**16.** B	**22.** B	**28.** C	**34.** C
5. B	**11.** C	**17.** A	**23.** B	**29.** D	**35.** C
6. C	**12.** B	**18.** B	**24.** D	**30.** D	

Glossary

A

Aberrant Deviating from the usual or natural type; atypical.

Abreaction Wedge-shaped area that typically occurs on the cervicofacial areas of teeth.

Abrasion The pathologic wearing away of tooth structure that results from repetitive mechanical habit.

Abscess Collection of pus that has accumulated in a cavity formed in the tissue.

Acantholysis Dissolution of the intercellular bridges of the prickle cell layer of the epithelium.

Acantholytic cells Cells detached from the epithelium that appear rounded. This process is caused by a loss of attachment between the epithelial cells. These cells are present with pemphigus vulgaris. Also known as *Tzanck cells.*

Acanthosis nigricans A skin condition characterized by hyperpigmented, velvety-textured plaques that appear symmetrically distributed in folds and creases of the body. It has been reported to be associated with type 2 diabetes mellitus and has been used as a clinical indicator when screening for it.

Acquired immune response A response by the body generated by the memory of past exposure to a foreign substance; this response is quicker than the initial immune response.

Acquired immunodeficiency syndrome A syndrome involving a defect in cell-mediated immunity that has a long incubation period, follows a protracted and debilitating course, manifests as opportunistic infections, and has a poor prognosis without treatment. It is caused by the retrovirus human immunodeficiency virus.

Acromegaly A condition caused by hyperfunction of the pituitary gland in adults.

Actinic Relating to or exhibiting chemical changes produced by radiant energy, especially the visible and ultraviolet parts of the spectrum; relating to exposure to the ultraviolet rays of sunlight.

Actinic cheilitis Degeneration of the tissue of the lips caused by sun exposure. Also called *solar cheilitis.*

Actinomycosis An infection caused by a filamentous bacterium called *Actinomyces israelii.* The most characteristic manifestation of the disease is the formation of abscesses that drain through fistulas.

Active immunity Immunity acquired naturally or artificially. It occurs naturally when a microorganism infects a person, causing disease to which immunity is then developed. It occurs artificially when a person is injected with or ingests either altered pathogenic microorganisms or products of those microorganisms.

Acute Of short duration or of short and relatively severe course.

Acute inflammation The initial phase of inflammation that is of short duration, lasting only a few days.

Acute lymphonodular pharyngitis An infectious disease caused by the coxsackievirus. It is characterized by fever, sore throat, and mild headache. Hyperplastic lymphoid tissue of the soft palate or tonsillar pillars appears as yellowish or dark pink nodules.

Acute necrotizing ulcerative gingivitis (ANUG) A painful erythematous gingivitis with necrosis and cratering of the interdental papillae. Presently called *necrotizing ulcerative gingivitis (NUG)* because it is not an acute condition.

Acute osteomyelitis An acute inflammation of the bone and bone marrow. Acute osteomyelitis of the jaws is most commonly a result of the extension of a periapical abscess. Other potential causes include fracture of the bone, surgery, and bacteremia.

Addison disease A condition characterized by insufficient production of adrenal steroids. Also known as *primary adrenal cortical insufficiency.*

Adenocarcinoma A nonspecific name for malignant tumors of glandular origin.

Adenoid cystic carcinoma A slow-growing malignant tumor of salivary gland origin that can originate from either the major or minor salivary gland tissue. It is unencapsulated and infiltrates surrounding tissue.

Adenoma A benign tumor that originates from glandular epithelium.

Adenomatoid Glandlike.

Adenomatoid odontogenic tumor An encapsulated, benign epithelial odontogenic tumor that has a distinctive age, sex, and site distribution. Seventy percent occur in females less than 20 years of age; 70% involve the anterior part of the jaws. May be associated with impacted teeth. Also known as an *odontogenic adenomatoid tumor.*

Adjuvants The agents that can be added to a vaccine to modify the immune response.

Agammaglobulinemia Lack of immunoglobulins.

Agranulocytosis A marked decrease in the number of granulocytes, particularly neutrophils.

Alleles Genes that are located at the same level or locus in the two chromosomes of a pair and that determine the same functions or characteristics.

Allergen Antigen producing a hypersensitivity or an allergic reaction.

Allergy A hypersensitive state acquired through exposure to a particular allergen. Reexposure to the same allergen elicits an exaggerated reaction.

Alveolar osteitis A postoperative complication of tooth extraction in which after extraction the blood clot breaks down and is lost before healing occurs. The socket appears empty, and the bone surface is exposed. Also known as *dry socket.*

Amalgam tattoo A flat, bluish-gray lesion of the oral mucosa resulting from the introduction of amalgam particles into the tissue.

Ameloblastic fibroma A nonencapsulated, benign odontogenic tumor of mixed tissue origin that is composed of strands and small islands of amelo-blast-like epithelial cells and mesenchymal cells that resemble the dental papilla. It occurs in young children and adults, and the most common location is the mandibular bicuspid and molar region. Most patients are asymptomatic, but bone expansion or swelling may be noted.

Ameloblastic fibro-odontoma A benign odontogenic tumor that has features of both an ameloblastic fibroma and an odontoma. It typically arises in the posterior jaws and is often asymptomatic.

Ameloblastoma A benign, slow-growing but locally aggressive epithelial odontogenic tumor that may arise in either the maxilla or the mandible. It is an unencapsulated tumor that infiltrates into surrounding tissue and can cause extensive destruction.

Amelogenesis The formation of enamel.

Amelogenesis imperfecta A broad group of conditions that affect the structural formation of enamel. The disease is divided into four main types: type I, hypoplastic; type II, hypocalcified; type III, hypomaturation; type IV, hypoplastic-hypomaturation.

Amenorrhea Abnormal temporary or permanent cessation of menstrual cycles.

Amino acid An organic compound containing the amino group NH_2. Amino acids are the main component of proteins.

Anaphylaxis A type of hypersensitivity or allergic reaction in which the exaggerated immunologic response results from the release of vasoactive substances such as histamine. The reaction occurs on reexposure to a foreign protein or other substance after sensitization.

Anaplastic A loss of differentiation of cells and their orientation to one another; a characteristic of malignant tumor tissue.

Anemia Reduction to less than the normal number of red blood cells, quantity of hemoglobin, or volume of packed red blood cells in the blood.

Aneuploid Any extra number of chromosomes that do not represent an exact multiple of the total chromosome complement (e.g., trisomy [a pair with an identical extra chromosome] and monosomy [a missing chromosome from a pair]).

Aneurysmal bone cyst A pseudocyst that consists of blood-filled spaces surrounded by multinucleated giant cells and fibrous connective tissue. The radiolucent lesion has a multilocular appearance that is often described as "honeycomb" or as "soap bubbles."

Angioedema A lesion that appears as a diffuse swelling of tissue caused by increased permeability of deeper blood vessels. The skin covering the swelling appears normal.

Angiogenesis The formation and differentiation of blood vessels.

Angular cheilitis Erythema or fissuring at the labial commissures. Angular cheilitis may be caused by factors such as nutritional deficiency; however, it most commonly results from *Candida* infection.

Ankyloglossia Extensive adhesion of the tongue to the floor of the mouth or the lingual aspect of the anterior portion of the mandible; caused by a short lingual frenum.

Ankylosed teeth Teeth in which bone has fused to cementum and dentin, preventing exfoliation of deciduous teeth and eruption of the underlying permanent tooth; ankylosed teeth typically appear submerged clinically.

Ankylosis Immobility of a joint because of fibrous or bony union between the articulating structures of the joint. Ankylosis can be classified by tissue type, location, and extent of fusion.

Anodontia Complete or almost complete congenital lack of teeth.

Anomaly Marked deviation from normal, especially as a result of a congenital or hereditary defect.

Anorexia nervosa An eating disorder characterized by a distorted perception of body image in addition to depression, intense fear of weight gain, and self-imposed starvation.

Anterior repositioning appliances Indicated for patients with temporomandibular joint dysfunction (TMJD) who have painful clicking or frequent locking; should be carefully monitored to prevent irreversible changes to occlusion.

Antibody A protein molecule, also called an *immunoglobulin,* which is produced by plasma cells and reacts with a specific antigen.

Antibody titer The specific level of an antibody in the blood. It can be measured by a laboratory test.

Antigen Any substance that is able to induce a specific immune response.

Antigenic determinate The portion of an antibody that recognizes and binds to the antigen.

Antigens Foreign substances against which the immune system defends the body.

Antinuclear antibody An antibody with an affinity for the cell nuclei.

Apertognathia Anterior open bite.

Aphthous ulcer Painful oral ulcers that frequently recur in episodes. There are three types of aphthous ulcers: minor, major, and herpetiform. Also known as *canker sore* or *aphthous stomatitis.*

Aplasia Lack of development.

Aplastic anemia A type of anemia in which patients experience a dramatic decrease in all the circulating blood cells (pancytopenia) because of a severe depression of bone marrow activity. Can be primary (cause unknown) or secondary (caused by a drug or chemical agent).

Arthralgia Severe pain in a joint.

Arthritis Inflammation of a joint. It is classified as either osteoarthritis or rheumatoid arthritis.

Arthrocentesis Surgical puncture of a joint, usually for the withdrawal of fluid, followed by lavage of the joint space.

Arthrography Radiography of a joint after injection of an opaque contrast material.

Arthroscopy A method for evaluating and manipulating a joint by the insertion of a camera and instruments.

Articular disk A pad of fibrocartilage or dense fibrous tissue present in some synovial joints (e.g., the temporomandibular joint).

Articulation A joint.

Aspirin burn A type of chemical injury that occurs when a patient places an aspirin tablet directly on mucosal tissue instead of swallowing it. The soft tissue becomes necrotic and appears white.

Atherosclerosis The process by which lipid accumulates within the walls of large and medium-sized arteries. It leads to reduced blood flow to and death of vital organs.

Atrophy The decrease in size and function of a cell, tissue, organ, or whole body.

Attenuate To reduce the severity of a disease or the virulence of a pathogenic agent, as is done in the development of certain vaccines.

Attrition The wearing away of tooth structure during mastication. Attrition occurs normally but may also be accelerated by teeth grinding.

Auscultation The act of listening to sounds within the body using a stethoscope.

Autoantibody An antibody that reacts against an antigenic constituent of the person's own tissues.

Autoimmune disease A disease characterized by tissue injury caused by a humoral or cell-mediated immune response against constituents of the body's own tissues.

Autoimmunity Immune-mediated destruction of the body's own cells and tissues; immunity against self.

Autosomal Related to nonsex chromosomes that are identical for males and females.

Autosomes (adjective, autosomal) The nonsex chromosomes that are identical for men and women.

Avascular Does not contain blood vessels.

B

B-cell lymphocyte A lymphocyte, also called a *B cell,* that matures without passing through the thymus and later can develop into a plasma cell that produces antibodies.

Barr body Condensed chromatin of the inactivated X chromosome, which is found at the periphery of the nucleus of cells in women.

Basal cell carcinoma A malignant skin tumor associated with excessive sun exposure that appears as a nonhealing ulcer with characteristic rolled borders. It does not occur in the oral cavity.

Behçet syndrome A chronic, recurrent, autoimmune disease consisting primarily of oral ulcers, genital ulcers, and ocular inflammation. The oral ulcers that appear are similar to aphthous ulcers.

Bell's palsy Acute, self-limiting loss of muscle control on one side of the face; also called *idiopathic facial paralysis* or *idiopathic facial nerve paralysis.*

Bence Jones proteins Fragments of immunoglobulins found in the urine of patients with multiple myeloma.

Benign A condition that, if untreated or treated symptomatically, will not become life threatening.

Benign cementoblastoma A cementum-producing tumor that is fused to the root or roots of a vital tooth. It typically occurs in young adults, and pain is a frequent symptom.

Benign cystic teratoma A lesion with a cystic component that resembles the dermoid cyst. In addition, teeth, bone, muscle, and nerve tissue may be found in the wall of this lesion.

Benign fibro-osseous lesion A benign lesion of bone characterized histologically by cellular fibrous connective tissue mixed with irregularly shaped bone trabeculae or cementoid material.

Benign mixed tumor The most common of the benign salivary gland tumors. Also known as a *pleomorphic adenoma.*

Benign mucous membrane pemphigoid A chronic autoimmune disease that affects the oral mucosa, conjunctiva, genital mucosa, and skin. It is also known as *mucous membrane pemphigoid* and *cicatricial pemphigoid.*

Benign tumor A tumor that is not malignant; favorable for treatment and recovery.

Biochemical mediators Chemicals in the body that activate responses.

Bleeding time A test that provides an assessment of the adequacy of platelet function. It measures how long it takes a standardized skin incision to stop bleeding by the formation of a temporary hemostatic plug or clot.

Botryoid odontogenic cyst When a lateral periodontal cyst is multilocular, it is called a *botryoid cyst;* microscopically, they are the same. A botryoid cyst has a greater potential for recurrence.

Brachydactyly Short fingers or toes or both.

Branchial arch One of a series of mesodermal bars located between the branchial clefts. During embryonic stages, the arch contributes to the formation of the face, jaws, and neck.

Brittle diabetes A term used to describe diabetes in patients who have blood glucose levels that are unstable or are not well controlled.

Brown tumor A lesion of bone identical to the central giant cell granuloma that occurs in patients with hyperparathyroidism.

Brush test A technique used to obtain information from oral mucosal epithelium. This technique uses a circular brush to obtain cells from the full thickness of the epithelium, including cells from the keratin layer through the basal layer.

Bruton disease A type of primary immunodeficiency in which B cells do not mature. Plasma cells are deficient throughout the body; T cells are normal. Also called *X-linked congenital agammaglobulinemia.*

Bruxism The habit of grinding and clenching of the teeth together for nonfunctional purposes.

Bulimia An eating disorder characterized by food binges, usually of high caloric intake, followed by self-induced vomiting. (Erosion is seen on the lingual aspects of maxillary anterior teeth.)

Bulla (adjective, *bullous;* plural, *bullae*) A circumscribed, elevated, fluid-filled lesion within or below the skin or mucous membranes that is greater than 5 mm in diameter and usually contains serous fluid.

Bullous lichen planus The type of lichen planus in which the epithelium separates from the connective tissue and erosions, bullae, or ulcers form.

Burning mouth disorder Disorder characterized by continuous burning sensation of the oral tissues; also called *stomatodynia.* Idiopathic or several local and systemic factors must be considered.

C

Café au lait Refers to a macular skin pigmentation that is the color of coffee with milk.

Café au lait spots Light-brown skin lesions.

Calcifying epithelial odontogenic tumor A benign epithelial odontogenic tumor in which the proliferating cells do not resemble odontogenic epithelium. The tumor is composed of islands and sheets of polyhedral (multisided) epithelial cells. It is also known as a *Pindborg tumor.*

Calcifying odontogenic cyst A nonaggressive cystic lesion lined by odontogenic epithelium with associated ghost cell keratinization.

Calcitonin A polypeptide secreted by the C cells of the thyroid gland.

Cancer Malignancy.

Candidal leukoplakia A type of candidiasis that appears as a white lesion that does not wipe off the mucosa. An important diagnostic feature of this type of candidiasis is that it responds to treatment with antifungal medication. Also called *chronic hyperplastic candidiasis* and *hypertrophic candidiasis.*

Candidiasis An overgrowth of the yeastlike fungus *Candida albicans.* It is the most common oral fungal infection. It can result from many different conditions, including antibiotic use, cancer, corticosteroid therapy, dentures, diabetes mellitus, and HIV infection. Also called *moniliasis* and *thrush*.

Capillary hemangioma A hemangioma that contains numerous small capillaries.

Capsulitis Inflammation; tenderness over the lateral pole of the condyle.

Carcinoma A malignant tumor of epithelial tissue origin.

Carcinoma arising in a pleomorphic adenoma Occurs when a pleomorphic adenoma undergoes malignant transformation.

Carrier In genetics, a heterozygous individual who is clinically normal but who can transmit a recessive trait or characteristic; also, a person who is homozygous for an autosomal-dominant condition with low penetrance.

Catabolism Component of metabolism that involves the breakdown of molecules with the concomitant release of energy.

Cavernous hemangioma A hemangioma containing large blood vessels.

Celiac disease A chronic disorder associated with sensitivity to dietary gluten, a protein found in wheat and wheat products. When gluten is ingested, injury to the intestinal mucosa results. Also called *celiac sprue* and *gluten-sensitive enteropathy*.

Cell-mediated immunity Immunity in which the predominant role is played by T lymphocytes.

Cementogenesis The formation of cementum.

Cementoma An apical lesion associated with the apices of teeth. It may present as a mass of fibrous connective tissue, fibrous connective tissue with spicules of cementum, or calcified mass resembling cementum and having few cellular elements. Also known as *periapical cemento-osseous dysplasia*.

Cemento-ossifying fibroma A tumor that has a mixture of globular calcifications resembling cementum and bone trabeculae that results from the potential of periodontal ligament cells to produce either cementum or bone.

Cementum Outermost layer of the root of the tooth.

Centimeter (cm) One hundredth of a meter. Equivalent to a little less than ½ inch (0.393 of an inch).

Central Occurring within the bone. In oral pathology, a lesion occurring within the maxilla or mandible.

Central cementifying fibroma A benign, well-circumscribed tumor classified as a fibro-osseous lesion. The calcifications are rounded and globular, resembling cementum. Affected patients may be asymptomatic or demonstrate bone expansion or facial asymmetry.

Central ossifying fibroma A benign, well-circumscribed tumor classified as a fibro-osseous lesion. The calcifications resemble bone trabeculae. Affected patients may be asymptomatic or demonstrate bone expansion or facial asymmetry.

Centromere The constricted portion of the chromosome that divides the short arms from the long arms.

Cervical lymphoepithelial cyst Located on the lateral neck at the anterior border of the sternocleidomastoid muscle. Also called *branchial cleft cyst*.

Chancre Lesion of the primary stage of syphilis. It is highly infectious and forms at the site at which the spirochete enters the body.

Chemotaxis The movement of white blood cells, directed by chemical mediators, to the area of injury.

Chemotherapy Cancer treatment that uses chemical agents to modify or destroy cancer cells.

Cherubism A disorder beginning in childhood characterized by progressive bilateral facial swelling that can occur in either the maxilla or mandible, with involvement of the mandible being most common. The swollen jaws and raised eyes give a "cherublike" appearance, and radiographs show multilocular radiolucent lesions.

Chiasmata The intercrossing of chromatids of the same or homologous chromosomes that takes place at metaphase of first meiosis for the purpose of genetic recombination.

Chickenpox A highly contagious disease caused by the varicella-zoster virus. It is characterized by vesicular and pustular eruptions of the skin and/or mucous membranes, along with systemic symptoms such as headache, fever, and malaise. It usually occurs in children.

Chondroma A benign tumor of cartilage.

Chondrosarcoma A malignant tumor of cartilage that can occur in either the maxilla or mandible.

Chromatid Either of the two vertical halves of a chromosome that are joined at the centromere.

Chromatin A general term used to refer to the material (DNA) that forms the chromosomes.

Chromosomes The small bodies in the nucleus of a cell that carry the chemical instructions for reproduction of the cell in addition to other cellular functions.

Chronic Persisting over a long time.

Chronic apical periodontitis A localized mass of chronically inflamed granulation tissue that forms at the opening of the pulp canal generally at the apex of a nonvital tooth. Also called *periapical granuloma* and *dental granuloma*.

Chronic atrophic candidiasis The most common type of candidiasis affecting the oral mucosa. This type of candidiasis presents as erythematous mucosa, but the erythematous change is limited to mucosa that is covered by a full or partial denture. Also called *denture stomatitis*.

Chronic hyperplastic candidiasis A type of candidiasis that appears as a white lesion that does not wipe off the mucosa. An important diagnostic feature of this type of candidiasis is that it responds to treatment with antifungal medication. Also called *candidal leukoplakia* and *hypertrophic candidiasis*.

Chronic hyperplastic pulpitis An excessive proliferation of chronically inflamed dental pulp tissue within the crown of a carious tooth. Also called *pulp polyp*.

Chronic inflammation Inflammation that may last weeks, months, or indefinitely.

Chronic mucocutaneous candidiasis A severe form of candidiasis that usually occurs in patients who are severely immunocompromised. Oral involvement may appear as pseudomembranous, erythematous, or hyperplastic candidiasis.

Chronic neutropenia A type of neutropenia in which the intraoral manifestations are similar to those of cyclic neutropenia but are constant. Also known as *Kostmann syndrome*.

Chronic osteomyelitis A long-standing inflammation of bone.

Chronic sclerosing osteomyelitis A condition that is characterized by an inflamed bone that has developed dense calcifications.

Cicatricial pemphigoid A chronic autoimmune disease that affects the oral mucosa, conjunctiva, genital mucosa, and skin. It is also known as *mucous membrane pemphigoid* and *benign mucous membrane pemphigoid*.

Cleft lip Congenital anomaly of the face caused by the failure of fusion between the embryonic maxillary and medial nasal processes.

Cleft palate Congenital anomaly of the oral cavity caused by the failure of fusion between the embryonic palatal shelves.

Cleidocranial dysplasia An inherited disease or congenital disorder characterized by slow or failed formation of the clavicles; delayed closure of the sutures and fontanels of the skull; and delayed eruption of teeth, with formation of supernumerary teeth. Characterized by underdevelopment of the maxillae, agenesis or aplasia of the clavicle, abnormalities in other skeletal bones and muscles, and irregularities of the dentition.

Clotting factors A cascade of circulating plasma proteins (made almost exclusively in the liver) that are necessary to convert precursor fibrinogen to fibrin. Also called *coagulation factors*.

Coagulation Formation of a clot.

Coagulation factors A cascade of circulating plasma proteins (made almost exclusively in the liver) that are necessary to convert precursor fibrinogen to fibrin. Also called *clotting factors*.

Coalescence The process by which parts of a whole join together, or fuse, to make one.

Codominance The full expression in a heterozygote of both alleles of a pair of chromosomes, with neither influenced by the other. A good example is the AB blood group.

Codon The sequence of three bases in DNA that encodes one amino acid.

Cold sore The most common type of recurrent oral herpes simplex infection that occurs on the vermilion border of the lips. Also called *herpes labialis* or *fever blister*.

Coloboma A cleft generally seen on the iris or the eyelids.

Colors Red, pink, salmon, white, blue-black, gray, brown, and black are the words used most frequently to describe the colors of oral lesions; they can be used to identify the specific lesions and may also be incorporated into general descriptions.

Commissural lip pits Epithelium-lined blind tracts located at the corners of the mouth. This is a relatively common developmental anomaly.

Commissure The site of union of corresponding parts (e.g., the corners of the lips).

Complete blood count A series of tests that examines the red blood cells, white blood cells, and platelets.

Complex odontoma An odontogenic tumor that radiographically consists of a mass of enamel, dentin, cementum, and pulp, which does not resemble a normal tooth. It commonly occurs in the posterior mandible.

Compound odontoma An odontogenic tumor that consists of a collection of numerous small teeth. They do not exhibit unlimited growth potential and therefore are more accurately classified as developmental lesions rather than true tumors. They are usually located in the anterior maxilla.

Concrescence A condition in dentistry in which two adjacent teeth are united by cementum.

Condensing osteitis A change in bone near the apices of teeth seen as a radiopacity; thought to be a reaction to low-grade infection.

Condyloma acuminatum A benign papillary lesion caused by human papilloma virus. Oral condylomas appear as papillary bulbous masses and can occur anywhere in the oral mucosa. They are considered a sexually transmitted disease.

Congenital Present at and existing from the time of birth.

Congenital disorder A disorder that is present at birth. It can be either inherited or developmental.

Congenital epulis A benign neoplasm composed of cells that closely resemble those seen in a granular cell tumor. The neoplasm most likely arises from a primitive mesenchymal cell. This tumor is present at birth and appears as a sessile or pedunculated mass on the gingiva and is seen predominantly in girls. Also known as *congenital epulis of the newborn*.

Congenital lip pit Congenital depression on the vermilion portion of the lower lip that may appear either unilaterally or bilaterally.

Congenital syphilis The type of syphilis that is transmitted from an infected mother to the fetus because the organism can cross the placenta and enter the fetal circulation.

Connective tissue disease Disease in which the body's recognition mechanism breaks down and certain body cells are no longer tolerated. The immune system treats body cells as antigens. Some conditions can also be known as *autoimmune diseases*.

Consanguinity Blood relationship. In genetics, the term is generally used to describe matings or marriages among close relatives.

Contact dermatitis Lesions resulting from the direct contact of an allergen with the skin.

Contact mucositis Lesions resulting from the direct contact of an allergen with the mucosa.

Cooley anemia The name of a group of inherited disorders of hemoglobin. Also called *thalassemia*.

Corrugated Having a surface that appears wrinkled.

Coxsackieviruses A group of viruses named for the town in New York where they were first discovered. Coxsackieviruses cause several different infectious diseases. Three of these diseases have distinctive oral lesions: herpangina, hand-foot-and-mouth disease, and acute lymphonodular pharyngitis.

C-reactive protein (CRP) A protein produced in the liver that becomes elevated during episodes of acute inflammation or infection.

Crepitus A dry, crackling sound.

Cretinism The presence of hypothyroidism during infancy and childhood.

Crossing over The exchange of segments between chromatids of the same or homologous chromosomes that takes place at metaphase of first meiosis. Crossing over results from the formation of chiasmata.

Cyclic neutropenia A hereditary disease characterized by a cyclic decrease in the number of circulating neutrophils. The cycles occur in intervals of 21 to 27 days, and the episodes of neutropenia persist for 2 to 3 days.

Cylindroma Another name for adenoid cystic carcinoma; so-called because of its microscopic appearance, which shows round and oval islands that represent cylinders of tumor.

Cyst An abnormal pathologic sac or cavity that is lined with epithelium and enclosed in a connective tissue capsule.

Cyst of the palatine papilla A cyst found in the incisive papilla.

Cytokines Chemical mediators produced by cells involved in the immune response.

Cytolysis The dissolution or destruction of a cell.

D

Dark-field microscopy Examination of a specimen by microscopy, in which illumination causes the specimen to appear to glow against a dark background. Used to identify the syphilis spirochete.

Delayed hypersensitivity The type of hypersensitivity in which there is a latent period between the antigen introduction and the reaction. Cellular reactions are mediated by T lymphocytes. It can be used to test for tuberculosis and is responsible for rejection of tissue grafts and transplanted organs.

Deletion In genetics, the loss of part of a chromosome.

Demastication When tooth wear is increased by chewing an abrasive substance.

Dendritic cell A type of white blood cell that acts as an antigen-presenting cell in the skin and mucosa.

Dens evaginatus An accessory enamel cusp found on the occlusal tooth surface. This developmental anomaly occurs most often on the mandibular premolars.

Dens in dente "A tooth within a tooth"; a developmental anomaly that results when the enamel organ invaginates into the crown of a tooth before mineralization. It is most commonly seen in the maxillary lateral incisor. Also called *dens invaginatus*.

Dens invaginatus "A tooth within a tooth"; a developmental anomaly that results when the enamel organ invaginates into the crown of a tooth before mineralization. Also called *dens in dente*.

Dental fluorosis A condition resulting from the ingestion of high concentrations of fluoride, causing the affected teeth to have a mottled discoloration of the enamel.

Dental granuloma A localized mass of chronically inflamed granulation tissue that forms at the opening of the pulp canal generally at the apex of a nonvital tooth. Also known as *periapical granuloma* and *chronic apical periodontitis*.

Dental papilla The mesenchymal tissue within a tooth germ. After dentin is produced, the dental papilla is called the *dental pulp*.

Dentigerous cyst A cyst that forms around the crown of an unerupted or developing tooth. Also called a *follicular cyst*.

Dentin Body of the tooth. It surrounds the pulp and underlies the enamel on the crown and the cementum on the root of teeth.

Dentin dysplasia A genetic disturbance of the dentin characterized by early calcification of the pulp chambers and root canals and root resorption. It is subdivided into radicular dentin dysplasia and coronal dentin dysplasia.

Dentinogenesis The formation of dentin.

Dentinogenesis imperfecta A disturbance of the dentin of genetic origin; characterized by early calcification of the pulp chambers and root canals, marked attrition, and an opalescent hue to the teeth. It is hereditary and associated with osteogenesis imperfecta, or it may occur in isolation.

Denture-associated inflammatory hyperplasia A lesion caused by an ill-fitting denture and generally located in the vestibule along the denture flange. Also called *denture-induced fibrous hyperplasia* and *epulis fissuratum*.

Denture-induced fibrous hyperplasia A lesion caused by an ill-fitting denture. It is located in the vestibule adjacent to the denture border. It is composed of dense fibrous connective tissue surfaced by stratified squamous epithelium. Commonly called *epulis fissuratum* or *inflammatory hyperplasia*.

Denture stomatitis The most common type of candidiasis affecting the oral mucosa. This type of candidiasis presents as erythematous mucosa, but the erythematous change is limited to the mucosa covered by a full or partial denture. Also called *chronic atrophic candidiasis*.

Deoxyribonucleic acid (DNA) A substance composed of a double chain of polynucleotides; both chains, coiled around a central axis, form a double helix. DNA is the basic genetic code or template for polypeptide formation.

Dermoid cyst A developmental cyst that is often present at birth or noted in young children. It is uncommon in the head and neck, but occurs in the anterior floor of the mouth. It is lined by orthokeratinized, stratified squamous epithelium surrounded by a connective tissue wall. The lumen is usually filled with keratin.

Desquamative gingivitis A clinical and descriptive term for gingival lesions that may be seen in lichen planus, pemphigus vulgaris, and mucous membrane pemphigoid. The gingival margin is ulcerated or eroded and shows loss of normal stippling.

Development The process by which an individual reaches maturity.

Developmental anomalies A failure or disturbance that occurs during the process of prenatal development that may result in a lack, excess, or deformity of a body part. Also known as *developmental disorder*.

Developmental disorder A failure or disturbance that occurs during the process of prenatal development that can result in a lack, excess, or deformity of a body part. Also called *developmental anomaly*.

Diabetes mellitus A chronic disorder of carbohydrate (glucose) metabolism that is characterized by abnormally high blood glucose levels (hyperglycemia). This is caused by a lack of the hormone insulin, defective insulin that does not work properly, or increased insulin resistance.

Differentiation The distinguishing of one thing from another.

Diffuse In the description of a lesion, the borders of the lesion are not well defined, and it is not possible to detect the exact parameters of the lesion.

DiGeorge syndrome A type of primary immunodeficiency in which the thymus is deficient or lacking; therefore T lymphocytes do not mature. Also called *thymic hypoplasia*.

Dilaceration An abnormal bend or curve in the root of a tooth.

Diploid Having two sets of chromosomes; the normal constitution of somatic cells.

Disk displacements Problems in which the disk of the temporomandibular joint (meniscus) is displaced.

Disk derangement Disk (meniscal) displacements, ankylosis, and hypermobility disorders related to the temporomandibular joint.

Dislocation Referring to the mandible, when one or both of the condyles translates anterior to the articular eminence, resulting in an open lock that the patient cannot reduce.

Disorder Derangement of function.

Distomolar A maxillary fourth molar; the second most common supernumerary tooth.

Dominant In genetics, a trait or characteristic that is manifested when it is carried by only one of a pair of homologous chromosomes.

Double helix The coiled structure of double-stranded DNA in which strands linked by hydrogen bonds form a spiral configuration.

Douloureux From the French meaning *painful tic or twitch*.

Down syndrome A type of abnormality in which three of chromosome 21 are found instead of two. This results in abnormal physical characteristics and mental impairment. Also called *trisomy 21*.

Dry socket A postoperative complication of tooth extraction. After extraction, the blood clot breaks down and is lost before healing occurs. The socket appears empty, and the bone surface is exposed. Also known as *alveolar osteitis*.

Duplication A chromosome that is larger than normal; the extra segment is identical to a segment of the normal chromosome.

Dysgeusia An alteration in taste.

Dysphasia Speech disorder that involves impaired ability to speak or communicate using language.

Dysphonia Impaired ability to speak or use phonation; also called *hoarse voice.*

Dysplasia Disordered growth; alteration in size, shape, and organization of adult cells or structures.

Dyspnea Difficult, labored, or gasping breathing (shortness of breath).

E

Ecchymosis A small, flat, hemorrhagic patch larger than a petechia on the skin or mucous membrane.

Ectopic geographic tongue A term used to described the condition of geographic tongue when it is found on mucosal surfaces other than the tongue.

Ectopic lingual thyroid nodule A mass of thyroid tissue located on the tongue, distant from the normal anatomic location of the thyroid gland. It is an uncommon developmental anomaly that results from the failure of the primitive thyroid tissue to migrate from its developmental location in the area of the foramen cecum on the posterior portion of the tongue to its normal position in the neck. Also called *lingual thyroid.*

Edema Excess plasma or exudate in the interstitial space of the tissues that causes swelling.

Ellis–Van Creveld syndrome A syndrome characterized by dwarfism, polydactyly, and possible retardation and congenital heart defects. Oral manifestations include fusion of the anterior portion of the maxillary gingiva to the upper lip from canine to canine. Most teeth have a conical shape and exhibit enamel hypoplasia.

Embedded teeth Teeth that do not erupt because of a lack of eruptive force.

Emigration The passage of white blood cells through the endothelium and wall of the microcirculation into an area of injured tissue.

Enamel Hard outer layer of the crown of a tooth.

Enamel hypocalcification A developmental anomaly that results in a disturbance of the maturation of the enamel matrix. It usually appears as a localized, chalky white spot on the middle third of smooth crowns, and the underlying enamel may be soft and susceptible to caries.

Enamel hypoplasia The incomplete or defective formation of enamel, resulting in the alteration of tooth form or color.

Enamel pearl A small, spherical enamel projection located on a root surface. Also called an *enameloma.*

Enameloma A small, spherical enamel projection located on a root surface. Also called an *enamel pearl.*

Encapsulated Surrounded by a capsule of fibrous connective tissue.

Endogenous Originating or produced within an organism or one of its parts.

Enucleation Surgical removal without cutting into the lesion; involves "scooping" out of a lesion along its peripheral borders.

Enzyme-linked immunosorbent assay (ELISA) A serologic laboratory procedure used to identify circulating antibodies. It is routinely used in HIV testing.

Eosinophilic granuloma of bone A solitary or chronic localized form of Langerhans cell disease. This form primarily affects older children and young adults. The skull and mandible are commonly involved with eosinophilic granuloma. The radiographic appearance varies, and the lesion may resemble periodontal disease or periapical inflammatory disease; or it may appear as a well-circumscribed radiolucency with or without a sclerotic border.

Epidemic parotitis A viral infection of the salivary glands caused by a paramyxovirus. The disease most commonly occurs in children and is characterized by painful swelling of the salivary glands, most commonly bilateral swelling of the parotid glands. Also called *mumps.*

Epidermal cyst A raised nodule in the skin. It is lined by keratinizing epithelium that resembles the epithelium of skin (epidermis). The cyst lumen is usually filled with keratin scales.

Epidermoid carcinoma A malignant tumor of the squamous epithelium. It is the most common primary malignancy of the oral cavity and, like other malignant tumors, can infiltrate adjacent tissues and metastasize to distant sites. Also known as *squamous cell carcinoma.*

Epidermoid cells Squamouslike epithelial cells.

Epilepsy A group of neurologic disorders characterized by recurrent episodes of convulsive seizures, sensory disturbances, abnormal behavior, and loss of consciousness.

Epistaxis Nosebleed.

Epithelial Pertaining to the epithelium.

Epithelialization The process of being covered with epithelium.

Epithelial dysplasia A histologic diagnosis that indicates disordered growth. It is considered a premalignant condition.

Epithelial tumor A tumor that develops from the epithelium. There are three types: (1) tumors derived from squamous epithelium, (2) tumors derived from glandular epithelium, and (3) tumors derived from odontogenic epithelium.

Epithelium The layer of cells that lines a body cavity.

Epstein-Barr virus A herpesvirus associated with several diseases that occur in the oral region, including infectious mononucleosis, nasopharyngeal carcinoma, Burkitt lymphoma, and hairy leukoplakia.

Epulis fissuratum A lesion caused by an ill-fitting denture located in the vestibule along the dental border. Also called *redundant tissue* and *denture-induced fibrous hyperplasia.*

Erosion The loss of tooth structure resulting from chemical action.

Erosive lichen planus The type of lichen planus in which the epithelium separates from the connective tissue and erosions or ulcers form.

Eruption cyst A cyst that forms in the soft tissue around the crown of an erupting tooth.

Erythema An abnormal redness of the skin or mucosa.

Erythema migrans See *geographic tongue.*

Erythema multiforme An acute, self-limited disease that affects the skin and mucous membranes. The cause is not clear, but some evidence exists that it is a hypersensitivity reaction.

Erythematous candidiasis A type of candidiasis characterized by an erythematous, often painful, mucosa. It may be localized to one area of the oral mucosa or be more generalized.

Erythroplakia A clinical term that is used to describe an oral mucosal lesion that appears as a smooth red patch or a granular red and velvety patch.

Euploid A cell or organism that has an integral multiple of the monoploid number of chromosomes.

Excision Surgical removal.

Exophthalmos Bulging eyes; an abnormal protrusion (bulging) of one or both eyeballs.

Exostosis (plural, *exostoses*) A small nodular excrescence of normal compact bone. Exostoses present as asymptomatic, bony, hard nodules on the buccal aspect of the maxillary or mandibular alveolar ridges.

Expressivity In genetics, the degree of clinical manifestation of a trait or characteristic.

External tooth resorption Resorption of a tooth structure beginning at the outside of the tooth. It usually involves the root of the tooth but may involve the crown of an impacted tooth.

Extramedullary plasmacytoma A localized tumor of plasma cells located in soft tissue.

Extraosseous cyst A cyst that occurs in the soft tissue.

Exudate Inflammatory fluid formed as a reaction to injury of tissues and blood vessels.

F

Facial hemihypertrophy Localized enlargement affecting one side of the orofacial structures.

Facies The appearance of the face.

Factor IX A factor that is active in the formation of intrinsic blood thromboplastin. A deficiency results in Christmas disease (hemophilia B), which is caused by a decrease in the amount of thromboplastin formed. Also called *plasma thromboplastin.*

Familial In genetics, something that affects more members of a family than would be expected by chance.

Fever An elevation of body temperature to greater than normal (98.6° F, or 37° C).

Fever blister The most common type of recurrent oral herpes simplex infection that occurs on the vermilion border of the lips. Also called *cold sore* or *herpes labialis.*

Fibrin An insoluble protein that is essential to the clotting of blood.

Fibroblasts The cells that form fibers as well as intercellular substance.

Fibroma A broad-based, persistent exophytic benign lesion composed of dense, scarlike connective tissue containing few blood vessels. It occurs as a result of chronic trauma or an episode of trauma. It is also known as an *irritation fibroma* or *traumatic fibroma.*

Fibroplasia The formation of fibrous tissue, as normally occurs in healing.

Fibrous dysplasia A benign fibro-osseous lesion composed of vascularized, cellular fibrous connective tissue interspersed with irregular trabeculae of bone emerging from the connective tissue. It is characterized by the replacement of bone with abnormal fibrous connective tissue interspersed with varying amounts of calcification.

First meiosis Step one to reduce and then maintain the normal number of human chromosomes. The new embryo must have 46 chromosomes per cell, as did its parents.

Fissure A cleft or groove, normal or otherwise, showing prominent depth.

Fissured Having surface clefting or grooves.

Fissured tongue Characterized by the dorsal surface of the tongue having deep fissures or grooves.

Fistula Formation of a drainage passage that bores through tissue, allowing drainage to the outside. It is formed at the expense of healthy, functioning tissue as the area that is lost becomes necrotic.

Fixed drug eruption A lesion that recurs at the same site with each exposure to a particular drug.

Flare Redness of the skin or mucosa around the area of exposure to an irritant.

Florid cemento-osseous dysplasia A fibro-osseous lesion characterized by disordered cementum and bone development. This lesion characteristically involves multiple quadrants in the maxilla and mandible. It is most common in middle-aged black women.

Focal cemento-osseous dysplasia An asymptomatic fibro-osseous lesion that typically arises in the posterior mandible. A characteristic feature is that it is composed of numerous gritty pieces of soft and hard tissue.

Focal epithelial hyperplasia A disease caused by a human papilloma virus (HPV) that is characterized by the presence of multiple whitish–to–pale-pink nodules distributed throughout the oral mucosa. Also known as *Heck disease.*

Focal palmplantar and gingival hyperkeratosis A syndrome characterized by areas of hyperkeratinization of the palms and soles and marked hyperkeratinization of the labial and lingual gingiva.

Folic acid A member of the vitamin B complex necessary for the normal production of red blood cells.

Follicular cyst A cyst that forms around the crown of an unerupted or developing tooth. Also called a *dentigerous cyst.*

Fordyce granules Clusters of ectopic sebaceous glands. They are most commonly seen on the lips and buccal mucosa. They are considered a variant of normal.

Frenectomy Surgical removal of a portion of the lingual frenum.

Frontal process Covering of the brain from which the forehead and other facial structures develop; located just above the stomodeum.

Fusion The union of two adjoining tooth germs.

G

Gamete Spermatozoon or ovum.

Gap 1 (G₁) phase The phase the cell enters after each cell division is completed and before the next division can occur.

Gap 2 (G₂) phase The phase that follows the S phase; it ends when mitotic division begins.

Gardner syndrome An inherited syndrome characterized by the presence of osteomas in various bones, especially in the frontal bones, mandible, and maxilla. Osteomas of the facial skeleton expand, obliterate the sinuses, and cause facial asymmetry. Intestinal polyps are also present, which become malignant after age 30 years. Also known as *familial colorectal polyposis.*

Gastrectomy Surgical removal of all or part of the stomach.

Gemination "Twinning"; when a single tooth germ attempts to divide, resulting in the incomplete formation of two teeth; the tooth usually has a single root and root canal.

Genes The hereditary units that are transmitted from one generation to another.

Genetic heterogeneity Having more than one inheritance pattern.

Geographic tongue A condition characterized by diffuse areas devoid of filiform papillae that develop on the dorsal and lateral borders of the tongue. These areas appear as erythematous patches surrounded by a white or yellow perimeter. The fungiform papillae are distinct within the erythematous patch.

Ghost cells Characteristic of a calcifying odontogenic cyst; exhibits a clear central area; thought to represent degenerating epithelial cells.

Ghost teeth A developmental anomaly in which one or several teeth in the same quadrant radiographically exhibit a marked reduction in radiodensity and a characteristic ghostlike appearance. Very thin enamel and dentin are present. Also called *regional odontodysplasia.*

Giant cell granuloma A lesion that contains many multinucleated giant cells and well-vascularized connective tissue. It occurs only in the jaws.

Gigantism Excessive growth caused by hyperpituitarism resulting in a stature larger than the range that is normal for age and race.

Gingival cyst A small bulge or swelling of the attached gingiva or interdental papillae. It exhibits the same type of epithelial lining as a lateral periodontal cyst and is located in the soft tissue of the same area.

Gingival fibromatosis An enlargement of the gingiva that results from the marked collagenization of the fibrous connective tissue. It is a component of many different inherited syndromes, is caused by certain drugs, or is idiopathic.

Gingival fibromatosis with hypertrichosis An inherited syndrome characterized by gingival fibromatosis and excessive growth of hair (hypertrichosis), especially of the eyebrows, extremities, genitals, and sacral region.

Gingival fibromatosis with multiple hyaline fibromas An inherited syndrome characterized by gingival fibromatosis; hypertrophy of the nail beds; and multiple hyaline fibrous tumors developing on the nose, chin, head, back, fingers, thighs, and legs. Also known as *Murray-Puretic-Drescher syndrome.*

Gingival hyperkeratosis A syndrome characterized by areas of hyperkeratinization of the palms and soles and marked hyperkeratinization of the labial and lingual gingiva.

Gingival hyperplasia Enlargement of the gingiva.

Globular process A pair of bulges formed from the median nasal process that grow downward, forming a portion of the upper lip.

Globulomaxillary cyst A cyst found between the roots of the maxillary lateral incisor and cuspid. It is characterized by well-defined, pear-shaped radiolucency and is believed to be of odontogenic epithelial origin. When it is large enough, divergence of the roots of adjacent teeth can result.

Gluten-sensitive enteropathy Hypersensitivity to gluten. Also called *celiac sprue* and *celiac disease.*

Granular cell tumor A benign tumor composed of large cells with a granular cytoplasm. It likely arises from a neural or primitive mesenchymal cell. It most often occurs on the tongue or buccal mucosa. The tumor appears as a painless, nonulcerated nodule.

Granulation tissue The initial tissue formed in the connective tissue portion of the injury. It is immature tissue with many capillaries and fibroblasts.

Granuloma A tumorlike mass of inflammatory tissue consisting of a central collection of macrophages, often with multinucleated giant cells, surrounded by lymphocytes.

Granulomatous disease A disease characterized by the formation of granulomas.

Granulomatous inflammation A distinctive form of chronic inflammation characterized by the formation of granulomas, which are collections of epithelioid histiocytes surrounded by a rim of lymphocytes.

Gumma A localized, noninfectious, destructive lesion that occurs during the tertiary stage of syphilis. The most common oral sites are the tongue and palate. The lesion appears as a firm mass that eventually becomes an ulcer.

H

Hairy leukoplakia An irregular, corrugated, white lesion that occurs almost exclusively on the lateral border of the tongue. Epstein-Barr virus has been identified in the epithelial cells of hairy leukoplakia and is considered to be the cause of the lesion.

Hairy tongue A condition in which the patient has elongated filiform papillae due to an increased accumulation of keratin. This results in either a light or dark "hairy" appearance.

Hand-foot-and-mouth disease An infectious disease caused by a coxsackievirus, characterized by painful vesicles and ulcers that can occur anywhere in the mouth. Multiple macules or papules occur on the skin, typically on the feet, toes, hands, and fingers. Usually occurs in epidemics in children less than 5 years of age.

Hand-Schüller-Christian disease A chronic disseminated or multifocal form of Langerhans cell disease. This form occurs in children, usually less than 5 years of age. All changes are caused by localized collections of Langerhans cells. The triad includes single to multiple well-defined or "punched-out" radiolucent areas in the skull (may also occur in the jawbones), unilateral or bilateral exophthalmos, and diabetes insipidus that is caused by collections of macrophages in the sella turcica area, affecting the pituitary gland.

Haploid A cell with a single set of chromosomes. A gamete is haploid.

Hemangioma A benign proliferation of capillaries. It is a common vascular lesion considered by many to represent a developmental lesion rather than a tumor. It may also occur in adults as a result of trauma.

Hematocrit The volume percentage of red blood cells in whole blood.

Hematoma A lesion that results from the accumulation of blood within tissue as a result of trauma.

Hemolysis The release of hemoglobin from red blood cells by destruction of the cells.

Hemophilia A disorder of blood coagulation that results in severely prolonged clotting time. The problem results from a deficiency of one of the plasma proteins involved in the coagulation cascade that is necessary for the conversion of fibrinogen to fibrin.

Hemostasis The stoppage or cessation of bleeding.

Hepatomegaly Enlargement of the liver.

Hereditary hemorrhagic telangiectasia A syndrome characterized by multiple capillary dilations of the skin and mucous membranes. The skin of the face shows numerous pinpoint and spiderlike telangiectasias, especially on the lips, eyelids, and around the nose. Telangiectasias of the oral mucosa are prominent on the tip and anterior dorsum of the tongue; the palate, gingiva, and buccal mucosa are often affected but to a lesser degree. Also known as *Osler–Rendu–Parkes Weber syndrome.*

Herpangina An infectious disease caused by a coxsackievirus, characterized by vesicles on the soft palate, along with fever, malaise, sore throat, and difficulty swallowing (dysphagia). An erythematous pharyngitis is also present.

Herpes labialis The most common type of recurrent oral herpes simplex infection that occurs on the vermilion border of the lips. Also called a *cold sore* or *fever blister.*

Herpes simplex Infections caused by herpesvirus types 1 and 2.

Herpes zoster A disease caused by the varicella-zoster virus that occurs in adults. It is characterized by a unilateral, painful eruption of vesicles along the distribution of a sensory nerve. Also called *shingles.*

Herpetic whitlow A painful infection of the fingers caused by the herpes simplex virus.

Herpetiform aphthous ulcer Tiny aphthous ulcers (1 to 2 mm) that resemble ulcers caused by the herpes simplex virus.

Hertwig epithelial root sheath An epithelial structure that proliferates to shape the root of the tooth and induce the formation of the root dentin.

Heterozygote (adjective, heterozygous) Individual with two different genes at the allele loci.

Highly active antiretroviral therapy (HAART) A combination of various types of antiretroviral (anti-HIV) drugs used in the management of HIV infection.

Hives Multiple areas of well-demarcated swelling of the skin, usually accompanied by itching. The lesions are caused by localized areas of vascular permeability in the superficial connective tissue beneath the epithelium. Also known as *urticaria*.

hnRNA Heterogenous nuclear RNA; the fourth type of RNA. It is found within the nucleus and is the precursor of mRNA.

Homozygote (adjective, homozygous) An individual having identical genes at the allele loci.

Hormone A chemical substance produced in the body that has a specific regulatory effect on certain cells or a certain organ or organs.

Human immunodeficiency virus (HIV) A retrovirus that causes acquired immunodeficiency syndrome (AIDS). It is transmitted through contact with an infected individual's blood, semen, cervical secretions, cerebrospinal fluid, or synovial fluid. It infects T-helper cells, dendritic cells, and macrophages of the immune system.

Human papilloma virus (HPV) A group of more than 150 related viruses. The papilloma viruses are attracted to and are able to live only in squamous epithelial cells. Low-risk types cause warts and papillomas. High-risk types are associated with malignant transformation of squamous cells.

Humoral immunity Immunity in which antibodies play the predominant role.

Hutchinson incisor Malformed incisor that results from the presence of congenital syphilis during tooth development. It is shaped like a screwdriver; broad cervically and narrow incisally, with a notched incisal edge.

Hyperacusia An increased sensitivity to normal environmental sound.

Hypercalcemia An excess of calcium in the blood.

Hypercementosis Excessive cementum on the roots of teeth.

Hyperchromic Staining more intensely than normal.

Hyperemia An excess of blood in a part of the body.

Hyperglycemia An excess of glucose in the blood.

Hypermobility An increase in the range of movement of a body part, especially a joint.

Hypermobility disorders Include **dislocation** and **subluxation**. See these terms elsewhere in this glossary.

Hyperparathyroidism A condition that results from excessive secretion of parathyroid hormone (parathormone or PTH), which is secreted by the parathyroid glands.

Hyperpituitarism Excess hormone production by the anterior pituitary gland.

Hyperplasia An abnormal increase in the number of normal cells in an organ or tissue.

Hypersensitivity A state of altered reactivity in which the body reacts to a foreign agent with an exaggerated immune response.

Hypertelorism A condition in which there is greater-than-normal distance between two paired organs. Orbital or ocular hypertelorism is a condition marked by a greater-than-normal distance between the eyes.

Hyperthermia Increased body temperature.

Hyperthyroidism A condition characterized by excessive production of thyroid hormone. Also called *thyrotoxicosis*.

Hypertrichosis The excessive growth of hair.

Hypertrophic candidiasis A type of candidiasis that appears as a white lesion that does not wipe off the mucosa. An important diagnostic feature of this type of candidiasis is that it responds to treatment with antifungal medication. Also called *chronic hyperplastic candidiasis* and *candidal leukoplakia*.

Hypertrophy An enlargement of a tissue or organ caused by an increase in size but not in the number of cells.

Hypochromic Staining less intensely than normal.

Hypodontia Partial anodontia. The lack of one or more teeth.

Hypoglycemia Low blood sugar.

Hypohidrosis Abnormally diminished secretion of sweat.

Hypohidrotic ectodermal dysplasia The most severe form of ectodermal dysplasia. Its major characteristics are hypodontia, hypotrichosis, and hypohidrosis.

Hyponatremia A deficiency of sodium in the blood.

Hypophosphatasia A syndrome characterized by a decrease in serum alkaline phosphatase levels with increased urinary and plasma levels of phosphoethanolamine. This can cause total or partial aplasia of the cementum, an abnormal periodontal ligament in the primary teeth, and a decreased phosphatase level that has been linked to premature loss of teeth.

Hypophosphatemia Deficiency of phosphates in the blood.

Hypophosphatemic vitamin D–resistant rickets A disorder characterized by low serum levels of phosphorus. This can be caused by low absorption of inorganic phosphate in the renal tubules, rickets, or osteomalacia. This condition demonstrates resistance to treatment with usual doses of vitamin D.

Hypoplasia The incomplete development of an organ or tissue.

Hypoplastic Underdeveloped.

Hyposalivation Decreased salivary flow.

Hypothyroidism A condition characterized by decreased output of thyroid hormone.

Hypotrichosis Presence of less than the normal amount of hair.

I

Iatrogenic Induced inadvertently by a medical/dental care provider or by medical treatment or a diagnostic procedure.

Icterus A condition characterized by an abnormal accumulation of bilirubin (red bile pigment) in the blood and manifested by a yellowish discoloration of the skin, mucous membranes, and cornea. Also called *jaundice*.

Idiopathic Relating to a disease or condition for which the cause is unknown.

Idiopathic leukoplakia A term used to emphasize that the specific cause of leukoplakia is unknown. See also **Leukoplakia**.

Idiopathic thrombocytopenic purpura A condition in which spontaneous bleeding occurs for an unknown reason.

Idiopathic tooth resorption Resorption that can involve the crown of an impacted tooth or roots of teeth. The cause cannot be identified.

Immune complex A combination of antibody and antigen.

Immunity The ability of an organism to resist or not be susceptible to injury or infection.

Immunization A process by which resistance to an infectious disease is induced. It lowers the risk of a microorganism causing disease because it prepares the immune system to fight future attacks by the disease-causing microorganism.

Immunodeficiency A deficiency of the immune response caused by hypoactivity or decreased numbers of lymphoid cells.

Immunoglobulin A protein, also called an *antibody*, synthesized by plasma cells in response to a specific antigen.

Immunologic tolerance The recognition and nonresponsiveness of the immune system to the body's own cells and tissues.

Immunomodulator A substance that alters the immune response by augmenting or reducing the ability of the immune system to produce antibodies or sensitized cells that recognize and react with the antigen that initiated their production.

Immunopathology The study of immune reactions involved in disease.

Impacted teeth Teeth that cannot erupt into the oral cavity because of a physical obstruction.

Impetigo A bacterial skin infection caused primarily by *Staphylococcus aureus* and occasionally by *Streptococcus pyogenes*. Impetigo most commonly involves lesions on the skin of the face or extremities.

Incisive canal cyst A developmental cyst located within the incisive canal or incisive papilla. It appears as a heart-shaped radiolucency. Also known as *nasopalatine canal cyst*.

Incubation period The period between the infection of an individual by a pathogen and the manifestation of the disease it causes.

Infectious mononucleosis An infectious disease caused by the Epstein-Barr virus. It is characterized by sore throat, fever, generalized lymphadenopathy, enlarged spleen, malaise, and fatigue. Palatal petechiae occur in infectious mononucleosis, usually appearing early in the course of the disease.

Inflammatory response (inflammation) A nonspecific response to injury that involves the microcirculation and its blood cells.

Inherited disorder A disorder caused by an abnormality in the genetic makeup (genes and chromosomes) of an individual that is transmitted from parent to offspring through the egg or sperm.

Injury Tissue damage caused by trauma or an alteration in the environment.

In situ Confined to the site of origin without invasion of neighboring tissues.

Insulin A peptide hormone produced in the pancreas by the beta cells in the islets of Langerhans. Insulin regulates glucose metabolism and is the major fuel-regulating hormone.

Insulin-dependent diabetes mellitus The type of diabetes that requires the administration of insulin to prevent ketosis. The onset is abrupt and may be characterized by polydipsia, polyuria, and polyphagia. Also called *type 1 diabetes*.

Insulin shock Profound hypoglycemia, or low blood sugar, that necessitates emergency intervention.

Interferon A family of glycoproteins that have immunoregulatory, antineoplastic, and antiviral activity; it is one of the cytokines.

Internal derangement Disk (meniscal) displacements, ankylosis, and hypermobility disorders related to the temporomandibular joint.

Internal tooth resorption Resorption usually involving a single tooth, often associated with an inflammatory response in the pulp. It can occur in any tooth.

International normalized ratio (INR) An expression of the ratio of prothrombin time (PT) to thromboplastin activity. It is a more accurate determination of PT.

Intraosseous cyst A cyst that occurs within bone.

Intrinsic Naturally occurring within; essential.

Intrinsic staining Tooth discoloration that occurs as a result of the deposition of substances circulating systemically during tooth development.

Invagination The infolding of one portion of a structure into another portion of the same structure.

Invasion The infiltration and active destruction of surrounding tissues.

Inversion In genetics, a portion of a chromosome arranged upside down.

Iron deficiency anemia A condition that occurs when an insufficient amount of iron is supplied to the bone marrow for red blood cell development.

Ischemia An inadequate blood supply to an organ or part of the body, especially the heart muscles.

J

Jaundice A condition characterized by an abnormal accumulation of bilirubin (bile pigment) in the blood and manifested by a yellowish discoloration of the skin, mucous membranes, and cornea. Also called *icterus*.

K

Kaposi sarcoma A malignant vascular tumor that may arise in multiple sites, including the skin and oral cavity. In HIV-positive patients, these lesions are often seen on the hard palate and gingiva, where they present as purple macules, plaques, or exophytic tumors.

Karyotype A photomicrographic representation of a person's chromosomal constitution arranged according to the Denver classification.

Keloid Excessive skin scarring that appears raised and extends beyond its original boundaries.

Keratin pearl Rounded concentric masses of epithelial cells and keratin found in some squamous cell carcinomas.

Keratoconjunctivitis sicca The eye damage that occurs in Sjögren syndrome caused by lack of tears.

Ketoacidosis A metabolic acidosis resulting from the accumulation of ketone bodies. It is most commonly a consequence of untreated type 1 diabetes mellitus.

Killed-type vaccines Vaccines that contain heat- or chemical-treated microorganisms; safe but may be less effective than attenuated vaccines.

Koplik spots Small erythematous macules with white necrotic centers seen intraorally in patients with measles.

L

Laband syndrome An inherited syndrome characterized by gingival fibromatosis, dysplastic or absent nails, malformed nose and ears, hepatosplenomegaly, and hypoplasia of terminal phalanges of the fingers and toes.

Labial melanotic macule A flat, well-circumscribed, brown lesion that occurs on the vermilion of the lip that darkens with exposure to sunlight.

Lack of penetrance The ability to carry a gene with a dominant effect without presenting any clinical manifestations.

Langerhans cell Specialized dendritic cell found in the skin and mucosa that is involved in the immune response.

Langerhans cell disease A disease formerly called *histiocytosis X*. Three entities traditionally grouped under the category of histiocytosis X are (1) Letterer-Siwe disease, (2) Hand-Schüller-Christian disease, and (3) solitary eosinophilic granuloma.

Langerhans cell histiocytosis See *Langerhans cell disease*.

Lateral nasal processes The processes that form the sides of the nose.

Lateral palatine processes The processes that develop from the maxillary tissues laterally and grow to the midline to form the palate.

Lateral periodontal cyst A cyst named for its location. It is most often seen in the mandibular cuspid and premolar area and presents as an asymptomatic, unilocular, or multilocular radiolucent lesion located on the lateral aspect of a tooth root. A thin band of stratified squamous epithelium that exhibits focal epithelial thickenings lines the cyst.

LE cell A cell that is a characteristic of lupus erythematosus and other autoimmune diseases. It is a mature neutrophil that has phagocytized a spherical inclusion derived from another neutrophil.

Leiomyoma A benign tumor of smooth muscle. When associated with blood vessels, it is called a *vascular leiomyoma*.

Letterer-Siwe disease An acute disseminated form of Langerhans cell disease that usually affects children younger than 3 years of age. The disease resembles a lymphoma in that it generally has a rapidly fatal course that sometimes responds to chemotherapy.

Leukemia A form of cancer characterized by an overproduction of atypical white blood cells. Can be acute or chronic.

Leukocyte See *white blood cell*.

Leukocytosis A temporary increase in the number of white blood cells circulating in the blood.

Leukoedema A condition that is a variant of normal and characterized by generalized opalescence of the buccal mucosa.

Leukopenia A decrease in white blood cells.

Leukoplakia A clinical term used to identify a white, plaquelike lesion of the oral mucosa that cannot be wiped off and cannot be diagnosed as any other disease on a clinical basis.

Lichen planus A benign, chronic disease affecting the skin and oral mucosa. The lesions have a characteristic pattern of interconnecting lines called *Wickham striae*.

Linea alba A white raised line that forms commonly on the buccal mucosa at the occlusal plane and is usually considered a variant of normal.

Linear gingival erythema A type of gingival disease that develops in patients with HIV infection. It has three characteristic features: (1) spontaneous bleeding, (2) punctate or petechia-like lesions on the attached gingiva and alveolar mucosa, and (3) a bandlike erythema of the gingiva that does not respond to therapy.

Lingual mandibular bone concavity A well-defined cystlike radiolucency in the posterior region of the mandible inferior to the mandibular canal that is caused by a lingual depression in the mandible, which contains normal salivary gland tissue. Also known as a *static bone cyst* or *Stafne bone cyst*. Often referred to as a *pseudocyst* because it is not a pathologic cavity and is not lined with epithelium.

Lingual thyroid Mass of thyroid tissue found on the dorsal tongue posterior to circumvallate papillae.

Lingual thyroid nodule A mass of thyroid tissue located on the tongue away from the normal anatomic location of the thyroid gland. It is an uncommon developmental anomaly that results from the failure of the primitive thyroid tissue to migrate from its developmental location in the area of the foramen cecum on the posterior portion of the tongue to its normal position in the neck. Also called *ectopic lingual thyroid nodule*.

Lingual varicosities Prominent lingual veins usually observed on the ventral and lateral surfaces of the tongue.

Lipoma A benign tumor of fat.

Lobule (adjective, lobulated) A segment or lobe that is part of a whole. Lobules sometimes appear fused together.

Local Confined to a limited part; not general or systemic.

Locus In genetics the position occupied by a gene on a chromosome.

Lymphadenopathy Any disease process that affects lymph nodes such that they become enlarged and palpable.

Lymphangioma A benign tumor of lymphatic vessels. The most common intraoral location is the tongue, where a lymphangioma presents as an ill-defined mass with a pebbly surface.

Lymphocytes The white blood cells involved in the immune response that have three major subsets: the B-cell lymphocyte, T-cell lymphocyte, and natural killer cell.

Lymphoepithelial cyst A cyst that is composed of a stratified squamous epithelial lining surrounded by a well-circumscribed component of lymphoid tissue. Also known as a *branchial cleft cyst* when located in the neck. The lymphoepithelial cyst occurs in the parotid gland and oral mucosa.

Lymphoid tissue Tissue composed of lymphocytes supported by a meshwork of connective tissue.

Lymphokines Cytokines produced by B-cell or T-cell lymphocytes in contact with antigens; mediators in an immune response.

Lymphoma A malignant tumor of lymphoid tissue.

Lyon hypothesis The hypothesis postulated by Mary Lyon that during the early period of embryonic development the genetic activity of one of the X chromosomes in each cell of a female embryo is inactivated.

Lysosomal enzyme An enzyme found in the granular cytoplasm of a neutrophil. Lysosomal enzymes destroy substances after the cell has engulfed them.

M

Macrodontia Abnormally large teeth.

Macrognathia Enlarged jaw.

Macrophage A large, mononuclear phagocyte derived from monocytes. Macrophages become mobile when stimulated by inflammation and interact with lymphocytes in an immune response.

Macrovascular disease Atherosclerosis of large- and medium-sized blood vessels.

Macule An area that is usually distinguished by a color different from that of the surrounding tissue; it is flat and does not protrude above the surface of the normal tissue. A freckle is an example of a macule.

Magnetic resonance imaging (MRI) A noninvasive diagnostic technique that uses radio waves to produce computerized images of internal body tissues.

Major aphthous ulcer A nonspecific aphthous ulcer that is greater than 1 cm in diameter, is deeper, and lasts longer than a minor aphthous ulcer. The presence of multiple major aphthous ulcers is known as *Sutton disease* or *periadenitis mucosa necrotica recurrens*.

Major histocompatibility complex Unique cell surface molecules that help T cells recognize antigen fragments.

Malaise A vague, indefinite feeling of discomfort, debilitation, or lack of health.

Malignant Resistant to treatment; able to metastasize and kill the host; describing cancer.

Malignant melanoma Malignant tumor of melanocytes that commonly arises on the skin as a result of exposure to sunlight.

Malignant tumor Cancer; a tumor that is resistant to treatment and may cause death; a tumor that has the potential for uncontrolled growth and dissemination or recurrence or both.

Mandibular process The first branchial arch divides into two maxillary processes and the mandibular process (or mandibular arch). It forms the lower part of the cheeks, the mandible, and part of the tongue.

Mandibular tori (singular, *torus*) Outgrowths of normal dense bone found on the lingual aspect of the mandible in the area of the premolars above the mylohyoid ridge. Also known as *torus mandibularis*.

Mandibulofacial dysostosis A syndrome characterized by developmental disturbance of the cranial bones and hypoplasia of the lower part of the face. The mandibular body is underdeveloped, and the eyes slant downward. The teeth are crowded and malposed. A high vaulted palate and deafness are other characteristic features. Also known as *Treacher Collins syndrome*.

Margination A process during inflammation in which white blood cells tend to move to the blood vessel walls.

Maxillary processes The first branchial arch divides into two maxillary processes and the mandibular process. The maxillary processes give rise to the upper part of the cheeks, the lateral portions of the upper lip, and part of the palate.

Measles A highly contagious disease, caused by paramyxovirus, with systemic symptoms and a skin rash. The disease occurs most commonly in childhood. Early in the disease, Koplik spots, which are small erythematous macules with white necrotic centers, may occur in the oral cavity.

Median mandibular cyst A rare cyst located in the midline of the mandible. It is characterized by a well-defined radiolucency that is seen below the apices of the mandibular incisors and is lined with squamous epithelium.

Median nasal process The process that forms the center and tip of the nose.

Median palatine cyst A cyst located in the midline of the hard palate. It is characterized by a well-defined, unilocular radiolucency and is lined with stratified squamous epithelium that is surrounded by dense fibrous connective tissue.

Median rhomboid glossitis A flat or slightly raised oval or rectangular erythematous area in the midline of the dorsal surface of the tongue, beginning at the junction of the anterior and middle thirds and extending posterior to the circumvallate papillae. It is devoid of filiform papillae; therefore its texture is smooth. It may be associated with *Candida albicans*.

Megaloblastic anemia A type of anemia characterized by hyperplastic bone marrow changes and maturation arrest resulting from a dietary deficiency, impaired absorption, impaired storage and modification, or impaired use of one or more hematopoietic factors.

Megaloblasts Red blood cells that are immature, abnormally large, and have nuclei. Megaloblasts are seen in high numbers in the bone marrow in megaloblastic anemia.

Meiosis The two-step cellular division of the original germ cells, which reduces the chromosomes from 4nDNA to 1nDNA. The two steps are called *first meiosis* and *second meiosis*.

Melanin The pigment that gives color to the skin, eyes, hair, mucosa, and gingiva.

Melanin pigmentation Discoloration of the oral tissues produced by the deposition of melanin.

Melanocytes Pigment-producing cells in the skin, hair, and eye that determine their color. The pigment that melanocytes make is called *melanin*.

Menorrhagia Abnormally heavy bleeding during menstruation.

Mental retardation A disorder characterized by certain limitations in a person's mental functioning and in skills such as communicating, taking care of himself or herself, and social skills.

Mesiodens The most common supernumerary tooth; found between the maxillary central incisors. It can be unerupted or erupted. The crown has a conical shape.

Metabolic Relating to the biochemical processes that occur in living organisms; metabolism.

Metaphase The phase of cellular division in which the chromosomes are lined up evenly along the equatorial plate of the cell; during this time, the chromosomes are most visible.

Metastasis (plural, *metastases*) The transport of neoplastic cells to parts of the body remote from the primary tumor and the establishment of new tumors in those sites.

Metastatic tumor A tumor formed by cells that have been transported from the primary tumor to a site not connected with the original tumor.

Methamphetamine A sympathomimetic amine related to amphetamine and ephedrine that stimulates central nervous system activity. It is used to treat obesity, minimal brain dysfunction, and attention deficit hyperactivity disorder. It is also used illicitly as a recreational drug.

Meth mouth The extensive and rapid destruction of teeth due to methamphetamine abuse.

Microcirculation Small blood vessels, including arterioles, capillaries, and venules.

Microcyte A red blood cell that is smaller than normal.

Microdontia Abnormally small teeth.

Microvascular disease Damage to small blood vessels.

Miliary tuberculosis The type of tuberculosis in which the bacteria are carried to widespread areas of the body and cause involvement of organs such as the kidneys and liver.

Millimeter (mm) One thousandth of a meter (1 m is equivalent to 39.3 inches). A periodontal probe is of great assistance in documenting the size or diameter of a lesion that can be measured in millimeters.

Minor aphthous ulcer The most commonly occurring type of aphthous ulcer. It appears as a discrete, round-to-oval ulcer that is up to 1 cm in diameter and exhibits a yellowish-white fibrin surface surrounded by a halo of erythema.

Mitochondria Cytoplasmic energy-producing organelles that have their own DNA in a circular chromosome.

Mitochondrial DNA DNA located in the mitochondria and needed for mitochondrial function; inherited maternally.

Mitosis The way in which somatic cells divide so that the two daughter cells receive the same number of identical chromosomes.

Mitotic cycle The part of the life span of a somatic cell when cellular division is achieved by mitosis.

Mitotic figures The microscopic appearance of cells during mitosis.

Molecular vaccine Vaccine developed using recombinant DNA techniques and containing antigenic determinants made of cloned bacteria, yeast, or synthetic peptides.

Moniliasis An overgrowth of the yeastlike fungus *Candida albicans*. It is the most common oral fungal infection. It can result from many different conditions, including antibiotic use, cancer, corticosteroid therapy, dentures, diabetes mellitus, and HIV infection. Also called *candidiasis* and *thrush*.

Monoclonal spike An elevation of a single type of immunoglobulin detected by immunoelectrophoresis; seen in patients with multiple myeloma.

Monokines Cytokines produced by monocytes or macrophages; mediators in an immune response.

Monomorphic adenoma A benign encapsulated salivary gland tumor composed of a uniform pattern of epithelial cells. It occurs most commonly in adult females, with a predilection for the upper lip and buccal mucosa.

Monostotic fibrous dysplasia The most common type of fibrous dysplasia. It is characterized by involvement of a single bone. The mandible and maxilla are commonly affected; the maxilla is more frequently involved than the mandible.

Mosaic bone A microscopic pattern seen in the involved bone of a patient with Paget disease of bone. It demonstrates prominent reversal lines that result from the resorption and deposition of bone.

mRNA Messenger RNA; the first type of RNA. It carries the message from the DNA to the ribosomes, where proteins are produced.

Mucocele A lesion that forms when a salivary gland duct is severed and the mucous salivary gland secretion spills into the adjacent connective tissue.

Mucoepidermoid carcinoma An unencapsulated and infiltrating malignant salivary gland tumor composed of a combination of mucous cells interspersed with squamouslike epithelial cells. Major gland tumors occur most often in the parotid gland. Minor gland tumors occur most commonly on the palate.

Mucormycosis A rare fungal infection caused by an organism that is a common inhabitant of soil and is usually nonpathogenic. Infection occurs in diabetic and debilitated patients and often involves the nasal cavity, maxillary sinus, and hard palate; it can present as a proliferating or destructive mass in the maxilla. Also called *phycomycosis*.

Mucositis Mucosal inflammation.

Mucous cyst (mucous retention cyst) An epithelium-lined cystic structure that occurs in association with a salivary gland duct. Most are not true cysts but dilated salivary gland ducts that develop as a result of obstruction.

Mucous membrane pemphigoid A chronic autoimmune disease that affects the oral mucosa, conjunctiva, genital mucosa, and skin. It is also known as *cicatricial pemphigoid* and *benign mucous membrane pemphigoid*.

Mucous patches Oral lesions that appear in the secondary stage of syphilis. They are characterized by multiple painless, grayish-white plaques covering ulcerated mucosa. They are very infectious.

Mucous retention cyst A mucosal swelling due to a dilated salivary gland duct that is caused by salivary duct obstruction.

Mulberry molar First molar with an irregularly shaped crown made up of multiple tiny globules of enamel instead of cusps, which imparts a berrylike appearance. Can be a manifestation of congenital syphilis.

Multifactorial conditions Conditions in which the phenotype results from a combination of genetic factors and environmental influences.

Multifactorial inheritance The type of hereditary pattern seen when there is more than one genetic factor involved and, sometimes, when there are also environmental factors participating in the causation of a condition.

Multilocular A term used to describe the radiographic appearance of multiple rounded compartments or locules. These can appear "soap bubble–like" or "honeycomb-like."

Multiple mucosal neuroma syndrome A syndrome composed of multiple mucosal neuromas, medullary carcinoma of the thyroid gland, and pheochromocytoma. Also termed *multiple endocrine neoplasia syndrome (MEN syndrome)*.

Multiple myeloma A systemic, malignant proliferation of plasma cells that causes destructive lesions in bone.

Mumps A viral infection of the salivary glands caused by a paramyxovirus. The disease most commonly occurs in children and is characterized by painful swelling of the salivary glands, most commonly bilateral swelling of the parotid glands. Also called *epidemic parotitis*.

Muscles of mastication The major muscles about the facial region that govern the movement of the mandible and chewing motions.

Mutation A permanent transmissible change in the genetic material, usually in a single gene.

Myalgia Muscle pain.

Myoepithelial cell A specific type of salivary gland cell with contractile properties.

Myofibroblasts A fibroblast that has some of the characteristics of smooth muscle cells, such as the ability to contract.

Myxedema The presence of hypothyroidism in older children and adults.

N

Nasolabial cyst A soft tissue cyst of the midlateral face with no alveolar bone involvement. It is lined with pseudostratified, ciliated columnar epithelium with multiple goblet cells. There is usually no associated radiographic change.

Nasopalatine canal cyst A cyst located within the nasopalatine canal or the incisive papilla. It arises from epithelial remnants of the embryonal nasopalatine ducts. Also known as an *incisive canal cyst*.

Natural killer cell (NK cell) A lymphocyte that is part of the body's initial innate immunity, which by unknown mechanisms is able to destroy cells recognized as foreign.

Natural passive immunity Passive immunity acquired by a developing fetus or newborn from its mother via the transfer of antibodies. These antibodies protect a newborn infant from disease while the infant's own immune system matures.

Necrosis The pathologic death of one or more cells or a portion of tissue or organ, resulting from irreversible damage.

Necrotizing sialometaplasia A benign condition of the minor salivary glands characterized by moderately painful swelling and ulceration in the area due to necrosis of the minor glands. Most common on the hard palate.

Necrotizing stomatitis A condition characterized by extensive focal areas of bone loss along with the features of necrotizing ulcerative periodontitis.

Necrotizing ulcerative gingivitis (NUG) A painful erythematous gingivitis with necrosis of the interdental papillae. Also formerly called *acute necrotizing ulcerative gingivitis* (ANUG).

Necrotizing ulcerative periodontitis A condition that resembles necrotizing ulcerative gingivitis in which patients experience pain, spontaneous gingival bleeding, interproximal necrosis, and interproximal cratering along with intense erythema and, most characteristically, extremely rapid bone loss.

Neoplasia New growth; the process of the formation of tumors by the uncontrolled proliferation of cells.

Neoplasm Tumor; a new growth of tissue in which the growth is uncontrolled and progressive.

Neoplastic Pertaining to the formation of tumors by the uncontrolled proliferation of cells.

Neurofibroma A benign tumor derived from Schwann cells and perineural fibroblasts, which are components of the connective tissue surrounding a nerve. The tongue is the most common intraoral location.

Neurofibromatosis of von Recklinghausen A syndrome characterized by multiple neurofibromas on the skin. Oral involvement is characterized by single or multiple tumors at any location in the oral mucosa. Café au lait skin pigmentation is common. Also called *von Recklinghausen disease*.

Neutropenia A diminished number of circulating neutrophils in the blood.

Neutrophil The first type of white blood cell to arrive at the site of injury and the primary cell involved in acute inflammation. The nucleus of this cell is multilobed. Also called a *polymorphonuclear leukocyte*.

Nevoid basal cell carcinoma syndrome A syndrome characterized by mild hypertelorism and mild prognathism, the appearance of basal cell carcinomas early in life, and multiple cysts of the jaws characterized histologically as odontogenic keratocysts. A variety of skeletal abnormalities may occur, including bifurcation of one or more ribs. Also known as *Gorlin syndrome*.

Nevus (plural, *nevi*) (1) A tumor of melanocytes (melanin-producing cells). (2) A pigmented congenital lesion (a lesion present at birth).

Nevus cells Melanocytes (melanin-producing cells).

Nicotine stomatitis A benign lesion on the hard palate typically associated with pipe and cigar smoking. It may also occur with cigarette smoking.

Nikolsky sign Seen in some bullous diseases such as pemphigus vulgaris and bullous pemphigoid; the superficial epithelium separates easily from the basal layer on exertion of firm sliding manual pressure.

Nodule A palpable, solid lesion in soft tissue that is up to 1 cm in diameter and may be above, level with, or beneath the skin or mucosal surface.

Nondisjunction In genetics, when chromosomes that are crossing over do not separate; therefore both migrate to the same cell.

Non–insulin-dependent diabetes mellitus The type of diabetes that is characterized by increased insulin resistance. It includes patients who can maintain proper blood sugar levels without the administration of insulin. However, insulin administration may be required. Also called *type 2 diabetes*.

Nonneoplastic Not neoplastic.

Nonodontogenic Not related to tooth development.

Nonpathogenic microorganisms Microorganisms that do not cause disease.

Nonthrombocytopenic purpuras Bleeding disorders that can result from either a defect in the capillary walls or disorders of platelet function.

Normal joint function The harmonious function of the temporomandibular joint and jaws.

Nucleotide A hydrolytic product of nucleic acid formed by a nitrogen-containing base, a five-carbon sugar (deoxyribose), and a phosphate.

O

Ocular hypertelorism A condition marked by a greater-than-normal distance between the eyes.

Odontogenesis Tooth development.

Odontogenic adenomatoid tumor An encapsulated, benign epithelial odontogenic tumor that has a distinctive age, sex, and site distribution. Seventy percent occur in females less than 20 years of age; 70% involve the anterior part of the jaws. May be associated with impacted teeth. Also known as an *adenomatoid odontogenic tumor*.

Odontogenic keratocyst An odontogenic developmental cyst with a unique histologic appearance. The lumen is lined by epithelium that is 8 to 10 cell layers thick and surfaced by parakeratin. The basal cell layer is palisaded and prominent; the interface between the epithelium and the connective tissue is flat. This cyst has a higher recurrence rate than many other odontogenic cysts.

Odontogenic myxoma A benign mesenchymal odontogenic tumor that occurs anywhere in the maxilla or mandible, with the mandible being more common. It may displace teeth and spread to other locations.

Odontogenic Arising from tooth-forming tissues.

Odontogenic tumor A tumor derived from tooth-forming tissues. It is most often benign.

Odontoma An odontogenic tumor composed of mature enamel, dentin, cementum, and pulp tissue. The odontoma is the most common of the odontogenic tumors, and there are two types: compound and complex.

Olfactory pits Two pits that mark the future openings of the nose that develop on the surface of the frontal process.

Oligodontia A subcategory of hypodontia in which six or more teeth are congenitally missing.

Oligogenic inheritance Characteristics or traits that are inherited by the participation of several genes.

Oncology The study of tumors or neoplasms.

Oogenesis The process of formation of female germ cells (ova).

Opacification The process of becoming opaque.

Open joint surgery Surgery used to perform disk repositioning, replacement or excision, and total joint reconstruction using a prosthetic device or autogenous graft.

Opportunistic infection A disease caused by a microorganism that does not ordinarily cause disease but becomes pathogenic under certain circumstances.

Opsonization The enhancement of phagocytosis.

Oral melanotic macule A flat, well-circumscribed, brown lesion of unknown cause. They are usually small and may require biopsy and histologic examination for diagnosis.

Oral submucous fibrosis Chronic oral mucosal disease associated with betel-quid and areca-nut chewing; oral mucosal tissues exhibit severe restriction of movement due to increased collagen deposition in the oral mucosa.

Orthokeratotic odontogenic cyst Odontogenic cyst lined by orthokeratin rather than parakeratin.

Osteoarthritis Characterized by degenerative changes of the articular cartilage with associated remodeling. It is the most common disease affecting the temporomandibular joint. It is also referred to as *degenerative joint disease*.

Osteoblast The cell that forms bone.

Osteogenesis imperfecta A congenital disorder characterized by abnormally formed bones that fracture easily. Other abnormalities include blue sclerae (mild cases), bowing of the legs, curvature of the spine, deformity of the skull, and shortening of arms and legs (severe cases). The oral manifestation of this syndrome is a dentinogenesis imperfecta–like condition.

Osteoma Benign tumor of normal compact bone.

Osteomalacia A disease of bone that develops over a long period as the result of a deficiency of calcium. When this disease occurs in young children, it is usually caused by a nutritional deficiency of vitamin D, and the associated disease is termed *rickets*.

Osteoporosis A hereditary disease marked by abnormally porous bone lacking normal density.

Osteoradionecrosis Necrosis of bone associated with radiation therapy.

Osteosarcoma A malignant tumor of the bone-forming tissue. Also known as *osteogenic sarcoma*.

Ovum (plural, *ova*) The mature female germ cell.

P

Paget disease of bone A chronic metabolic bone disease characterized by resorption, osteoblastic repair, and remineralization of the involved bone. It typically involves the pelvis and spinal column. Also called *osteitis deformans* and *leontiasis ossea*.

Palatal papillomatosis A form of denture stomatitis. Also called *papillary hyperplasia of the palate*.

Palatal torus An inherited exophytic growth of normal compact bone in the midline of the hard palate. Also known as *torus palatinus*.

Palatine processes Processes formed during development from the maxillary processes that fuse with the premaxilla to form the palate.

Palisaded encapsulated neuroma (PEN) A benign lesion that presents as a mucosal nodule. It appears microscopically as a well-circumscribed lesion composed of nerve tissue partially surrounded by a fibrous tissue capsule.

Pallor Paleness of the skin or mucosal tissues.

Palpation The evaluation of a lesion by feeling it with the fingers to determine the texture of the area; the descriptive terms for palpation are *soft, firm, semifirm,* and *fluid-filled;* these terms also describe the consistency of a lesion.

Pancytopenia A dramatic decrease in all the circulating blood cells.

Papillary Describing a small nipple-shaped projection or elevation; usually found in clusters.

Papillary cystadenoma lymphomatosum A unique type of monomorphic adenoma characterized by an encapsulated tumor composed of two types of tissue: epithelial and lymphoid. It presents as a painless, soft, compressible, or fluctuant mass, usually located in the parotid gland. It is also called a *Warthin tumor*.

Papillary hyperplasia of the palate A form of denture stomatitis. Also called *palatal papillomatosis*.

Papilloma A benign tumor of squamous epithelium that presents as a small, exophytic, pedunculated, or sessile growth. It is often described as cauliflower-like in appearance and occurs most often on the soft palate or tongue.

Papillon-Lefèvre syndrome An inherited disease characterized by marked destruction of the periodontal tissues of both dentitions, with premature loss of teeth and hyperkeratosis of the palms of the hands and soles of the feet.

Papule A small circumscribed lesion usually less than 1 cm in diameter that protrudes above the surface of normal surrounding tissue.

Paramedian lip pit A congenital lip pit that occurs near the midline of the vermilion border of the lower lip.

Paramyxovirus A member of a family of viruses that include the organisms that cause influenza, mumps, and some respiratory infections.

Parathormone Parathyroid hormone.

Parenteral Administered by injection.

Paresthesia An abnormal alteration of touch sensation often perceived as numbness, prickling, or tingling.

Partial thromboplastin time A test that measures the effectiveness of clot formation. It is performed by measuring the time it takes for a clot to form after the addition of kaolin, a surface-activating factor, and cephalin, a substitute platelet factor, to the patient's plasma.

Passive immunity The type of immunity in which antibodies produced by another person are used to protect an individual against infectious disease. This type of immunity can occur naturally or be acquired.

Pathogenic microorganism A microorganism that causes disease.

Pavementing Adherence of white blood cells to the walls of a blood vessel during inflammation.

Pedunculated Attached by a stemlike or stalklike base.

Pegged Resembling a small peg.

Pegged/absent maxillary lateral incisors A condition characterized by a lateral incisor that is small and peg shaped or congenitally lacking, either unilaterally or bilaterally. Both primary and secondary dentitions can be affected, but mostly the latter.

Pemphigus vulgaris A severe, progressive autoimmune disease that affects the skin and mucous membranes. It is characterized by intraepithelial blister formation that results from breakdown of the cellular adhesion between epithelial cells (acantholysis).

Penetrance In genetics, the prevalence of individuals with a given genotype who manifest clinically the phenotype associated with that trait.

Periapical abscess An abscess composed of pus and surrounded by connective tissue containing neutrophils and lymphocytes. The abscess may develop directly from the inflammation in the pulp or in an area of previously existing chronic inflammation.

Periapical cemento-osseous dysplasia A relatively common disease of unknown cause that affects periapical bone. It is commonly seen in the anterior mandible.

Periapical cyst A true cyst that is associated with the root of a nonvital tooth and consists of a pathologic cavity lined by squamous epithelium that is surrounded by inflamed fibrous connective tissue.

Periapical granuloma A localized mass of chronically inflamed granulation tissue that forms at the opening of a pulp canal, generally at the apex of a nonvital tooth root.

Periapical inflammation Inflammation at or around the root of a tooth.

Pericoronitis An inflammation of the mucosa around the crown of a partially erupted tooth. Usually the result of infection by bacteria that are part of the normal oral flora.

Peripheral Occurring outside of bone.

Peripheral ameloblastoma Ameloblastoma that occurs solely in the gingiva and not in the bone.

Peripheral giant cell granuloma A reactive lesion that occurs on the gingival or alveolar mucosa,

typically anterior to the molars. It is usually a result of local irritating factors.

Peripheral ossifying fibroma A well-demarcated sessile or pedunculated lesion that appears to originate from the gingival interdental papilla and is most likely derived from cells of the periodontal ligament.

Pernicious anemia Anemia caused by impaired vitamin B_{12} absorption, resulting from a deficiency of intrinsic factor, a substance secreted by the parietal cells of the stomach.

Petechia (plural, *petechiae*) A minute red spot on the skin or mucous membranes resulting from escape of a small amount of blood.

Peutz-Jeghers syndrome Syndrome characterized by multiple melanotic macular pigmentations of the skin and mucosa, which are associated with gastrointestinal polyposis. The polyps are usually benign.

Phagocytosis A process of ingestion and digestion by cells.

Pharyngitis Inflammatory condition of the tonsils and pharyngeal mucosa caused by many different organisms. Clinical features include sore throat, fever, tonsillar hyperplasia, and erythema of the oropharyngeal mucosa and tonsils.

Phenotype The physical and clinical visible characteristics of an individual. Genotype is the genetic composition; phenotype is its observable appearance.

Pheochromocytoma A benign neoplasm that generally develops in ganglia around the adrenal glands. The tumor is often bilateral and is responsible for night sweats, high blood pressure, and episodes of severe diarrhea.

Philadelphia chromosome A genetic abnormality of chromosome 22 in which part of chromosome 9 is transferred to chromosome 22.

Philtrum The vertical groove in the midline of the upper lip.

Phycomycosis A rare fungal infection caused by an organism that is a common inhabitant of soil and is usually nonpathogenic. Infection occurs in diabetic and debilitated patients. It often involves the nasal cavity, maxillary sinus, and hard palate and can present as a proliferating or destructive mass in the maxilla. Also called *mucormycosis*.

Pituitary adenoma A benign tumor of the pituitary gland. Often causes hyperpituitarism.

Plasma cell A lymphoid or lymphocyte-like cell found in the bone marrow, connective tissue, and sometimes blood. It has the ability to produce immunoglobulins and is derived from B cells.

Plasma thromboplastin A factor that is active in the formation of intrinsic blood thromboplastin. A deficiency results in Christmas disease (hemophilia B), which is caused by a decrease in the amount of thromboplastin formed. Also called *factor IX*.

Platelet A disk-shaped structure, also called a *thrombocyte*, found in the blood, which plays an important role in blood coagulation.

Platelet count A quantitative or numeric evaluation of platelets.

Pleomorphic Occurring in various forms.

Pleomorphic adenoma The most common of the benign salivary gland tumors. It is also called a *benign mixed tumor*.

Polycythemia An increase in the total red blood cell mass in the blood.

Polydactyly The presence of extra fingers or toes or both.

Polydipsia Chronic excessive thirst and intake of fluid. A possible sign of type 1 diabetes.

Polymorphonuclear leukocyte The most prevalent of the white blood cells containing a multilobed nucleus; also called a *neutrophil*.

Polyostotic fibrous dysplasia A type of fibrous dysplasia characterized by involvement of more than one bone. The skull, clavicles, and long bones are commonly affected.

Polyphagia Excessive appetite. A possible sign of type 1 diabetes.

Polyploid Three (triploid) or four (tetraploid) complete sets of chromosomes. This has been occasionally described in humans and is incompatible with life.

Polyuria Excessive urination. A possible sign of type 1 diabetes.

Postinflammatory melanosis Melanin pigmentation of the oral mucosa that occurs after an inflammatory response.

Postprandial After a meal.

Precocious Early.

Predilection A disposition in favor of something; preference.

Pregnancy tumor A pyogenic granuloma that may occur in pregnant women. They may be caused by changing hormonal levels and increased response to plaque.

Premaxilla The area of the palate that develops from the globular process. It forms the anterior part of the maxillae.

Pretrigeminal neuralgia Dull ache and burning sensation located on the face near the trigeminal nerve that serves as precursor to trigeminal neuralgia.

Primary adrenal cortical insufficiency A condition characterized by an insufficient production of adrenal steroids. Also known as *Addison disease.*

Primary dental lamina A band of ectoderm in each jaw on which proliferations of epithelial cells develop, which become the early enamel organs for each of the primary teeth.

Primary herpetic gingivostomatitis Oral disease caused by initial infection with the herpes simplex virus. It is characterized by painful, erythematous, and swollen gingiva and multiple tiny vesicles on the perioral skin, vermilion border of the lips, and oral mucosa. Patients also experience malaise and cervical lymphadenopathy.

Primary immunodeficiencies Immunodeficiencies of developmental or genetic origin that can involve B cells, T cells, or both. They provide information about the functions of the various immunologic responses and are extremely rare.

Primary Sjögren syndrome Lacrimal and salivary gland involvement without the presence of another autoimmune disease.

Primary tumor The original tumor; the source of metastasis.

Primordial cyst A cyst that develops in place of a tooth.

Proliferation The multiplication of cells.

Prothrombin time A test that measures the patient's ability to form a clot. It is performed by measuring the time it takes for a clot to form when calcium and a tissue factor are added to the patient's plasma.

Pruritus Itching.

Pseudoanodontia A condition in which normal teeth cannot erupt due to interference, such as in cleidocranial dysplasia.

Pseudocyst An abnormal cavity that resembles a true cyst but is not a pathologic cavity and is not lined with epithelium.

Pseudomembranous candidiasis A type of candidiasis in which a white curdlike material is present on the mucosal surface. When the material is wiped off, the underlying mucosa is erythematous.

Pulp polyp An excessive proliferation of chronically inflamed dental pulp tissue. Also called *chronic hyperplastic pulpitis.*

Purified protein derivative An antigen used to test whether an individual has been exposed to and infected with *Mycobacterium tuberculosis.*

Purpura A group of disorders characterized by purplish or brownish-red discolorations caused by bleeding into the skin or tissues.

Purulent Containing or forming pus.

Purulent exudate An exudate containing or forming pus.

Pustule A variably sized, circumscribed, pus-filled, elevated lesion.

Pyogenic granuloma A commonly occurring intraoral lesion characterized by a proliferation of connective tissue containing numerous blood vessels and inflammatory cells. It occurs in response to injury. The lesion does not produce pus and is not a true granuloma.

Pyrogens The fever-inducing substances produced from either white blood cells or pathogenic microorganisms.

R

Radiation The process of emitting radiant energy in the form of waves or particles.

Radiation therapy The treatment of a disease or condition with a type of radiation.

Radicular Pertaining to the root of a tooth.

Radicular cyst A cyst with a wall of fibrous connective tissue and a lining of stratified squamous epithelium that is attached to the root apex of a tooth with a necrotic pulp or a defective root canal filling.

Radiolucent The black or dark areas in a radiograph that result from the ability of radiant energy to pass through the structure. Less dense structures (e.g., the pulp) are radiolucent.

Radiolucent and radiopaque Terms used to describe a mixture of light and dark areas within a lesion, usually denoting a stage in the development of the lesion; for example, in a stage I periapical cemento-osseous dysplasia (cementoma), the lesion is radiolucent; in stage II, it is radiolucent and radiopaque.

Radiopaque The white or clear appearance in a radiograph that results from the inability of radiant energy to pass through a structure. The more dense the structure (e.g., amalgam restorations), the whiter it appears in a radiograph.

Ranula A large mucocele-like lesion that forms unilaterally on the floor of the mouth. It is associated with the sublingual and submandibular glands. It is caused by a sialolith or trauma to the major duct.

Raynaud phenomenon A disorder that affects the fingers and toes. Cold and emotional stress trigger a reaction, which is characterized by an initial pallor of the skin that results from vasoconstriction and reduced blood flow. The initial pallor is followed by cyanosis, which occurs because of the decreased blood flow.

Reactive arthritis (Reiter syndrome) A chronic disease that classically comprises the triad of three features: (1) arthritis, (2) urethritis, and (3) conjunctivitis. An antigenic marker called *HLA-B27* is present in most patients with this condition, suggesting a strong genetic influence.

Reactive connective tissue hyperplasia Proliferating exuberant granulation tissue and dense fibrous connective tissue resulting from overzealous repair.

Receptor A cell surface protein to which a molecule can bind; such binding leads to biochemical events.

Recessive In genetics a trait or characteristic manifested clinically with a double gene dose in autosomal chromosomes or with a single dose in males if the trait is X-linked.

Recontouring Shaped to fit the outline or contour.

Recurrent aphthous ulcer Painful oral ulcer of unknown cause; substantial evidence indicates that aphthous ulcers have an immunologic pathogenesis.

Recurrent herpes simplex infection Herpes simplex virus that persists in a latent state, usually in the nerve tissue of the trigeminal ganglion, and causes localized recurrent infections. Recurrent infections are often produced by stimuli such as sunlight, menstruation, or stress.

Regeneration The process by which injured tissue is replaced with tissue identical to that present before the injury.

Regional odontodysplasia A developmental problem in which one or several teeth in the same quadrant radiographically exhibit a marked reduction in radiodensity and a characteristic ghostlike appearance. Very thin enamel and dentin are present. Also called *ghost teeth.*

Repair The restoration of damaged or diseased tissues.

Residual cyst A cyst that forms when a tooth is removed and all or part of a periapical cyst is left behind.

Reticular lichen planus The most common form of lichen planus. The lesions are composed of Wickham striae along with white, slightly raised plaquelike areas.

Retrocuspid papilla A sessile nodule on the gingival margin of the lingual aspect of the mandibular cuspids.

Rhabdomyoma A benign tumor of striated muscle that has been reported to occur on the tongue.

Rhabdomyosarcoma A malignant tumor of striated muscle that grows rapidly and is destructive. It is the most common malignant soft tissue tumor of the head and neck in children.

Rheumatic fever A childhood disease that follows a group A β-hemolytic streptococcal infection, usually tonsillitis and pharyngitis. Characterized by an inflammatory reaction involving the heart, joints, and central nervous system.

Rheumatoid arthritis An inflammatory autoimmune disorder of the joints.

Rheumatoid factor An antibody against IgG found in serum and detectable on laboratory tests. It is associated with rheumatoid arthritis and other autoimmune diseases.

Ribonucleic acid (RNA) Single strands of polynucleotides found in all cells; different types of RNA have different functions in the production of proteins by the cell.

Ribosome The cytoplasmic organelles in which proteins are formed on the basis of the genetic code provided by an RNA template.

Root resorption Observed radiographically when the apex of the tooth appears shortened or blunted and irregularly shaped. It occurs as a response to stimuli, which can result from a cyst, tumor, or trauma.

rRNA Ribosomal RNA; the third type of RNA. It combines with several polypeptides to form ribosomes.

S

S phase The phase in which the replication of DNA takes place.

Sarcoma A malignant tumor of connective tissue.

Scalloping around the root The radiographic appearance of a radiolucent lesion that extends between the roots of multiple teeth, as seen in a traumatic bone cyst.

Scarlet fever Contagious childhood disease caused by group A β-hemolytic Streptococcus. Characterized by a red rash, strawberry tongue, sore throat, fever, enlarged lymph nodes, and prostration.

Schirmer test A test that measures lacrimal gland flow by placing special filter paper strips inside the lower eyelid for 5 minutes.

Schwannoma A benign tumor derived from Schwann cells, a component of the connective tissue surrounding nerves. The tongue is the most common intraoral location.

Scoliosis Lateral curvature of the spine.

Scrofula Pertaining to tuberculosis, the enlargement of the submandibular and cervical lymph nodes. Also known as *tuberculous lymphadenitis.*

Second meiosis Second stage of meiosis that is essentially a mitotic division in which each chromosome splits longitudinally. Replication of DNA occurs in second meiosis.

Secondary immunodeficiencies Immunodeficiencies that occur as a result of an underlying disorder. They are more common than the primary immunodeficiency disorders.

Secondary Sjögren syndrome The combination of another autoimmune disease with salivary and lacrimal gland involvement.

Secondary thrombocytopenic purpura The condition of thrombocytopenic purpura secondary to an existing disease or condition.

Serous A substance having a watery consistency; relating to serum.

Serous exudate An exudate that has a watery consistency. The consistence resembles that of serum.

Serum sickness A delayed allergic response after exposure to some antibiotics or antiserum. It is caused by an antibody reaction to an antigen in the donor serum. Symptoms include fever, painful swelling of the joints, renal disturbance or failure, edema around the eyes, carditis, and skin lesions.

Sessile Broad based.

Severe combined immunodeficiency A genetic disorder in which both B cells and T cells of the immune system are crippled, leaving the patient extremely vulnerable to infectious diseases.

Shingles A disease caused by the varicella-zoster virus that occurs in adults. It is characterized by a unilateral, painful eruption of vesicles along the distribution of a sensory nerve. Also called *herpes zoster.*

Sialadenitis A painful swelling of a salivary gland that may be caused by obstruction or infection. It can be acute or chronic.

Sialolith A salivary gland stone.

Sicca syndrome A combination of dry mouth and dry eyes.

Sickle cell anemia An inherited disorder of the blood that is found predominantly in black individuals and those of Mediterranean origin. It occurs as a result of an abnormal type of hemoglobin in red blood cells that causes the cells to develop a sickle shape in the presence of decreased oxygen.

Sickle cell trait People who are heterozygous for sickle cell anemia.

Sign Objective evidence of disease that can be observed by a health care provider.

Simple bone cyst A pathologic cavity in bone that is not lined with epithelium. Also known as a *traumatic bone cyst.*

Single-gene inheritance Characteristics that are governed by the action of one gene.

Sjögren syndrome An autoimmune disease that affects the salivary and lacrimal glands, resulting in a decrease in saliva and tears.

Smokeless tobacco–associated keratosis A white lesion that develops in the oral mucosa in the area where smokeless tobacco is habitually placed. Also known as *smokeless tobacco keratosis* and *tobacco pouch keratosis.*

Smoker's melanosis (smoking-associated melanosis) A type of melanosis in which the melanin pigmentation is associated with smoking and the intensity is related to the amount and duration of smoking.

Solar cheilitis Degeneration of the tissue of the lips caused by sun exposure. Also called *actinic cheilitis.*

Somatic cells All the cells of the human body with the exception of the primitive germ cells (oogonia and spermatogonia).

Smooth, rough, folded Terms used to describe the surface of a lesion.

Speckled leukoplakia An oral mucosal lesion that shows a mixture of red and white areas.

Spermatogenesis The process of formation of spermatozoa (sperm).

Spermatozoon The mature masculine germ cell.

Spina bifida A defect in the spine caused by a lack of the vertebral arches through which the spinal cord protrudes.

Spina bifida occulta Similar to spina bifida, but with little or no protrusion of the spinal cord.

Splenomegaly Enlargement of the spleen.

Squamous cell carcinoma A malignant tumor of squamous epithelium. It is the most common primary malignancy of the oral cavity and, like other malignant tumors, can infiltrate adjacent tissues and metastasize to distant sites. Also known as *epidermoid carcinoma.*

Stabilization appliances A treatment modality used in the management of certain temporomandibular joint disorders that consists of the fabrication of occlusal appliances.

Stafne bone defect Often referred to as a pseudocyst because it is not a pathologic cavity and is not lined with epithelium. It is characterized by a well-defined radiolucency in the posterior region of the mandible inferior to the mandibular canal, which is caused by a lingual depression in the mandible containing normal salivary gland tissue. Also known as a *lingual mandibular bone concavity* or *static bone cyst.*

Static bone cyst Often referred to as a *pseudocyst* because it is not a pathologic cavity and is not lined with epithelium. It is characterized by a well-defined radiolucency in the posterior region of the mandible inferior to the mandibular canal, which is caused by a lingual depression in the mandible containing normal salivary gland tissue. Also known as a *lingual mandibular bone concavity* or *Stafne bone cyst.*

Stevens-Johnson syndrome A severe form of erythema multiforme characterized by oral, ocular, and genital involvement.

Stomatodynia Burning mouth.

Stomodeum The embryonic invagination that becomes the oral cavity.

Strawberry tongue Oral manifestation of scarlet fever in which the fungiform papillae are red and prominent, with the dorsal surface of the tongue exhibiting either a white coating or erythema.

Striae Streaks or interconnecting lines.

Subclinical infection An infectious disease not detectable by the usual clinical signs.

Subluxation Hypermobility in which the patient is able to relocate the mandible back into the glenoid fossa.

Succedaneous Replacing or substituting for something else; often used when referring to the permanent teeth.

Supernumerary In excess of the normal or regular number, as in teeth or roots.

Supernumerary roots More than the normal number of roots. Supernumerary roots tend to occur in teeth in which roots form after birth.

Supernumerary teeth Extra teeth found in the dental arches.

Symblepharon Fibrous adhesion between the eyeball and conjunctiva.

Symptom Subjective evidence of disease or a physical disorder that is observed by the patient.

Syndactyly Soft tissue or bone fusion or both of fingers and toes.

Syndrome A set of signs or symptoms or both occurring together.

Synovial fluid The transparent viscous fluid that is secreted by the synovial membrane and found in joint cavities.

Synovial membrane Tissue that forms a portion of the lining of some joints (e.g., the temporomandibular joint).

Syphilis A disease caused by the spirochete *Treponema pallidum.* The organism is transmitted from one person to another by direct contact. It occurs in three stages: (1) primary, (2) secondary, and (3) tertiary.

Systemic Pertaining to or affecting the body as a whole.

Systemic lupus erythematosus An acute and chronic inflammatory autoimmune disease of unknown cause. It includes a wide spectrum of disease activity and signs and symptoms.

T

T-cell lymphocyte A lymphocyte that passes through the thymus before migrating to tissues. The T lymphocyte, also called a *T cell,* is responsible for cell-mediated immunity and may modulate the humoral immune response.

Talon cusp An accessory cusp located in the area of the cingulum of a maxillary or mandibular permanent incisor.

Taurodontism A condition characterized by very large, pyramid-shaped molars with large pulp chambers and short roots.

Temporomandibular disorders (TMDs) Abnormalities in the functioning of the temporomandibular joint or associated structures.

Thalassemia A group of inherited disorders of hemoglobin synthesis. Also called *Mediterranean* or *Cooley anemia.*

Thalassemia major The homozygous form of thalassemia in which genes on both chromosomes are involved.

Thalassemia minor The heterozygous form of thalassemia in which only one gene locus is involved.

Thrombocyte A platelet.

Thrombocytopenia Decrease in the number of platelets in circulating blood. It is sometimes called *immune thrombocytopenia* because an autoimmune type of process has been identified.

Thrombocytopenic purpura A bleeding disorder that results from a severe reduction in circulating platelets.

Thrush An overgrowth of the yeastlike fungus *Candida albicans.* It is the most common oral fungal infection. It can result from many different conditions, including antibiotic use, cancer, corticosteroid therapy, dentures, diabetes mellitus, and HIV infection. Also called *candidiasis* and *moniliasis.*

Thymic hypoplasia A type of primary immunodeficiency in which the thymus is deficient or lacking;

therefore T lymphocytes do not mature. Also called *DiGeorge syndrome.*

Thymus A lymphoid organ situated in the chest. It reaches maximal development at about puberty and then undergoes gradual involution.

Thyroglossal tract (duct) cyst A cyst that forms along the same tract that the thyroid gland follows in development, from the area of the foramen cecum to its permanent location in the neck. Most occur below the hyoid bone. The epithelial lining varies from stratified squamous to ciliated columnar epithelium.

Thyrotoxicosis A condition characterized by excessive production of thyroid hormone. Also called *hyperthyroidism.*

TNM staging system A staging and classification system of malignant tumors. T: tumor size; N: lymph nodes involved; M: presence of metastasis.

Tobacco pouch keratosis A lesion caused by tobacco chewing; typically located in the mucobuccal fold.

Tonsillitis Inflammatory condition of the tonsils and pharyngeal mucosa caused by many different organisms. Clinical features include sore throat, fever, tonsillar hyperplasia, and erythema of the oropharyngeal mucosa and tonsils.

Torus (plural, *tori*) A benign lesion composed of normal compact bone.

Torus mandibularis An exophytic growth of bone occurring on the lingual aspect of the mandible in the area of the premolars. Also known as *mandibular tori.*

Torus palatinus An exophytic growth of bone occurring in the midline of the hard palate. Also known as *palatal torus.*

Translocation In genetics, a portion of a chromosome attached to another chromosome.

Transudate The fluid component of blood that normally passes through the endothelial cell walls of the microcirculation.

Traumatic bone cyst A pathologic cavity in bone that is not lined with epithelium. Also known as a *simple bone cyst.*

Traumatic fibroma A broad-based, persistent, exophytic mucosal lesion that is composed of dense, scarlike, fibrous connective tissue surfaced by stratified squamous epithelium. Also known as *irritation fibroma, fibroma,* and *focal fibrous hyperplasia.*

Traumatic granuloma A hard, raised, ulcerated lesion resulting from persistent trauma.

Traumatic injury A disease process that results from injury that causes tissue damage.

Traumatic neuroma A lesion caused by injury to a peripheral nerve.

Traumatic ulcer An ulcer that occurs from some form of trauma such as biting the cheek, lip, or tongue; irritation from a denture; and injury from the sharp edge of food.

Trigeminal neuralgia A neurologic condition of the trigeminal nerve characterized by paroxysms of flashing, stablike, usually unilateral pain radiating along the maxillary branch (most often) of the nerve.

"Trigger point" A specific area on the face in which a touch or temperature change can trigger an episode of trigeminal neuralgia.

Trismus Inability to open the mouth fully due to one of many causes.

Trisomy A pair of chromosomes with an identical extra chromosome.

Trisomy 21 A type of abnormality in which three instances of chromosome 21 are found instead of two. This results in abnormal physical characteristics and mental impairment. Also called *Down syndrome.*

tRNA Transfer RNA; the second type of RNA. It transfers amino acids from the cytoplasm and matches them to the mRNA, positioning amino acids in the proper sequence to form polypeptides and proteins.

Tuberculosis An infectious chronic granulomatous disease usually caused by the organism *Mycobacterium tuberculosis.* The chief form of the disease is a primary infection of the lung.

Tuberculous lymphadenitis Pertaining to tuberculosis, the enlargement of the submandibular and cervical lymph nodes. Also known as *scrofula.*

Tumor A neoplasm; also a swelling or enlargement.

Turner tooth A permanent tooth showing enamel hypoplasia resulting from infection or trauma to the deciduous tooth.

Type 1 diabetes The type of diabetes that is characterized by profound insulin deficiency. It includes patients requiring the administration of insulin to prevent ketosis. The onset is abrupt and may be characterized by polydipsia, polyuria, and polyphagia. Also called *insulin-dependent diabetes mellitus.*

Type 2 diabetes The type of diabetes that is characterized by increased insulin resistance. It includes patients who can maintain proper blood sugar levels without the administration of insulin. Obesity is a common finding. Also called *non–insulin-dependent diabetes mellitus.*

Tzanck cells (1) Detached rounded cells caused by a loss of attachment between epithelial cells. Also known as *acantholytic cells.* These cells are present with pemphigus vulgaris. (2) Enlarged, multinucleated epithelial cells that occur as a result of infection with herpes simplex or varicella-zoster virus.

U

Undifferentiated Absence of normal differentiation; anaplasia; a characteristic of malignant tumor tissue.

Unilocular A term used to describe the radiographic appearance of a single rounded compartment or locule.

Urticaria Multiple areas of well-demarcated swelling of the skin, usually accompanied by itching. The lesions are caused by localized areas of vascular permeability in the superficial connective tissue beneath the epithelium. Also known as *hives.*

V

Varicella-zoster virus (VZV) The virus that causes both chickenpox (varicella) and shingles (herpes zoster).

Vascular leiomyoma A benign tumor of smooth muscle that may occur in association with blood vessels. They occur occasionally in the oral cavity.

Verruca vulgaris A white, papillary, exophytic lesion caused by a human papilloma virus. It is a common skin lesion. The lips are one of the most common intraoral sites for this lesion.

Verrucous carcinoma A specific type of squamous cell carcinoma that appears as a slow-growing, exophytic tumor with a pebbly white and red surface, usually in the vestibule or buccal mucosa. Often associated with the use of smokeless tobacco.

Vesicle A small, elevated, fluid-filled lesion on the epithelium that is less than 1 cm in diameter.

Vitamin B$_{12}$ A vitamin that contains cobalt and is essential for the maturation of red blood cells.

von Willebrand disease An inherited disorder of platelet function. It is the most common hereditary coagulation anomaly in humans.

W

Waldeyer's ring The ring of lymphatic tissue formed by the two palatine tonsils, the pharyngeal tonsil, the lingual tonsil, and intervening lymphoid tissue.

Well circumscribed Used to describe the borders of a lesion that are specifically defined; the exact margins and extent of the lesion can be clearly seen.

Western blot test A confirmatory test for HIV infection that identifies antibodies to HIV proteins and glycoproteins.

Wheal A localized swelling of tissue caused by edema during inflammation; often accompanied by severe itching.

White blood cells The cells within the blood and surrounding tissue, also called *leukocytes,* that are involved in the inflammatory and immune responses.

White sponge nevus An inherited disorder characterized by a white, corrugated, soft folding of the oral mucosa. The buccal mucosa is always affected, and in most patients the lesions are bilateral. A thick layer of keratin, which at times desquamates and leaves a raw mucosal surface, produces the whitening. Also called *Cannon disease* or *familial white folded mucosal dysplasia.*

Whitlow An infection involving the distal phalanx of a finger.

X

Xerophthalmia Abnormal dryness of the eyes caused by decreased lacrimal flow.

Xerostomia Dryness of the mouth caused by a decrease in salivary flow.

X-linked congenital agammaglobulinemia A type of primary immunodeficiency in which B cells do not mature. Plasma cells are deficient throughout the body; T cells are normal. Also called *Bruton disease.*

Index

Page numbers followed by "*f*" indicate figures,
"*t*" indicate tables, and "*b*" indicate boxes.